Infectious Disease

Retroviral Immunology

Immune Response and Restoration

Edited by

Giuseppe Pantaleo, MD
Hospital de Beaumont, Lausanne, Switzerland

and

Bruce D. Walker, MD
Harvard Medical School, Boston, MA

Humana Press **Totowa, New Jersey**

Softcover reprint of the hardcover 1st edition 2001
999 Riverview Drive, Suite 208
Totowa, New Jersey 07512

This publication is printed on acid-free paper. ∞
ANSI Z39.48-1984 (American Standards Institute) Permanence of Paper for Printed Library Materials.

Cover design by Patricia F. Cleary.

Production Editor: Mark J. Breaugh.

For additional copies, pricing for bulk purchases, and/or information about other Humana titles, contact Humana at the above address or at any of the following numbers: Tel: 973-256-1699; Fax: 973-256-8341; E-mail: humana@humanapr.com, or visit our Website: http://humanapress.com

Library of Congress Cataloging in Publication Data

Retroviral Immunology : immune response and restoration / edited by Giuseppe Pantaleo and Bruce D. Walker.
p. ; cm. -- (Infectious disease)
Includes bibliographical references and index.
ISBN 978-1-61737-128-8 ISBN 978-1-59259-110-7 (eBook)
DOI 10.1007/978-1-59259-110-7

1. Retrovirus infections--Immunological aspects. 2. HIV infections--Immunological aspects. I. Pantaleo, G. (Giuseppe) II. Walker, Bruce D., 1952- III. Series.
[DNLM: 1. Retroviridae Infections--immunology. 2. HIV Infections--immunology. 3. Major Histocompatibility Complex--immunology. WC 502 R438 2001]
QR201 .R47 R465 2001
616'.0194--dc21 00-054274

Retroviral Immunology

Infectious Disease

SERIES EDITOR: *Vassil St. Georgiev*
National Institute of Allergy and Infectious Diseases
National Institutes of Health

Retroviral Immunology: *Immune Response and Restoration,* edited by ***Giuseppe Pantaleo,*** *MD* and ***Bruce D. Walker,*** *MD,* 2001

Antimalarial Chemotherapy: *Mechanisms of Action, Resistance and New Directions in Drug Discovery*, edited by ***Philip J. Rosenthal,*** *MD*, 2001

Drug Interactions in Infectious Diseases, edited by ***Stephen C. Piscitelli,*** *PharmD* and ***Keith A. Rodvold,*** *PharmD,* 2000

Management of Antimicrobials in Infectious Diseases: *Impact of Antibiotic Resistance,* edited by ***Arch G. Mainous III,*** *PhD* and ***Claire Pomeroy,*** *MD*, 2000

Infectious Disease in the Aging: *A Clinical Handbook,* edited by ***Thomas T. Yoshikawa,*** *MD* and ***Dean C. Norman,*** *MD*, 2000

Infectious Causes of Cancer: *Targets for Intervention,* edited by ***James J. Goedert,*** *MD*, 2000

Preface

Although there have been many books on HIV and AIDS, surprisingly little has been published that focuses on the immunology of retroviral infections in general, and HIV in particular. *Retroviral Immunology: Immune Response and Restoration* is the first book of its kind to address the most important aspects of the immunology of retroviruses, including not only the virus-specific immune responses, but also genetic and virologic factors modulating these responses.

The book also deals directly with the emerging concept of immune restoration in retroviral infections, a particularly important subject to the thousands of clinicians who deal with this problem on a daily basis. With the advent of highly effective antiviral drug regimens to slow down the replication of HIV and the progression of AIDS, new challenges and opportunities are arising. Restoration of general immune function has brought with it not only complications of immune restoration-mediated disease, but also the realistic hope for meaningful restoration of the ability to control HIV replication with the immune system.

Leading scientists in the field have summarized the most current information regarding experimental and clinical aspects of retroviral infections. *Retroviral Immunology: Immune Response and Restoration* should prove an important point of reference for basic scientists and clinicians in this area of research. We are indebted to all of our authors for their excellent contributions.

Giuseppe Pantaleo, MD
Bruce D. Walker, MD

Contents

Contributors

HANS ACHA-ORBEA, PhD • *Ludwig Institute for Cancer Research, Lausanne Branch and Institute of Biochemistry, University of Lausanne, Epalinges, Switzerland*

R. PAT BUCY, MD, PhD • *Departments of Pathology, Microbiology, and Medicine, Center for AIDS Research, University of Alabama at Birmingham School of Medicine, Birmingham, AL*

DANIELA FINKE, MD• *Ludwig Institute for Cancer Research, Lausanne Branch and Institute of Biochemistry, University of Lausanne, Epalinges, Switzerland*

BRIAN FOLEY, PhD• *Theoretical Biology and Biophysics, Los Alamos National Laboratory, Los Alamos, NM*

BRIAN GASCHEN, MS • *Theoretical Biology and Biophysics, Los Alamos National Laboratory, Los Alamos, NM*

MARIE-CLAIRE GAUDUIN, PhD • *Harvard Medical School, Boston, MA; Department of Immunology, New England Regional Primate Research Center, Southborough, MA*

JAAP GOUDSMIT, MD, PhD • *Department of Human Retrovirology, Academic Medical Center, University of Amsterdam, Amsterdam, Netherlands*

STEVEN JACOBSON, PhD • *Viral Immunology Section, National Institute of Neurological Disorders and Stroke, National Institute of Health, Bethesda, MD*

R. PAUL JOHNSON, MD • *Harvard Medical School, Boston, MA, Department of Immunology, New England Regional Primate Research Center, Southborough, MA, and Infectious Disease Unit, Massachusetts General Hospital, Boston, MA*

RICHARD A. KASLOW, MD, MPH • *Departments of Epidemiology and International Health, Medicine, and Microbiology, Center for AIDS Research, University of Alabama at Birmingham Schools of Public Health and Medicine, Birmingham, AL*

AMITINDER KAUR, MD • *Harvard Medical School, Boston, MA, Department of Immunology, New England Regional Primate Research Center, Southborough, MA*

KRISHNA V. KOMANDURI, MD • *Section of Transplant Immunology, Department of Blood and Marrow Transplantation, University of Texas M.D. Anderson Cancer Center, Houston, TX*

BETTE T. KORBER, PhD • *Theoretical Biology and Biophysics, Los Alamos National Laboratory, Los Alamos, NM*

CARLA KUIKEN, PhD • *Theoretical Biology and Biophysics, Los Alamos National Laboratory, Los Alamos, NM*

GABRIELLE KUSCHERT, PhD • *Center for Immunology and Inflammatory Diseases, Division of Rheumatology, Allergy, and Immunology, Partners AIDS Research Center, Massachusetts General Hospital and Harvard Medical School, Boston, MA*

H. CLIFFORD LANE, MD • *Laboratory of Immunoregulation, National Institute of Allergy and Infectious Diseases, National Institutes of Health, Bethesda, MD*

FREDERICK S. LEE, MD, PhD • *Center for Immunology and Inflammatory Diseases, Division of Rheumatology, Allergy, and Immunology, Partners AIDS Research Center, Massachusetts General Hospital and Harvard Medical School, Boston, MA*

VLADIMIR V. LUKASHOV, MD, PhD • *Department of Human Retrovirology, Academic Medical Center, University of Amsterdam, Amsterdam, Netherlands*

ANDREW D. LUSTER, MD, PhD • *Center for Immunology and Inflammatory Diseases, Division of Rheumatology, Allergy, and Immunology, Partners AIDS Research Center, Massachusetts General Hospital and Harvard Medical School, Boston, MA*

ARAM MANGASARIAN, PhD, MBA • *Department of Genetics and Microbiology, Centre Médical Universitaire, Geneva, Switzerland*

JOSEPH M. MCCUNE, MD, PhD • *Gladstone Institute of Virology and Immunology, Departments of Medicine and of Microbiology and Immunology, University of California, San Francisco, CA*

DAVID C. MONTEFIORI, PhD • *Department of Surgery, Duke University Medical Center, Durham, NC*

GIUSEPPE PANTALEO, MD • *Department of Infectious Diseases, Centre Hospitaliere, Universitaire Vaudois, Lausanne, Switzerland*

GUIDO POLI, MD • *AIDS Immunopathogenesis Unit, San Raffaele Scientific Institute, Milan, Italy*

SCOTT SEELEY, BS • *Laboratory of Immunoregulation, National Institute of Allergy and Infectious Diseases, National Institutes of Health, Bethesda, MD*

SAMANTHA S. SOLDAN, BA, MS • *Viral Immunology Section, National Institute of Neurological Disorders and Stroke, National Institutes of Health, Bethesda, MD; Institute for Biomedical Sciences, Department of Genetics, George Washington University, Washington, DC*

HUGO SOUDEYNS, PhD • *Departments of Microbiology and Immunology, and Pediatrics, Faculty of Medicine, University of Montreal, Montreal, Canada*

DIDIER TRONO, MD • *Department of Genetics and Microbiology, Centre Médical Universitaire, Geneva, Switzerland*

BRUCE D. WALKER, MD • *Harvard Medical School, Partners AIDS Research Center, Massachusetts General Hospital, Boston, MA*

OTTO O. YANG, MD • *AIDS Institute, Infectious Diseases Division, Department of Medicine, UCLA School of Medicine, Los Angeles, CA*

1

Epidemiological and Immunological Implications of the Global Variability of HIV-1

Bette T. Korber, Brian Foley, Brian Gaschen, and Carla Kuiken

INTRODUCTION

Human immunodeficiency virus (HIV) is an extraordinarily variable virus. This is in part a result of a lack of a proofreading mechanism and the consequential high error rate, a feature shared by all RNA viruses (0.2–2 mutations per genome per cycle) *(1)*, a high replication rate, as well as an apparent high tolerance and selection for change. As a result of this variability, HIV is a particularly formidable opponent for those who seek ways to counter it. While any given HIV infection generally starts out with a relatively homogeneous virus population *(2)*, over the course of the infection viruses that have mutated to alter more than 10% of their genetic information can arise *(3–6)*. The variants that emerge in an individual (together considered a quasispecies) can differ in biological properties such as drug sensitivity *(7–9)*, coreceptor specificity *(10–12)*, and immunological susceptibility *(13–15)*. The viral quasispecies in a single individual is capable of eluding virtually any antiviral medication given as monotherapy (but not combination therapy *16*), and of slipping past the host's immune response.

As different variants are transmitted from one person to the next, the epidemic within a given population includes ever more diverse viral strains *(17)*. Very rapidly spreading epidemics, such as those in Thailand in the early 1990s *(18,19)*, and Kaliningrad in the late 1990s *(20)*, show very little variability as every virus sequenced is sampled close in time to the shared ancestral sequence, or founder virus, of the epidemic. Older HIV epidemics, such as one in the Central African Republic that is related to a newer epidemic in Thailand, show more diversity *(21)*, as would be expected. If very different viral forms are cocirculating in the same population, coinfections can result and recombination between distant forms can provide a volatile mechanism for genetic diversification *(22,23)*. In our search for effective vaccines, we must ultimately consider the spectrum of variability, the speed with which variation accumulates in populations, and the breadth of the immune response to the vaccine. The diversity and potential for change inherent in HIV suggest there may never be a single vaccine to answer global needs, and therefore our technology will need to adapt in step with the virus.

In this chapter we first briefly consider the place of HIV in the broad evolutionary context of primate lentiviruses. Both HIV-1 and HIV-2 are thought to have been transmitted from primates to humans (from chimpanzee and sooty mangabey, respectively)

From: *Retroviral Immunology: Immune Response and Restoration*
Edited by: Giuseppe Pantaleo and Bruce D. Walker © Humana Press Inc., Totowa, NJ

based on the relationships of viral genetic sequences *(24–26)*. There is evidence suggesting that multiple cross-species transmission events may have occurred in establishing both HIV-1 and HIV-2 in humans. A troubling but logical extension of this is that it highlights the potential for novel as yet unimagined viruses to make the cross-species jump from primate (or other animals) to humans *(27)*. Other primate viruses have made the cross-species leap from nonhuman primate to human, for example, the potentially lethal Herpesvirus Simiae *(28,29)*.

We then focus on the range of diversity within HIV-1. HIV-1 has been subdivided into three major groups based on genetic relatedness that gives rise to phylogenetic tree clustering patterns. Sequence-based phylogenetic trees are an attempt to reconstruct the past through contemporary genetic sequence data, by determining the relationships between viruses according to sequence similarities analyzed in the context of an evolutionary model. When these methods are applied to HIV-1, clear and distinctive lineages emerge (Fig. 1). HIV-1 is divided into three very distinctive groups: group M, responsible for the global epidemic; group O, a less common form most often found in West Africans *(30,31)*; and group N, an even rarer form, so far found in only a few individuals in Cameroon *(32)*. These groups have genetic sequence distances of >40% in some coding regions, and are likely to have been introduced into humans by independent cross-species transmission events (zoonoses). The M group has been further divided into genetically defined subtypes A–J *(33)*. The genetic distance in envelope, one of the most variable genes, ranges from 20–30% between subtypes to <15% within a subtype (Fig. 1). Some potential biological differences have been noted that correlate with subtypes, including differences in mutational patterns, drug sensitivity, and trends in coreceptor usage and SI/NSI phenotypes. Analysis of HIV genetic variation by subtype also provides a basis for global molecular epidemiology and tracking. HIV-2 is also divided into subtypes, that in terms of the genetic distances, are more similar to the groups of HIV-1 than to the subtypes.

Finally, the implications of variation for vaccine design and immunity are considered. There is evidence that escape mutations in HIV occur in response to all three arms of the immune response: Cytolytic T lymphocytes (CTLs), T-helper cells, and B cells. Different vaccine strategies are being considered to contend with variation. We make a case that a hypothetical ancestor or consensus sequences should be considered for vaccine prototypes along with the more standard strategy of selecting specific strains. Also, genetic subtype considerations may be critical for vaccines directed at generating cross-reactive T-cell immunity.

HIV AND PRIMATE LENTIVIRUSES

Relationship of HIV-1 Group M and Group O to the N and SIV–CPZ Isolates

Of all of the primate lentiviruses, HIV-1 sequences are most closely related to the virus found in the chimpanzee subspecies *Pan troglodytes troglodytes (Ptt) (24,34)*. The complete genomes of three viruses from chimpanzees have been sequenced. The chimpanzees carrying these viruses appear to be healthy. CPZUS (AF103818) is from "Marilyn," an African-born Ptt chimpanzee that was kept in captivity in the USA, and died in 1985 giving birth to stillborn twins *(24)*. CPZGAB (X52154) is from another *Ptt* chimpanzee that was captured in Gabon *(34)*. CPZANT (U42720) is from a *Pan troglodytes schweinfurthii (Pts)* chimpanzee, "Noah," originally captured in the Democratic Republic of Congo (formerly Zaire) *(35)*. The sequences from *Ptt* chimpanzees

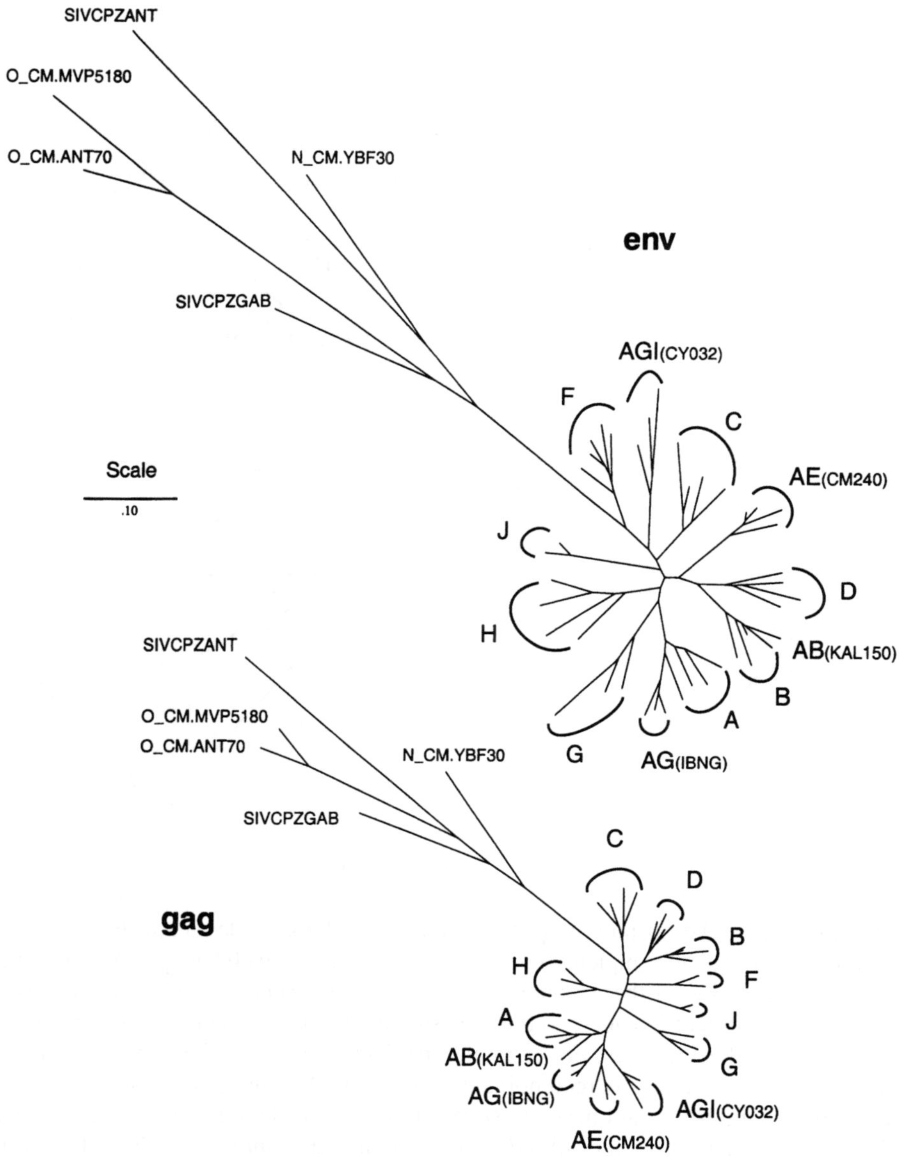

Fig. 1. The subtype reference set from the 1998 database. These *gag* and *env* trees include the reference sequences from the 1998 database *(33)*. The subtypes and the circulating recombinant forms are both included. The scale is the same for both *env* and *gag* trees, to illustrate the greater divergence of *env*.

are more similar to HIV-1 group M sequences than HIV-1 group M are to HIV-1 group O. The HIV-1 group N sequence is a mosaic with some regions more similar to CPZUS, and some more similar to HIV-1 group M, suggesting an early recombination event may have occurred between an ancestral sequence of the M group and of the CPZUS sequence. The CPZANT sequence is a relatively distant outlier. This combined evidence suggests that HIV-1 groups are derived from three independent *Ptt*-to-human cross-species transmission events *(24)*.

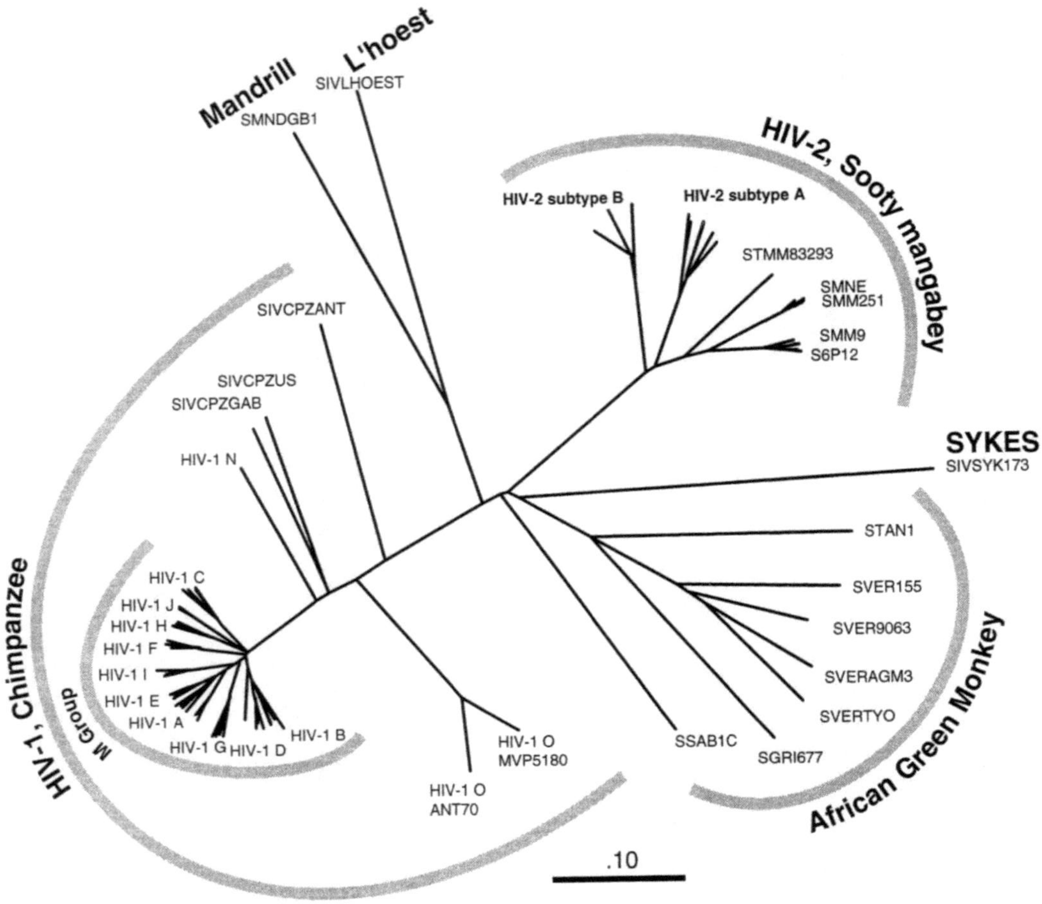

Fig. 2. Phylogenetic relationships of primate lentivirus. This phylogenetic tree was constructed from an alignment of complete genomes available at: hiv-web.lanl.gov/ALIGN under the "other SIV" menu. Some of the genomes are known to represent recombinants or mosaics between two or more different lineages, so this tree should not be assumed to represent the true phylogenetic history of these viruses. For example, the SAB1C genome from the *sabaeus* subspecies of African green monkeys is recombinant between an African green monkey lentiviral lineage and a sooty mangabey viral lineage *(43)*. When the AGM-like regions of its genome are used to build a phylogenetic tree, the SAB1C lineage shares the same major branch with the other AGM lineages. Given these limitations, the tree is still useful for graphically representing the diversity and relationships between these viruses. It is readily apparent that HIV-2 is related to Sooty mangabey virus, and HIV-1 to chimpanzee virus. The AGM subspecies are *grivet (gri), vervet (ver), tantalus (tan),* and *sabaeus (sab)* and the subspecies of origin is indicated in the sequence name. CPZANT is from the chimpanzee subspecies *Pan troglodytes schweinfurthii (Pts),* and CPZGAB and CPZUS are from *Pan troglodytes troglodytes (Ptt).* Phylogenetic analysis was done after gapstripping (any column in the alignment for which any sequence is represented by a gap was removed). The tree was constructed using PHYLIP DNADIST with maximum likelihood distance estimation and a transition/transversion ratio of 1.6. The DNADIST output was then used to create a neighbor-joining tree using the WEIGHBOR program (the PHYLIP neighbor program gave similar results). WEIGHBOR is available for UNIX, Mac, and PC platforms at http://synapse.lanl.gov/~billb/weighbor/index.html.

Multiple transmissions from *Ptt* to human is the simplest interpretation of the sequence data currently available coupled with the geographic data. The two full-length *Ptt* CPZ sequences are quite distant from each other (Fig. 2), however, and only a few chimpanzees have been found to be infected with virus, suggesting that the story is not completely closed. New discoveries resulting from the ongoing search for new viruses in all of the four chimpanzee subspecies and in other primates, as well as improvements in analytical methods, may ultimately allow us to better understand the historical origins of this epidemic. The diversity of sequences recovered from *Ptt* chimpanzees suggests that this subspecies of chimpanzee could also harbor other, equally diverse strains of SIV–CPZ, some of which may be more similar to HIV-1 groups. If a specific band of *Ptt* chimpanzees carried the HIV-1 M group ancestor, it may not be available for sampling today, owing to habitat loss or hunting pressures. Alternative scenarios that have previously been considered to explain an HIV introduction into humans are that a single primate to human event was followed by diversification of the three major groups within the human host, which seems unlikely given the available data *(24),* or that there is an additional, as yet unidentified natural reservoir for the virus that was the source of infections in both human and chimpanzee.

Relationship of HIV-2 Subtypes to SIV-SM Isolates

HIV-2 has been subclassified into subtypes A–E based on reasoning similar to that used to subdivide the HIV-1 M group into subtypes *(36–38).* It seems likely that the HIV-1 M group subtypes evolved from a common ancestor within humans after a single primate to human transmission event *(39).* In contrast, it seems likely that HIV-2 subtypes evolved from a common ancestor in sooty mangabeys (SM) *(Cercocebus torquatus atys)* followed by a separate sooty mangabey to human transmission event for each HIV-2 subtype; the evidence for this is that in phylogenetic analysis, some HIV-2 subtypes are found more closely associated with divergent SIVSM strains than with other HIV-2 subtypes *(26,40,41),* and there is geographic overlap between the sources of related HIV-2 and SIVSM samples *(41).*

Only subtype A of HIV-2 is common in humans, with subtype B being fairly rare and subtypes C–E being found in very few individuals. The phylogenetic distance between HIV-2 subtypes A and B is greater than the distance between HIV-1 M group subtypes, and more similar to the distance between the HIV-1 groups M, N, and O (Fig. 2). There has been extensive sampling of the sooty mangabey natural host, and similar to the situation in chimpanzees, SIV is essentially nonpathogenic in this host *(42).* Like the HIV-1/SIV–CPZ diversity, there is a great deal of diversity between HIV-2/SIV–SM isolates, with no sooty mangabey isolate being clearly related to HIV-2 subtypes A or B *(41,42).*

SIV and their Hosts: Ancient Lineages

The highly divergent viruses found in the chimpanzee subspecies *Pts* and *Ptt* may be contemporary representatives of virus in a long standing natural reservoir that originated in chimpanzees prior to the divergence of the two subspecies, a separation thought to have occurred several hundred thousand years ago *(24).* The geographic isolation of African Green Monkey (AGM) subspecies, and distinctive viral phylogenetic clustering patterns within them, suggest similar long-standing viral–host relationships *(43).* Phylogenetic analysis of envelope sequences from viruses sampled from four subspecies of AGM show that all SIVAGM strains cluster together, so originated in

AGM, but that viruses from any given subspecies are more closely related to other SIVAGMs from the same subspecies *(43)* (Fig. 2). The relationships between virus and subspecies described here superficially suggest a rather simple situation, but cross-species transmission and recombination have been well documented in wild primates, and SIV relationships are complex *(40,43–45)*.

In contrast, the HIV epidemic seems to have it origins in the not too distant past, probably some time in the first half of this century *(39,46)*. This does not mean that the cross-species transmission event occurred then, but rather that the group M virus that fuels the global epidemic had an ancestral sequence that originated in that time frame, and that the current global diversity of group M took only a half century to accrue.

DIVERSITY WITHIN HIV-1

HIV-1 Groups

As previously discussed, within HIV-1, three major groups have been defined, designated HIV-1 group M (for Main), group O (for Outlier), and group N (for Not-M, Not-O) *(32,47,48)*. Phylogenetically defined subtypes have also been recognized for both HIV-1 group M *(49–51)*, and for HIV-2 *(37,38,40)*. Distinctive clades in HIV-1 group O have also be distinguished, and it has been suggested that these clades should also be given subtype designations *(52,53)*. The variability of group O sequences, coupled with the fact that the first documented HIV-1 group O infections date back to the early 1960s (in Norway) *(54)*, provide clear evidence that the group O epidemic is not new. The oldest group O sample is roughly comparable to the oldest HIV-1 M group sequence, dating from a sample collected in 1959 in The Democratic Republic of the Congo *(39)*. It is not known why the group O epidemic is limited found to a relatively small number of West Africans or people who have an association with individuals from that geographic region *(30)*, while the group M epidemic has spread globally, with HIV-1 currently infecting approx 33.4 million people, and leaving 13.9 million dead in its wake (UNAIDS surveillance 1998, at: www.unaids.org). N group viral infections are very rare *(32)*, and may represent a cross-species transmission event from chimp to human that was not able to establish itself readily in the human host population.

What Constitutes a Subtype?

The HIV-1 subtype classification system has existed since 1992; five subtypes were initially identified for *env* (A–E) and four for *gag* (A–D). Since then, the classification system has been continually updated as new viral isolates were sequenced and new data became available; the yearly publication of the "Human Retroviruses and AIDS" Compendium, published in Los Alamos, provides a historical overview of the changes, and a set of subtyping reference sequences that is updated annually *(33)* (Fig. 1). Sequencing technology has greatly improved through the last decade, resulting a natural extension of the minimum sequence requirements for defining a new subtype, from *env,* to *env* plus *gag,* and now finally, full-length genomes have become a reasonable minimal requirement *(55)*. Through 1998, subtypes A–J have been identified, but several of these subtypes are represented only in fragments of mosaic genomes, based on the complete genome subtype reference sequences currently available (E, I, and possibly G). Subtypes A, B, C, D, F, H, and J each have full-length nonrecombinant representative sequences available. Subtype G is controversial in the literature, as all

Gs sequenced to date appear to have some A-like regions *(33,55,56)*. Subtype F has recently been broken down into three clusters F1, F2, and F3 *(57)*, but F3 will been reclassified as subtype K based on the outcome of full genome analysis (Martine Peeters, personal communication).

At present, we suggest the following criteria could be used as a practical guide to determine when a new subtype could be proclaimed:

- The identification of at least three epidemiologically unrelated isolates that cluster together phylogenetically and are well separated from established genotypes.
- The availability of full-length genome sequences (>8000 bases) from the three reference strains.
- Establishing that the distinctive phylogenetic association is not simply due to recombination of fragments of preexisting subtypes.

The extension of the subtype classification does not always proceed smoothly. For example, in 1995, an article appeared that described the discovery of a new HIV-1 subtype, called subtype I *(58)*. However, the samples on which the announcement was based were from two epidemiologically related infections in Cyprus, and the only available sequences were short fragments. More recently, epidemiologically unrelated samples were discovered that were very similar to the original subtype I isolates, and longer sequences were obtained *(59)*. From these, it appears that the first designated subtype I genomes are a mosaic of fragments of subtypes A and G, and unclassifiable fragments *(55,60)*. No complete subtype I has been found. The HIV research community is still unresolved about how to handle such cases. Currently the subtype I containing genomes are listed as recombinant forms AGI or ADI in the Los Alamos HIV database (http://hiv-web.lanl.gov/).

It should be emphasized that the present subtype classification system is to some extent a historical accident. For example, if the subtype I mosaic had been sequenced before subtypes A and G, it might now be regarded as a "pure" subtype, and subtypes A and G would now both be termed "recombinants," as they contain parts similar to subtype I and parts that do not resemble the subtype I genome. Therefore the basic reason subtype I, not subtype A, is called a recombinant is that A was discovered first. It is reasonable to assume, however, that an overwhelmingly more common subtype with broad geographic distribution (as subtype A is compared to I) is more likely to represent the parental subtype. Thus, although the distinction between pure subtypes and recombinants is somewhat artificial, it may be appropriate for the case of subtypes A and I. The most critical thing that the subtype nomenclature conveys is genetic similarity: that regions in an AGI mosaic (such as 94CY032.3 *55*) closely resemble other established subtypes (A and G), while other regions (I regions) are very diverged from both A and G, yet similar to one another. Thus subtyping nomenclature system is an attempt to develop conventions to distinguish similar forms of the virus that are important and genetically distinctive epidemic strains. Describing and tracking the divergence of viral strains is a critical function as we do not yet understand the consequences of genetic variability for vaccines.

Intersubtype Recombination

There have always been isolates that did not fit the subtype classification system very well. Some of these turned out to be the first representatives of a new subtype, such as the first mention of subtype F *(61)*. Others were later found to be recombinants.

One of the fruits of the subtype classification system is that it yielded a convenient handle to detect and label recombinants *(22,61,62)*, and many have been identified using this strategy. Some recombinants (most notably the MAL isolate) were identified before the subtypes were introduced *(63,64)*. It is likely, however, that recombination research would have proceeded much more slowly without the simple classification system that the subtype taxonomy provided. To date, some within-subtype recombinants have been studied *(65,66)*, but their number is far smaller than between-subtype recombinants, probably because they are harder to detect with certainty, not because they are rare. Computational methods for recombination identification are summarized at a web site maintained at l'Agence Nationale de Recherches sur le SIDA (http://igs-server.cnrs-mrs.fr/anrs/phylogenetics/RAP). As a word of warning, evidence for recombination requires careful study, and while distance measures are very useful and provide rapid preliminary screens to identify nonrecombinants, we have found that the outcome can be sensitive both to the reference strains selected and to the input alignment (Brian Foley, unpublished observations).

The discovery of increasing numbers of between-subtype recombinants has inevitably (and appropriately) muddled the once simple subtype classification system. The classification of recombinants is a complicated problem even to formulate, and it shifts continuously as new recombinants are found that "break the rules." It is unsatisfying to group recombinant sequences between the same two subtypes as one amorphous group, because there are clear shared patterns in some sequences. For example, the pattern of A/G interspersion is different in many of the A/G recombinant strains, but some strains do share the same pattern, and are similar to each other in that they cluster together within a portion of the genome that has been defined to have originated in a particular subtype. It was recently proposed *(56)* to group these recombinants and name them after the first available full-length sequence representing the group. The term "circulating recombinant form" (CRF) has been coined to designate variants that are not "pure" subtypes, but that do form epidemiologically relevant variants because they are found in large numbers of geographically distinct infections *(33)*. The Thai subtype E, or CRF AE (CM240) in the new nomenclature, is the best known example *(67,68)*. The AG recombinant strain IbNG and its relatives *(33)* are another example, and are called CRF AG (IbNG). Sequences that resemble IbNg are currently spreading in parts of Northern Africa *(23)*. Similarly, the CRF AB (KAL153) is spreading very rapidly among IVDUs in Russia *(20)*. A major disadvantage of the CRF nomenclature is that it is best applied when the genome has been fully sequenced; otherwise, although most of the genome may share recombination breakpoints and have similar sequences, additional recombination sites may be present in the remaining unsequenced stretches. This problem is shared, however, with subtyping of any fragments; if only a fragment is sequenced it may in fact be embedded in a recombinant genome. And the overwhelming majority of HIV sequences are fragments; approximately half the HIV sequences in the Los Alamos Database (and GenBank) are <300 bases long.

Recombination between more distant sequences has also been documented. A recombinant between HIV-2 subtypes has been found *(26)*. At least one of the SIV-SM sequences also appears to be recombinant between two diverse sequences and there is evidence for an ancient recombination event involving African green monkey SIVs *(25,43)*. Recently, a recombinant form of M and O group viruses was discovered in a

Cameroonian woman *(69)*. Recombination of such distant viral forms could provide a mechanism for rapid acquisition of new biological properties.

Biological Differences Between Subtypes

There are two possible causes for the existence of viral subtypes. First, they may be the result of a "founder effect": certain variants of the virus become founders of a subepidemic because they happen to be involved in an extensive transmission chain. In this scenario, the subtypes can be biologically equivalent even though they are genetically very different. An alternative explanation is that the subtypes have certain characteristics that allowed them to out-compete less fit viral variants. This presupposes biological differences between the subtypes. These two are not mutually exclusive: founder effects may have established the subtypes, but the virus that emerges to dominate a given lineage may do so as a result of distinct selective pressures, and thus subtypes or lineages within a subtype could potentially display different phenotypic characteristics.

Since the existence of subtypes was first established, the hunt has been on for biological differences between them. In 1996, a biological distinction was reported in susceptibility of Langerhans cells to infection, which were suggested to make viruses of Thai subtype E more easily transmissible via heterosexual intercourse than Thai subtype B *(70,71)*. UNAIDS devoted an expert meeting to discussion of the possible implications and to developing a course of action *(72)*. Later studies, however, did not reproduce this result, and found instead that while isolates can differ in their ability to infect Langerhans cells, and thus presumably in their transmissibility through heterosexual intercourse, no correlation with viral subtype was observed *(73,74)*.

Ongoing studies are attempting to examine the rate of T-cell decline as indicator of immune dysfunction and predictor of the onset of acquired immune deficiency syndrome (AIDS) in individuals infected with different subtypes. Cohorts with two (or more) subtypes cocirculating in the same population and well documented incident cases are ideal study groups for attempting to answer this kind of question. So far, however, the data from these cohorts are limited. A study of 126 infected individuals living in Sweden infected with subtypes A–D found no evidence for subtype specific differences in viral load or rate of CD4 T cell decline *(75)*. A study in Senegal found the opposite, that subtype A infections progressed more slowly than others *(76)*. In addition, mortality due to HIV-2 has been correlated with HIV-2 genotype *(77)*. Although subtyping provides a handle for seeking biological distinctions that could correlate with genotype, a potential concern is that subtypes could also act as a blinder so real differences in specific, but unnamed, sublineages may be missed and contradictory results obtained. There is a need for further study in this area.

Despite the lack of clear correlations between subtypes and overt biological characteristics, other more subtle phenotypic distinctions have been reported, which may have biological importance if confirmed. There are several recent studies suggesting there may be patterns of coreceptor usage that relate to subtype. Some background information is necessary to explain this phenomenon. HIV-1 requires two receptors to enter a target cell, the CD4 molecule and a chemokine receptor, usually either CCR5 or CXCR4. The coreceptor functions of these proteins are inhibited by their natural chemokine ligands (for a review see *10*), and a homozygous deletion in the CCR5 gene confers resistance to HIV-1 infections *(78)*. Examples of viruses that use either CCR5 or CXCR4 (called R5 or X4 viruses, respectively *79*), have been found in all group M subtypes tested, group O viruses *(80,81)*, and HIV-2 *(82)*. Viruses that use CCR5 are generally not syncytium inducing (NSI), and are frequently referred to as macrophage-tropic viruses. Viruses that can use CXCR4 for viral entry usually retain their ability to use CCR5, and thus are dual tropic R5X4 viruses *(11)*. These viruses are generally syncytium inducing (SI), and can grow and cause syncytia in MT2 cells, which lack the CCR5 receptor. The in vitro SI capacity of HIV-1 isolates is associated with disease progression *(83,84)*, as is appearance of R5X4 or X4 virus *(12)*.

There is growing evidence that the C subtype has a preponderance of R5, or NSI, virus and relative lack of X4, or SI viruses *(85–88)* although it is clearly possible for C subtype viruses to occasionally be X4 or SI *(81)*. Other studies that predict SI phenotype based on positive charge in the V3 loop *(89,90)* yield a consistent story, with predicted SI virus rarely found among C subtype isolates *(91,92)*. There may be other interesting coreceptor-related distinctions between subtypes. It appears that subtype D isolates, if they use the CXCR4 coreceptor, tend to use that coreceptor exclusively, while viruses of other subtypes that use CXCR4 are usually also capable of using the CCR5 receptor (X4 vs R5X4) *(85)*. It has also been suggested that E subtype (CRF AE (CM240) infections may tend to shift more rapidly to SI viral forms *(86)*.

A second property associated with subtypes was noted by Gao et al., who have found a distinctive RNA secondary structure in the important transcriptional regulatory domain TAR that is unique to the A and AE mosaic subtypes *(68)*. The TAR element is a conserved, stable stem-loop structure required for Tat-mediated transactivation of HIV-1 gene expression, and the level of activity of this system may influence the rate of disease progression *(93)*. In addition, distinct numbers of *cis*-acting transcriptional activator NF-κB binding sites have been observed in the long terminal repeats (LTRs) of C subtypes sequences, which may also influence the level of viral gene expression *(67,68,94)*. A third potentially distinctive property is drug susceptibility. Some subtype F samples may be less susceptible to a non-nucleoside reverse transcriptase inhibitor *(95)*, and subtype G may have a decreased sensitivity to protease inhibitors *(96)*. There are also some biological differences associated with more distant HIV-1 genotypes. Group O does not not require the incorporation of cyclophilin A to produce infectious virions, while group M does *(97)*. In addition, group O viruses are naturally resistant to non-nucleoside reverse transcriptase inhibitors *(98,99)*. There are also pragmatic concerns related to genetic distinctions: RNA quantitation kits *(100)* and serology based diagnostic kits *(101)* have both required modification to cope with HIV-1 group and subtype variation.

Another potential difference between subtypes is reflected in subtype specific patterns of genetic variation *(102,103)*; some of these observations are directly related to receptor usage and phenotype *(88)*. There is an elevated rate of nonsynonymous (amino acid altering) substitutions in the third variable (V3) loop of subtype D viruses *(102,103)*, and apparently in a subset of subtype E viruses, compared with other subtypes (Fig. 3). The sequences from the V3 loop of subtype D are highly variable, in contrast to the highly conserved V3 loop sequences of subtype C (Fig. 3). The amino acid sequences flanking the V3 loop are comparable in subtypes A, B, C, and D; however, subtype E is very conserved in the flanking region, in accord with the phylogenetic similarity of most available subtype E sequences (Fig. 3). A subset of CRF AE V3 loops is almost as radically divergent as subtype D, despite the conservation of the flanking sequences. Serological studies have further indicated that the V3 loop of the D subtype is the most diverse *(104)*. The V3 loop is a functionally important domain of the viral envelope. Positively charged amino acids in certain positions in the V3 loop correlate with a syncytium-inducing phenotype in culture *(89,90)*, and the V3 loop strongly influences coreceptor usage *(105–108)*. Although the V3 loop is one of the more variable regions of the Env protein, a highly conserved form of the V3 loop is found in many C subtype viruses and a subset of A subtype viruses *(102)* (Fig. 3). This common conserved form of the V3 loop is probably the reason that A and C subtype viruses are difficult to distinguish by V3 peptide serology, which can be used with some success to discriminate between other subtypes *(104,109)*, and furthermore is probably related to the dominance of R5 viruses among C subtype sequences.

HIV-1 Subtypes and Molecular Epidemiology

The prevalence of the different HIV-1 group M subtypes varies in different geographic locations. Subtype B is by far the most common strain in the Americas, most of Europe, Australia, and Eastern Asia (Japan, Korea, Taiwan), while it is rare in Africa, the region that is widely regarded as the origin of the HIV epidemic. Of 2077 African sequences with known subtype in the HIV database in Los Alamos, only 20 (1%) are subtype B; 15 of these are from South Africa, and these include infections that can be traced back directly to imports from the United States or Western Europe. In the rest of Africa, subtypes A, C, and D are prevalent, while in West-Central Africa, almost all group M subtypes as well as groups N and O viruses can be found. Globally, the C subtype accounts for the majority of new infections. (See the UNAIDS website for updates concerning the global epidemic: www.unaids.org.)

The subtype distribution also changes with time. For example, in the early days of the HIV epidemic in Thailand (1985–1990), the subtype B variant B′ and subtype E (or CRF AE [CM240]) cocirculated; subtype B′ was mostly found among intravenous (IV) drug users, and subtype E most common among heterosexually acquired infections. Interestingly, there were also a small number of early (1986–87) infections with the Western subtype B, as opposed to B′, among Thai prisoners who mostly identified themselves as IVDU *(110)*. It has been found that most infections among homosexual men are caused by the Western subtype B *(111)*, suggesting that this branch of the epidemic results from imports rather than local transmissions. CRF AE (CM240) strains have also been found in the Central African Republic, showing that it was imported into the Far East from Africa. CRF AE (CM240) has gained ground rapidly, and is now responsible for most new infections among Thai IV drug users *(112,113)*. Both subtype B′ and subtype AE have spread to most other countries in Southeast Asia *(21,114–118)*.

Recently, several Korean datasets (Nef and V3 sequences) were published, consisting of samples from patients infected through heterosexual and homosexual contact and infected blood products. In one study, 41 of 46 isolates were subtype B *(119)*; infections with other subtypes were invariably associated with heterosexual transmission and could usually be

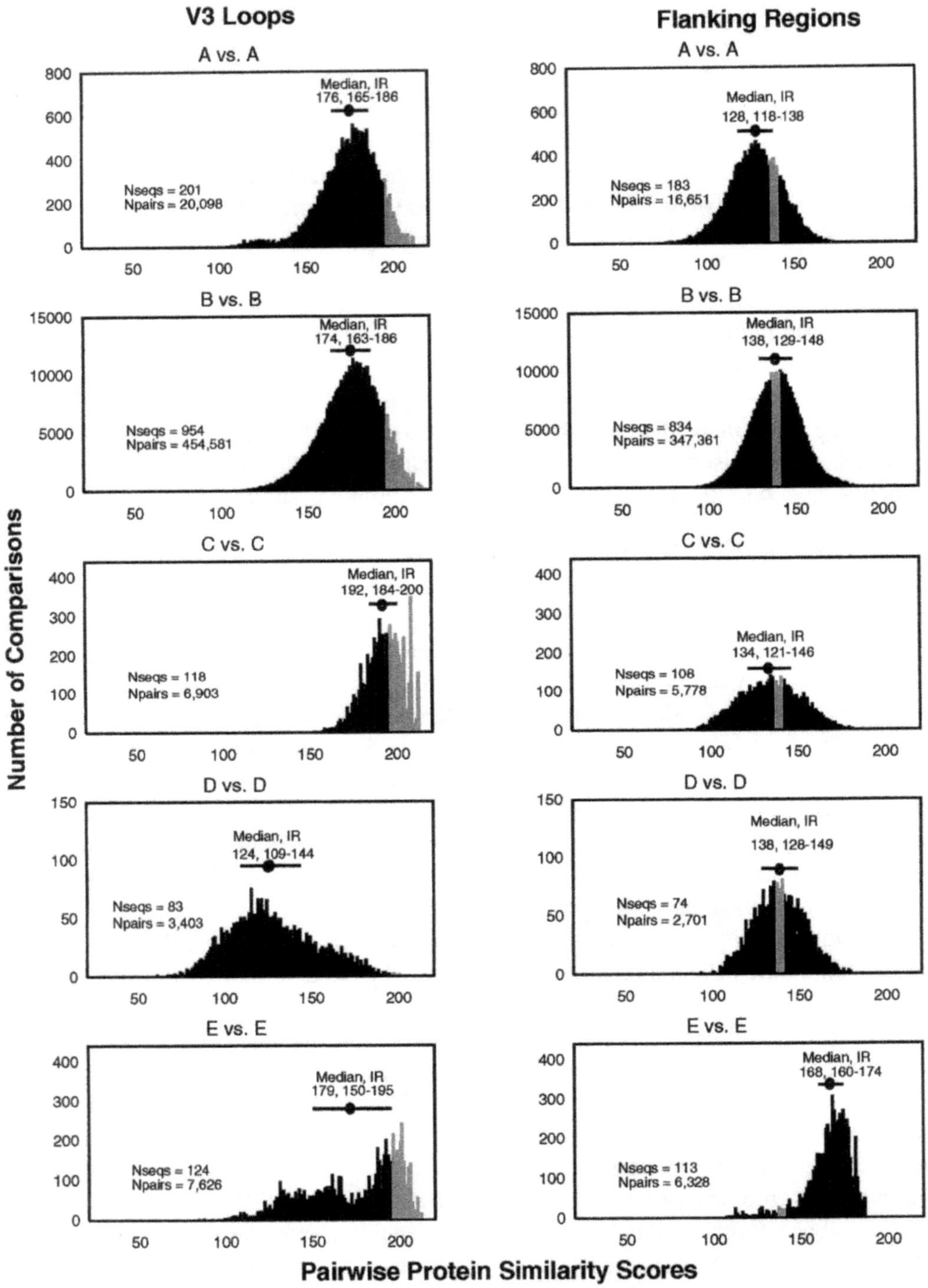
V3 Loops
Flanking Regions
A vs. A
Median, IR 176, 165-186
Nseqs = 201
Npairs = 20,098
A vs. A
Median, IR 128, 118-138
Nseqs = 183
Npairs = 16,651
B vs. B
Median, IR 174, 163-186
Nseqs = 954
Npairs = 454,581
B vs. B
Median, IR 138, 129-148
Nseqs = 834
Npairs = 347,361
C vs. C
Median, IR 192, 184-200
Nseqs = 118
Npairs = 6,903
C vs. C
Median, IR 134, 121-146
Nseqs = 108
Npairs = 5,778
D vs. D
Median, IR 124, 109-144
Nseqs = 83
Npairs = 3,403
D vs. D
Median, IR 138, 128-149
Nseqs = 74
Npairs = 2,701
E vs. E
Median, IR 179, 150-195
Nseqs = 124
Npairs = 7,626
E vs. E
Median, IR 168, 160-174
Nseqs = 113
Npairs = 6,328
Number of Comparisons
Pairwise Protein Similarity Scores

Fig. 3. Subtype-specific differences in the pattern of variability accumulating in the HIV-1 envelope protein V3 region. This figure is a modified version of an analysis of V3 loop variability included in the 1997 sequence database *(103)*. The compilation of V3 region sequences used for this study includes just one sequence per patient or group of epidemiologically linked patients, thus eliminating the bias of multiple sequences from the same patient. Patients representing the spectrum of every stage of disease development are included in each subtype. The sequences were divided into two regions: the V3 loop, typically including 35 amino acid residues including two cysteine residues which form a disulfide bond to produce the loop; and 35 amino acids flanking the loop, including 20 amino acids immediately adjacent to the amino-terminal side of the loop (e.g., NFTDNARVIIVQLNESVEIN) and 15 amino acids immediately adjacent to the carboxy-terminal side of the loop (e.g., NLSSTKWNNLTKQIT). Each of the two regions was scored for pairwise similarity using optimal pairwise alignments using a modified version of the PIMA software package *(191)* that incorporates protein similarity scores based on amino acid substitution matrices from protein blocks *(192,193)*. For the V3 loops, gray bars indicate highly conserved pairs with scores of 195 or greater, highlighting both the large percentage of subtype C isolates with conserved amino acid sequence, and the lack of highly similar sequences among subtype D isolates. For the flanks, gray columns were included at the position of the subtype B median (from 136 to 140) to highlight the similarity of distributions in subtypes A–D, and the relative conservation of subtype E. The flanks serve as an internal control, showing that outside the V3 loop the level of protein divergence is roughly comparable for subtypes A–D, and far less for subtype E. Subtype E sequences were predominantly from the early part of the 1990s in Asia, and were generally closely related; the tail of divergent flanking sequences were from the Central African Republic. Further studies have confirmed these comparisons using more up-to-date larger data sets with several hundred individuals represented in each of subtypes A, C, and D (BK and BF, *manuscript in preparation*).

traced to foreign contacts. Sequences in all three Korean studies show the presence of a founder effect in Korea *(119,120)*; the Korean variant of subtype B is quite distinct from the worldwide consensus. The "Western" subtype B is also found in Korea, but in a minority of cases (5/23 in the Kim study, 6/41 in the Kang study) (Fig. 4).

A subdivision within a subtype similar to the B/B′ distinction has also been reported for subtype A *(56)*. There appear to be at least three distinct sublineages of subtype A at present. The first is composed of isolates from Central and East Africa. The second consists of the A-like segments in the CRF AG (IbNG), and is found mainly in West Africa (Ivory Coast, Liberia) and in Djibouti, possibly introduced by soldiers of the French Foreign Legion who had contracted the infection in West Africa. The third subtype A lineage is the A-like segments of CRF AE (CM240), of which the subtype A sections always cluster together, separate from the other subtype A sequences (Fig. 4). It is not surprising that CRFs cluster together, as the CRFs all have a common ancestor, the original recombinant strain. Similarly sequences that were originally designated subtype F also were broken down into three sub-clusters: F1, which included sequences originating in Brazil and Finland; F2, with sequences from Cameroon; and F3, including sequences from the Democratic Republic of the Congo and Cameroon *(57)*.

In general, finding an exotic HIV-1 subtype (i.e., one that is not endemic to the region under study) can be traced to foreign travel or risk activity with a foreign person *(121,122)*. However, a few cases of spread of exotic subtypes that could not be traced to a foreign source have been reported Canada *(59,123,124)*. In the future, a further global mixing of HIV-1 subtypes is inevitable. As subtypes cocirculate and become increasingly

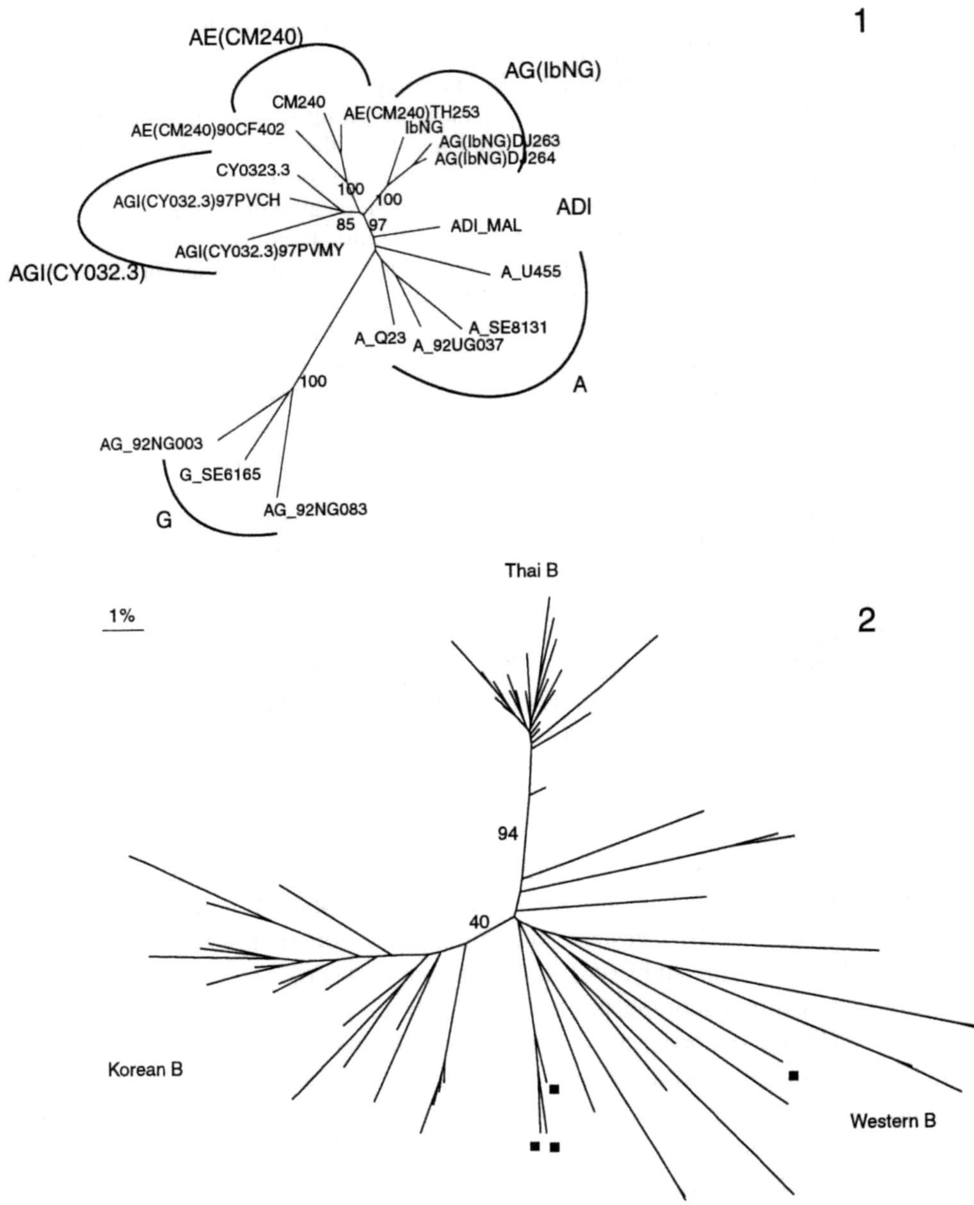

Fig. 4. Neighbor-joining trees illustrating subtype subclusters. The subtype A subclusters are shown in panel 1, based on sequences from the 1000 nucleotide gag region alignment, where all mosaics included are characterized as subtype A. Subtype B subclusters are shown in panel 2, and are based on 300 nucleotide V3 sequence alignments. A scale is shown next to the trees. Blocks in panel 2 represent "Western" sequences from Korea. Bootstrap values (% of 500 replicates) are shown next to each cluster.

prevalent in multiple populations, the opportunity for intersubtype recombination will increase, and consequently, the problems for targeted vaccine design will also.

In many European countries (Sweden, Germany, Great Britain, The Netherlands), it has been shown that HIV-1 isolated from homosexuals is different from the virus found in IV drug users *(125,126)*. A recent dataset of 12 V3 sequences from Greece *(127)* had the same distinguishing signature differentiating IV drug users from others that was first found in The Netherlands *(125)*. It has been suggested that the HIV-1 variant found in European IV drug users originated in the United States, where about half the infected IV drug users from a Baltimore cohort were found to be infected with a similar variant *(121)*.

Even when the locally prevalent subtype is different from subtype B, HIV in samples obtained from homosexuals often tend to belong to subtype B. The distinction has been reported in the former Soviet Union *(128)*, the Baltic states *(129)*, South Africa *(130)*, and Thailand *(111)*. These results suggest that the HIV epidemic among homosexual men is generally spreading separately from that among IV drug users and heterosexual infections not only in the West, but also in other parts of the world. Even before the phylogenetic difference between the HIV variants was known, it was suggested that the homosexual-associated HIV epidemic in South Africa was probably imported from Europe or the United States *(131)*. The propagation of different subtypes across the world can be used as a means to trace the epidemic, but even on a smaller geographical scale, clues can be found by studying variation within one subtype. In fact, the variability of the virus even makes it possible to trace individual transmission events on the basis of genetic analysis *(19,132,133)*.

Traditional epidemiological studies have suggested that most likely source of infection for the heterosexual population in the Western world (at least those who are infected through local sexual contact) is the IV drug user population. In a modeling study based on US data, it was estimated that approx 1% of infections in heterosexual women result from sex with bisexual men *(134)*. Studies based on self-report data from HIV-1–infected bisexual men in San Francisco show very infrequent risk contacts with women *(135)*. Similarly, in the Dutch cohort study of homosexual men, very few participants indicated ever having had sex with a woman, and most of those always used condoms *(136)*. In this light, molecular epidemiology studies give surprising results. More than half of a group of heterosexually infected women in The Netherlands carried the "homosexual" variant *(137)*. Based on comparisons of samples taken over a period of 10 yr, the prevalence of the IVDU variant in Dutch drug users does not seem to be declining *(125)*. The "homosexual" variant, however, forms the vast majority of subtype B sequences collected. It may be that this variant forms the majority in the present-day HIV-1 heterosexuals in the United States, and that some of the Dutch infections are imported from abroad. Alternatively, the frequency of unprotected bisexual contacts may be underestimated by traditional methods.

THE IMMUNOLOGICAL IMPLICATIONS OF DIVERSITY

Immune Protection: Reasons for Hope

A handful of people have been identified who remain persistently HIV negative in spite of frequent HIV exposure, who have a T-cell immune response to HIV-1 *(138–141)*. In a particularly interesting study, in a cohort of Nairobi prostitutes with a seroprevalence of 90–95%, (indicative of their intense HIV exposure), a small number of women have been seronegative for 12 yr of follow-up *(139)*. No behavioral distinctions have been found that would account for their long-term seronegativity. Some of these long-term seronegative women have clear anti-HIV CTL bulk responses, and some have HIV-specific T helper-1 (Th1) responses *(139)*. Similarly there is a group of Gambian prostitutes who carry the HLA-B35 allele and are persistently seronegative *(138)*. Both HIV-1 and HIV-2 circulate in this geographic region, and HIV-1/HIV-2 cross-reactive B35 epitopes were identified that could elicit HIV specific CTLs from three of six repeatedly exposed but uninfected sex workers who carry the HLA-B35 allele. In addition, HIV CTL have been found in a significant fraction of CCR5 wild-type, high-risk sexual partners of HIV-1 positive individuals *(140,141)*.

There also are rare (<1%) of HIV-1–positive individuals that are clearly infected, but that control viremia without the aid of medications. These individuals can be infected and healthy for up to 20 yr (as long as they have been followed to date). HIV-specific T helper (Th) responses were generally believed to be eliminated after the early stages of infection in most HIV-1–infected individuals *(142)*, but a strong CTL and *gag*-specific Th response was found in some of the individuals that controlled viremia *(143,144)*. A recent study using a sensitive assay employing flow cytometric detection of antigen-induced intracellular cytokines, indicated that *gag* specific, Th1 memory T cells were more common in HIV-1–infected people than was previously believed *(145)*, but the long-term survivors may have had a stronger than typical response. These cell frequencies declined with antiretroviral therapy, suggesting vaccination may need to become part of long-term HIV-1 control strategies for continued immunologic participation.

T-Cell Immune Escape

Some studies have clearly shown examples of CTL HIV epitope-specific mutations selected to fixation, as well as adaptive CTL responses in vivo *(13–15,146,147)*. There are other studies, however, that have found little evidence for escape mutations in specific epitopes that elicited an immunodominant response *(148,149)*. Escape mutations have also been observed to arise in conjunction with progression to AIDS *(150)*, and to be more common in mothers that transmit virus to their infants *(151)*. CTL responses to conserved epitopes may slow the rate of disease progression, and thus some HLA alleles may be more protective. For example, some human HLA types (in particular class I B27, B51, B57 *(152)*, B14 and C8 *(153)*, and class II DR13 *154*) have been associated with slow disease progression. In the case of HLA*B5101, it was found that several epitopes capable of stimulating CTL responses are located in highly conserved regions *(155)*. Tomiyama and colleagues suggest that HLA alleles associated with slow progression generally tend to present more conserved epitopes than those associated with rapid progression *(155)*. Interestingly, HLA class I homozygosity, thus a more limited repertoire of potential CTL viral responses, is associated with accelerated disease progression *(156)*.

Helper T-cell HIV escape variants have been documented in two asymptomatic individuals who had proliferative responses to HIV antigens. Some of the antigenic variants found in vivo failed to stimulate autologous $CD4^+$ Th cell clones that could be stimulated by an index peptide. Furthermore, the index peptide could stimulate fresh uncultured cells, but the variants could not. While the ability of the virus to evade an immune response is discouraging, it focuses attention for vaccines on T-cell responses to epitopes in conserved regions of proteins with functional constraints that do not easily accommodate mutation and allow escape *(157,158)*. HIV escape from antibodies is also well documented. There are multiple studies documenting shifts in autologous viral neutralization, and serum tends to be poor at neutralization of contemporaneous viral isolates *(159–161)*.

Glycosylation and Immune Evasion

HIV Env is among the most heavily glycosylated proteins known, and the number of Env *N*-linked glycosylation sites varies widely from strain to strain of HIV-1. *N*-linked glycolsylation sites require an asparagine, followed by any amino acid, followed by either serine or threonine (N-X-[S or T]). The rapid acquisition and loss of glycosylation sites in hypervariable domains such as the V1, V2, V4, and V5 domains of gp120 constitutes one of the most striking aspects of HIV variation, and this kind of variability is not captured in phylogenetic trees. These regions are extremely difficult to align, and the variation in these domains is often the product of insertions and deletions, so even seemingly unambiguous alignments in these regions may not be appropriate for the mutational models that are the basis of the phylogenetic trees. As such regions contribute heavily to the overall variability, and can confound the ability to discern evolutionary relationships, they are usually excluded. This results in general underestimates of HIV envelope variability, but better phylogenetic reconstructions of viral relationships.

Glycosylation mutations can influence antibody responses *(162)* and can also alter CTL responses *(163)*. The recently obtained crystal structure of a modified HIV-1 HXB2 envelope revealed a remarkable "armor" of carbohydrate, with a concentration of glycosylation sites on what is believed to be the outward face of the trimeric envelope spike, shielding it from host antibodies *(164,165)*. The antibody 2G12 is interesting in that it is broadly neutralizing, it binds to a rarely immunogenic region on the glycosylated face of gp120, and its binding is dependent on glycosylation *(164,165)*. An unexpected facet of glycosylation is the role of deglycosylation in CTL epitope processing. A recent study found an Env epitope that contains a glycosylation site that requires a deglycosylation step that converts asparagine (N) to aspartic acid (D) for presentation, and it is the D that is critical for CTL recognition of the epitope *(163)*. Thus the loss of the glycosylation site means no N to D conversion occurs, and the epitope is not properly processed to allow CTL recognition.

Vaccines and Variation

There are many approaches to HIV vaccines, including naked DNA vaccines, canarypox and vaccinia constructs containing HIV protein coding regions, liposomes and purified recombinant proteins, as well as serial combinations, for example, a DNA vaccine with a protein boost (for recent reviews, see *166,167*). A vaccine that includes multiple conserved antigenic sites, and is capable of eliciting anti-HIV CTL, T helper cells, and neutralizing antibodies, is obviously most desirable, and it is hoped that newer vaccine technologies will be able to evoke stronger immune responses of longer duration.

Several strategies are being considered for eliciting broad CTL responses to vaccines. The most straightforward involves including conserved proteins, like reverse transcriptase, and conserved domains of variable proteins, in vectors designed to stimulate an HIV specific CTL response (e.g., see *168–170*). Alternatively, several groups are developing multiepitope minigenes that incorporate conserved epitopes that can be presented in the context of multiple dominant HLA molecules *(171,172)*. When a string of 20 human, 3 macaque, and 1 mouse epitopes were delivered in a combined gun DNA and recombinant vaccinia virus Ankara (MVA) vaccination regimen in macaques, high frequencies of circulating CTL were observed *(172)*. Such a multiepitope strategy would allow great flexibility, and one could pick the most conserved epitopes presented by the most common HLA alleles of a target population.

Whatever strategy of vaccine design is used, the question of what strain or strains on which to base the vaccine on arises. For example, should one use a contemporary R5 primary isolate for a vaccine strain? As discussed earlier, the diversity of HIV in a population increases over time, with viruses growing ever more distant from one another. This suggests it may be logical to use an artificial construct based on either a consensus or hypothetical ancestral sequence, as such a sequence would be the most similar to the most strains. Phylogenetic methods such as parsimony and maximum likelihood allow one to create a predicted "most parsimonious" or "most likely" ancestral sequence at virtually any interior node in a phylogenetic tree (many programs have this capability, including Joe Felsenstein's PHYLIP package at http://evolution.genetics.washington.edu/phylip.html). This strategy could either be applied to a vaccine intended for a single subtype (such as subtype B in the United States), where the consensus or ancestral sequence of the B clade would be used, or it could be applied in a setting where multiple subtypes are cocirculating. In a multiple-subtype setting one might optimize coverage by including either a cocktail of subtype consensus sequences or a hypothetical ancestor to all subtypes circulating in the target region. Such a global ancestral sequence would be genetically as close to contemporary sequences of any subtype as within-subtype contemporary sequences are to each other. Although this has advantages for T-cell linear epitopes, such an unnatural protein may not fold properly and so may be less useful for eliciting antibodies. Conformational studies would be a critical first step in such a strategy.

Eliciting neutralizing antibodies is thought to be a desirable, if not essential, goal for vaccine design, but results in animal models have been somewhat mixed. There are only three broadly reactive neutralizing monoclonal antibodies identified to date: IgG1b12, 2G12, and 2F5 *(173)*. These antibodies, delivered in combination and in high concentration, are ineffective in controlling established infections, in hu-PBL-SCID mice *(174)*. IgG1b12 alone at high dose, however, is able to completely protect hu-PBL-SCID mice even when given several hours after viral challenge, which is promising in terms of vaccine or antibody-based post-exposure prophylaxis *(175)*. Neutralizing serum or monoclonal antibodies protect macaques against parenterally delivered simian–human immunodeficiency virus (SHIV) infection *(176,177)*, but fail to protect against mucosally inoculated virus *(176)*. Finally, some gp120 vaccines elicit antibodies that can neutralize only T cell line adapted (TCLA) virus *(178)*; for example an R5, E subtype gp120 vaccine tested in baboons *(179)* elicits antibodies that can neutralize both subtype E and B TCLA virus, but not primary isolates.

Are Subtypes an Important Consideration for Vaccine Design?

Whereas some CTL epitopes are conserved and elicit responses across clades, others tend to be highly clade specific *(169,170,180–185)*. Most CTL responses have been defined in individuals in the United States Europe where the B-clade infections dominate, and the reagents and clones used to define CTL epitopes are generally based on B-clade viruses. Thus the implications of global viral diversity for CTL are just beginning to be understood. Whether a vaccine is being considered for a geographic area with predominantly one subtype so intraclade diversity it the main issue, or for an area with many subtypes cocirculating so interclade diversity is important, it is logical to attempt to provide multiple epitopes that are as conserved as possible.

In an attempt to compare approaches to vaccine candidates, we determined the subtype-specific variation within experimentally defined epitopes relative to different potential vaccine candidate sequences. For our "vaccine-candidates," we compared HXB2, a B consensus, a C consensus, and a consensus of the consensus sequences from subtypes A–G, using a basic strategy developed for Cao et al. *(182)*. First, we optimized the alignments of protein sequences with respect to every well-defined epitope. "Well-defined" epitopes were those for which 8–10 amino acid optimal reactive peptides have been defined, with known HLA presenting molecules. Most of these are defined using B-clade reagents and CTL from B-clade infections, and we are making the assumption that the majority of these motifs will be functional epitopes in the context of other clades, although we are not assuming they will be cross-reactive. We asked the question of how similar each of the vaccine candidates were to the optimally aligned motifs from each clade (Fig. 5). Each well-defined epitope in the Los Alamos 1998 HIV Immunology database was incorporated into the analysis of the protein which includes it, as well as all full-length protein sequences available in the Los Alamos database as of January 1999. Only full-length sequences, limited to one sequence per individual, were included in the analysis. Only those clades with four or more sequences available (A, B, C, D, and AE) were included. We tallied the number of epitopes that were identical, had one substitution, two substitutions, or more than two substitutions relative to the "vaccine strain." Figure 5 shows the of percentage of epitope sequences that fall into each category.

Our conclusions are as follows:

- There is extensive potential for intersubtype cross-reactivity for most reagents and proteins, particularly if one or two amino acid substitutions can usually be tolerated *(182)*. But there are definitely strategies that can optimize that potential.
- Gag p24 contains the greatest proportion of conserved epitopes of the five proteins compared, closely followed by RT. gp120, not surprisingly, has the fewest conserved epitopes.
- There is only a slight benefit conferred by using a B subtype consensus rather than a specific B subtype strain (HXB2 in this case), when comparing known epitope sequences to within-subtype, B subtype sequence diversity. The most pronounced benefit was found for the Nef protein.
- There was a definite increase in perfectly preserved epitopes and well-preserved epitopes when comparing the C subtype consensus to to C subtype sequences, and the B subtype consensus to B subtype sequences. This strongly suggests that subtype-specific vaccines should be considered for CTL vaccines. To emphasize this point, we have extracted data from the complicated Fig. 5, and created an easier to interpret Fig. 6. Figure 6 compares the proportion of identical epitope sequences relative to the B and C subtype consensus sequences, in sequences derived from subtypes A–D. Within subtype comparisons have greater than twofold more epitope perfect matches than the between-subtype comparisons.
- The genetic association between B and D subtypes is reflected in epitope conservation; D subtype viruses are most likely to cross-react with B strains than are other subtypes.
- Using an artificial protein sequence that is the consensus of all subtypes, as would be predicted, gives moderate between-subtype conservation, falling somewhere between intrasubtype conservation and interclade conservation. This consensus is identical to about half the epitope sequences (40–60%) in every protein, in every clade.

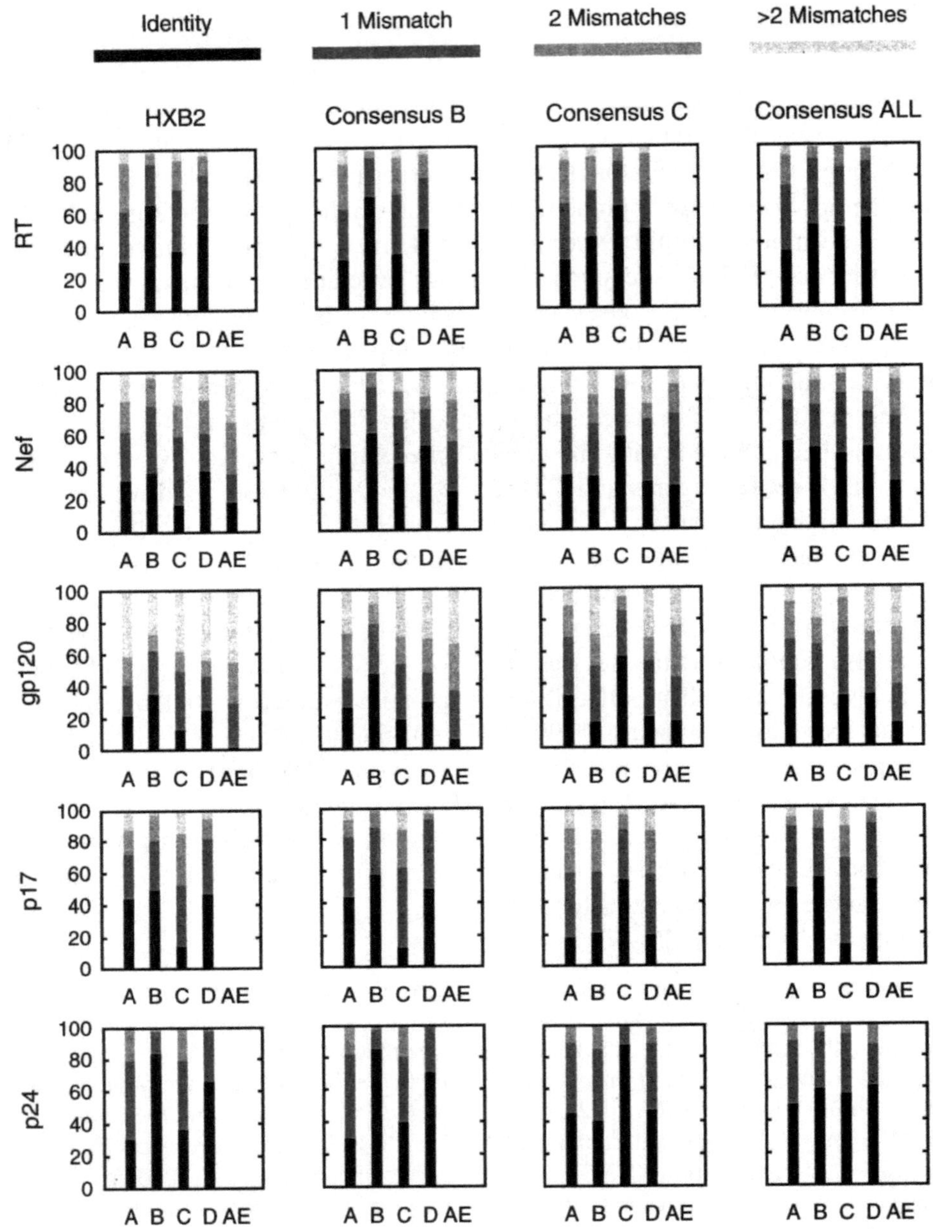

Fig. 5. Subtype-specific conservation of well-defined CTL epitopes in five HIV proteins, compared to potential vaccine strains. Here we compare the variation in known epitopes to potential vaccine candidates: HXB2, a B consensus sequence, a C consensus sequence, and a consensus sequence of all subtype consensus sequences (A–G). Optimal alignments for every well-defined epitope in the 1998 Los Alamos HIV immunology database for the HIV-1 proteins RT, Nef, gp120, p17, and p24 were generated, starting from the protein sequence alignments the 1998 Los Alamos HIV sequence database website. To preclude bias, these alignments include only full-length proteins, and only one representative sequence from any given HIV-infected individual. For a subtype to be included in this figure, a minimum of four sequences representing that subtype were required. Because the purpose of this figure is to present a global view of the implications of variability, the epitopes are grouped by protein. There were 29 well-defined epitopes in Nef, 33 in RT, 23 in gp120, 15 in p17, and 29 in p24. We will use the comparison of HXB2 to A subtype in Nef as an example. There were 29 well-defined, distinct CTL epitopes described in Nef, listed in the 1998 database. There are eight A subtype sequences. Therefore,

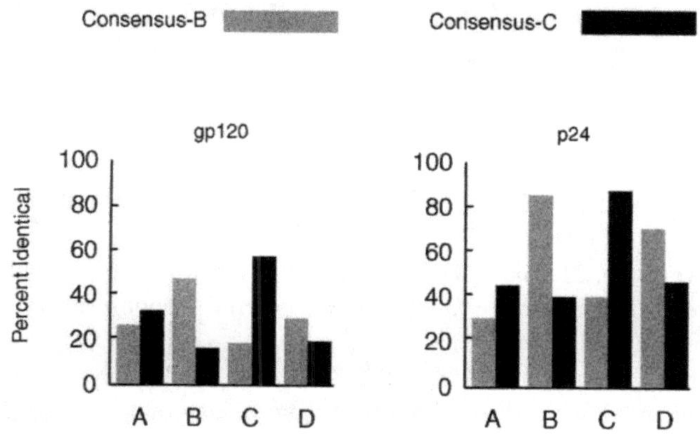

Fig. 6. Percentage of CTL epitopes from gp120 and p24 (subtypes A, B, C, and D) with no mismatches when compared to epitopes from a B consensus sequence and a C consensus sequence. This figure contains elements from Fig. 5, selected to highlight the potential benefit of subtype-appropriate vaccines for eliciting CTL responses. The *y*-axis indicates the percentage of identical epitope sequences in a comparison of either the B subtype consensus or the C subtype consensus, to sequences from subtype A–D. While it is obvious that the B subtype consensus would be more similar to B sequences, and likewise C consensus to C sequences, the relative importance of within-subtype conservation for defined epitope sequences, which are motifs of 8–10 amino acids, is less obvious. As is illustrated here, the number of identical epitope sequences relative to a subtype-appropriate potential vaccine is more than twofold greater than the number of identities with a vaccine from a different subtype. p24 and gp120 were selected for this figure as they represent extremes, the most conserved and least conserved of the proteins analyzed.

Neutralizing serotypes generally do not correlate well with genotype *(186–188);* hence subtype-specific vaccine reagents may be generally less important for antibodies than for linear T-cell epitopes. For antibody stimulation, studies directed toward discovery of reagents better able to generate breadth of response *(179,189,190)* may ultimately be more fruitful than efforts to develop subtype-appropriate reagents. For example, an innovative vaccine approach that shows promise for stimulating broadly reactive antibodies was capable of eliciting antibodies in mice that could neutralize 23 of 24 primary HIV isolates, reacting with clades A–E *(190).* The strategy involves forcing the envelope protein into a vulnerable "fusion-competent" conformation, which exposes antigenic domains by using formaldehyde-fixed whole-cell vaccines *(190).*

there are subtype A, Nef epitope sequences. 32% of these epitope sequences were identical to HXB2 spanning the appropriate motif (the black bar in the figure), 30% had one amino acid mismatch (dark gray), 19% had two mismatches (medium gray), and 19% had more than two mismatches (white). It is very likely that the identical epitope sequences would be cross-reactive, possible that one or two mismatches could be tolerated, and unlikely that more than two mismatches would be tolerated *(182).* The number of sequences available for each subtype for these comparisons is as follows: Nef: A = 8, B = 166, C = 20, D = 4, AE = 22; RT: A = 8, B = 26, C = 7, D = 5; gp120 A = 16, B = 98, C = 22, D = 14, AE = 9; p17: A = 8, B = 30, C = 8, D = 5; and p24: A = 8, B = 30, C = 8, D = 5)

Using strategies to create vaccines that elicit broadly reactive neutralizing antibodies, coupled with CTL and Th immunogens that are tailored for the sequences circulating in a given area, may be an optimal approach.

REFERENCES

1. Drake JW. Rates of spontaneous mutation among RNA viruses. Proc Natl Acad Sci USA 1993; 90:4171–5.
2. Zhang LQ, MacKenzie P, Cleland A, Holmes EC, Leigh Brown AJ, Simmonds P. Selection for specific sequences in the external envelope protein of HIV-1 upon primary infection. J Virol 1993; 67:3345–56.
3. Wolinsky S, Korber B, Neumann A, Daniels M, Kuntsman K, Whetsell A, et al. Adaptive evolution of human immunodeficiency virus type 1 during the natural course of infection. Science 1996; 277:537–42.
4. Shankarappa R, Gupta P, Learn GH Jr, Rodrigo AG, Rinaldo CR Jr, Gorry MC, et al. Evolution of human immunodeficiency virus type 1 envelope sequences in infected individuals with differing disease progression profiles. Virology 1998; 241:251–9.
5. Lukashov VV, Kuiken CL, Goudsmit J. Intrahost human immunodeficiency virus type 1 evolution is related to length of the immunocompetent period. J Virol 1995; 69:6911–6.
6. Ganeshan S, Dickover R, Korber B, Bryson Y, Wolinsky S. Human immunodeficiency virus type 1 genetic evolution over time in children with different rates of development of disease. J Virol 1997; 71:663–7.
7. Condra JH. Resistance to HIV protease inhibitors. Haemophilia 1998; 4:610–5.
8. Wong JK, Ignacio CC, Torriani F, Havlir D, Fitch NJ, Richman DD. In vivo compartmentalization of human immunodeficiency virus: evidence from the examination of pol sequences from autopsy tissues. J Virol 1997; 71:2059–71.
9. Hammond J, Calef C, Larder B, Schinazi R, Mellors JW. Mutations in retroviral genes associated with resistance. In: Korber B, Kuiken C, Foley B, Hahn B, McCutchan F, Sodroski JWMJ (eds). Human Retroviruses and AIDS 1998. Los Alamos, NM: Los Alamos National Laboratory, 1998, pp. III 10–9.
10. Paxton WA, Dragic T, Koup R, Moore JP. Perspective: The beta-chemokines, HIV type 1 second receptors, and unexposed uninfected persons. AIDS Res Hum Retrovir 1996; 18:1687–91.
11. Lu Z, Berson JF, Chen Y, Turner JD, Zhang T, Sharron M, et al. Evolution of HIV-1 coreceptor usage through interactions with distinct CCR5 and CXCR4 domains. Proc Natl Acad Sci USA 1997; 94:6426–31.
12. Connor RI, Sheridan KE, Ceradini D, Choe S, Landau NR. Change in coreceptor use coreceptor use correlates with disease progression in HIV-1–infected individuals. J Exp Med 1997; 185:621–8.
13. Borrow P, Lewicki H, Wei X, Horwitz MS, Peffer N, Meyers H, et al. Anti-viral pressure exerted by HIV-1-specific cytotoxic T lymphocytes (CTLs) during primary infection demonstrated by rapid selection of CTL escape virus. Nat Med 1997; 3:205–11.
14. Price DA, Goulder PJ, Klenerman P, Sewell AK, Easterbrook PJ, Troop M, et al. Positive selection of HIV-1 cytotoxic T lymphocyte escape variants during primary infection. Proc Natl Acad Sci USA 1997; 94:1890–5.
15. Van Baalen CA, Schutten M, Huisman RC, Boersand PH, Gruters RA, Osterhaus AD. Kinetics of Antiviral Activity by Human Immunodeficiency Virus Type 1-Specific Cytotoxic T Lymphocytes (CTL) and Rapid Selection of CTL Escape Virus in Vitro. J Virol 1998; 72:6852–7.
16. Colgrove R. A combinatorial ledge: reverse transcriptase fidelity, total body viral burden, and the implications of multiple-drug HIV therapy for the evolution of antiviral resistance. Antivir Res 1999; 41:45–56.

17. Kuiken C, Lukashov V, Baan E, Dekker J, Leunissen J, Goudsmit J. Evidence for limited intra-subject evolution of the V3 domain of the HIV-1 envelope in the Amsterdam population. AIDS 1996; 10:31–7.
18. McCutchan FE, Hegerich PA, Brennan TP, Phanuphak P, Singharaj P, Jugsudee A, et al. Genetic variants of HIV-1 in Thailand. AIDS Res Hum Retrovir 1992; 8:1887–95.
19. Ou C, Clesieisky CA, Myers G, Bandes CI, Luo CC, Korber BTM. Molecular epidemiology of HIV transmission in a dental practice. Science 1992; 256:1165–71.
20. Liitsola K, Tashkinova I, Laukkanen T, Korovina G, Smolskaja T, Momot O, et al. HIV-1 genetic subtype A/B recombinant strain causing an explosive epidemic in injecting drug users in Kaliningrad. AIDS 1998; 12:1907–19.
21. McCutchan F, Artenstein A, Sanders-Buell E, Salminen M, Carr J, Mascola J, et al. Diversity of the envelope glycoprotein among human immunodeficiency virus type 1 isolates of clade E from Asia and Africa. J Virol 1996; 70:3331–8.
22. Robertson DL, Sharp PM, McCutchan FE, Hahn BH. Recombination in HIV-1. Nature 1995; 374:124–6.
23. McCutchan F, Carr J, Bajani M, Sanders-Buell E, Harry T, Stoeckli T, et al. Subtype G and multiple forms of A/G intersubtype recombinant human immunodeficiency virus type 1 in Nigeria. Virology 1999; 254:226–34.
24. Gao F, Bailes E, Robertson DL, Chen Y, Rodenburg CM, Michael SF, et al. Origin of HIV-1 in the chimpanzee *Pan troglodytes troglodytes.* Nature 1999; 397:436–41.
25. Chen Z, Telfier P, Gettie A, Reed P, Zhang L, Ho DD, Marx PA. Genetic characterization of new West African simian immunodeficiency virus SIVsm: geographic clustering of household-derived SIV strains with human immunodeficiency virus type 2 subtypes and genetically diverse viruses from a single feral sooty mangabey troop. J Virol 1996; 70:3617–27.
26. Gao F, Yue L, White A, Pappas P, Barchue J, Hanson A, et al. Human infection by genetically-diverse SIVsm-related HIV-2 in West Africa. Nature 1992; 358:495–9.
27. Weiss R. From pan to pandemic. Nature 1999; 397:385–6.
28. Brown DW. Threat to humans from virus infections of non-human primates. Rev Med Virol 1997; 7:239–46.
29. Ostrowski S, Leslie MJ, Parrott T, Abelt S, Piercy PE. B-virus from pet macaque monkeys: an emerging threat in the United States? Emerg Infect Dis 1998; 4:117–21.
30. Loussert-Ajaka I, Chaix M, Korber B, Letourneur F, Gomas E, Ly T, et al. The variability of HIV type 1 group O strains isolated from Cameroonian patients living in France. J Virol 1995; 69:5640–49.
31. Korber B, Loussert-Ajakai I, Blouin J, Saragosti S. A comparison of HIV-1 group M and group O functional and immunogenic domains in the Gag p24 protein and the C2V3 region of the envelope protein. In: Myers G, Korber B, Foley B, Jeang K, Mellors JW, Wain-Hobson S (eds). Human Retroviruses and AIDS 1996. Los Alamos, NM: Los Alamos National Laboratory: Theoretical Biology and Biophysics, 1996, pp. III 41–56.
32. Simon F, Mauclere P, Roques P, Loussert-Ajaka I, Muller-Trutwin MC, Saragosti S, et al. Identification of a new human immunodeficiency virus type 1 distinct from group M and group O. Nat Med 1998; 4:1032–7.
33. Carr JK, Foley BT, Leitner T, Salminen M, Korber B, McCutchan F. Reference sequences representing the principal genetic diversity of HIV-1 in the pandemic. In: Korber B, Kuiken C, Foley B, Hahn B, McCutchan F, Sodroski JWMJ (eds). Human Retroviruses and AIDS 1998. Los Alamos NM: Los Alamos National Laboratory: Theoretical Biology and Biophysics, 1998, pp. III 10–9.
34. Huet T, Cheynier R, Meyerhans A, Roelants G, Wain-Hobson S. Genetic organization of a chimpanzee lentivirus related to HIV-1. Nature 1990; 345:356–9.

35. vanden Haesevelde MM, Peeters M, Jannes G, Janssens W, van der Groen G, Sharp PM, Saman E. Sequence analysis of a highly divergent HIV-1 related lentivirus isolated from a wild captured chimpanzee. Virology 1996; 221:346–50.
36. Sharp PM, Robertson DL, Gao F, Hahn BH. Origins and diversity of human immunodeficiency viruses. AIDS: 1994 A Year in Review 1994; 8:S27–S43.
37. Gao F, Yue L, Robertson DL, Hill SC, Hui H, Bigger RJ et al. Genetic diversity of human immunodeficiency virus type 2: evidence for distinct sequence subtypes with differences in virus biology. J Virol 1994; 68:7433–47.
38. Korber B, Allen E, Farmer AD, Myers G. Heterogeneity of HIV-1 and HIV-2. AIDS 1995; 9(Suppl A):S5–S18.
39. Zhu T, Korber BT, Nahmias AJ, Hooper E, Sharp PM, Ho DD. An African HIV-1 sequence from 1959 and implications for the origin of the epidemic. Nature 1998; 391:594–6.
40. Sharp PM, Robertson D, Hahn B. Cross-species transmission and recombination of AIDS viruses. Philos Trans R Soc Lond B Biol Sci 1995; 349:41–7.
41. Chen A, Luckay A, Sodora DL, Telfer P, Reed P, Gettie A, et al. Human immunodeficiency virus type 2 (HIV-2) seroprevalence and characterization of a distinct HIV-2 genetic subtype from the natural range of simian immunodeficiency virus-infected sooty mangabeys. J Virol 1997; 71:3953–60.
42. Rey-Cuille MA, Berthier JT, Chaduc MCBY, Montagnier L, Hovanessian AG, Chakrabarti LA. Simian immunodeficiency virus replicates to high levels in sooty mangabeys without inducing disease. J Virol 1998; 72:3872–86.
43. Jin MJ, Hui H, Robertson DL, Muller MC, Barre-Sinoussi F, Hirsch VM, et al. Mosaic genome structure of simian immunodeficiency virus from west African green monkeys. EMBO J 1994; 13:2935–47.
44. Hirsch VM, Campbell BJ, Bailes E, Goeken R, Brown C, Elkins WR, et al. Characterization of a novel simian immunodeficiency virus (SIV) from L'Hoest monkeys (Cercopithecus l'hoesti): implications for the origins of SIVmnd and other primate lentiviruses. J Virol 1999; 73:1036–45.
45. Jin MJ, Rogers J, Phillips-Conroy JE, Allan JS, Desrosiers RC, Shaw GM, et al. Infection of a yellow baboon with simian immunodeficiency virus from african green monkeys: evidence for cross-species transmission in the wild. J Virol 1994; 68:8454–60.
46. Korber B, Theiler J, Wolinsky S. Limitations of a Molecular Clock Applied to Considerations of the Origins of HIV-1. Science 1998; 280:1868–71.
47. de Leys R, Vanderborght B, vanden Haesevelde M, Heyndrickx L, van Geel A, Wauters C, et al. Isolation and partial characterization of an unusual human immunodeficiency retrovirus from two persons of west-central African origin. J Virol 1990; 64:1207–16.
48. Gurtler LG, Hauser PH, Eberle J, von Brunn A, Knapp S, Zekeng L, et al. A new subtype of human immunodeficiency virus type 1 (MVP-5180) from Cameroon. J Virol 1994; 68:1581–5.
49. Louwagie J, Janssens W, Mascola J, Hendrickx L, Hegerich P, van der Groen G, McCutchan F, Burke D. Genetic diversity of the envelope glycoprotein from human immunodeficiency virus type-1 (HIV-1) isolates of Africa origin. J Virol 1995; 69:263–71.
50. Louwagie J, McCutchan FE, Peeters M, Brennan TP, Buell E, Eddy GA, et al. Phylogenetic analysis of gag genes from 70 international HIV-1 isolates provides evidence for multiple genotypes. AIDS 1993; 7:769–80.
51. Gao F, Morrison SG, Robertson DL, Thornton CL, Craig S, Karlsson G, et al. Molecular cloning and analysis of functional envelope genes from human immunodeficiency virus type 1 sequence subtypes A through G. J Virol 1996; 1651–7.
52. Quinones-Mateu ME, Albright JL, Mas A, Soriano V, Arts EJ. Analysis of pol gene heterogeneity, viral quasispecies, and drug resistance in individuals infected with group O strains of human immunodeficiency virus type 1. J Virol 1998; 72:9002–15.

53. Janssens W, Heyndrickx L, Van der Auwera G, Nkengasong J, Beirnaert E, Vereecken K, et al. Interpatient genetic variability of HIV-1 group O. AIDS 1999; 13:41–8.
54. Jonassen T, Stene-Johansen K, Berg ES, Hungnes O, Lindboe CF, Grinde B. HIV-1 group O infection in Norwegian patients in the 1960s. Virology 1997; 231:43–47.
55. Gao F, Robertson DL, Carruthers CD, Morrison SG, Jian B, Chen Y, et al. A comprehensive panel of near-full-length clones and reference sequences for non-subtype B isolates of human immunodeficiency virus type 1. J Virol 1998; 72:5680–98.
56. Carr JK, Salminen MO, Albert J, Sanders-Buell E, Gotte D, Birx DL, McCutchan FE. Full genome sequences of human immunodeficiency virus type 1 subtypes G and A/G intersubtype recombinants. Virology 1998; 247:22–31.
57. Triques K, Bourgeois A, Saragosti S, Vidal N, Mpoudi-Ngole E, Nzilambi N, et al. High diversity of HIV-1 subtype F strains in Central Africa. Virology 1999; 259:99–109.
58. Kostrikis L, Bagdades E, Cao Y, Zhang L, Dimitriou D, Ho DD. Genetic analysis of human immunodeficiency virus type 1 strains from patients in Cyprus: identification of a new subtype designated subtype I. J Virol 1995; 69:6122–30.
59. Nasioulas G, Paraskevis D, Paparizos V, Lazanas M, Karafoulidou A, Hatzakis A. Genotypic characterization of human immunodeficiency virus type 1 in Greece. Multicentre Study on HIV-1 Heterogeneity. AIDS Res Hum Retrovir 1998; 14:685–90.
60. Robertson DL, Gao F, Hahn BH. Intersubtype recombinant HIV-1 sequences. In: Korber B, Hahn B, Foley B, Mellors J, Leitner T, Myers G, et al. (eds). Human Retroviruses and AIDS 1997. Los Alamos, NM: Los Alamos National Laboratory: Theoretical Biology and Biophysics, 1997, pp. III 41–56.
61. Potts KE, Kalish ML, Bandea CI, Orloff GM, St. Louis M, Brown C, et al. Genetic diversity of human immunodeficiency virus type 1 strains in Kinshasa, Zaire. AIDS Res Hum Retrovir 1993; 9:613–8.
62. Sabino E, Shpaer E, Morgado M, Korber B, Diaz R, Bongertz V, et al. Identification of human immunodeficiency virus type 1 envelope genes recombinant between subtypes B and F in two epidemiologically linked individuals from Brazil. J Virol 1994; 68:6340–6.
63. Myers G. In: Human Retroviruses and AIDS 1987. Myers G, Robson A, Josephs S, and Smith T, eds. Los Alamos, NM: Los Alamos National Laboratory, 1987, Part I, Theoretical Biology and Biophysics.
64. Li W-H, Tanimura M, Sharp PM. Rates and dates of divergence between AIDS virus nucleotide sequences. Mol Biol Evol 1988; 5:313–30.
65. Zhu T, Wang N, Carr A, Wolinsky S, Ho DD. Evidence for coinfection by multiple strains of human immunodeficiency virus type 1 subtype B in an acute seroconvertor. J Virol 1995; 69:1324–7.
66. Diaz R, Sabino E, Mayer A, Mosley J, Busch M. Dual human immunodeficiency virus type 1 infection and recombination in a dually exposed transfusion recipient. J Virol 1995; 69:3273–81.
67. Carr JK, Salminen MO, Koch C, Gotte D, Artenstein AW, Hegerich PA, et al. Full-length sequence and mosaic structure of a human immunodeficiency virus type 1 isolate from Thailand. J Virol 1996; 70:5935–43.
68. Gao F, Robertson DL, Morrison SG, Hui H, Craig S, Decker J, et al. The heterosexual human immunodeficiency virus type 1 epidemic in Thailand is caused by an intersubtype (A/E) recombinant of African origin. J Virol 1996; 70:7013–29.
69. Takehisa J, Zekeng L, Ido E, Yamaguchi-Kabata Y, Mboudjeka I, Harada Y, et al. Human immunodeficiency virus type 1 intergroup (M/O) recombination in Cameroon. J Virol 1999; 73:6810–20.
70. Soto-Ramirez LE, Renjito B, McLane MF, Marlink R, O'Hara C, Sutthent R, Wasi C, et al. HIV-1 Langerhans' cell tropism associated with heterosexual transmission of HIV. Science 1996; 271:1291–3.
71. Essex M, Soto-Ramirez LE, Renjifo E, Wang WK, Lee T. Genetic variation within human immunodeficiency viruses generates rapid changes in tropism, virulence, and transmission. Leukemia 1997; 11:93–4.

72. The European Commission and the Joint United Nations Programme on HIV/AIDS. HIV-1 subtypes: implications for epidemiology, pathogenicity, vaccines and diagnostics. AIDS 1997; 11:17–36.
73. Dittmar MT, Simmons G, Hibbitts S, O'Hare M, Louisirirotchanakul S, Beddows S, et al. Langerhans cell tropism of HIV-1 subtype A through F isolates derived from different transmission groups. J Virol 1997; 71:8008–13.
74. Pope M, Frankel SS, Mascola JR, Trkola A, Isdell F, Birx DL, et al. HIV-1 strains from subtypes B and E replicate in cutaneous dendritic cell-T cell mixtures without displaying subtype-specific tropism. J Virol 1997; 71:8001–7.
75. Alaeus A, Lidman K, Bjorkman A, Giesecke J, Albert J. Similar rate of disease progression among individuals infected with HIV-1 genetic subtypes A–D. AIDS 1999; 13:901–7.
76. Kanki PJ, Hamel DJ, Sankale JL, Hsieh CC, Thior I, Barin F, et al. Human immunodeficiency virus type 1 subtypes differ in disease progression. J Infect Dis 1999; 179:68–73.
77. Grassly NC, Xiang Z, Ariyoshi K, Aaby P, Jensen H, van der Loeff MS, et al. Mortality among human immunodeficiency virus type 2-positive villagers in rural Guinea-Bissau is correlated with viral genotype. J Virol 1998; 72:7895–9.
78. Huang Y, Paxton WA, Wolinsky SM, et al. The role of a mutant CCR5 allele in HIV-1 transmission and disease progression. Nat Med 1996; 2:1240–3.
79. Berger EA, Doms RW, Fenyo E, Korber B, Littman DR, Moore JP, et al. A new classification for HIV-1. Nature 1998; 391:240–1.
80. Zhang L, Huang Y, He T, Cao Y, Ho DD. HIV-1 subtype and second-receptor use. Nature 1996; 383:768.
81. Doms RW, Edinger AL, Moore JP. Coreceptor use by primate lentiviruses. In: Korber B, Kuiken C, Foley B, Hahn B, McCutchan F, Sodroski JWMJ (eds). Human Retroviruses and AIDS 1998. Los Alamos, NM: Los Alamos National Laboratory: Theoretical Biology and Biophysics, 1998, pp. III 10–9.
82. Morner A, Bjorndal A, Albert J, Kewalramani VN, Littman DR, Inoue R, et al. Primary human immunodeficiency virus type 2 (HIV-2) isolates, like HIV-1 isolates, frequently use CCR5 but show promiscuity in coreceptor usage. J Virol 1999; 73:2343–9.
83. Tersmette M, Gruters RA, de Wolf F, de Goede REY, Lange JMA, Schellekens PTA, et al. Evidence for a role of virulent human immunodeficiency virus (HIV) variants in the pathogenesis of Acquired Immunodeficiency Syndrome: studies on sequential HIV isolates. J Virol 1989; 63:2118–25.
84. Tersmette M, Lange JMA, de Goede REY, de Wolf F, Schattenkerk JKME, Schellekens PTH, et al. Association between biological properties of human immunodeficiency virus variants and risk for AIDS and AIDS mortality. Lancet 1989; i:983–5.
85. Tscherning C, Alaeus A, Fredriksson R, Bjorndal A, Deng H, Littman DR, et al. Differences in chemokine coreceptor usage between genetic subtypes of HIV-1. Virology 1998; 241:181–8.
86. Peeters M, Vincent R, Perret JL, Lasky M, Patrel D, Liegeois F, et al. Evidence for differences in MT2 cell tropism according to genetic subtypes of HIV-1: syncytium-inducing variants seem rare among subtype C HIV-1 viruses. J Acquir Immune Defic Syndr Hum Retrovirol 1999; 20:115–21.
87. Bjorndal A, Sonnerborg A, Tscherning C, Albert J, Fenyo EM. Phenotypic characteristics of human immunodeficiency virus type 1 subtype C isolates of Ethiopian AIDS patients. AIDS Res Hum Retrovir 1999; 15:647–53.
88. Ping L, Nelson JA, Hoffman IF, Schock J, Lamers SL, Goodman M, et al. Characterization of V3 sequence heterogeneity in subtype C human immunodeficiency virus type 1 isolates from Malawi: underrepresentation of X4 variants. J Virol 1999; 73:6271–81.
89. de Jong JJ, Goudsmit J, Keulen W, Klaver B, Krone WJA, Tersmette M, de Ronde A. Human immunodeficiency virus type 1 clones chimeric for the envelope V3 domain differ in syncytium formation and replication capacity. J Virol 1992; 66:757–65.

90. de Wolf F, Hogervorst E, Goudsmit J, Fenyo E, Rubsamen-Waigmann H, et al. Syncytium inducing (SI) and non-syncytium inducing (NSI) capacity of human immunodeficiency virus type 1 (HIV-1) subtypes other than B: phenotypic and genotypic characteristics. AIDS Res Hum Retrovir 1994; 10:1387–400.
91. Van Harmelen JH, Van der Ryst E, Loubser AS, York D, Madurai S, Lyons S, et al. A predominantly HIV type 1 subtype C-restricted epidemic in South African urban populations. AIDS Res Hum Retrovir 1999; 15:395–408.
92. Abebe A, Kuiken CL, Goudsmit J, Valk M, Messele T, Sahlu T, et al. HIV type 1 subtype C in Addis Ababa, Ethiopia. AIDS Res Hum Retrovir 1997; 13:1071–5.
93. Kirchhoff F, Greenough TC, Hamacher M, Sullivan JL, Desrosiers RC. Activity of human immunodeficiency virus type 1 promoter/TAR regions and *tat1* genes derived from individuals with different rates of disease progression. Virology 1997; 232:319–31.
94. Montano MA, Novitsky VA, Blackard JT, Cho NL, Katzenstein DA, Essex M. Divergent transcriptional regulation among expanding human immunodeficiency virus type 1 subtypes. J Virol 1997; 71:8657–65.
95. Apetrei C, Descamps D, Collin G, Loussert-Ajaka I, Damond F, Duca M, et al. Human immunodeficiency virus type 1 subtype F reverse transcriptase sequence and drug susceptibility. J Virol 1998; 72:3534–8.
96. Descamps D, Apetrei C, Collin G, Damond F, Simon F, Brun-Vezinet F. Naturally occurring decreased susceptibility of HIV-1 subtype G to protease inhibitors. AIDS 1998; 12:1109–11.
97. Braaten D, Franke EK, Luban J. Cyclophilin A is required for the replication of the group M human immunodeficiency virus type 1 (HIV-1) and simian immunodeficiency virus SIVcpz-GAB but not group O HIV-1 or other primate immunodeficiency viruses. J Virol 1996; 70:4420–7.
98. Descamps D, Collin G, Loussert-Ajaka I, Saragosti S, Simon F, Brun-Vezinet F. HIV-1 group O sensitivity to antiretroviral drugs. AIDS 1995; 9:977–8.
99. Descamps D, Collin G, Letourneur F, Apetrei C, Damond F, Loussert-Ajaka II, et al. Susceptibility of HIV-1 group O isolates to antiviral agents: in vitro phenotypic and genotypic analyses. J Virol 1997; 71:8893–8.
100. Alaeus A, Lilja E, Herman S, Spadoro J, Wang J, Albert J. Assay of plasma samples representing different HIV-1 genetic subtypes: an evaluation of new versions of the amplicor HIV-1 monitor assay. AIDS Res Hum Retrovir 1999; 15:889–94.
101. Gurtler L. Difficulties and strategies of HIV diagnosis. Lancet 1996; 348:176–9.
102. Korber BTM, MacInnes K, Smith R, Myers G. Mutational trends in V3 loop protein sequences observed in different genetic lineages of human immunodeficiency virus type-1. J Virol 1994; 68:6730–44.
103. Dighe PK, Korber B, Foley BT. Global Variation in the HIV-1 V3 Region. In: Korber B, Hahn B, Foley B, Mellors J, Leitner T, Myers G, et al. (eds). Human Retroviruses and AIDS 1997. Los Alamos, NM: Los Alamos National Laboratory: Theoretical Biology and Biophysics, 1997, pp. III 74–206.
104. Barin F, Lahbabi Y, Lejeune LBB, Baillou-Beaufils A, Denis F, Mathiot C, et al. Diversity of antibody binding to V3 peptides representing consensus sequences of HIV type 1 genotypes A to E: an approach for HIV type 1 serological subtyping. AIDS Res Hum Retrovir 1996; 12:1279–89.
105. Cocchi E, DeVico AL, Garzino-Demo A, Cara A, Gallo RC, Lusso P. The V3 domain of the HIV-1 gp120 envelope glycoprotein in critical for chemokine-mediated blockage of infection. Nature Med 1996; 270:1811–15.
106. Bieniasz PD, Fridell RA, Aramori I, Ferguson SS, Caron MG, Cullen BR. HIV-1-induced cell fusion is mediated by multiple regions within both the viral envelope and the CCR-5 co-receptor. EMBO J 1997; 16:2599–609.

107. Kato K, Sato H, Takebe Y. Role of naturally occurring basic amino acid substitutions in the human immunodeficiency virus type 1 subtype E envelope V3 loop on viral coreceptor usage and cell tropism. J Virol 1999; 73:5520–6.
108. Verrier F, Borman AM, Brand D, Girard M. Role of the HIV type 1 glycoprotein 120 V3 loop in determining coreceptor usage. AIDS Res Hum Retrovir 1999; 15:731–43.
109. Hoelscher M, Hanker S, Barin F, Cheingsong-Popov R, Dietrich U, Jordan-Harder B, et al. HIV type 1 V3 serotyping of Tanzanian samples: probable reasons for mismatching with genetic subtyping. AIDS Res Hum Retrovir 1998; 14:139–49.
110. Kalish ML, Luo CC, Weniger BG, Limpakarnjanarat K, Young N, Ou CY, Schochetman G. Early HIV type 1 strains in Thailand were not responsible for the current epidemic. AIDS Res Hum Retrovir 1994; 10:1573–5.
111. Ubolyam S, Ruxrungtham K, Sirivichayakul S, Okuda K, Phanuphak P. Evidence of three HIV-1 subtypes in subgroups of individuals in Thailand. Lancet 1994; 344:485–6.
112. Kalish ML, Baldwin A, Raktham S, Wasi C, Luo CC, Schochetman G, et al. The evolving molecular epidemiology of HIV-1 envelope subtypes in injecting drug users in Bangkok, Thailand: implications for HIV vaccine trials. AIDS 1995; 9:851–7.
113. Subbarao S, Limpakarnjanarat K, Mastro TD, Bhumisawasdi I, Warachit P, Jayavasu C, et al. HIV type 1 in Thailand, 1994–1995: persistence of two subtypes with low genetic diversity. AIDS Res Hum Retrovir 1998; 14:319–27.
114. Kusagawa S, Sato H, Watanabe S, Nohtomi K, Kato K, Shino T, et al. Genetic and serologic characterization of HIV type 1 prevailing in Myanmar (Burma). AIDS Res Hum Retrovir 1998; 14:1379–85.
115. Brown TM, Robbins KE, Sinniah M, Saraswathy TS, Lee V, Hooi LS, et al. Human immunodeficiency virus type 1 subtypes in Malaysia include BC, and E. AIDS Res Hum Retrovir 1996; 12:1655–7.
116. Nerurkar V, Nguyen H, Woodward C, Hoffmann P, Dashwood W, Long H, et al. Sequence and phylogenetic analyses of HIV-1 infection in Vietnam: subtype E in commercial sex workers (CSW) and injection drug users (IDU). Cell Mol Biol 1997; 43:959–68.
117. Porter K, Mascola J, Hupudio H, Ewing D, VanCott T, Anthony R, et al. Genetic, antigenic and serologic characterization of human immunodeficiency virus type 1 from Indonesia. J Acquir Immune Defic Syndr Hum Retrovirol 1997; 14:1–6.
118. Menu E, Truong T, Lafon M, Nguyen T, Muller-Trutwin M, Nguyen T, et al. HIV type 1 Thai subtype E is predominant in South Vietnam. AIDS Res Hum Retrovir 1996; 12:629–33.
119. Kang M, Cho Y, Chun J, Kim Y, Lee I, Lee H, et al. Phylogenetic analysis of the nef gene reveals a distinctive monophyletic clade in Korean HIV-1 cases. J Acquir Immune Defic Syndr Hum Retrovirol 1998; 17:58–68.
120. Kim E, Cho Y, Maeng S, Kang C, Nam J, Lee J. Characterization of V3 loop sequences from HIV type 1 subtype B in South Korea: predominance of the GPGS motif. AIDS Res Hum Retrovir 1999; 15:681–6.
121. Lukashov VV, Kuiken CL, Boer K, Goudsmit J. HIV type 1 subtypes in the Netherlands circulating among women originating from AIDS endemic regions. AIDS Res Hum Retrovir 1996; 12:951–3.
122. Alaeus A, Leitner T, Lidman K, Albert J. Most HIV-1 genetic subtypes have entered Sweden. AIDS 1997; 11:199–202.
123. Montpetit M. HIV-1 subtype A in Canada. AIDS Res Hum Retrovir 1995; 11:1421–2.
124. Charneau P, Borman AM, Quillent C, Guetard D, Chamaret S, Cohen J, et al. Isolation and evelope sequence of a highly divergent HIV-1 isolate: definition of a new HIV-1 group. Virology 1994; 205:247–53.
125. Kuiken CL, Cornelissen MT, Zorgdrager F, Hartman S, Gibbs AJ, Goudsmit J. Consistent risk group-associated differences in human immunodeficiency virus type 1 vpr, vpu and V3 sequences despite independent evolution. J Gen Virol 1996; 77:783–92.

126. Leigh-Brown A, Lobidel D, Wade C, Rebus S, Phillips A, Brettle R, et al. The molecular epidemiology of human immunodeficiency virus type 1 in six cities in Britain and Ireland. Virology 1997; 235:166–77.
127. Adwan G, Papa A, Kouidou S, Alexiou S, Malissiovas N, Ntoutsos I, et al. HIV type 1 sequences with GGC substitution in injecting drug users in Greece. AIDS Res Hum Retrovir 1999; 15:679–80.
128. Lukashov VV, Cornelissen MT, Goudsmit J, Papuashvilli MN, Rytik PG, Khaitov RM, et al. Simultaneous introduction of distinct HIV-1 subtypes into different risk groups in Russia, Byelorussia and Lithuania. AIDS 1995; 9:435–9.
129. Liitsola K, Laukkanen T, Denisova A, Grishkevichius A, Smolskaja T, Ustina V, et al. Genetic characterization of HIV-1 strains in the Baltic countries and Russia. Scand J Infect Dis 1996; 28:537–41.
130. van Harmelen J, Wood R, Lambrick M, Rybicki EP, Williamson AL, Williamson C. An association between HIV-1 subtypes and mode of transmission in Cape Town, South Africa. AIDS 1997; 11:81–7.
131. Sher R. HIV infection in South Africa, 1982–1988—a review. S Afr Med J 1989; 76:314–8.
132. Holmes EC, Zhang LQ, Simmonds P, Leigh Brown AJ. Molecular investigation of human immunodeficiency virus HIV infection in a patient of an HIV-infected surgeon. J Infect Dis 1993; 167:1411–4.
133. Wolfs TFW, Zwart G, Bakker M, Goudsmit J. HIV-1 genomic RNA diversification following sexual and parenteral virus transmission. Virology 1992; 189:103–10.
134. Kahn JG, Gurvey J, Pollack LM, Binson D, Catania JA. HIV-1 strains specific for Dutch injecting drug users in heterosexually infected individuals in The Netherlands. AIDS 1997; 12:635–41.
135. Ekstrand ML, Coates TJ. Maintenance of safer sexual behaviors and predictors of risky sex: the San Francisco Men's Health Study. Am J Public Health 1990; 80:973–7.
136. Krijnen P, van den Hoek JA, Coutinho RA. Do bisexual men play a significant role in the heterosexual spread of HIV. Sex Transm Dis 1994; 21:24–5.
137. Lukashov V, Op de Coul E, Coutinho R, Goudsmit J. HIV-1 strains specific for Dutch injecting drug users in heterosexually infected individuals in The Netherlands. AIDS 1998; 12:635–41.
138. Rowland-Jones S, Sutton J, Ariyoshi K, Dong T, Gotch F, McAdam S, et al. HIV-specific cytotoxic T-cells in HIV-exposed but uninfected Gambian women. Nat Med 1995; 1:59–64.
139. Rowland-Jones S, Dong T, Dorrell L, Ogg G, Hansasuta P, Krausa P, et al. Broadly cross-reactive HIV-specific cytotoxic T-lymphocytes in highly-exposed persistently seronegative donors. Immunol Lett 1999; 66:9–14.
140. Bernard N, Yannakis C, Lee J, Tsoukas C. Human immunodeficiency virus (HIV)-specific cytotoxic T lymphocyte activity in HIV-exposed seronegative persons. J Infect Dis 1999; 179:538–47.
141. Goh W, Markee J, Akridge R, Meldorf M, Musey L, Karchmer T, et al. Protection against human immunodeficiency virus type 1 infection in persons with repeated exposure: evidence for T cell immunity in the absence of inherited CCR5 coreceptor defects. J Infect Dis 1999; 179:548–57.
142. Pontesilli O, Carlesimo M, Varani A, Ferrara R, Guerra E, Bernardi M, et al. HIV-specific lymphoproliferative responses in asymptomatic HIV-infected individuals. Clin Exp Immunol 1995; 100:419–24.
143. Rosenberg E, Walker B. HIV type 1-specific helper T cells: a critical host defense. AIDS Res Hum Retrovir 1998; 14: Suppl 2:S143–7.
144. Rosenberg E, Billingsley J, Caliendo A, Boswell S, Sax P, Kalams S, Walker B. Vigorous HIV-1-specific $CD4^+$ T cell responses associated with control of viremia. Science 1997; 278:1447–50.
145. Pitcher C, Quittner C, Peterson D, Connors M, Koup R, Maino V, Picker L. HIV-1-specific $CD4^+$ T cells are detectable in most individuals with active HIV-1 infection, but decline with prolonged viral suppression. Nat Med 1999; 5:518–25.

146. Couillin I, Culmann-Penciolelli B, Gomard E, Choppin J, Levy J, Guillet JG, Sarasgosti S. Impaired cytotoxic T lymphocyte recognition due to genetic variations in the main immunogenic region of the human immunodeficiency virus 1 NEF protein. J Exp Med 1994; 180:1129–34.
147. Goulder P, Sewell A, Lalloo D, Price D, Whelan J, Evans J, et al. Patterns of immunodominance in HIV-1-specific cytotoxic T lymphocyte responses in two human histocompatibility leukocyte antigens (HLA)-identical siblings with HLA-A*0201 are influenced by epitope mutation. J Exp Med 1997; 8:1423–33.
148. Meyerhans A, Dadaglio G, Vartanian JP, Langlade-Demoyen P, Frank R, Asjo B, et al. In vivo persistence of an HIV-1-encoded HLA-B27-restricted cytotoxic T lymphocyte epitope despite specific in vitro reactivity. Eur J Immunol 1991; 21:2637–40.
149. Brander C, Hartman KE, Trocha AK, Jones NG, Johnson RP, Korber B, et al. Lack of strong immune selection pressure by the immunodominant, HLA-A*0201-restricted cytotoxic T lymphocyte response in chronic human immunodeficiency virus-1 infection. J Clin Invest 1998; 101:2559–66.
150. Goulder PJR, Phillips RE, Colbert RA, McAdam S, Ogg G, Nowak MA. Late escape from an immunodominant cytotoxic T-lymphocyte response associated with progression to AIDS. Nat Med 1997; 3:212–6.
151. Wilson C, Brown R, Korber B, Wilkes B, Ruhl D, Sakamoto D, et al. Detection of escape from cytotoxic T lymphocyte recognition in perinatal HIV-1 transmission. J Virol 1999; 73:3975–85.
152. Kaslow RA, Carrington M, Apple R, Park L, Munoz A, Saah AJ, et al. Influence of combinations of MHC genes on the course of HIV-1 infection. Nat Med 1996; 2:405.
153. Hendel H, Caillat-Zucman S, Lebuanec H, Carrington M, O'Brien S, Andrieu JM, et al. New class I and II HLA alleles strongly associated with opposite patterns of progression to AIDS. J Immunol 1999; 162:6942–6.
154. Chen Y, Winchester R, Korber B, Gagliano J, Bryson Y, Hutto C, et al. Influence of HLA alleles on the rate of progression of vertically transmitted HIV infection in children: association of several HLA-DR13 alleles with long-term survivorship and the potential association of HLA-A*2301 with rapid progression to AIDS. Hum Immunol 1997; 55:154–62.
155. Tomiyama H, Sakaguchi T, Miwa K, Oka S, Iwamoto A, Kaneko Y, Takiguchi M. Identification of multiple HIV-1 CTL epitopes presented by HLA-B*5101 molecules. Hum Immunol 1999; 60:177–86.
156. Tang J, Costello C, Keet I, Rivers C, Leblanc S, Karita E, et al. HLA class I homozygosity accelerates disease progression in human immunodeficiency virus type 1 infection. AIDS Res Hum Retrovir 1999; 15:317–24.
157. Wagner R, Leschonsky B, Harrer E, Paulus C, Weber C, Walker B, et al. Molecular and functional analysis of a conserved CTL epitope in HIV-1 p24 recognized from a long-term nonprogressor: constraints on immune escape associated with targeting a sequence essential for viral replication. J Immunol 1999; 162:3727–34.
158. van der Burg S, Kwappenberg K, Geluk A, van der Kruk M, Pontesilli O, Hovenkamp E, et al. Identification of a conserved universal Th epitope in HIV-1 reverse transcriptase that is processed and presented to HIV-specific $CD4^+$ T cells by at least four unrelated HLA-DR molecules. J Immunol 1999; 162:152–60.
159. Bradney AP, Scheer S, Crawford J, Buchbinder S, Montefiori D. Neutralization escape in human immunodeficiency virus type 1-infected long-term nonprogressors. Infect Dis 1999; 179:1264–7.
160. Pilgrim A, Pantaleo G, Cohen O, Fink L, Zhou J, Zhou J, et al. Neutralizing antibody responses to human immunodeficiency virus type 1 in primary infection and long-term-nonprogressive infection. J Infect Dis 1997; 176:924–32.
161. Moog C, Fleury H, Pellegrin I, Kirn A, Aubertin A. Autologous and heterologous neutralizing antibody responses following initial seroconversion in human immunodeficiency virus type 1-infected individuals. J Virol 1997; 71:3734–41.

162. Cheng-Mayer C, Brown A, Harouse J, Luciw PA, Mayer AJ. Selection for neutralization resistance of the simian human immunodeficiency virus SHIVSF33A variant in vivo by virtue of sequence changes in the extracellular envelope glycoprotein that modify N-linked glycosylation. J Virol 1999; 73:5294–300.
163. Ferris RL, Hall C, Sipsas NV, Safrit JT, Trocha A, Koup RA, et al. Processing of HIV-1 envelope glycoprotein for Class I-restricted recognition: dependence on TAP1/2 and mechanisms of cytosolic localization. J Immunol 1999; 162:1324–32.
164. Wyatt R, Kwong PD, Desjardins E, Sweet RW, Robinson J, Hendrickson WA, Sodroski JG. The antigenic structure of the HIV gp120 envelope glycoprotein. Nature 1998; 393:705–11.
165. Wyatt R, Sodroski J. The HIV-1 envelope glycoproteins: fusogens, antigens, and immunogens. Science 1998; 280:1884–8.
166. Frey S. HIV vaccines. Infect Dis Clin North Am 1999; 13:95–112.
167. Wagner R, Shao Y, Wolf H. Correlates of protection, antigen delivery and molecular epidemiology: basics for designing an HIV vaccine. Vaccine 1999; 17:1706–10.
168. Evans T, Keefer M, Weinhold K, Wolff M, Montefiori D, Gorse GJ, et al. A canarypox vaccine expressing multiple human immunodeficiency virus type 1 genes given alone or with rgp120 elicits broad and durable $CD8^+$ cytotoxic T lymphocyte responses in seronegative volunteers. J Infect Dis 1999; 180:290–8.
169. Boyer JD, Chattergoon M, Shah A, Ginsberg R, MacGregor RR, Weiner DB. HIV-1 DNA based vaccine induces a CD8 mediated cross-clade CTL response. Dev Biol Stand 1998; 95:147–53.
170. Lynch JA, deSouza M, Robb MD, Markowitz L, Nitayaphan S, Sapan CV, et al. Cross-clade cytotoxic T cell response to human immunodeficiency virus. J Infect Dis 1998; 178:1040–6.
171. Ishioka GY, Fikes J, Hermanson G, Livingston B, Crimi C, Qin M, et al. Utilization of MHC class I transgenic mice for development of minigene DNA vaccines encoding multiple HLA-restricted CTL epitopes. J Immunol 1999; 162:3915–25.
172. Hanke T, McMichael A. Pre-clinical development of a multi-CTL epitope-based DNA prime MVA boost vaccine for AIDS. Immunol Lett 1999; 66:177–81.
173. D'Souza P, Livnat D, Bradac JA, Bridges SH, the AIDS Clinical Trials Group Antibody Selection Working Group and Collaborating Investigators. Evaluation of monoclonal antibodies to human immunodeficiency virus type 1 primary isolates by neutralization assays: performance criteria for selecting candidate antibodies for clinical trials. J Infect Dis 1997; 175:1056–62.
174. Poignard P, Sabbe R, Picchio GR, Wang M, Gulizia RJ, Katinger H, et al. Neutralizing antibodies have limited effects on the control of established HIV-1 infection in vivo. Immunity 1999; 10:431–8.
175. Gauduin MC, Parren PW, Weir R, Barbas CF, Burton DR, Koup RA. Passive immunization with a human monoclonal antibody protects hu-PBL-SCID mice against challenge by primary isolates of HIV-1. Nat Med 1997; 3:1389–93.
176. Joag S, Li Z, Wang C, Foresman L, Jia F, Stephens EB, et al. Passively administered neutralizing serum that protected macaques against infection with parenterally inoculated pathogenic simian-human immunodeficiency virus failed to protect against mucosally inoculated virus. AIDS Res Hum Retrovir 1999; 15:391–4.
177. Mascola J, Lewis M, Stiegler G, DHD, VanCott T, Hayes D, et al. Protection of macaques against pathogenic simian/human immunodeficiency virus 89.6PD by passive transfer of neutralizing antibodies. J Virol 1999; 73:4009–18.
178. Moore JP, Ho DD. HIV-1 neutralization: the consequences of adaptation to growth on transformed T-cells. AIDS 1995; 9: Suppl A:S117–36.
179. VanCott T, Mascola J, Loomis-Price L, Sinangil F, Zitomersky N, McNeil J, et al. Cross-subtype neutralizing antibodies induced in baboons by a subtype E gp120 immunogen based on an R5 primary human immunodeficiency virus type 1 envelope. J Virol 1999; 73:4640–50.

180. Dorrell L, Dong T, Ogg G, Lister S, McAdam S, Rostron T, et al. Distinct recognition of non-clade B human immunodeficiency virus type 1 epitopes by cytotoxic T lymphocytes generated from donors infected in Africa. J Virol 1999; 73:1708–14.

181. Wilson SE, Pedersen SL, Kunich JC, Wilkins VL, Mann DL, Mazzara GP, et al. Cross-clade envelope glycoprotein 160-specific $CD8^+$ cytotoxic T lymphocyte responses in early HIV type 1 clade B infection. AIDS Res Hum Retrovir 1998; 14:925–37.

182. Cao H, Kanki P, Sankale JL, Dieng-Sarr A, Mazzara GP, Kalams S, et al. CTL cross-reactivity among different HIV-1 clades: Implications for vaccine development. J Virol 1997; 71:8615–23.

183. Betts MR, Krowka J, Santamaria C, Balsamo K, Gao F, Mulundu G, et al. Cross-clade human immunodeficiency virus (HIV)-specific cytotoxic T-lymphocyte responses in HIV-infected Zambians. J Virol 1997; 71:8908–11.

184. Buseyne F, Chaix ML, Fleury B, Manigard O, Burgard M, Blanche S, et al. Cross-clade-specific cytotoxic T lymphocytes in HIV-1–infected children. Virology 1998; 250:316–24.

185. Durali D, Morvan J, Letourneur F, Schmitt D, Guegan N, Dalod M, et al. Cross-reactions between the cytotoxic T-lymphocyte responses of human immunodeficiency virus-infected African and European patients. J Virol 1998; 72:3547–53.

186. Nyambi P, Nkengasong J, Lewi P, Andries K, Janssens W, Fransen K, et al. Multivariate analysis of human immunodeficiency virus type 1 neutralization data. J Virol 1996; 70:6235–43.

187. Moore JP, Cao Y, Leu J, Qin L, Korber B, Ho DD. Inter- and intra-subtype neutralization of human immunodeficiency virus type 1: the genetic subtypes do not correspond to neutralization serotypes but partially correspond to gp120 antigenic serotypes. J Virol 1995; 70:427–44.

188. Kostrikis LG, Cao Y, Ngai H, Moore JP, Ho DD. Quantitative analysis of serum neutralization of human immunodeficiency virus type 1 from subtypes A, B, C, D, E, F, and I: lack of direct correlation between neutralization serotypes and genetic subtypes and evidence for prevalent serum-dependent infectivity enhancement. J Virol 1996; 70:445–8.

189. Devico AL, Rahman R, Welch J, Crowley R, Lusso P, Sarngadharan MG, Pal R. Monoclonal antibodies raised against covalently crosslinked complexes of human immunodeficiency virus type 1 gp120 and CD4 receptor identify a novel complex-dependent epitope on gp120. Virology 1995; 211:583–8.

190. LaCasse R, Follis K, Trahey M, Scarborough JD, Littman DR, Nunberg J. Fusion-competent vaccines: broad neutralization of primary isolates of HIV. Science 1999; 283:357–62.

191. Smith RF, Smith TF. Pattern-induced multi-sequence alignment (PIMA) algorithm employing secondary structure-dependent gap penalties for use in comparative protein modeling. Protein Engng 1992; 5:35–41.

192. Henikoff S, Henikoff JG. Amino acid substitution matrices from protein blocks. Proc Natl Acad Sci USA 1992; 89:10915–9.

193. Henikoff S, Henikoff JG. Performance evaluation of amino acid substitution matrices. Proteins Struct Funct Gene 1993; 17:49–61.

2

Role of Chemokines and Their Receptors in the Pathogenesis of HIV Infection

Frederick S. Lee, Gabriele Kuschert, Otto O. Yang, and Andrew D. Luster

INTRODUCTION

The chemokines comprise a rapidly expanding group of *chemo*tactic cyto*kines* now known to play a critical role in regulating leukocyte trafficking during development and in homeostasis, inflammation, and infection. In the brief period since the original description of platelet factor 4 (PF4) *(1)* and interferon-inducible protein of 10 kDa (IP-10) *(2)* this family has grown to more than 50 members. Numerous studies now link chemokines to the pathogenesis of a wide range of inflammatory processes including asthma, atherosclerosis, pneumonia, meningitis, psoriasis, rheumatoid arthritis, inflammatory bowel disease, and sarcoidosis, among others *(3)*. Many also play roles in angiogenesis, hematopoiesis, and fetal development.

Chemokine and chemokine receptor genes have also been pirated by pathogens. Many herpes viruses encode chemokine-like molecules as well as functional chemokine receptors. In addition, several intracellular pathogens such as *Plasmodium vivax (4)*, Poxviruses *(5)* and HIV-1 *(6)* utilize chemokine receptors to gain access to the cytoplasm of leukocytes. The recent discovery that HIV-1 uses chemokine receptors together with CD4 to enter cells has been a major advance in understanding the pathogenesis of HIV-1 infection and has revealed an entirely new class of therapeutic targets. In this chapter, we briefly review general aspects of chemokine biology *(3,7,8)*, and then examine in detail the role of chemokines and their receptors in the pathogenesis of HIV-1 disease.

CHEMOKINES AND CHEMOKINE RECEPTORS

Structure

Chemokines are 8–10-kDa proteins sharing 20–95% amino acid homology (reviewed in *3,7,8*). They are divided into families based on the arrangement of four conserved cysteine residues. In the α-chemokines, the first two cysteines are separated by a single amino acid (cysteine–X amino acid–cysteine, or CXC). In the β-family, these two cysteines are adjacent (cysteine–cysteine, or CC). Lymphotactin, a "C" chemokine, is homologous to CC members but lacks the first and third canonical

From: *Retroviral Immunology: Immune Response and Restoration*
Edited by: Giuseppe Pantaleo and Bruce D. Walker © Humana Press Inc., Totowa, NJ

cysteines *(9)*. Fractalkine contains a unique CX3C motif and may represent a new class in which the chemokine moiety sits atop a membrane-anchored mucin-like stalk *(10)*. While a soluble cleavage product of the chemokine domain is chemotactic for T cells and monocytes, the membrane-bound form of fractalkine is expressed on activated endothelial cells and mediates leukocyte adhesion *(11)*.

Several generalizations can be made with respect to the chemokine families. The CC or β-chemokines represent the largest group and generally attract monocytes, lymphocytes, basophils, and eosinophils but not neutrophils. The monocyte chemoattractant proteins (MCPs 1–5) and the eotaxin molecules (eotaxin 1–3) form a closely related subfamily within the β-chemokines *(12)*. Members of the α-family containing the sequence glutamic acid–leucine–arginine amino (N)-terminal to the CXC motif (E-L-R-C-X-C) are chemotactic for neutrophils (e.g., interleukin-8 [IL-8], GRO), while those lacking this ELR sequence attract lymphocytes (e.g., interferon-induced protein 10 [IP-10], stromal cell-derived factor [SDF-1α]. Many chemokines bind multiple receptor molecules, often overlapping with one another. Some, however, are presently known to bind only a single receptor (e.g., eotaxin and CCR3, MIP-1β, and CCR5, and SDF-1α and CXCR4). CC and CXC chemokines do not share common receptors.

The chemokine receptors belong to the seven-transmembrane G protein-coupled receptor (GPCR) group, which includes a diverse array of 1000–2000 signaling molecules constituting >1% of the vertebrate genome *(13)*. While the families lack sequence homology, they share a common seven transmembrane core (TMI–VII) with three intracellular (i1–i3) and extracellular (e1–e3) loops. Two conserved cysteines in e1 and e2 are disulfide bonded. The TMI–VII domains are thought to form a circle in the cell membrane, with grouping of the corresponding ectodomains to generate chemokine-binding site(s). Ligand interaction changes the receptor core conformation, exposing G protein binding sites by which further signaling occurs. These models await confirmation by high-resolution structural analyses.

Chemokine Signaling and Function

Chemokines mediate diverse biological effects including chemotaxis, activation of integrins and adhesion, coordinated lymphocyte and dendritic cell trafficking, and selective recruitment of polarized lymphocyte subsets *(3,7,8,14)*. These functions play a central role in inflammatory and immune responses, as well as in pathologic states such as autoimmune disease, and are tightly regulated at numerous levels, for example, temporal–spatial control of ligand–receptor gene expression, chemokine binding by extracellular matrix, modulation of receptor signaling pathways, and interaction with other signaling pathways, for example stem cell factor/kit ligand (SCF/KL)/c-*kit (15)*.

The intracellular events linking receptor activation to effector function are only beginning to be unraveled. Numerous biochemical phenomena have been described; however, the causal relationships among these remain to be fully defined. Chemokine receptors are coupled to the Gi subfamily of G proteins. Pertussis toxin (PTX), which ADP-ribosylates and irreversibly inactivates the Gα subunit of the i class, inhibits the majority of chemokine-induced effects on leukocytes, including chemotaxis, calcium flux, and integrin activation *(16)*. Other signaling events triggered by the majority of chemokine receptors include the activation of phospholipase C (PLC) leading to generation of inositol triphosphate, intracellular calcium release, and protein kinase C (PKC) activation. Phorbol myristate acetate (PMA) activation of integrins implicates PKC as a potential mediator by which chemokines activate integrins. Inhibition of chemokine-induced chemotaxis by wortmannin implicates phosphatidylinositol 3-kinase (PI3K) in chemokine receptor signal transduction. Chemokine signaling also leads to guanine nucleotide exchange on Rho, indicating the latter's activation *(17)*. Rac and Rho are small GTP binding proteins involved in controlling cell locomotion via actin cytoskeletal rearrangement, membrane ruffling, and pseudopod formation.

Agonist-stimulated receptors also activate G protein receptor kinases (GRKs), which in turn phosphorylate serine and threonine residues in the tail of GPCRs *(18)*. Receptor phosphorylation is followed by binding of arrestins and uncoupling from G proteins (desensitization). In addition, the arrestins function as adaptor molecules leading to clathrin-mediated endocytosis (internalization). These internalized receptors are either dephosphorylated by phosphatases and recycled to the cell surface or targeted for degradation. Desensitization and recycling of chemokine receptors may be an important mechanism by which leukocytes maintain their ability to sense a chemoattractant gradient during an inflammatory response, whereas degradation of chemokine receptors may lead to termination of migration. Thus, chemokine receptors activate multiple signaling pathways that regulate the intracellular machinery necessary to propel the cell in its chosen direction.

CHEMOKINE RECEPTORS ARE OBLIGATE CORECEPTORS AND DETERMINE HIV-1 TROPISM

Soon after the initial isolation of HIV-1 in the mid-1980s, its tropism for CD4-bearing cells rapidly led to the identification of CD4 as a viral entry receptor. Several early observations, however, suggested that the CD4 molecule by itself was insufficient for entry. For example, nonhuman cells transfected with CD4 still required a human-specific cofactor to support membrane fusion.

In addition, a single-receptor model could not explain the phenomenon of viral tropism. It was found that different isolates of human immunodeficiency virus type 1 (HIV-1) could be broadly classified into three phenotypic groups. Although all isolates could infect primary $CD4^+$ lymphocytes, they differed in their ability to infect primary monocytes and immortalized laboratory T cell lines such as MT-2 cells. Viral strains could be phenotypically grouped as M tropic (able to infect primary monocytes), T tropic (able to infect laboratory T cell lines), or dual tropic (able to infect both), and this specificity was found to be determined by the V3 loop of the gp120 envelope molecule. These observations strongly suggested that there must be another receptor for HIV-1 in addition to the CD4 molecule.

In a landmark experiment, Berger and co-workers *(19)* used an expression cDNA cloning strategy to isolate "fusin," a seven-transmembrane G protein coupled receptor, which when coexpressed with CD4, permitted T-tropic (but not M-tropic) Env-mediated fusion and infection of nonhuman cells. At the time, fusin was an "orphan receptor" with homology to the receptor for CXC chemokine IL-8. These observations prompted speculation that the known inhibitory activity of RANTES on M-tropic HIV-1 *(20)* might occur via a CC chemokine receptor functioning as a fusion cofactor for M- but not T-tropic virus. In short order, five groups reported that CCR5—a receptor for MIP-1α, MIP-1β, and RANTES—functioned as a coreceptor for M-tropic HIV-1 *(21–25)*. "Fusin" was subsequently found to be a receptor for the CXC chemokine SDF-1 and renamed CXCR4. HIV-1 strains are now designated "R5" (CCR5), "X4" (CXCR4), or "R5X4" (CCR5/CXCR4 dual tropic) depending on coreceptor usage *(26)*. In general, R5 strains are M tropic while X4 strains are T tropic.

Although CCR5 and CXCR4 are believed to be the primary cofactors for viral entry in vivo, numerous reports have shown that other chemokine receptors can function similarly. Thus, the dual-tropic primary HIV-1 isolate 89.6 uses CXCR4, CCR5, CCR3, and CCR2 *(24)*—an unexpectedly broad repertoire (while CCR5 shares 76% identity with CCR2, only 21% of its extracellular amino acids are homologous to CXCR4). Using an env-complementation assay, Choe et al. *(25)* found that CCR3 enhanced infection (9–32-fold) by viruses with ADA and YU2, but not BR20-4 or HXBc2 envelope glycoproteins. This effect was abolished by addition of CCR3 ligand eotaxin (60 n*M*). Other investigators have demonstrated coreceptor function for CCR8 *(27)*, CX3CR1 *(28,29)*, the orphan chemokine-like receptors STRL33/Bonzo *(30,31)*, gprl *(32,33)*, gpr15/BOB *(31,34)*, ChemR23 *(35)*, D6 *(36)*, and the angiotensin receptor-related Apj *(36,37)*. By contrast, the Duffy blood group antigen, a seven-transmembrane GPCR with 20% homology to CXCR4, does not support membrane fusion by HIV-1 89.6, IIIB, or JR-FL env proteins *(24)*.

How are we to interpret these in vitro data? The clinical relevance of experiments using laboratory strains of HIV-1 or cell fusion assays is unclear. While in vivo genetic analysis has underscored the critical importance of CCR5 (see later), other coreceptors expressed in specific target tissues, such as CCR3 on microglia in the central nervous system, may play a critical role in the pathogenesis of HIV-1 infection. However, these hypotheses await definitive experimental validation.

STRUCTURE–FUNCTION STUDIES REVEAL CONFORMATIONALLY COMPLEX INTERACTIONS BETWEEN SPECIFIC HIV-1 STRAINS AND CORECEPTORS

As described in the preceding section, CD4 and chemokine coreceptors and viral Env protein are the main components involved in HIV entry into target cells. The HIV-1 Env protein complex is initially produced as a gp160 precursor, which is then proteolytically cleaved into two subunits: (1) The external gp120 subunit, which is heavily glycosylated and contains the CD4 and coreceptor binding sites; and (2) the membrane-spanning gp41 subunit, which is derived from the C-terminal portion of the precursor and contains an N-terminal, hydrophobic peptide directly involved in the fusion process. These two subunits remain noncovalently associated and oligomerize as trimers on the virion surface.

The mechanism of viral entry has been examined intensively, with the following overall mechanism now generally accepted *(6,38)*: CD4 interaction with the gp120 subunit induces conformational changes, which presumably create, stabilize, or expose the coreceptor binding site on gp120. This is followed by binding of gp120 to coreceptor, conformational changes in the Env protein, and activation of gp41. Fusion of the viral membrane with the target cell membrane is mediated by exposing and extending the gp41 fusion peptide, allowing it to insert into the plasma membrane of the target cell. In support of this model, complexes of CD4, gp120 and coreceptor have been isolated *(39),* and mutational, antigenic, and X-ray crystallographic studies *(40–42)* have confirmed conformational changes in gp120.

Chemokine function is mediated by coupling of their receptors to G proteins, initiating a complex array of intracellular signaling pathways. Although soluble Env protein can induce signaling via CCR5 and CXCR4 *(43),* it is now generally accepted, that Env-mediated fusion can occur independently from G protein coupled signaling *(44–47).*

The domains of the coreceptor involved in the interaction with gp120 have been extensively investigated. Mutational studies, receptor chimeras, antireceptor antibodies and other methods have yielded complex and sometimes contradictory results *(6,48–51).* The N-terminus and extracellular loops of the coreceptors seem to be important for gp120 binding and subsequent viral entry, whereas the intracellular loops and the so-called DRY motif required for G protein coupled signaling, do not seem to play an important role in coreceptor function. It should be noted that coreceptor modifications can have variable effects for different Env proteins.

gp120 contains 5 variable loops (V1–V5) interspersed with five relatively conserved regions (C1–C5). The V3 loop is critical for viral fusion and tropism, as well as coreceptor binding and specificity. X-ray crystallographic, mutational, and antigenic studies *(40–42)* suggest that the coreceptor interacts with the V3 loop, a "bridging sheet" of the V1/V2 stem, and an antiparallel, four-stranded structure including parts of the C4 domain.

The CD4-dependent interaction of gp120/CD4/coreceptor is undoubtedly the main mechanism for HIV-1 entry and fusion. However, certain Env proteins can interact with coreceptor in the absence of CD4 resulting in fusion and entry, as first described for HIV-2, and later for SIV and HIV-1 *(52–58).* However, this pathway is less efficient, and addition of CD4 in most cases enhances binding of gp120 and coreceptor. The biological relevance of this CD4-independent pathway is unclear. Nevertheless, the ability to select for CD4-independent strains of HIV-1 and simian immunodeficiency virus (SIV) in vitro, as well as the natural CD4-independence of feline immunodeficiency virus, suggest that chemokine receptors are probably the key receptors for viral entry.

CHEMOKINE RECEPTORS ARE MAJOR HOST GENETIC FACTOR IN INFECTION AND DISEASE PROGRESSION

Numerous host factors including determinants of innate and adaptive immune function (e.g., major histocompatibility alleles, chemokine/cytokine expression levels, mucosal immunity) as well as coreceptor mutations have been linked to disease susceptibility and progression. The complex interplay of these factors is only beginning to be unraveled *(59,60).* In the following sections, we focus on the recent findings regarding mutations/polymorphisms in chemokines and their receptors (Table 1).

CCR5 Δ32

Studies of individuals who remained uninfected despite multiple high-risk exposures to HIV-1 ("exposed-uninfected" or "EU" individuals) demonstrated that in some cases, their CD4$^+$ T cells were resistant to infection in vitro *(61).* Analysis of two such individuals showed that (1) T cells were resistant to M-tropic but not T-tropic virus; (2) approx 10-fold higher levels of β-chemokines were secreted by T cells from one EU

Table 1
Inherited Polymorphisms in Chemokine and Chemokine Receptor Genes that Affect Susceptibility to HIV-1 Infection and Progression

					Genotypes		
Molecule	Polymorphism	Sites	Type	Freq	–/–	+/–	Mechanism
CCR5	CCR5 Δ32	ORF	Del	10%	R	DP	Truncation
	m303	ORF	SNP	1%	R	ND	Truncation
	59029G/A	Prom	SNP	50%	DP	—	ND
CCR2	CCR2-64I	ORF	SNP	10%	ND	DP	ND
SDF-1	SDF-1 3′ A	3′ UTR	SNP	21%	DP	—	ND

Abbreviations: Freq, Allelic frequency; –/–, homozygous for the given allele; +/–, heterozygous for the given allele; ORF, open reading frame; SNP, single nucleotide polymorphism; Del, deletion; Prom, promoter; 3′ UTR, 3′ untranslated region of the mRNA; R, HIV-1 resistance; DP, delayed progression to AIDS relative to other genotypes; ND, not determined, NE, no effects.

Table (including allelic frequencies) adapted from Berger et al. *(6)*.

compared to controls *(62);* and *(3)* both individuals were homozygous for a 32-bp deletion in the second extracellular loop of the CCR5 gene. This so-called Δ32 mutation resulted in a frameshift and premature translation termination with consequent failure of the truncated receptor to reach the cell surface *(63)*. Similar results were reported by other investigators *(64–66)*. Of note, no obvious clinical effect of the Δ32/Δ32 genotype was seen implying that CCR5 is nonessential, which has important therapeutic implications.

Heterozygosity for the Δ32 deletion also appears to be beneficial, reducing cell surface coreceptor expression by gene dosage as well as heterodimerizing with wild-type CCR5 and trapping it in the endoplasmic reticulum *(67)*. In vitro, using the M-tropic SF162 strain, Liu et al. *(63)* found that although EU $CD4^+$ T cells (Δ32/Δ32) did not support viral replication, parental (heterozygous) cells permitted an intermediate level of replication. Patients homozygous for the Δ32 mutation were not found in an HIV-1–infected cohort of Caucasian subjects, and heterozygotes were 35% less frequent in this group compared to the general population *(64)*. Analysis of 1955 patients from six acquired immune deficiency syndrome (AIDS) cohort studies showed that while heterozygosity did not appear to confer reduced susceptibility to infection, the Δ32/+ genotype was associated with delayed progression to AIDS in infected subjects *(65)*. Similarly, in studies of vertical transmission, heterozygosity in the child was not protective but may be associated with slower development of HIV-related disease *(68–71)*. It should be noted that these effects were not consistently seen in all patient groups *(72–74)*.

The Δ32 allele is found almost exclusively among Caucasions, and exhibits a north-to-south geographic cline across Eurasia *(75–77)*. In a screen of 3342 individuals, the frequency of this deletion was 20.93% (Ashkenazi), 14.71 (Iceland), 11.13 (Britain), 9.78 (Russia: Udmurtia), 8.62 (Spain), 2.94 (Pakistan), 2.07 (Saudi Arabia), 0.50 (Thailand), 0.45 (Nigeria) *(77)*. The near absence of the mutation in native African, American Indian and East Asian ethnicities suggests a recent and unique origin, which has been estimated at ~1200 AD by haplotype analysis *(76)*. The current high allele frequency of 5–15% as well as the recent finding that other naturally occuring CCR5 mutations are predominantly codon altering (nonsynonymous; *78*) suggest a positive selective force for these alleles. Given the estimated origin of Δ32 approx 700 yr, ago, some speculate that this allele might have conferred a protective effect during the Black Death (1346–1352 AD) or against other widespread pathogens targeting macrophage (e.g., *Shigella, Salmonella, Mycobacterium tuberculosis*) *(76)*.

Homozygosity for the Δ32 deletion provides nearly complete protection against the M-tropic isolates studied thus far, implying that CCR5 is in fact the critical coreceptor in HIV-1 infection. The identification of rare HIV-1$^+$ Δ32/Δ32 individuals, however, indicates that other routes of viral entry in vivo exist. In one such patient with hemophilia A, a homogenous SI, T-tropic quasispecies was found. This individual's viral isolates used CXCR4 exclusively as coreceptor during the period of observation, which began 4 yr postinfection *(79,80)*. Consistent with the increased virulence of X4 virus, relatively rapid CD4 loss was reported (see also *81,82*). These observations together with a Danish study showing decreased survival after diagnosis of AIDS in Δ32 carriers *(83)* have raised concern that CCR5 antagonists may be detrimental.

Other Disease-Modifying Receptor Mutation/Polymorphisms

The CCR5 Δ32 allele is present in only a fraction of EU individuals. Moreover, Δ32/+ heterozygous long-term nonprogressors do not appear to differ significantly from wild-type nonprogressors with respect to immunologic and virologic parameters *(84)*. These observations imply the existence of additional genetic or epigenetic factors that influence susceptibility to infection and disease course. The complexity of such interacting factors has made direct comparison of cohorts problematic and reduced the likelihood of identifying single-gene effects. Nevertheless, a number of additional disease-modifying mutations/polymorphisms have been discovered (see *6*):

- *CCR5 m303:* One EU heterozygous for the Δ32 allele was found to have a T→A mutation at position 303 of CCR5 on the other allele (i.e., genotype CCR5 m303/CCR5 Δ32) *(85)*. The m303 mutation results in premature translation termination and lack of functional receptor expression. Its precise frequency in the general population is not known.
- *CCR5 59029 A/G* promoter polymorphism: McDermott et al. *(86)* identified an A/G polymorphism at position 59029 in the CCR5 promoter. In an in vitro CAT assay system, the 59029-G promoter was 45% less active than 59029-A, although this site is not part of a known transcription factor binding element. Patients with genotype 59029-G/G progressed to AIDS significantly more slowly than those homozygous for 59029-A. CCR5 transcription is complex—consisting of at least two promoters, multiple start sites, complex alternative splicing, and polymorphisms in regulatory as well as other 5′ noncoding sequences *(87)*. Consistent with this, other possible disease-modifying promoter polymorphisms are beginning to be reported *(88,89)*.
- *CCR2-V64I:* A conservative valine → isoleucine change in the first transmembrane domain of CCR2 delayed disease progression in some *(90–93)*, but not all *(94,95)* cohorts studied. These results were unexpected, as few HIV-1 strains use CCR2 as coreceptor. In vitro studies of CCR2b, the major CCR2 isoform, showed that the V64I mutation is expressed comparably to wild-type protein and retains coreceptor function. In addition, this polymorphism did not affect MCP-1 induced calcium mobilization, or expression/coreceptor activity of CCR5 or CXCR4 in cotransfected cell lines *(96)*. The V64I polymorphism was associated with a small decrease in CXCR4 levels in unstimulated peripheral blood mononuclear cells (PBMCs). Recently, it has been reported that CCR2-V64I is in complete linkage disequilibrium with a CCR5 promoter mutation (position 59653) *(92,97)* but not associated with decreased CCR5 expression.

Table 2
Chemokine Receptors Known to Support HIV-1 Entry and Blocking Ligands

Receptor	Ligands	Virus
CCR2	MCP-1, MCP-2, MCP-3, MCP-4	R5X4
CCR3	RANTES, MCP-2, MCP-3, MCP-4, Eotaxin-1, Eotaxin-2, Eotaxin-3	R5X4
CCR5	RANTES, MIP-1α, MIP-1β, MCP-2	R5, R5X4, HIV-2
CCR8	I-309	R5X4, HIV-2
CXCR4	SDF-1α, SDF-1β	X4, R5X4
CX3CR1	Fractalkine	R5X4, HIV-2
APJ	(Unknown)	R5X4
ChemR23	(Unknown)	
GPR15/Bob	(Unknown)	R5X4
STRL33/Bonzo	(Unknown)	R5X4
D6	(Unknown)	
US28 (cytomegalovirus)	RANTES, MIP-1α, MIP-1β	R5X4

The preceding discussion attests to the complexity of identifying disease-modifying genetic factors in heterogenous populations. While the dominant role played by CCR5 in disease pathogenesis is clear, analyses of other polymorphisms/mutations have not been completely concordant. This may reflect numerous factors including tight linkage of CCR1, CCR3, CCR4, CCR8, and CXCR1 *(98)*, sampling bias (e.g., use of seroprevalent versus seroincident cohorts), statistical power, and epigenetic phenomena, among other possibilities.

CHEMOKINES ARE POTENT INHIBITORS OF HIV-1 ENTRY

The existence of cytokine inhibitors of HIV-1 replication was first proposed in 1986, when it was found that CD8+ T lymphocytes could mediate viral suppression in vitro at least in part through released soluble factors *(99,100)*. The first such factors to be isolated from CD8+ T cells were MIP-1α, MIP-1β, and RANTES *(20)*. These chemokines could inhibit M-tropic but not T-tropic strains of HIV-1 in vitro, suggesting that they might bind a common receptor used by M-tropic HIV-1 strains. As noted above, this indeed proved to be the case. Soon thereafter, the orphan chemokine receptor CXCR4 was identified as the specific "coreceptor" for T-tropic strains of virus. The discovery of MIP-1α, MIP-1β, and RANTES as ligands of CCR5 that block R5 strains of HIV-1 in vitro, and the identification of SDF-1 as a CXCR4 ligand that blocks entry of X4 but not R5 virus confirmed the hypothesis that chemokine receptor ligands are specific antagonists of viral entry *(101,102)*.

Although all strains of HIV-1 are classifiable as R5, X4, or R5X4 a growing list of other chemokine receptors aside from CCR5 and CXCR4 have been found to serve as entry receptors for HIV-1 in vitro (Table 1). Their specific chemokine ligands generally block viral entry. Because of the epidemiological evidence regarding the critical importance of CCR5 in disease transmission and the fact that CCR5 and/or CXCR4 are found on monocytes, dendritic cells, and CD4+ T lymphocytes, the predominant primary cell types known to be infected in vivo, it is unclear what role these other receptors and their ligands might play in the pathogenesis of infection.

A possible exception to the specific mechanism of chemokine blockade of specific chemokine receptors involved in viral entry is the chemokine MDC. This chemokine, which is a ligand for CCR4 and not CCR5 or CXCR4, has been reported to block entry of both R5 and X4 strains of HIV-1 through an undetermined mechanism *(103)*. This activity remains controversial, however, as several other studies have failed to validate these findings *(104)*.

MECHANISM OF CHEMOKINE-MEDIATED INHIBITION OF HIV-1

Chemokines have been postulated to inhibit HIV-1 entry into cells by (1) direct competition with HIV-1 envelope for chemokine receptor binding and (2) induction of chemokine receptor internalization. Experimental evidence suggests that both can contribute to suppression of viral entry, and clearly these mechanisms are not mutually exclusive. Because chemokine action involves binding to receptor followed by receptor activation, phosphorylation and internalization, chemokines may potentially suppress viral entry through both pathways.

Support for simple competitive inhibition of HIV-1 entry comes from experiments using peptide (e.g., T22 *105,* ALX40-4C *106*) and small molecule (e.g., AMD3100 *([107,108])* antagonists of CXCR4. Several such compounds are capable of binding CXCR4 without signaling through the receptor (and presumably not downregulating it), and have been found to inhibit entry of X4 strains of HIV-1 into cells. This suggests that binding of a receptor by a ligand alone is enough to compete with viral entry. Furthermore, a study of varying N-terminal truncated forms of SDF-1 indicated that CXCR4 binding affinity was inversely correlated with ability to antagonize viral entry, again suggesting that receptor binding can compete with viral entry *(109)*.

Other data indicate an important role for receptor downregulation as the mechanism of chemokine-mediated inhibition of HIV-1 entry. Studies of N-terminal modified RANTES and SDF-1 have revealed that downregulation of chemokine receptors has a potent effect on viral entry *(110–112)*. Modifications of these chemokines which enhance receptor downregulation (presumably through more efficient internalization and/or impaired receptor recycling to the cell surface) markedly increase viral blocking activity. This increase in activity can be observed even in the absence of Gi-mediated signaling, as noted for aminooxypentane–RANTES, or decreased receptor affinity, as in the case of methionine–SDF, indicating that downregulation of the chemokine receptor is the key factor in the enhanced antiviral activity of these compounds. In addition, a small molecule inhibitor of HIV-1 cell fusion (NSC 651016) was shown to downregulate CCR5 and CXCR4 *(113)*. Furthermore, carboxy (C)-terminal nonsignaling truncation mutants of CXCR4 while able to support viral entry were not inhibitable by the addition of SDF-1, its natural ligand *(114,115)*. Thus, although chemokine receptor signaling is not required for viral entry, it is required for chemokine-induced inhibition of HIV-1 entry.

The chemokines are basic proteins and bind avidly to negatively charged heparin and heparan sulfate *(116–119)*. Heparan sulfate proteoglycans serve to capture chemokines in the extracellular matrix and on the surface of cells, which may serve to establish a local concentration gradient from the point source of chemokine secretion *(116)*. In addition, proteoglycans can influence the biological activity of chemokines, and several studies have demonstrated that they play an important role in chemokine-induced inhibition of HIV-1 entry *(120–122)*. Because chemokines are secreted from HIV-1-specific CTL bound to proteoglycans this interaction is likely to be relevant in vivo.

CHEMOKINE LIGANDS AS HOST GENETIC FACTOR IN INFECTION AND DISEASE PROGRESSION

Despite evidence that numerous chemokine ligands can inhibit HIV-1 entry via their receptors in vitro, the in vivo relevance of this phenomenon remains unclear. Whether chemokines serve a directly antiviral role in vivo is debatable, in contrast to the well-established clinical impact of CCR5 mutations on susceptibility to infection and disease progression. Clinical correlations of chemokine levels in HIV-1 infection have provided circumstantial evidence that chemokines may have roles both in protection from infection as well as affecting the rate of disease progression (reviewed in *123*).

Although some heavily HIV-1-exposed yet uninfected individuals are resistant to infection by virtue of CCR5 Δ32 mutation homozygosity, the vast majority are not of this genotype. One proposed immunologic mechanism is protection by MIP-1α, MIP-1β, and RANTES. This is based upon the observation of higher production of these CC chemokines by mitogen-activated PBMCs from highly exposed yet uninfected homosexuals *(124)* and hemophiliacs *(125)*, as compared to other seronegative controls. Similarly, $CD4^+$ lymphocytes from highly EU individuals with wild-type receptors for CCR5 were found be more sensitive to the HIV inhibitory effects of β-chemokines *(124)*. Long-term nonprogressing infected individuals appear to have increased production of MIP-1α, MIP-1β, and RANTES as well, indicating that these chemokines may affect the rate of disease progression (*125a*). Although these results correlate apparent protection from infection and disease progression with increased chemokine production by PBMCs, it is not clear whether protection is mediated by the chemokines themselves or an associated factor such as the activated T cells that produce them.

Further indirect evidence for an impact of chemokines on the course of disease includes a correlation of a polymorphism in the 3′ untranslated region of SDF-1. This is a G to A transition at bp 809 of the 3′ untranslated region of the mRNA of SDF-1β, also designated SDF-1 3′A (this is found only with SDF-1β, and not in SDF-1α, which is a splice variant of the same gene). An initial report suggested a statistically significant correlation of homozygosity for this polymorphism with delayed progression to AIDS, particularly in patients infected for longer periods *(126)*. The postulated mechanism was an effect of this polymorphism on posttranscriptional modulation of SDF-1 levels; however, this has never been demonstrated. A second study failed to confirm the association. In fact, in this second cohort, 3′ A homozygosity was associated with more rapid progression to death *(97)*. The reasons for this discrepancy are unclear, and the precise molecular effect(s) of the 3′UTR mutation remains to be determined.

THERAPEUTIC IMPLICATIONS

The discovery that HIV requires a chemokine coreceptor to invade host cells and that chemokines can inhibit HIV-1 entry into cells has prompted many investigations into therapeutic strategies that target these receptors in an attempt to block HIV entry. The concept that blocking HIV-1 entry into cells is a useful drug strategy was sup-

Table 3
Anti-HIV Therapeutic Strategies Based on Chemokine Receptors

Strategy	Therapy	Target
Immune restoration	Downregulation of CCR5 on $CD4^+$ T cells	CCR5
Gene therapy	Antisense	CCR5, CXCR4
	Ribozymes	CCR5, CXCR4
	Single chain mAbs	CCR5, CXCR4
	Intrakines	CCR5, CXCR4
Immunotherapy	mAbs	CCR5, CXCR4
Chemokines	MIP-1 α, MIP-1β, RANTES	CCR5
	SDF-1	CXCR4
Chemokine analogs	Met–RANTES	CCR5
	AOP–RANTES	CCR5
	Met-SDF-1	CXCR4
Peptide antagonists	T22	CXCR4
	ALX40-4C	CXCR4
Small molecule antagonists	AMD3100	CXCR4
	NSC 651016	CCR5, CXCR4

Adapted from Cairns et al. *(128)*.

ported by studies using a peptide T-20 that inhibits the interaction of gp41 with the cell membrane *(127)*. This inhibitor was able to significantly reduce viral load in HIV infected patients and revealed that blocking HIV entry could complement existing anti-retroviral drug therapy *(127)*. We briefly summarize some approaches being developed (Table 3), which have also been reviewed by Cairns et al. *(128)*.

Novel strategies are being developed to sequester or prevent the expression of chemokine receptors in order to make cells resistant to HIV. These include inducing CCR5 downregulation or gene therapy approaches to prevent chemokine receptor expression. Activation of $CD4^+$ T cells with monoclonal antibodies (mAbs) to the cell surface receptors CD3 and CD28 results in downmodulation of CCR5 and the production of soluble factors that inhibit R5 as well as X4 virus replication *(129,130)*. These $CD4^+$ T cells are resistant to R5 viruses but are still susceptible to X4 viruses. Resistance of stimulated cells to HIV-1 infection is short lived in vitro, with reacquisition of HIV infectability occurring within one week after the stimuli are removed. However, these findings illustrate that CCR5 levels can be experimentally manipulated and support studies to explore this concept further.

Gene therapy approaches are also being explored and are based on the premise that insertion of anti-HIV genes into target cells will render them resistant to HIV infection and/or replication. In current gene therapy strategies, cells are taken from the donor and transduced with a vector capable of expressing genes that interfere with chemokine receptor function. Several different types of gene therapy vectors can be developed that affect levels of a specific gene in unique ways. For example, these vectors can encode antisense RNA to arrest translation of chemokine receptors, ribozymes (enzymatic RNA molecules) designed to specifically recognize and cleave other RNAs, intrakines (modified chemokines) designed to be retained intracellularly and trap chemokine receptors in the endoplasmic reticulum, or single chain mAbs designed to bind and prevent expression and function of chemokine receptors.

Other anti-HIV strategies are designed to more directly interfere with the chemokine receptor HIV gp120 interaction. These approaches include blocking mAbs, natural chemokine receptor ligands, peptide antagonists and small molecule inhibitors. In addition to its potential benefit for chronically infected individuals, passive immunization with anti-CCR5 mAbs may also be useful as post-exposure prophylaxis and for the prevention of maternal–fetal transmission.

Because of their ability to inhibit HIV-1 entry into cells, chemokines are being explored as therapeutic agents. In addition, modified chemokines with more potent HIV inhibitory activities, such as AOP–RANTES and Met–SDF-1 are promising compounds particularly since some of these (e.g., AOP–RANTES) lack inflammatory activity. Two peptides that specifically block CXCR4–HIV interaction are T22 *(130)* and ALX40–4C *(106)*. T22 is an 18 amino acid peptide isolated from the horseshoe crab and ALX40-4C is a cationic peptide containing nine arginines. These peptides block X4 envelope as well as SDF-1 interactions with CXCR4.

Because of issues of bioavailability and expense, much effort has been focused on the discovery of small molecule chemokine receptor inhibitors. The biopharmaceutical industry has significant experience in developing small molecule antagonists for seven transmembrane spanning G protein coupled receptors and the industry is actively trying to develop such molecules for the chemokine receptors. Recent reports *(107,108,131)* describe the feasibility of using a small molecule, AMD3100, to block HIV entry. AMD3100 is a member of the heterocyclic family of compounds called bicyclins. AMD3100 binds to CXCR4 and inhibits the interaction between X4 envelope and CXCR4 as well as the interaction of SDF-1 and CXCR4. In vivo studies of AMD3100 in the severe combined immunodeficiency (SCID)-human mouse model have shown that it is nontoxic, and efficacious steady state levels can be maintained by subcutaneous injections or implantable minipump administration. However, its poor oral bioavailability may limit clinical development. Small molecule antagonists of CCR5 have also been developed by several companies and are now registered in the patent database. The identification of such agents capable of inhibiting the interaction of HIV-1 with CXCR4 and CCR5 establishes "proof of principle" for this approach, and provides a basis for rational drug design. If such inhibitors can be developed with adequate oral bioavailability and acceptable toxicity, they could prove to be invaluable additions to our current pharmacologic armamentarium.

SUMMARY

The discovery that chemokine receptors are obligate coreceptors for HIV-1 entry into cells, hailed by the journal *Science* in 1998 as the discovery of the year, has without a doubt been a major advance in our understanding of the pathogenesis of HIV-1 infection. Intense investigation in this area has revealed that chemokine receptors determine viral cell tropism, and that CCR5 is a major genetic determinant of disease susceptibility and progression. In addition, we have learned much about the structural requirements for HIV-1 entry into cells and have shown that chemokine and chemokine analogs are potent inhibitors of viral entry. All of this has underscored the exciting possibility that chemokine receptor antagonists or molecules that interfere with the HIV-1 gp120 chemokine receptor interaction will prove to be novel and welcome additions to our armamentarium of antiretroviral agents.

REFERENCES

1. Deuel TF, Keim PS, Farmer M, Heinrikson RL. Amino acid sequence of human platelet factor 4. Proc Natl Acad Sci USA 1977; 74:2256–8.
2. Luster AD, Unkeless JC, Ravetch JV. Gamma-interferon transcriptionally regulates an early-response gene containing homology to platelet proteins. Nature 1985; 315:672–6.
3. Luster AD. Chemokines: chemotactic cytokines that mediate inflammation. N Engl J Medicine 1998; 388:436–45.
4. Horuk R, Chitnis CE, Darbonne WC, Colby TJ, Rybicki A, Hadley TJ, et al. A receptor for the malarial parasite *Plasmodium vivax:* the erythrocyte chemokine receptor. Science 1993; 261:1182–4.
5. Lalani AS, Masters J, Zeng W, Barrett J, Pannu R, Everett H, et al. Use of chemokine receptors by poxviruses. Science 1999; 286:1968–71.
6. Berger EA, Murphy PM, Farber JM. Chemokine receptors as HIV-1 coreceptors: roles in viral entry, tropism, and disease. Annu Rev Immunol 1999; 17:657–700.
7. Locati M, Murphy P. Chemokines and chemokine receptors: biology and clinical relevance in inflammation and AIDS. Annu Rev Med 1999; 50:425–40.
8. Baggiolini M. Chemokines and leukocyte traffic. Nature 1998; 392:565–8.
9. Kelner GS, Kennedy J, Bacon KB, Kleyensteuber S, Largaespada DA, Jenkins NA, et al. Lymphotactin: a cytokine that represents a new class of chemokine. Science 1994; 266:1395–9.
10. Bazan JF, Bacon KB, Hardiman G, Wang W, Soo K, Rossi D, et al. A new class of membrane-bound chemokine with a CX3C motif. Nature 1997; 385:640–4.
11. Haskell C, Cleary M, Charo I. Molecular uncoupling of fractalkine-mediated cell adhesion and cignal transduction. Rapid flow arrest of CX3CR1-expressing cells is independent of G-protein activation. J Biol Chem 1999; 274:10053–8.
12. Luster AD, Rothenberg ME. The role of the monocyte chemoattractant protein and eotaxin subfamily of chemokines in allergic inflammation. J Leuk Biol 1997; 62:620–33.
13. Bockaert J, Pin JP. Molecular tinkering of G protein-coupled receptors: an evolutionary success. EMBO J 1999; 18:1723–9.
14. Cyster JG. Chemokines and the homing of dendritic cells to the T cell areas of lymphoid organs [comment]. J Exp Med 1999; 189:447–50.
15. Dutt P, Wang JF, Groopman JE. Stromal cell-derived factor-1 alpha and stem cell factor/kit ligand share signaling pathways in hemopoietic progenitors: a potential mechanism for cooperative induction of chemotaxis. J Immunol 1998; 161:3652–8.
16. Becknew S. G-protein activation by chemokines. In: Horuk R (ed). Methods in Enzymology, Chemokine Receptors. San Diego: Academic Press, 1997, pp. 309–26.
17. Laudanna C, Campbell JJ, Butcher EC. Role of Rho in chemoattractant-activated leukocyte adhesion through integrins. Science 1996; 271:981–3.
18. Richmond A, Mueller S, White JR, Schraw W. C-X-C chemokine receptor desensitization mediated through ligand-enhanced receptor phosphorylation on serine residues. In: Horuk R (ed). Methods in Enzymology, Chemokine Receptors. San Diego: Academic Press, 1997, pp. 3–15.
19. Feng Y, Broder CC, Kennedy PE, Berger EA. HIV-1 entry cofactor: functional cloning of a seven-transmembrane, G protein-coupled receptor. Science 1996; 272:872–7.

20. Cocchi F, DeVico AL, Garzino-Demo A, Arya SK, Gallo RC, Lusso P. Identification of RANTES, MIP-1α, and MIP-1β as the major HIV-suppressive factors produced by CD8+ T cells. Science 1995; 270:1811–5.
21. Deng H, Liu R, Ellmeier W, Choe S, Unutmaz D, Burkhart M, et al. Identification of a major co-receptor for primary isolates of HIV-1. Nature 1996; 381:661–6.
22. Dragic T, Litwin V, Allaway GP, Martin SR, Huang Y, Nagashima KA, et al. HIV-1 entry into CD4+ cells is mediated by the chemokine receptor CC-CKR-5. Nature 1996; 381:667–73.
23. Alkhatib G, Combadiere C, C. BC, Feng Y, Kennedy PE, Murphy PM, et al. CC CKR5: a RANTES, MIP-1alpha, MIP-1 beta receptor as a fusion cofactor for macrophage-tropic HIV-1. Science 1996; 272:1955–8.
24. Doranz BJ, Rucker J, Yi Y, Smyth RJ, Samson M, Peiper SC, et al. A dual-tropic primary HIV-1 isolate that uses fusin and the β-chemokine receptors CKR-5, CKR-3, and CKR-2b as fusion cofactors. Cell 1996; 85:1149–58.
25. Choe H, Farzan M, Sun Y, Sullivan N, Rollins B, Ponath PD, et al. The β-chemokines receptors CCR3 and CCR5 facilitate infection by primary HIV-1 isolates. Cell 1996; 85:1135–48.
26. Berger EA, Doms RW, Fenyo EM, Korber BT, Littman DR, Moore JP, et al. A new classification for HIV-1. Nature 1998; 391:240.
27. Horuk R, Hesselgesser J, Zhou Y, Faulds D, Halks-Miller M, Harvey S, et al. The CC chemokine I-309 inhibits CCR8-dependent infection by diverse HIV-1 strains. J Biol Chem 1998; 273:386–91.
28. Combadiere C, Salzwedel K, Smith ED, Tiffany HL, Berger EA, Murphy PM. Identification of CX3CR1. A chemotactic receptor for the human CX3C chemokine fractalkine and a fusion coreceptor for HIV-1. J Biol Chem 1998; 273:23799–804.
29. Rucker J, Edinger AL, Sharron M, Samson M, Lee B, Berson JF, et al. Utilization of chemokine receptors, orphan receptors, and herpesvirus-encoded receptors by diverse human and simian immunodeficiency viruses. J Virol 1997; 71:8999–9007.
30. Liao F, Alkahatib G, Peden KWC, Sharma G, Berger EA, Farber JM. STRL33, a novel chemokine receptor-like protein, functions as a fusion cofactor for both macrophage-tropic and T cell line-tropic HIV-1. J Exp Med 1997; 185:2015–23.
31. Deng H, Unutmaz D, Kewalramani VN, Littman DR. Expression cloning of new receptors used by simian and human immunodeficiency viruses. Nature 1997; 388:296–300.
32. Edinger AL, Hoffman TL, Sharron M, Lee B, O'Dowd B, Doms RW. Use of GPR1, GPR15, and STRL33 as coreceptors by diverse human immunodeficiency virus type 1 and simian immunodeficiency virus envelope proteins. Virology 1998; 249:367–78.
33. Shimizu N, Soda Y, Kanbe K, Liu HY, Jinno A, Kitamura T, et al. An orphan G protein-coupled receptor, GPR1, acts as a coreceptor to allow replication of human immunodeficiency virus types 1 and 2 in brain-derived cells. J Virol 1999; 73:5231–9.
34. Farzan M, Choe H, Martin K, Marcon L, Hofmann W, Karlsson G, et al. Two orphan seven-transmembrane segment receptors which are expressed in CD4-positive cells support simian immunodeficiency virus infection. J Exp Med 1997; 186:405–11.
35. Samson M, Edinger AL, Stordeur P, Rucker J, Verhasselt V, Sharron M, et al. ChemR23, a putative chemoattractant receptor, is expressed in monocyte-derived dendritic cells and macrophages and is a coreceptor for SIV and some primary HIV-1 strains. Eur J Immunol 1998; 28:1689–700.
36. Choe H, Farzan M, Konkel M, Martin K, Sun Y, Marcon L, et al. The orphan seven-transmembrane receptor apj supports the entry or primary T-cell-line-tropic and dualtropic human immunodeficiency virus type 1. J Virol 1998; 7:6113–8.
37. Edinger AL, Hoffman TL, Sharron M, Lee B, Yi Y, Choe W, et al. An orphan seven-transmembrane domain receptor expressed widely in the brain functions as a coreceptor for human immunodeficiency virus type 1 and simian immunodeficiency virus. J Virol 1998; 72:7934–40.
38. Wyatt R, Sodroski J. The HIV-1 envelope glycoproteins: fusogens, antigens, and immunogens. Science 1998; 280:1884–8.

39. Lapham CK, Ouyang J, Chandrasekhar B, Nguyen NY, Dimitrov DS, Golding H. Evidence of cell-surface association between fusin and the CD4-gp120 complex in human cell lines. Science 1996; 274:602–5.
40. Kwong PD, Wyatt R, Robinson J, Sweet RW, Sodroski J, Hendrickson WA. Structure of an HIV gp120 envelope glycoprotein in complex with the CD4 receptor and a neutralizing human antibody. Nature 1998; 393:648–59.
41. Rizzuto CD, Wyatt R, Hernandez-Ramos N, Sun Y, Kwong PD, Hendrickson WA, et al. A conserved HIV gp120 glycoprotein structure involved in chemokine receptor binding. Science 1998; 280:1949–53.
42. Wyatt R, Kwong PD, Desjardins E, Sweet RW, Robinson J, Hendrickson WA, et al. The antigenic structure of the HIV gp120 envelope glycoprotein. Nature 1998; 393:705–11.
43. Weissman D, Rabin RL, Arthos J, Rubbert A, Dybul M, Swofford R, et al. Macrophage-tropic HIV and SIV envelope proteins induce a signal through the CCR5 chemokine receptor. Nature 1997; 389:981–5.
44. Alkhatib G, Locati M, Kennedy PE, Murphy PM, Berger EA. HIV-1 coreceptor activity of CCR5 and its inhibition by chemokines: independence from G protein signaling and importance of coreceptor downmodulation. Virology 1997; 234:340–8.
45. Gosling J, Monteclaro FS, Atchison RE, Arai H, Tsou C-L, Goldsmith MA, et al. Molecular uncoupling of C-C chemoking receptor 5-induced chemotaxis and signal transduction from HIV-1 coreceptor activity. Proc Natl Acad Sci USA 1997; 94:5061–6.
46. Aramori I, Ferguson SS, Bieniasz PD, Zhang J, Cullen B, Cullen MG. Molecular mechanism of desensitization of the chemokine receptor CCR-5: receptor signaling and internalization are dissociable from its role as an HIV-1 co-receptor. EMBO J 1997; 15:4606–16.
47. Hu H, Shioda T, Hori T, Moriya C, Kato A, Sakai Y, et al. Dissociation of ligand-induced internalization of CXCR-4 from its co-receptor activity for HIV-1 Env-mediated membrane fusion. Arch Virol 1998; 143:851–61.
48. Rucker J, Samson M, Doranz BJ, Libert F, Berson JF, Yi Y, et al. Regions in beta-chemokine receptors CCR5 and CCR2b that determine HIV-1 cofactor specificity. Cell 1996; 87:437–46.
49. Alkhatib G, Ahuja SS, Light D, Mummidi S, Berger EA, Ahuja SK. CC chemokine receptor 5-mediated signaling and HIV-1 co-receptor activity share common structural determinants. Critical residues in the third extracellular loop support HIV-1 fusion. J Biol Chem 1997; 272:19771–6.
50. Lu Z, Berson JF, Chen Y, Turner JD, Zhang T, Sharron M, et al. Evolution of HIV-1 coreceptor usage through interactions with distinct CCR5 and CXCR4 domains. Proc Natl Acad Sci USA 1997; 94:6426–31.
51. Rabut GE, Konner JA, Kajumo F, Moore JP, Dragic T. Alanine substitutions of polar and nonpolar residues in the amino- terminal domain of CCR5 differently impair entry of macrophage- and dualtropic isolates of human immunodeficiency virus type 1. J Virol 1998; 72:3464–8.
52. Endres MJ, Clapman PR, Marsh M, Ahuja M, et al. CD4-independent infection by HIV-2 is mediated by Fusin/CXCR4. Cell 1996; 87:745–56.
53. Reeves JD, McKnight A, Potempa S, Simmons G, Gray PW, Power CA, et al. CD4-independent infection by HIV-2 (ROD/B): use of the 7-transmembrane receptors CXCR-4, CCR-3, and V28 for entry. Virology 1997; 231:130–4.
54. Martin KA, Wyatt R, Farzan M, Choe H, Marcon L, Desjardins E, et al. CD4-independent binding of SIV gp 120 to rhesus CCR5. Science 1997; 278:1470–3.
55. Hesslegesser J, Halks-Miller M, DelVecchio V, Peiper SC, Hoxie J, Kolson DL, et al. CD4-independent association between HIV-1 gp120 and CXCR4: functional chemokine receptors are expressed in human neurons. Curr Biol 1997; 7:112–21.
56. Bandres JC, Wang QF, O'Leary J, Baleaux F, Amara A, Hoxie JA, et al. Human immunodeficiency virus (HIV) envelope binds to CXCR4 independently of CD4, and binding can be enhanced by interaction with soluble CD4 or by HIV envelope deglycosylation. J Virol 1998; 72:2500–4.

57. Potempa S, Picard L, Reeves JD, Wilkinson D, Weiss RA, Talbot SJ. CD4-independent infection by human immunodeficiency virus type 2 strain ROD/B: the role of the N-terminal domain of CXCR-4 in fusion and entry. J Virol 1997; 71:4419–24.
58. Reeves JD, Schulz TF. The CD4-independent tropism of human immunodeficiency virus type 2 involves several regions of the envelope protein and correlates with a reduced activation threshold for envelope-mediated fusion. J Virol 1997; 71:1453–65.
59. Fauci AS. Host factors and the pathogenesis of HIV-induced disease. Nature 1996; 384:529–34.
60. Simonsen JN, Fowke KR, MacDonald KS, Plummer FA. HIV pathogenesis: mechanisms of susceptibility and disease progression. Curr Opin Microbiol 1998; 1:423–9.
61. Paxton WA, Martin SR, Tse D, O'Brien TR, Skurnick J, VanDevanter NL, et al. Relative resistance to HIV-1 of CD4 lymphocytes from persons who remain uninfected despite multiple high-risk sexual exposures. Nat Med 1996; 2:412–7.
62. Dragic T, Litwin V, Allaway GP, Martin SR, Huang Y, Nagashima KA, et al. HIV-1 entry into $CD4^+$ cells is mediated by the chemokine receptor CC- CKR-5 [see comments]. Nature 1996; 381:667–73.
63. Liu R, Paxton WA, Choe S, Ceradini D, Martin SR, Horuk R, et al. Homozygous defect in HIV-1 coreceptor accounts for resistance of some multiply-exposed individuals to HIV-1 infection. Cell 1996; 86:367–77.
64. Samson M, Libert F, Doranz BJ, Rucker J, Liesnard C, Farber C-M, et al. Resistance to HIV-1 infection in caucasion individuals bearing mutant alleles of the CCR-5 chemokine receptor gene. Nature 1996; 332:722–5.
65. Dean M, Carrington M, Winkler C, Huttley GA, Smith MW, Allikmets R, et al. Genetic restriction of HIV-1 infection and progression to AIDS by a deletion allele of the CKR5 structural gene. Science 1996; 273:1856–62.
66. Zimmerman PA, Buckler-White A, Alkhatib G, Spalding T, Kubofcik J, Combadiere C, et al. Inherited resistance to HIV-1 conferred by an inactivating mutation in CC chemokine receptor 5: studies in populations with contrasting clinical phenotypes, defined racial background, and quantified risk. Mol Med 1997; 3:23–36.
67. Benkirane M, Jin D, Chun RF, Koup RA, Jeang K. Mechanism of transdominant inhibition of CCR5-mediated HIV-1 infection by ccr5Δ32. Biol Chem 1997; 272:30603–6.
68. Misrahi M, Teglas JP, N'Go N, Burgard M, Mayaux MJ, Rouzioux C, et al. CCR5 chemokine receptor variant in HIV-1 mother-to-child transmission and disease progression in children. French Pediatric HIV Infection Study Group [see comments]. JAMA 1998; 279:277–80.
69. Mangano A, Prada F, Roldan A, Picchio G, Bologna R, Sen L. Distribution of CCR-5 delta32 allele in Argentinian children at risk of HIV-1 infection: its role in vertical transmission [letter]. AIDS 1998; 12:109–10.
70. Shearer WT, Kalish LA, Zimmerman PA. CCR5 HIV-1 vertical transmission. Women and Infants Transmission Study Group [letter]. J AIDS Hum Retrovirol 1998; 17:180–1.
71. Rousseau CM, Just JJ, Abrams EJ, Casabona J, Stein Z, King MC. CCR5del32 in perinatal HIV-1 infection. J AIDS Hum Retrovirol 1997; 16:239–42.
72. Huang Y, Paxton WA, Wolinsky SM, Neumann AU, Zhang L, He T, et al. The role of a mutant CCR5 allele in HIV-1 transmission and disease progression. Nat Med 1996; 2:1240–3.
73. Hoffman TL, MacGregor RR, Burger H, Mick R, Doms RW, Collman RG. CCR5 genotypes in sexually active couples discordant for human immunodeficiency virus type 1 infection status. J Infect Dis 1997; 176:1093–6.
74. Garred P. Chemokine-receptor polymorphisms: clarity or confusion for HIV-1 prognosis? [comment]. Lancet 1998; 351:2–3.
75. Libert F, Cochaux P, Beckman G, Samson M, Aksenova M, Cao A, et al. The deltaccr5 mutation conferring protection against HIV-1 in Caucasian populations has a single and recent origin in Northeastern Europe. Hum Mol Genet 1998; 7:399–406.

76. Stephens JC, Reich DE, Goldstein DB, Shin HD, Smith MW, Carrington M, et al. Dating the origin of the CCR5-delta32 AIDS-resistance allele by the coalescence of haplotypes. Am J Hum Genet 1998; 62:1507–15.
77. Martinson JJ, Chapman NH, Rees DC, Liu YT, Clegg JB. Global distribution of the CCR5 gene 32-basepair deletion. Nat Genet 1997; 16:100–3.
78. Carrington M, Kissner T, Gerrard B, Ivanov S, O'Brien SJ, Dean M. Novel alleles of the chemokine-receptor gene CCR5. Am J Hum Genet 1997; 61:1261–7.
79. O'Brien TR, Winkler C, Dean M, Nelson JA, Carrington M, Michael NL, et al. HIV-1 infection in a man homozygous for CCR5 delta 32. Lancet 1997; 349:1219.
80. Michael NL, Nelson JA, KewalRamani VN, Chang G, O'Brien SJ, Mascola JR, et al. Exclusive and persistent use of the entry coreceptor CXCR4 by human immunodeficiency virus type 1 from a subject homozygous for CCR5 delta32. J Virol 1998; 72:6040–7.
81. Biti R, Ffrench R, Young J, Bennetts B, Stewart G, Liang T. HIV-1 infection in an individual homozygous for the CCR5 deletion allele. Nat Med 1997; 3:252–3.
82. Theodorou I, Meyer L, Magierowska M, Katlama C, Rouzioux C. HIV-1 infection in an individual homozygous for CCR5 delta 32. Seroco Study Group. Lancet 1997; 349:1219–20.
83. Garred P, Eugen-Olsen J, Iversen AK, Benfield TL, Svejgaard A, Hofmann B. Dual effect of CCR5 delta 32 gene deletion in HIV-1-infected patients. Copenhagen AIDS Study Group [letter] [see comments]. Lancet 1997; 349:1884.
84. Cohen OJ, Vaccarezza M, Lam GK, Baird BF, Wildt K, Murphy PM, et al. Heterozygosity for a defective gene for CC chemokine receptor 5 is not the sole determinant for the immunologic and virologic phenotype of HIV-infected long-term nonprogressors. J Clin Invest 1997; 100:1581–99.
85. Quillent C, Oberlin E, Braun J, Rousset D, Gonzalez-Canali G, Metais P, et al. HIV-1-resistance phenotype conferred by combination of two separate inherited mutations of CCR5 gene [see comments]. Lancet 1998; 351:14–8.
86. McDermott DH, Zimmerman PA, Guignard F, Kleeberger CA, Leitman SF, Murphy PM. CCR5 promoter polymorphism and HIV-1 disease progression. Multicenter AIDS Cohort Study (MACS). Lancet 1998; 352:866–70.
87. Mummidi S, Ahuja SS, McDaniel BL, Ahuja SK. The human CC chemokine receptor 5 (CCR5) gene. Multiple transcripts with 5′-end heterogeneity, dual promoter usage, and evidence for polymorphisms within the regulatory regions and noncoding exons. J Biol Chem 1997; 272:30662–71.
88. Martin MP, Dean M, Smith MW, Winkler C, Gerrard B, Michael NL, et al. Genetic acceleration of AIDS progression by a promoter variant of CCR5. Science 1998; 282:1907–11.
89. Easterbrook PJ, Rostron T, Ives N, Troop M, Gazzard BG, Rowland-Jones SL. Chemokine Receptor Polymorphisms and Human Immunodeficiency Virus Disease Progression. J Infect Dis 1999; 180:1096–105.
90. Smith MW, Dean M, Carrington M, Winkler C, Huttley GA, Lomb DA, et al. Contrasting genetic influence of CCR2 and CCR5 variant on HIV-1 infection and disease progression. Science 1997; 277:959–65.
91. Rizzardi GP, Morawetz RA, Vicenzi E, Ghezzi S, Poli G, Lazzarin A, et al. CCR2 polymorphism and HIV disease. Nat Med 1998; 4:252–3.
92. Kostrikis LG, Huang Y, Moore JP, Wolinsky SM, Zhang L, Guo Yl, et al. A chemokine receptor CCR2 allele delays HIV-1 disease progression and is associated with a CCR5 promoter mutation. Nat Med 1998; 4:350.
93. Anzala AO, Ball TB, Rostron T, O'Brien SJ, Plummer FA, Rowland-Jones SL. CCR2-64I allele and genotype association with delayed AIDS progression in African women. University of Nairobi Collaboration for HIV Research [letter]. Lancet 1998; 351:1632–3.
94. Michael NL, Louie LG, Rohrbaugh AL, Schultz KA, Dayhoff DE, Wang CE, et al. The role of CCR5 and CCR2 polymorphisms in HIV-1 transmission and disease progression [see comments]. Nat Med 1997; 3:1160–2.

95. Eugen-Olsen J, Iversen AK, Benfield TL, Koppelhus U, Garred P. Chemokine receptor CCR2b 64I polymorphism and its relation to CD4 T⁻ cell counts and disease progression in a Danish cohort of HIV-infected individuals. Copenhagen AIDS cohort. J AIDS Hum Retrovirol 1998; 18:110–6.
96. Lee B, Doranz BJ, Rana S, Yi Y, Mellado M, Frade JM, et al. Influence of the CCR2-V64I polymorphism on human immunodeficiency virus type 1 coreceptor activity and on chemokine receptor function of CCR2b, CCR3, CCR5, and CXCR4. J Virol 1998; 72:7450–8.
97. Mummidi S, Ahuja SS, Gonzalez E, Anderson SA, Santiago EN, Stephan KT, et al. Genealogy of the CCR5 locus and chemokine system gene variants associated with altered rates of HIV-1 disease progression. Nat Med 1998; 4:786.
98. Samson M, Soularue P, Vassart G, Parmentier M. The genes encoding the human CC-chemokine receptors CC-CKR1 to CC-CKR5 (CMKBR1-CMKBR5) are clustered in the p21.3-p24 region of chromosome 3. Genomics 1996; 36:522–6.
99. Walker CM, Levy JA. A diffusible lymphokine produced by $CD8^+$ T lymphocytes suppresses HIV replication. Immunology 1989; 66:628–30.
100. Walker CM, Moody DJ, Stites DP, Levy JA. $CD8^+$ lymphocytes can control HIV infection in vitro by suppressing virus replication. Science 1986; 234:1563–6.
101. Bleul CC, Farzan M, Choe H, Parolin C, Clark-Lewis I, Sodroski J, et al. The lymphocyte chemoattractant SDF-1 is a ligand for LESTR/fusin and blocks HIV-1 entry. Nature 1996; 382:829–33.
102. Oberlin E, Amara A, Bachelerie F, Bessia C, Virelizier J-L, Arenzana-Seisdedos F, et al. The CXC chemokine SDF-1 is the ligand for LESTR/fusin and prevents infection by T-cell-line-adapted HIV-1. Nature 1996; 382:833–5.
103. Pal R, Garzino-Demo A, Markham PD, Burns J, Brown M, Gallo RC, et al. Inhibition of HIV-1 infection by the β-chemokine MDC. Science 1997; 278:695–8.
104. Lee B, Rucker J, Doms RW, Tsang M, Hu X, Dietz M, et al. β-chemokine MDC and HIV-1 infection. Science 1998; 281(Technical Comments):487a.
105. Murakami T, Nakajima T, Koyanagi Y, Tachibana K, Fujii N, Tamamura H, et al. A small molecule CXCR4 inhibitor that blocks T cell line-tropic HIV-1 infection. J Exp Med 1997; 186:1389–93.
106. Doranz BJ, Grovit-Ferbas K, Sharron MP, Mao S-H, Goetz MB, Daar ES, et al. A small-molecule inhibitor directed against the chemokine receptor CXCR4 prevents its use as an HIV-1 coreceptor. J Exp Med 1997; 186:1395–400.
107. Schols D, Struyf S, Van Damme J, Este JA, Henson G, De Clercq E. Inhibition of T-tropic HIV strains by selective antagonization of the chemokine receptor CXCR4. J Exp Med 1997; 186:1383–8.
108. Donzella GA, Schols D, Lin SW, Este JA, Nagashima KA, Maddon PJ, et al. AMD3100, a small molecule inhibitor of HIV-1 entry via the CXCR4 co-receptor. Nature Medicine 1998; 4:72–7.
109. Heveker N, Montes M, Germeroth L, Amara A, Trautmann A, Alizon M, et al. Dissociation of the signalling and antiviral properties of SDF-1-derived small peptides. Curr Biol 1998; 7:369–76.
110. Mack M, Luckow B, Nelson PJ, Cihak J, Simmons G, Clapham PR, et al. Aminooxypentane-RANTES induces CCR5 internalization but inhibits recycling: a novel inhibitory mechanism of HIV infectivity. J Exp Med 1998; 187:1215–24.
111. Simmons G, Clapham P, Picard L, Offord RE, Rosenkilde MM, Schwarta TW, et al. Potent inhibition of HIV-1 infectivity in macrophages and lymphocytes by a novel CCR5 antagonist. Science 1997; 276:276–9.
112. Yang OO, Swanberg SL, Lu Z, Dziejman M, McCoy J, Luster AD, et al. Enhanced inhibiton of HIV-1 by Met-SDF-1β correlates with down-modulation of CXCR4. J Virol 1999; 73:4582–9.
113. Howard OMZ, Korte T, Tarasova NI, Grimm M, Turpin JA, Rice WG, et al. Small molecule inhibitor of HIV-1 cell fusion blocks chemokine receptor-mediated function. J Leuk Biol 1998; 64:6–13.

114. Signoret N, Oldridge J, Pelchen-Matthews A, Klasse PJ, Tran T, Brass LF, et al. Phorbol esters and SDF-1 induce rapid endocytosis and down modulation of the chemokine receptor CXCR4. J Cell Biol 1997; 139:651–64.
115. Amara A, Le Gall S, Schwartz O, Salamero J, Montes M, Loetscher P, et al. HIV coreceptor downregulation as antiviral principle: SDF-1α-dependent internalization of the chemokine receptor CXCR4 contributes to inhibition of HIV replication. J Exp Med 1997; 186:139–46.
116. Tanaka Y, Adams DH, Hubscher S, Hirano H, Siebenlist U, Shaw S. T-cell adhesion induced by proteoglcan-immobilized cytokine MIP-1β. Nature 1993; 361:79–82.
117. Rot A. Endothelial cell binding of NAP-1/IL-8: role in neutrophil emigration. Immunol Today 1992; 13:291–4.
118. Luster AD, Greenberg S, Leder P. The IP-10 chemokine binds to a specific cell surface heparan sulfate site shared with platelet factor 4 and inhibits endothelial cell proliferation. J Exp Med 1995; 182:219–31.
119. Middleton J, Neil S, Wintle J, Clark-Lewis I, Moore H, Lam C, et al. Transcytosis and surface presentation of IL-8 by venular endothelial cells. Cell 1997; 91:385–95.
120. Wagner L, Yang OO, Garcia-Zepeda EA, Ge Y, Kalams S, Walker BD, et al. β-Chemokines are released from HIV-1 specific cytolytic T-cell granules complexed to proteoglycans. Nature 1998; 391:908–11.
121. Oravez T, Pall M, Wang J, Roderiquez G, Ditto M, Norcross MA. Regulation of anti-HIV-1 activity of RANTES by heparan sulfate proteoglycans. J Immunol 1997; 159:4587–92.
122. Burns JM, Gallo RC, DeVico AL, Lewis GK. A new monoclonal antibody, mAb 4A12, identifies a role for the glycosaminoglycan (GAG) binding domain of RANTES in the antiviral effect against HIV-1 and intracellular $Ca2^+$ signaling. J Exp Med 1998; 188:1917–27.
123. Gallo RC, Garzino-Demo A, DeVico AL. HIV infection and pathogenesis: what about chemokines? J Clin Immunol 1999; 19:293–9.
124. Paxton WA, Liu R, Kang S, Wu L, Gingeras TR, Landau NR, et al. Reduced HIV-1 infectability of $CD4^+$ lymphocytes from exposed-uninfected individuals: association with low expression of CCR5 and high production of beta-chemokines. Virology 1998; 25:66–73.
125. Zagury D, Lachgar A, Chams V, Fall LS, Bernard J, Zagury JF, et al. C-C chemokines, pivotal in protection against HIV type 1 infection. Proc Natl Acad Sci USA 1998; 7:3857–61.
125a. Saja K, Bentsman G, Chess L, and Volsky DJ. Endogenous production of β-chemokines by $CD4^+$ but not $CD8^+$, T-cell clones correlates with the clinical state of human immunodeficiency virus type I (HIV-I). Infected individuals and may be responsible for blocking infection with nonsynctium-inducing HIV-I in vitro. J Virol 1998; 876–81.
126. Winkler C, Modi W, Smith MW, Nelson GW, Wu X, Carrington M, et al. Genetic restriction of AIDS pathogenesis by an SDF-1 chemokine gene variant. Science 1998; 279:389–93.
127. Kilby J, Hopkins S, Venetta T, DiMassimo B, Cloud G, Lee J, et al. Potent suppression of HIV-1 replication in humans by T-20, a peptide inhibitor of gp41-mediated virus entry. Nat Med 1998; 4:1302–7.
128. Cairns JS, D'Sousa MP. Chemokines and HIV-1 second receptors: the therapeutic connection. Nat Med 1998; 5:563–8.
129. Levine BL, Mosca JD, Riley JL, Carroll RG, Vahey MT, Jagodzinski LL, et al. Antiviral effect and ex vivo $CD4^+$ T cell proliferation in HIV-positive patients as a result of CD28 costimulation. Science 1996; 272:1939–43.
130. Carroll RG, Riley JL, Levine BL, Feng Y, Kaushal S, Ritchey DW, et al. Differential regulation of HIV-1 fusion cofactor expression by CD28 costimulation of $CD4^+$ T cells. Science 1997; 276:273–6.
131. De Clercq E, Yamamoto N, Pauwels R, Balzarini J, Witvrouw M, De Vreese K, et al. Highly potent and selective inhibition of human immunodeficiency virus by the bicyclam derivative JM3100. Antimicrob Agents Chemother 1994; 38:668–74.

3
Cytokines and Chemokines in HIV Infection

Guido Poli

INTRODUCTION: CYTOKINE DETERMINATION IN VIVO AND EX VIVO

Primary human immunodeficiency virus (HIV) infection is associated with a profound activation of the immune system resulting in strong cellular and humoral immune response within a few weeks from the moment of infection *(1,2)*. At the clinical level this may be associated with a mononucleosis-like syndrome with lymph node enlargement and constitutional symptoms. Accordingly, several cytokines are upregulated and detectable during this initial stage of infection, usually enduring for a few weeks and stabilizing within a few months in the majority of individuals, a stage corresponding to a clinically asymptomatic phase. This second period spans several years and is associated with relatively stable levels of plasma-associated HIV RNA (viremia) and slow erosion of peripheral $CD4^+$ T cell counts. Finally, in most individuals, opportunistic infections or tumors mark the transition to the acquired immune deficiency syndrome (AIDS) stage resulting in the death of the individual in the absence of potent antiviral agents *(2)*. These three distinct although interconnected stages of disease have been substantially changed in recent years since the introduction of potent antiretroviral regimens known as highly aggressive antiretroviral therapy (HAART) based on combinations of protease inhibitors and inhibitors of the virion-associated reverse transcriptase enzyme *(3)*. Therefore, it is quite difficult at present to investigate the natural history of the disease in industrialized countries, where combination therapy is available, whereas it remains possible in developing countries where antiviral agents are poorly or not accessible at all. It is important to underscore that individuals from the less developed areas of the world, and particularly from Sub-Saharan Africa, are frequently affected by other important infectious diseases and in conditions (i.e., malnutrition) that may profoundly affect cytokine expression *(4)*. In addition, a heterogeneous distribution of viral subtypes may differ in terms of both susceptibility to cytokines for their replication, as suggested by difference in their long terminal repeat (LTR) configuration *(5,6)* and, potentially for their ability to induce or modulate cytokine expression.

With these considerations in mind, an important point in the attempt to provide a consistent view of the relevance of cytokines in HIV disease derives from the observation that there are multiple ways to investigate their expression and perturbation in

From: *Retroviral Immunology: Immune Response and Restoration*
Edited by: Giuseppe Pantaleo and Bruce D. Walker © Humana Press Inc., Totowa, NJ

vivo. Cytokines can be directly measured in body fluids, such as plasma/serum, urine, lung bronchoalveolar lavages, and cerebrospinal fluid. However, these methods of detection in most cases underestimate the actual levels of cytokine expression, in that cytokines are frequently complexed to their soluble receptors, acting as specific carrier molecules that prolong the cytokine half-life and prevent its degradation *(7)*. Soluble cytokine receptors had been described earlier as cytokine inhibitors, at least in vitro *(7,8)*. In general, by considering a cytokine and its related receptor as a system rather than as distinct molecules, the determination of the fluid levels of soluble cytokine receptors is a more reliable approach for monitoring the perturbation of a specific cytokine system. The simultaneous determination of free and circulating receptor-bound cytokines may provide a more comprehensive understanding of the involvement of these molecules in the condition or disease under investigation. In addition to the direct detection and quantitation of cytokines, several other approaches can be utilized for investigating cytokine expression in vivo. Cytokine mRNAs have been investigated in several diseases, including HIV infection *(9)*, as sensitive correlates of cytokine expression, particularly if analyzed after amplification by qualitative or quantitative polymerase chain reaction (PCR) *(10)* or RNAse protection assays. It should be underscored, however, that the expression of most cytokines is regulated by UA-rich regions present in their 3′ untranslated region that affect the stability of their mRNA *(11)*. Therefore, accumulation of a given cytokine mRNA may not necessarily translate into a linear and parallel secretion of the related protein, particularly by sensitive PCR-based assays. Posttranslational modifications are frequently important for cytokine biological activity. Interleukin-1β (IL-1β) is cleaved into its mature form by a membrane-associated protein known as IL-1 converting enzyme *(7)*, whereas transforming growth factor β (TGF-β) needs to be dissociated from an inhibitory molecule after cell secretion *(12)* (Fig. 1).

One of the most consolidated methods consists of cytokine determination is the cultivation of peripheral blood mononuclear cells (PBMCs) in the presence or absence of stimuli such as bacterial lypopolysaccaride or mitogens such as phytohemagglutinin. Finally, it has become recently feasible to investigate cytokine production at the cellular level by use of the fluorescence-activated cell sorter (FACS) on permeabilized cells that have been maximally stimulated in the presence of inhibitors of protein secretion such as brefeldin A *(13)*. As in the case of cytokine detection in the culture supernatants of cells stimulated with mitogens or bacterial endotoxin, this last methodology provides information on the potential rather than actual expression of cytokines.

CYTOKINE PERTURBATIONS AFTER HIV INFECTION IN VIVO

Our current knowledge of the alterations of the cytokine network in in vivo HIV infection can be summarized in the following points:

1. The expression of several pro-inflammatory cytokines, such as tumor necrosis factor-α (TNF-α), interferon-γ (IFN-γ), and interleukin-6 (IL-6), and/or their receptors is elevated in the infectious process, from primary infection to the last stages of disease. Their levels in plasma/serum or expression in cells and tissue have been frequently linked to disease activity and clinical progression *(14–16)*. In particular, at the peripheral level, both plasma-associated TNF-α and its receptors (in particular sTNFRII) have been linked to disease progression, although they are usually weaker

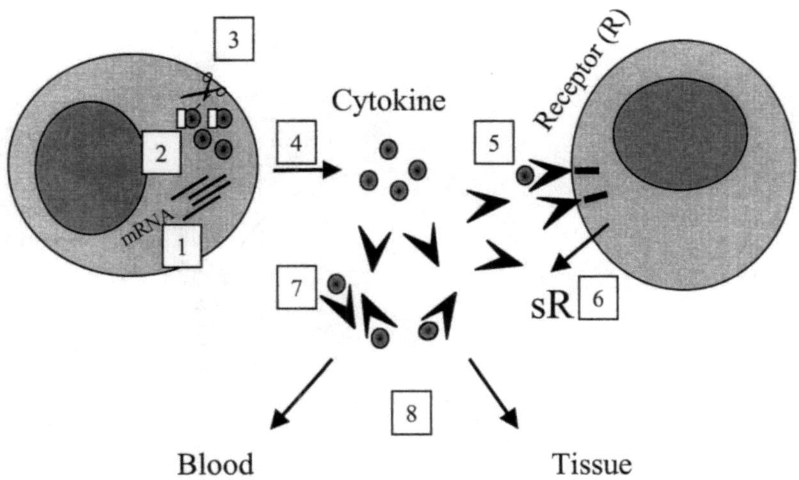

Fig. 1. Multiple levels of cytokine/cytokine receptor biology useful for monitoring their levels of expression in vivo and ex vivo. The levels of cytokine mRNA expression [1] can be investigated by Northern blotting, qualitative or quantitative PCR, and RNase protection assay, whereas intracytoplasmic cytokine protein levels can be analyzed by FACS after cell activation and treatment with brefeldin A to prevent their secretion [2]. Certain cytokines are processed as immature proteins by enzymes such as interleukin-1 converting enzyme (ICE) [3]. Cytokines can be detected by enzyme-linked immunosorbent assay (ELISA) in fluids, including culture supernatants, plasma, urine, and cerebrospinal fluid [4]. Released and cell surface cytokines can bind to cell surface receptors on target cells whose levels can be determined by either FACS analysis or binding studies [5]. Cytokine receptors are often shed abundantly in response to cell activation by their related cytokine [6] or by other forms of cell stimulation, and can be easily detected in body fluids, whole blood, or culture supernatants. Soluble, receptor-bound cytokines can be detected by some ELISAs [7], whereas cytokine and cytokine receptor expression or presence in tissue can be studied by *in situ* hybridization and immunocytochemistry, respectively.

correlates if compared to $CD4^+$ T cell counts and/or viremia *(17–20)*. In this regard, a recent study suggested that in advanced patients with fewer than 200 $CD4^+$ T-cell counts per microliter, both TNF-α and sTNFRII are better correlates of disease evolution than $CD4^+$ T-cell counts and viremia, respectively *(21)*. Analogous considerations can been drawn for IFN-γ *(21–23)*. These investigations imply that the relative importance of immunologic or virologic markers may change as a function of the disease stage and, perhaps, antiviral therapy. In addition to its role in systemic infection, TNF-α is likely to play a key pathogenic role in organ diseases such as those involving the lungs *(15)*, and, particularly, the brain, where several studies have directly related its levels of expression to those of HIV *(24–27)* (Fig. 2).

Structurally and functionally related to the TNF/TNFR families, also the Fas/Apo-1 antigen (CD95) and its ligand as well as CD30/CD30-ligand, both as membrane-bound and soluble proteins or in soluble form, have been indicated as a markers of disease progression during both primary and chronic infection, respectively *(28,29)*. As previously described for TNF receptors, CD30 transduces an HIV-activating signal *(30,31)*, as discussed further, whereas CD95 engagement leads to apoptotic cell death, as reviewed in *(32)*.

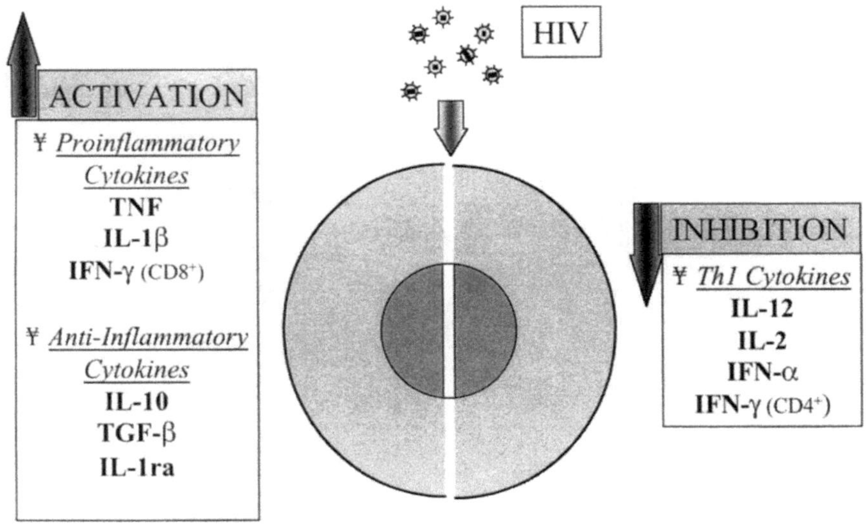

Fig. 2. Effect of HIV infection and/or interaction of its proteins on target immune cells. Several cytokines, including both pro- and antiinflammatory cytokines, are upregulated in their expression after in vitro infection, particularly in macrophages. Other cytokines are, in contrast, downregulated by HIV infection; of note is the fact that these molecules belong to the Th1 activation pathway of differentiation of $CD4^+$ T lymphocytes. Among HIV-encoded proteins, gp120 Env, Tat, and Nef have been reported to be capable of modulating cytokine expression.

Expression of cytokines is an essential component of immune and inflammatory responses. Therefore, several patterns of cytokine expression described in HIV-infected individuals are common to other infectious or autoimmune diseases. In this scenario, however, expression of IFN-γ in the enlarged germinal centers of the lymph nodes is a peculiar feature of HIV infection not observed in other diseases, as first described by immunostaining studies *(33),* and then confirmed by other approaches, including reverse transcriptase (RT)-PCR *(10).* Of interest, IFN-γ expression was by and large accounted for by infiltration of $CD8^+$ cells in the germinal centers *(33).* Surrogates of IFN-γ expression are neopterin *(23,34)* and interferon-inducible protein of 10 -kDA (IP-10) *(35),* a CXC chemokine, that, indeed, has been found elevated in HIV-infected individuals. Finally, IFN-γ is a major component of the so-called "acid-labile" IFN-α *(36)* detected earlier in HIV-infected individuals in analogy with other immune disorders *(22,23)* (Fig. 2).

2. As for inflammatory cytokines, the expression of antiinflammatory molecules, such as TGF-β *(27,37)*, IL-10 *(16,38,39)*, and of the IL-1 receptor antagonist IL-12a *(7,40)* is increased (Fig. 2). This feature likely indicates that the immune system is profoundly perturbed in its attempt to control the ongoing infection and that counter-regulatory cytokines aimed at turning off a chronic inflammatory state are activated as well. In addition, the possibility that some of these features are the results of either direct infection of immune cells by HIV and/or the consequence of cell stimulation by HIV proteins, including gp120 Env, Nef, or VpR *(41,42),* is sustained by both in vitro results, as discussed further, and by the fact that these viral proteins are incorporated into newly formed viral particles (virions) circulating in blood and diffusing in several tissues and organs.

Increased expression of IL-10, in particular, has been highlighted by several studies *(10,16,33,43)*, and it has been considered by some investigators evidence of a Th2 dominance in HIV-infected individuals *(44,45)*, implying an impaired ability to mount a protective cell-mediated immune response carried out by cytotoxic T lymphocytes *(46)*. It should be underscored, however, that IL-10 production, at least in humans, is not restricted, as for IL-4, to Th2-polarized CD4+ T cells or CD8+ Tc2 cells, but it is equally associated with both Th1 and Th0 cell activation *(47)*. In addition, expression of IL-10 in infected individuals is mostly accounted for by non-T lymphocytic antigen presenting cells *(10)*. As in other species, IL-10 maintains in humans an important role as a potent downregulator of cytokine expression and immune responses, acting via interference with costimulatory molecules such as B7.1 and B7.2 *(48,49)*.

3. Th1-related cytokines, such as IL-2 and IL-12, are downregulated in HIV infection (Fig. 2). In contrast to a general scenario of cytokine upregulation, IL-2 production has been described earlier as suppressed in infected individuals *(14,50–52)*, although this general observation was confuted by a study conducted at the single cell level *(53)*. An overall deficit of IL-2 is likely to contribute to the progressive immunodeficiency typical of HIV-infected individuals and represents one of the rationales for the administration of exogenous IL-2 as immunotherapeutic agent, as discussed further. Similar considerations can be made for IL-12 *(54)*, a crucial cytokine in the development of Th1-dependent immune responses *(55)*, although its clinical use is prudently explored because of concerns of serious toxicity. IFN-α has been reported to be downregulated in vivo, although the observations of increased levels of a related "acid-labile" form have generated a substantial confusion in regard, as mentioned previously. IFN-α possesses clear antiviral and antiretroviral activities in vitro *(56–59)* as well as in vivo *(60)* and it has been successfully used for the treatment of AIDS-associated Kaposi's sarcoma in individuals with a relatively well preserved immune system *(23,60)*. Although IFN-γ and/or IFN-γ-related molecules are usually found elevated in HIV-infected individuals, this feature is likely accounted for mostly by expression from CD8+ T and natural killer cells *(33)*. In contrast, CD4+ T cells are usually impaired in their ability to express IFN-γ, a finding that has been correlated to downregulation by HIV-1 *nef* gene product, as discussed later *(61)*, and to the methylation of its promoter *(62)*.

These and other studies, including the observation of T helper-1 (Th1)-related responses, such as secretion of IL-2 after in vitro stimulation with peptides derived from HIV-1 Env, have suggested that infection by HIV represents the failure of the immune system to defend the host as reflected by a loss of protective Th1 responses and prevalence of a useless and even harmful Th2-response *(44–46)*. Evidence both in support of *(13,46,61,63)* and against *(10,64–66)* this hypothesis have been reported. Of interest, efficient replication of HIV in Th0 and Th2, but not Th1 cell clones was observed earlier *(64)*, an observation that has been recently correlated with a positive effect of IL-4 and negative effect of IFN-γ on the cell surface levels of the CXCR4 HIV coreceptor *(67–69)*.

CYTOKINE PERTURBATIONS AFTER HIV INFECTION IN VITRO

Supporting the complex picture emerging from several in vivo studies, the ability of HIV to modulate cytokine expression after either productive in vitro infection or cell stimulation by some of its proteins has been broadly demonstrated. Infection of monocyte-derived macrophages (MDMs) as well as their stimulation by HIV-1 gp120 Env or monoclonal antibodies (mAbs) interacting with its binding to the CD4 molecule, such as Leu-3a or OKT4a, have been correlated to production of TNF-α and IL-1β *(70,71)*, and, more recently, with the activation of different signaling pathways including p56Lck and Raf-1 *(72)* and the MEK/ERK signaling pathway *(73–75)*. Earlier studies underscored that only some gp120 Env possess cytokine-inducing activity *(76)*. In partial contrast to an earlier report *(77)*, our laboratory has recently demonstrated that most HIV-infected individuals show a constitutive activation of the Janus kinase/signal transducer and activator of transcription (JAK/STAT) pathway in their $CD4^+$ PBMC. In particular STAT1 and a carboxy (C)-terminus truncated isoform of STAT5 were found phosphorylated in unstimulated cells *(78)*. Given the fact that multiple cytokines and interferons utilize this signal transduction pathway *(79)*, these findings are independent proof of the state of immune activation caused by HIV infection.

In addition to gp120 Env, Nef and Tat, two regulatory gene products translated from the 2-kb multiply spliced mRNA, have been shown to affect cytokine expression. Expression of Nef has been associated to either down- or upregulation of IL-2 and IFN-γ *(61,80,81)*. Tat has been shown to interact and activate transcription of IL-6 *(82)*, and TNF-β/lymphotoxin-α *(83)*. Induction of TGF-β via exogenously added Tat has been also reported *(84)*, providing a potential mechanism of functional impairment of bone marrow derived precursor cell maturation. In addition, exogenous Tat has been also reported to upregulate the secretion of MCP-1, a prototypic CC chemokine, both in astrocytic cells *(85)* and MDM *(86)*, as well as interacting with some chemokine receptors, particularly CXCR4 *(87,88)*. Although not via direct interference with cytokines, VpR, like Nef *(89)*, is incorporated into the virion and can mediate important cellular functions such as cell cycle arrest in the G_2/M phase *(41,42)*.

PRO- AND ANTIINFLAMMATORY CYTOKINES REGULATE HIV REPLICATION

The observation that TNF-α and IL-1β were upregulated in HIV-infected individuals stimulated interest in understanding their role during infection. Although initially considered an anti-HIV agent *(90)*, on the basis of a protective activity exerted against other viral infections *(91)*, TNF-α soon became the paradigm of HIV inductive cytokines *(71,92)* (Fig. 3). Its mechanism of action was elegantly shown to depend on activation of the cellular transcription factor NF-κB *(93–95)*, a dimeric protein complex residing inactively in the cytoplasm conjugated to the I-κB inhibitory molecule *(96)*. Activation of NF-κB involves its dissociation from I-κB followed by nuclear translocation of a dimer usually composed of p50 and p65 subunits (or by equivalent molecules) encompassing both DNA recognition specificity and transactivating capacity *(96)*. Two sites specifically binding NF-κB are present in the enhancer region of the U3 LTR of HIV-1 (only one site in HIV-2 and SIV) in close proximity to the +1 start site *(93–95)* (Fig. 3). Therefore, TNF-induced NF-κB activation can either initiate or potentiate HIV transcription and expression both in $CD4^+$ T cells *(93)* and macrophages *(94)*, whereas viruses either lacking NF-κB binding sites or containing mutated sequences lose the capacity of being transactivated by TNF *(97)*. Similar conclusions have been drawn for IL-1β *(95)*, although NF-κB–dependent activation of viral expression was not observed in the chronically infected promonocytic U1 cell line

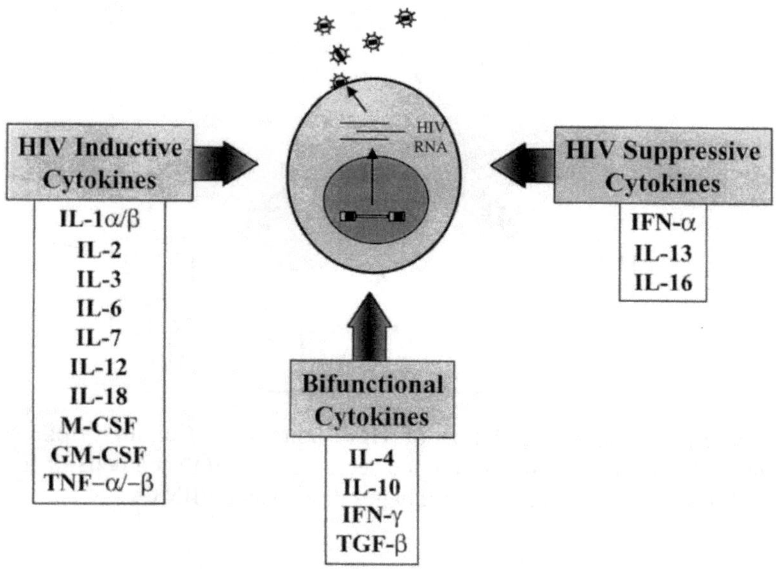

Fig. 3. Cytokines regulate HIV replication. Several cytokines, mostly associated with a pro-inflammatory role, have been shown to enhance virus production in different model systems. Only a few cytokines have been associated with a clear-cut suppressive effect, whereas others can either upregulate or downregulate HIV expression as a function of the experimental conditions.

(98), one of the most utilized in vitro models for studying HIV reactivation from latency *(99).* More recently, a functional transcriptional interaction between NF-κB and AP-1 consequent to activation of ERK-1 and ERK-2 mitogen-activated protein (MAP) kinases was described in U1 cells stimulated with different cytokines *(100).*

Other pro-inflammatory cytokines have been associated with the augmentation of HIV expression, including IL-2, IL-6, and IFN-γ, as reviewed in *(99),* and, more recently, IL-18 *(101).* In the case of IL-6, a posttranscriptional mechanism of enhanced protein and virion expression has been reported in U1 cells *(102),* whereas IFN-γ both directly induced and modulated the production of new progeny virions in phorbol myristate acetate (PMA) activated U1 cells undergoing monocytic differentiation, with the effect of shifting the major site of particle production from the plasma membrane to intracytoplasmic vacuoles of Golgi origin *(103).*

Of note is the fact that autocrine/paracrine induction of HIV replication by cytokines has been demonstrated both in primary cells and cell lines for IL-1β, IL-6, TNF-α, and IFN-γ *(104–107)* (Fig. 4).

Several aspects of transcriptional regulation of HIV expression have been highlighted recently, including the cooperation between cytokine induced NF-κB and other cellular transcription factors or coactivators, such as NF-IL 6, p300, and the viral transcriptional activator Tat *(108–110).*

When antiinflammatory cytokines such as TGF-β and IL-10 were studied for their effect on HIV replication, the results have not been univocal. For both cytokines, evidence supporting their role as enhancers or suppressors of HIV production were obtained in different model systems, including mitogen-stimulated PBMCs and MDMs, as a function of whether cells were pretreated with the cytokine before vs after

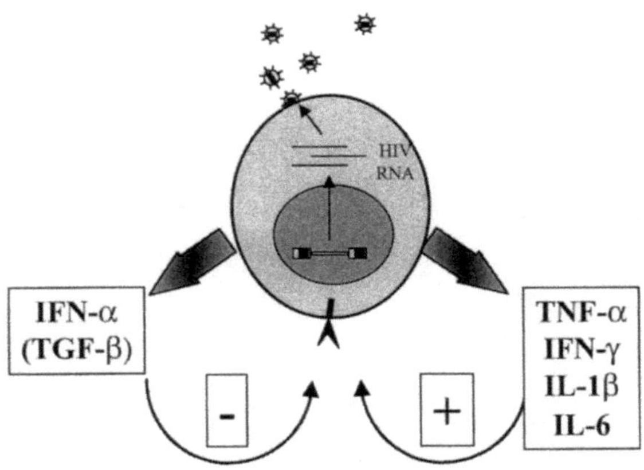

Fig. 4. Autocrine/paracrine regulation of HIV expression. Certain cytokines have been shown to control the levels of expression once secreted from infected cells or from bystander cells both in cell lines and in primary macrophages or activated PBMCs.

infection, respectively *(111)*. In IL-10–stimulated MDMs, inhibition of HIV production was observed at concentrations effectively suppressing secretion of HIV-inductive cytokines (i.e., TNF-α and IL-6) *(106),* whereas enhancement occurred at lower concentrations of IL-10 *(112,113)*. Enhancement of HIV replication by TGF-β has been independently reported in both MDMs *(114)* and T-cell blasts that had been treated with cocaine *(115)*. Opposite effects on viral replication have been also reported in the case of IL-4 *(116–119)* and IFN-γ *(120),* whereas inhibition of HIV replication by IL-13 has been observed in MDMs but not in activated PBMCs *(121)* (Figs. 3 and 4).

It is likely that several conflicting reports regarding the effect of cytokines in modulating HIV replication may be explained by differential effects played on different steps of the virus life cycle, including the possibility of inducing HIV-inhibitory chemokines and/or regulating chemokine receptors, as discussed further in detail. In this regard, pretreatment of cells with TNF-α and IFN-γ has been reported to interfere with entry of HIV into MDMs *(122),* although the precise mechanism involved has not been clarified. More importantly, in vivo chronic inflammatory conditions and concurrent mycobacterial infections, often associated with HIV infection *(123–126),* have been correlated to increased levels of viremia and accelerated disease progression.

CHEMOKINES AND THEIR RECEPTORS

Two independent lines of research have brought to a major breakthrough in HIV research: the discovery of HIV entry coreceptors. Indirect evidence that molecules additional to CD4 needed to be expressed on the cell surface to allow HIV to efficiently enter and infect cells were obtained after the engineering of mice transgenic for human CD4. Cells from these animals perfectly expressed the human molecule and bound HIV with affinity comparable to that of human CD4+ cells; they were decorated by the virus particles, but remained poorly infectable *(127,128)*. After a decade and many false successes, a previously identified molecule was shown to confer fusogenic properties and in vitro infectibility to mouse cells by T-cell tropic HIV strains *(129)*. This molecule, temporarily renamed "fusin," showed a seven-transmembrane domain structure typical of chemokine receptors and other molecules, although its ligand(s) was unknown.

Ten years earlier, CD8+ T cells of infected individuals, in addition to being cytotoxic precursors and effectors against HIV-infected cells, were shown to secrete a nonlytic inhibitor(s) of viral expression and replication *(130)*. The nature of this/these soluble factors has remained elusive for several years, and it has been negatively defined by considering that several cytokines were not responsible for the effect *(130)*, until the identification of two independent factors was announced at the end of 1995. One team reported that three β-chemokines—regulated upon activation normal T cell expressed and secreted (RANTES), macrophage inflammatory protein-1α (MIP-1α), and MIP-1β—were released by transformed and activated CD8+ T lymphocytes and potently inhibited the infection of a T-cell line, PM-1, with a relative selectivity for macrophage-tropic viruses *(131)*. A second group simultaneously reported that IL-16, a natural ligand of CD4 *(132)*, a notion however, recently challenged *(133)*, was responsible for the original soluble "CD8 antiviral factor" activity *(134)*. Subsequent studies on IL-16 supported the original claim *(135–137)*. Although IL-16 better fitted the characteristics of the original CD8-release antiviral factor (CAF), substantial more attention has been devoted to the role of chemokines in HIV disease because of their competition for the HIV entry coreceptors. Indeed, the discovery of fusin as a receptor for T-cell tropic viruses in 1996 indicated that chemokines and their receptors were likely important factors for HIV infection of CD4+ human cells. The three HIV-inhibitory chemokines shared the binding to CCR5, in addition to other chemokine receptors, which was rapidly identified as the major receptor for macrophage-tropic strains *(138,139)*. Fusin was renamed CXCR4 and its ligand was identified in the CXC (or "α") chemokine stromal cell derived factor-1 (SDF-1) *(140,141)*. Both CCR5 and CXCR4 were found to be the major HIV coreceptors allowing entry of the virus in CD4+ cells, whereas their related chemokines inhibited the penetration and thus the subsequent cycle of infection of HIV, as reviewed in *(142,143)* (Fig. 5). The discovery of the role of chemokine receptors and the related inhibitory effects of chemokines demonstrate that all the fundamental steps of the HIV life cycle, from viral entry to release of progeny virions, are influenced by the cytokine network, at least in vitro *(99)* (Fig. 5). In addition to a better understanding of the pathogenic process in vivo, this information is potentially important for designing new antiviral agents acting on the target cell rather than the rapidly mutating virus. With specific regard to chemokines and their receptors, a number of analogs of chemokines directly to either CXCR4 or CCR5 have been already shown to exert potent antiviral effects in vitro *(144–147)*, and their potential clinical use is under intense investigation.

The molecular interactions occurring when virions infect CD4+ cells seem to involve first the binding of gp120 Env to CD4 and a subsequent recognition of the chemokine receptor after a conformational change of some regions of the viral envelope involving the hypervariable V3 loop *(148–151)*. As a consequence, the fusogenic component (gp41 Env) can spring and insert itself into the target cell membrane, starting the infection process by allowing the injection of the viral nucleoprotein complex *(143)*.

In addition to CCR5 and CXCR4, a number of other chemokine receptors and related molecules have been shown to act as entry receptors for HIV-1, HIV-2 or SIV *(143)*, although their in vivo relevance is questioned *(152–154)*. Among these, CCR3

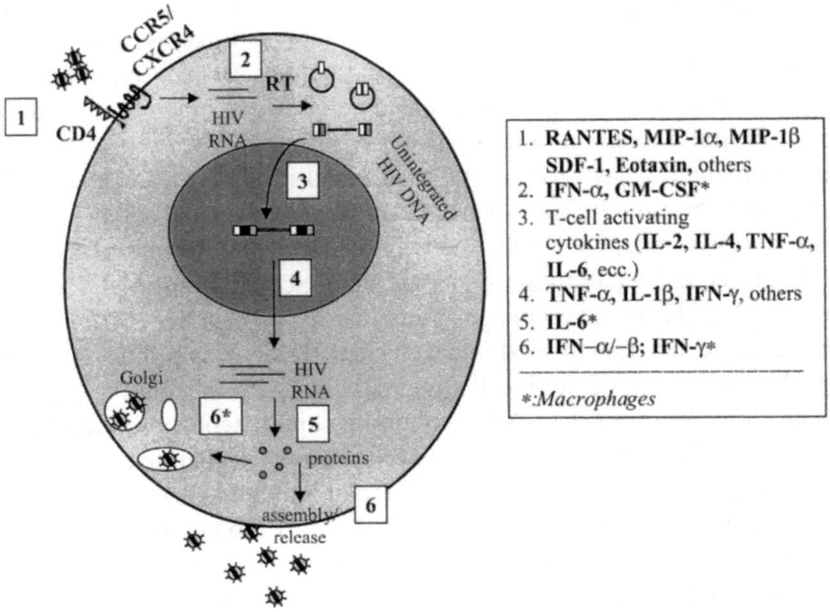

Fig. 5. Multiple steps of the HIV life cycle are affected by chemokines and/or cytokines. [1] Entry; [2] reverse transcription; [3] integration; [4] *ex novo* transcription of HIV mRNA; [5] translation of viral proteins; [6] assembly and release of new progeny virions. This last process is accomplished in macrophages in Golgi-derived vacuoles in addition to budding from the plasma membrane that represents the only site of virion production for T lymphocytes.

appears to be of peculiar relevance for infection of microglial cells, the main target cells of infection in the brain *(155)*.

The importance of chemokine receptors, and of their ligands, in vivo has been highlighted by studying highly HIV-exposed but uninfected individuals, including male and female prostitutes, intravenous drug users, and partners of seropositive individuals *(156,157)*. A substantial fraction of these individuals is characterized by a homozygous deletion of 32 bp in the *CCR5* gene leading to the synthesis of an imperfect protein incapable of being expressed at the cell surface *(158)*. The cells of these individuals are resistant to infection by macrophage-tropic HIV strains, recently renamed "R5" *(159)*, although they maintain susceptibility to infection by T-cell tropic (X4) viruses (Fig. 6). Only a few exceptions have been reported in relationship to this finding *(160,161)*. The almost absolute resistance of Δ32-CCR5 homozygotes to HIV infection highlights the previous observation that only macrophage-tropic viruses, i.e. R5 strains *(159)*, efficiently spread after transmission, regardless of the dominant viral quasispecies of the donor *(150,162)*. The reasons for this strong selection are still not completely understood, but are explained, at least in the cases of sexual transmission, by a relatively poor expression of CXCR4 on the surface of mucosal Langherans' dendritic cells *(163,164)*. In addition, R5 viruses appear capable of replication in quiescent *(165)* or semiquiescent *(166)* T lymphocytes, a functional feature that may confer them a selective advantage over X4 strains.

The mechanism(s) by which chemokines inhibit HIV infection are constantly refined. The relatively simple "mechanistic" model whereby chemokines, via bind-

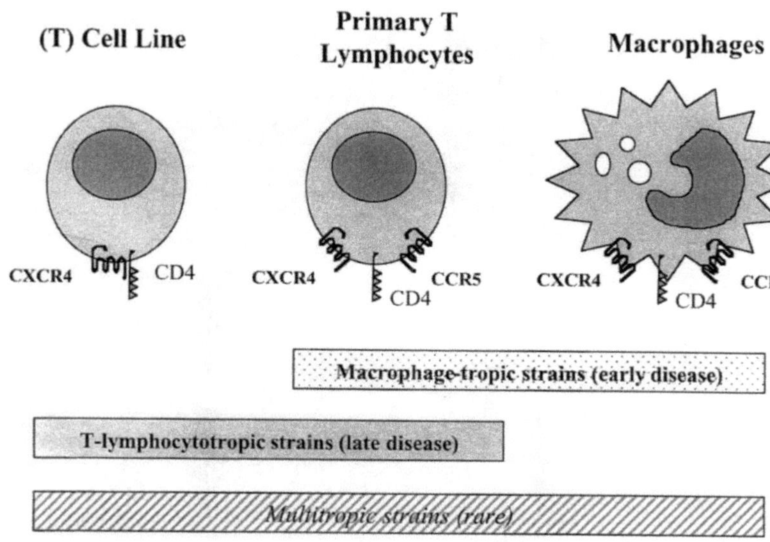

Fig. 6. HIV cell tropisms. HIVs have been classified as a function of their preferential or restricted replicative capacity into either human macrophages (macrophage-tropic strains, also unable to spread and form syncytia in the MT-2 T-cell line, and therefore referred to as nonsyncytia inducing (NSI) viruses are characterized by use of CCR5 or other CC chemokine receptors), activated primary T lymphocytes, or cell lines. These latter viruses usually were SI in MT-2 cells and have also been called T-lymphotropic viruses. Rare strains have been isolated from individuals in advanced stages of disease that were capable of replication in all these cell types. Of note is the fact that macrophage tropic strains are also capable of replication in activated primary PBMCs (which express CCR5) and predominate in the early phase of infection. In contrast, usage of CXCR4, causing the NSI→SI switch and partial changes in in vitro cell tropisms, occurs in approx 50% of individuals infected with the clade B HIV subtype before the onset of AIDS.

ing to portions of the chemokine receptor distinct from those recognized by HIV, sterically interfere and compete with the virus without the requirement of signaling through the chemokine receptor *(167)* is challenged by recent observations. In particular, chemokine-like inhibition of viral entry by the B-oligomeric portion of pertussis toxin has been correlated to its disruptive effect on the cocapping of CCR5 and CD4 in activated T lymphocytes *(168)*, as discussed in detail by others *(169)*. Of interest, the B oligomer possesses an additional and broader post-entry anti-HIV activity that is exerted against cells both acutely *(170)* and chronically infected with X4 HIV-1 *(170a)*.

In addition to classical inhibition of viral entry, macrophage–derived chemokine (MDC), binding to CCR4, a chemokine receptor not utilized as entry coreceptor by HIV has been described as a potent inhibitor of both R5 and X4 virus replication in T lymphocytes *(171)*. Although others have not reproduced this finding *(172,173)*, we have recently observed a potent inhibitory activity for R5 HIV replication in MDMs, but not in T cells. Of interest, MDC inhibited virus replication in macrophages at a post-entry level *(174)*. An interesting aspect of MDC is the fact that, as other chemokines *(175)*, it is subject to truncation at the amino (N)-terminus by a proteolytic process. Truncated forms of MDC, such as the molecules that were utilized in the orig-

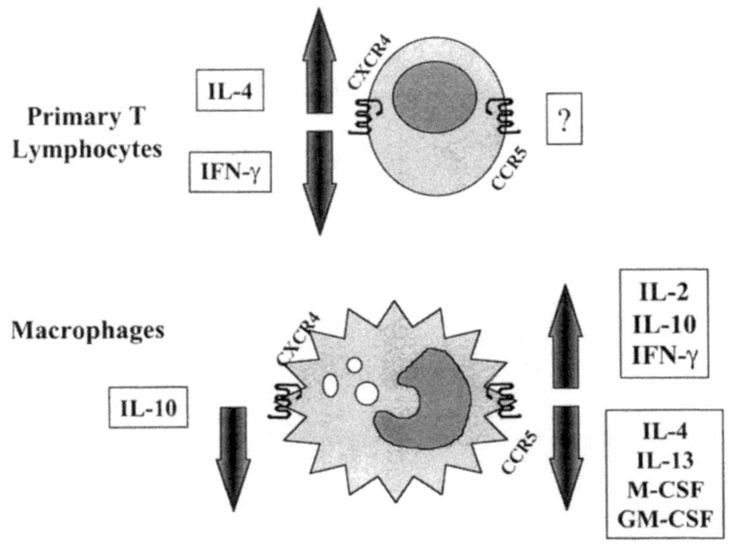

Fig. 7. Cytokine regulation of HIV coreceptors in T cells and macrophages. CXCR4 expression on the surface of T lymphocytes is regulated by Th1 (IFN-γ)/Th2 (IL-4) cytokines in an opposite manner *(69)*. Concerning CCR5, IL-2 upregulates CCR5 *(229,230)* as well as other chemokine receptors *(231)* on T lymphocytes, whereas IL-10 exerts a negative effect *(232)*. Several cytokines either up- or downregulate CCR5 expression on human macrophages.

inal description of its antiviral activity *(171)*, appear more potent inhibitors of HIV replication than the full-length chemokine, although they lose the capacity of binding specifically to CCR4 *(176)*. Whether a specific unknown receptor is involved in the anti-HIV effect of MDC is currently unknown.

A growing body of evidence suggests that chemokines can also enhance HIV replication as a function of the experimental conditions and target cells. The possibility that signaling through the chemokine receptor results in the activation of the infected cells and enhanced virus expression was reported both in MDM *(177,178)* and then in activated T cells and PBMCs *(179,180)*. Whether β-chemokine enhancement of HIV replication may influence the in vivo selection of T-cell tropic variants (usually characterized by dual use of CCR5 and CXCR4), an event occurring in approx 50% of individuals infected with clade B HIV-1 before or during the onset of AIDS *(181)*, is debated.

The functional interaction between cytokines and chemokines and/or their receptors in relationship to HIV infection and spreading has been recently studied and promises to be a fertile area of investigation. IL-2, IL-4, IL-10, IL-13, macrophage and granulocyte-macrophage colony stimulating factors (M-CSF and GM-CSF, respectively) have been reported to modulate CCR5 expression and, consequently, HIV infection in primary monocytes or MDM *(182,183)* (Fig. 7). Similar findings have been reported in terms of upregulation of several CC chemokine receptors, but not CXCR4, in U937 promonocytic cells by IFN-γ *(184)*; CXCR4 was instead upregulated by the myeloid differentiating agent vitamin D_3 in a family of clones of the U937 cell lines *(185)*. Regarding T lymphocytes, it has been recently shown that polarization toward either Th1 or Th2 phenotypes is associated with a differential or preferential expression of certain chemokine receptors that may serve as entry coreceptors for HIV. CCR3, CCR8, and CXCR4 are preferentially expressed on Th2 cells, whereas CCR5 is more abundant on the Th1 cell surface *(186–188)*. The relevance of these findings for HIV infection and spreading has not been yet fully clarified, although initial reports do not indicate a substantial impact of differential chemokine receptor expression on HIV replication *(166,189)*, with the possible exception of IL-4–induced upregulation of CXCR4 *(67–69)*.

Finally, the release of HIV-inhibitory chemokine by cytotoxic T lymphocytes as well as their activation by RANTES *(190–193)* illustrate other modalities and roles played by chemokines in the immune response against HIV infection.

CYTOKINES FROM THE BENCH TO THE BEDSIDE

The possibility of complementing the pharmacological approach to HIV disease, currently based on potent cocktails of antivirals, with cell-based immunotherapy has been previously discussed in general terms *(194)*, and it has become a feasible approach at least in the case of IL-2. Although many other experimental approaches targeting the host rather than the virus are being pursued, including the use of hydroxyurea *(195,196)*, mycophenolic acid *(197)*, G-SCF *(198)* and GM-CSF *(199–201)*, IL-12 *(202,203)*, and vaccination by either inactivated HIV *(204)* or HIV subunits *(205)*, IL-2 has gained a special place in the therapeutical armamentarium under current scrutiny. Two fundamental approaches have been taken into account in terms of using IL-2 in HIV-infected individuals: an "ultralow dose" (<1 millions of international units [MIU] per die) continuous administration, mostly aimed at the potentiation of certain immune responses against HIV *(206–209)* and a "high-dose" (usually 9–15 MIU per die) intermittent administration. This second approach has shown in multiple independent studies that IL-2 can induce a stable raise in $CD4^+$ cell counts of infected individuals up to normal or near normal levels, an end-point rarely matched by the best retroviral combinations, including HAART *(210–214)*. The mechanisms triggered by in vivo IL-2 administration to infected individuals are certainly multiple and essentially unknown, but they ultimately result in increased numbers of memory T cells playing an important role in the defense against common pathogens and opportunistic agents *(215,216)*. Increased numbers of naive T cells in concomitance with decreased levels of PBMC-associated HIV DNA under IL-2 therapy also has been reported *(217,218)*.

Regarding the effect of IL-2 on virus replication, it has been initially observed that administration of this cytokine was associated with transient increases in plasma-associated virus, that rapidly returned to baseline *(210)*. This latter phenomenon has been recently correlated to the downmodulation of transcriptional repressors *(219)*. Therefore, IL-2 is usually administered in the presence of potent antivirals. Finally, the efficacy of antiviral treatments is clearly not antagonized by IL-2 administration.

A more recent use of IL-2 and other immune-based agents such as anti-CD3 monoclonal antibodies (mAbs), aimed at activating most T lymphocytes, has been recently proposed as a strategy for attempting to eradicate HIV from latently infected cells *(220)*. In support to this approach, patients' cells activated ex vivo by either anti-CD3 mAb or by a cocktail of cytokines, such as IL-2 plus IL-6 and TNF-α, a combination of cytokines previously shown capable of activating naive T lymphocytes *(221)*, in the presence of antivirals decreased the efficiency of recovery of replication competent HIV *(222)*. However, it is important to underscore that potent rebounds of viremia were almost univocally observed after therapy suspension, both in the presence and absence of IL-2 although there is debate on whether viral emergence from a different tissue reservoir may be responsible for the observed phenomenon *(223,224)*.

CONCLUSIONS

Cytokines, and more recently chemokines, have been long studied as tools for investigating the replicative properties of HIV both in chronically infected cell lines and primary cells. This information is of great importance in light of current investigations on the clinical use of cytokines either directly in vivo, as in the case of G-CSF or IL-2, or ex vivo with the goal of purging immune cells of HIV infection. The possibility of investigating the effect and the role of cytokines, both endogenously released and therapeutically administered, must stimulate the search for new and better markers for evaluating their antiviral efficacy and effects on the immunologic reconstitution of infected individuals. Cytokines, chemokines, and their receptors will influence both the short- and long-term control of HIV replication and the size of the viral reservoirs. In addition, restoration of immune functions may help in preventing opportunistic infections and cytokine–mediated tumors during recently introduced protocols of structured therapy interruption *(225–228)*.

REFERENCES

1. Pantaleo G, Graziosi C, Fauci AS. New concepts in the immunopathogenesis of human immunodeficiency virus infection. N Engl J Med 1993; 328:327–35.
2. Fauci AS. Host factors and the pathogenesis of HIV-induced disease. Nature 1996; 384:529–34.
3. Autran B, Carcelain G, Li TS, Blanc C, Mathez D, Tubiana R, et al. Positive effects of combined antiretroviral therapy on $CD4^+$ T cell homeostasis and function in advanced HIV disease. Science 1997; 277:112–6.
4. Bentwich Z, Kalinkovich A, Weisman Z. Immune activation is a dominant factor in the pathogenesis of African AIDS. Immunol Today 1995; 16:187–91.
5. Montano MA, Nixon CP, Essex M. Dysregulation through the NF-kappaB enhancer and TATA box of the human immunodeficiency virus type 1 subtype E promoter. J Virol 1998; 72:8446–52.
6. Montano MA, Nixon CP, Ndung'u T, Bussmann H, Novitsky VA, Dickman D, Essex M. Elevated tumor necrosis factor-alpha activation of human immunodeficiency virus type 1 subtype C in Southern Africa is associated with an NF-kappaB enhancer gain-of-function. J Infect Dis 2000; 181:76–81.
7. Dinarello CA. Interleukin-1, interleukin-1 receptors and interleukin-1 receptor antagonist. Int Rev Immunol 1998; 16:457–99.
8. Eliaz R, Wallach D, Kost J. Long-term protection against the effects of tumour necrosis factor by controlled delivery of the soluble p55 TNF receptor. Cytokine 1996; 8:482–7.
9. Esser R, Glienke W, Andreesen R, Unger RE, Kreutz M, Rubsamen-Waigmann H, von Briesen H. Individual cell analysis of the cytokine repertoire in human immunodeficiency virus-1-infected monocytes/macrophages by a combination of immunocytochemistry and in situ hybridization. Blood 1998; 91:4752–60.
10. Graziosi C, Pantaleo G, Gantt KR, Ortin J-P, Demarest JF, Cohen OJ, et al. Lack of evidence for the dichotomy of TH1 and TH2 predominance in HIV-infected individuals. Science 1994; 265:248–52.

11. Revel M, Groner Y. Post-transcriptional and translational controls of gene expression in eukaryotes. Annu Rev Biochem 1978; 47:1079–126.
12. Letterio JJ, Roberts AB. Regulation of immune responses by TGF-beta. Annu Rev Immunol 1998; 16:137–61.
13. Klein SA, Dobmeyer JM, Dobmeyer TS, Pape M, Ottmann OG, Helm EB, et al. Demonstration of the Th1 to Th2 cytokine shift during the course of HIV-1 infection using cytoplasmic cytokine detection on single cell level by flow cytometry. AIDS 1997; 11:1111–8.
14. Scott-Algara D, Vuillier F, Marasescu M, De Saint Martin J, Dighiero G. Serum levels of IL-2, IL-1, TNF-α, and soluble receptor of IL-2 in HIV-1-infected patients. AIDS Res Hum Retrovir 1991; 7:381–6.
15. Agostini C, Zambello R, Trentin L, Cerutti A, Enthammer C, Facco M, et al. Expression of TNF receptors by T cells and membrane TNF-alpha by alveolar macrophages suggests a role for TNF-alpha by regulation of the local immune responses in the lung of HIV-1-infected patients. J Immunol 1995; 154:2928–38.
16. Clerici M, Piconi S, Balotta C, Trabattoni D, Capetti A, Fusi ML, et al. Pentoxifylline improves cell-mediated immunity and reduces human immunodeficiency virus (HIV) plasma viremia in asymptomatic HIV-seropositive persons. J Infect Dis 1997; 175:1210–5.
17. Kalinkovich A, Engelmann H, Harpaz N, Burstein R, Barak V, Kalickman I, et al. Elevated serum levels of soluble tumour necrosis factor receptors (sTNF-R) in patients with HIV infection. Clin Exp Immunol 1992; 89:351–5.
18. Barcellini W, Rizzardi GP, Poli G, Tambussi G, Velati C, Meroni PL, et al. Cytokines and soluble receptor changes in the transition from primary to early chronic HIV type 1 infection. AIDS Res Hum Retrovir 1996; 12:325–31.
19. Salazar-Gonzalez JF, Martinez-Maza O, Aziz N, Kolberg JA, Yeghiazarian T, Shen LP, Fahey JL. Relationship of plasma HIV-RNA levels and levels of TNF-alpha and immune activation products in HIV infection. Clin Immunol Immunopathol 1997; 84:36–45.
20. Hestdal K, Aukrust P, Muller F, Lien E, Bjerkeli V, Espevik T, Froland SS. Dysregulation of membrane-bound tumor necrosis factor-alpha and tumor necrosis factor receptors on mononuclear cells in human immunodeficiency virus type 1 infection: low percentage of p75-tumor necrosis factor receptor positive cells in patients with advanced disease and high viral load. Blood 1997; 90:2670–9.
21. Fahey JL, Taylor JM, Manna B, Nishanian P, Aziz N, Giorgi JV, Detels R. Prognostic significance of plasma markers of immune activation, HIV viral load and CD4 T-cell measurements. AIDS 1998; 12:1581–90.
22. Rinaldo CR Jr, Armstrong JA, Kingsley LA, Zhou S, Ho M. Relation of alpha and gamma interferon levels to development of AIDS in homosexual men. J Exp Pathol 1990; 5:127–32.
23. Krown SE, Niedzwiecki D, Bhalla R, Flomerberg B, Bundow D, Chapman D. Relationship and prognostic value of endogenous interferon-α, β2-microglobulin, and neopterin serum levels in patients with Kaposi's sarcoma and AIDS. J AIDS Hum Retrovir 1991; 4:871–80.
24. Genis P, Jett M, Bernton EW, Boyle T, Gelbard HA, Dzenko K, et al. Cytokines and arachidonic metabolites produced during human immunodeficiency virus (HIV)-infected macrophage-astroglia interactions: implications for the neuropathogenesis of HIV disease. J Exp Med 1992; 176:1703–18.
25. Koka P, He K, Zack JA, Kitchen S, Peacock W, Fried I, et al. Human immunodeficiency virus 1 envelope proteins induce interleukin 1, tumor necrosis factor alpha, and nitric oxide in glial cultures derived from fetal, neonatal, and adult human brain. J Exp Med 1995; 182:941–51.
26. Tan SV, Guiloff RJ, Henderson DC, Gazzard BG, Miller R. AIDS-associated vacuolar myelopathy and tumor necrosis factor-alpha (TNF alpha). J Neurol Sci 1996; 138:134–44.
27. McManus CM, Brosnan CF, Berman JW. Cytokine induction of MIP-1 alpha and MIP-1 beta in human fetal microglia. J Immunol 1998; 160:1449–55.

28. Pizzolo G, Vinante F, Morosato L, Nadali G, Chilosi M, Gandini G, et al. High serum levels of the soluble form of CD30 molecule in the early phase of HIV-1 infection as an independent predictor of progression to AIDS. AIDS 1994; 8:741–5.
29. Rizzardi GP, Barcellini W, Tambussi G, Lillo F, Malnati M, Perrin L, Lazzarin A. Plasma levels of soluble CD30, tumour necrosis factor (TNF)-alpha and TNF receptors during primary HIV-1 infection: correlation with HIV-1 RNA and the clinical outcome. AIDS 1996; 10:F45–50.
30. Biswas P, Smith CA, Goletti D, Hardy EC, Jackson RW, Fauci AS. Cross-linking of CD30 induces HIV expression in chronically infected T cells. Immunity 1995; 2:587–96.
31. Maggi E, Annunziato F, Manetti R, Biagiotti R, Giudizi MG, Ravina A, et al. Activation of HIV expression by CD30 triggering in $CD4^+$ T cells from HIV-infected individuals. Immunity 1995; 3:251–5.
32. Kaplan D, Sieg S. Role of the Fas/Fas ligand apoptotic pathway in human immunodeficiency virus type 1 disease. J Virol 1998; 72:6279–82.
33. Emilie D, Peuchmaur MC, Maillot MC, Crevon N, Brousee JF, Delfraissy J, et al. Production of interleukins in human immunodeficiency virus-1-replicating lymphnodes. J Clin Invest 1990; 86:148–59.
34. Fuchs D, Hansen A, Reibnegger G, Werner ER, Dierich MP, Watcher H. Neopterin as a marker for activated cell-mediated immunity: application in HIV infection. Immunol Today 1988; 9:150–5.
35. Buhl R, Jaffe HA, Holroyd KJ, Borok Z, Roum JH, Mastrangeli A, et al. Activation of alveolar macrophages in asymptomatic HIV-infected individuals. J Immunol 1993; 150:1019–28.
36. Capobianchi MR, Mattana P, Mercuri F, Conciatori G, Ameglio F, Anke H, Dianzani F. Acid lability is not an intrinsic property of interferon-alpha induced by HIV-infected cells. J Interferon Res 1992; 12:431–8.
37. Wahl SM, Allen JB, McCartney-Francis N, Morganti-Kossmann MC, Kossmann T, Ellingsworth L, et al. Macrophage- and astrocyte-derived transforming growth factor beta as a mediator of central nervous system dysfunction in acquired immune deficiency syndrome. J Exp Med 1991; 173:981–91.
38. Gallo P, Sivieri S, Rinaldi L, Yan XB, Lolli F, De Rossi A, Tavolato B. Intratechal synthesis of interleukin-10 (IL-10) in viral and inflammatory diseases of the central nervous system. J Neurol Sci 1994; 126:49–53.
39. Muller F, Aukrust P, Nordøy I, Frøland SS. Possible role of interleukin-10 (IL-10) and CD40 ligand expression in the pathogenesis of hypergammaglobulinemia in human immunodeficiency virus infection: modulation of IL-10 and Ig production after intravenous Ig infusion. Blood 1998; 92:3721–9.
40. Kreuzer KA, Dayer JM, Rockstroh JK, Sauerbruch T, Spengler U. The IL-1 system in HIV infection: peripheral concentrations of IL- 1beta, IL-1 receptor antagonist and soluble IL-1 receptor type II. Clin Exp Immunol 1997; 109:54–8.
41. Ayyavoo V, Mahboubi A, Mahalingam S, Ramalingam R, Kudchodkar S, Williams WV, et al. HIV-1 Vpr suppresses immune activation and apoptosis through regulation of nuclear factor kappa B. Nat Med 1997; 3:1117–23.
42. Poon B, Grovit-Ferbas K, Stewart SA, Chen ISY. Cell cycle arrest by Vpr in HIV-1 virions and insensitivity to antiretroviral agents. Science 1998; 281:266–9.
43. Than S, Hu R, Oyaizu N, Romano J, Wang X, Sheikh S, Pahwa S. Cytokine pattern in relation to disease progression in human immunodeficiency virus-infected children. J Infect Dis 1997; 175:47–56.
44. Clerici M, Shearer GM. A TH1→TH2 switch is a critical step in the etiology of HIV infection. Immunol Today 1993; 14:107–11.
45. Clerici M, Shearer GM. The Th1-Th2 hypothesis of HIV infection: new insights. Immunol Today 1994; 15:575–81.

46. Shearer GM. HIV-induced immunopathogenesis. Immunity 1998; 9:587–93.
47. Del Prete G, De Carli M, Almerigogna F, Giudizi MG, Biagiotti R, Romagnani S. Human IL-10 is produced by both type 1 helper (Th1) and type 2 helper (Th2) T cell clones and inhibits their antigen-specific proliferation and cytokine production. J Immunol 1993; 150:353–60.
48. Ozawa H, Aiba S, Nakagawa S, Tagami H. Interferon-gamma and interleukin-10 inhibit antigen presentation by Langerhans cells for T helper type 1 cells by suppressing their CD80 (B7-1) expression. Eur J Immunol 1996; 26:648–52.
49. Hasegawa A, Ueno Y, Yamashita M, Nakayama T, Tada T. Regulation of T cell autoreactivity to MHC class II by controlling CD80 (B7-1) expression on B cells. Int Immunol 1998; 10:147–58.
50. Murray HW, Rubin BY, Masur H, Roberts RB. Impaired production of lymphokines and immune (gamma) interferon in the acquired immunodeficiency syndrome. N Engl J Med 1984; 310:883–9.
51. Rook AH, Hooks JJ, Quinnan GV, Lane HC, Manischewitz J F, Macher AM, et al. Interleukin 2 enhances the natural killer cell activity of acquired immunodeficiency syndrome patients through a gamma-interferon-independent mechanism. J Immunol 1985; 134:1503–7.
52. Honda M, Kitamura K, Matsuda K. Soluble IL-2 receptor in AIDS. Correlation of its serum level with the classification of HIV-induced diseases and its characterization. J Immunol 1989; 142:4248–55.
53. Lane HC, Depper JM, Greene WC, Whalen G, Waldmann TA, Fauci AS. Qualitative analysis of immune function in patients with the acquired immunodeficiency syndrome. Evidence for a selective defect in soluble antigen recognition. N Engl J Med 1985; 313:79–84.
54. Chehimi J, Starr SE, Frank I, D' Andrea A, Ma X, MacGragor RR, et al. Impaired interleukin-12 production in human immunodeficiency virus-infected patients. J Exp Med 1994; 179:1361–6.
55. Trinchieri G. Interleukin-12 and its role in the generation of TH1 cells. Immunol Today 1993; 14:335–8.
56. Ho DD, Hartshorn KL, Rota TR, Andrews CA, Kaplan JC, Schooley RT, Hirsch MS. Recombinant human interferon alpha-A suppresses HTLV-III replication in vitro. Lancet 1985; i:602–4.
57. Poli G, Orenstein JM, Kinter A, Folks TM, Fauci AS. Interferon-alpha but not AZT suppresses HIV expression in chronically infected cell lines. Science 1989; 244:575–7.
58. Shirazi Y, Pitha PM. Alpha interferon inhibits early stages of the human immunodeficiency virus type 1 replication cycle. J Virol 1992; 66:1321–8.
59. Honda Y, Rogers L, Nakata K, Zhao BY, Pine R, Nakai Y, et al. Type I interferon induces inhibitory 16-kD CCAAT/enhancer binding protein (C/EBP)beta, repressing the HIV-1 long terminal repeat in macrophages: pulmonary tuberculosis alters C/EBP expression, enhancing HIV-1 replication. J Exp Med 1998; 188:1255–65.
60. Lane HC, Kovacs JA, Feinberg J, Herpin B, Davey V, Walker R, et al. Anti-retroviral effects of interferon-α in AIDS-associated Kaposi's sarcoma. Lancet 1988; ii:1218–22.
61. Collette Y, Chang HL, Cerdan C, Chambost H, Algarte M, Mawas C, et al. Specific Th1 cytokine down-regulation associated with primary clinically derived human immunodeficiency virus type 1 *Nef* gene-induced expression. J Immunol 1996; 156:360–70.
62. Mikovits JA, Young HA, Vertino P, Issa JP, Pitha PM, Turcoski-Corrales S, et al. Infection with human immunodeficiency virus type 1 upregulates DNA methyltransferase, resulting in de novo methylation of the gamma interferon (IFN-gamma) promoter and subsequent downregulation of IFN-gamma production. Mol Cell Biol 1998; 18:5166–77.
63. Gazzinelli RT, Bala S, Stevens R, Baseler M, Wahl L, Kovacs J, Sher A. HIV infection suppresses type 1 lymphokine and IL-12 responses to Toxoplasma gondii but fails to inhibit the synthesis of other parasite-induced monokines. J Immunol 1995; 155:1565–74.
64. Maggi E, Mazzetti M, Ravina A, Annunziato F, de Carli M, Piccinni MP, et al. Ability of HIV to promote a TH1 to TH0 shift and to replicate preferentially in TH2 and TH0 cells. Science 1994; 265:244–8.

65. Graziosi C, Gantt KR, Vaccarezza M, Demarest JF, Daucher M, Saag MS, et al. Kinetics of cytokine expression during primary human immunodeficiency virus type 1 infection. Proc Natl Acad Sci USA 1996; 93:4386–91.
66. Fakoya A, Matear PM, Filley E, Rook GA, Stanford J, Gilson RJ, et al. HIV infection alters the production of both type 1 and 2 cytokines but does not induce a polarized type 1 or 2 state. AIDS 1997; 11:1445–52.
67. Jourdan P, Abbal C, Nora N, Hori T, Uchiyama T, Vendrell J-P, et al. Cutting Edge: IL-4 induces functional cell-surface expression of CXCR4 on human T cells. J Immunol 1998; 160:4153–7.
68. Galli G, Annunziato F, Mavilia C, Romagnani P, Cosmi L, Manetti R, et al. Enhanced HIV expression during Th2-oriented responses explained by the opposite regulatory effect of IL-4 and IFN-gamma of fusin/CXCR4. Eur J Immunol 1998; 28:3280–90.
69. Valentin A, Lu W, Rosati M, Schneider R, Albert J, Karlsson A, Pavlakis GN. Dual effect of interleukin 4 on HIV-1 expression: implications for viral phenotypic switch and disease progression. Proc Natl Acad Sci USA 1998; 95:8886–91.
70. Merrill JE, Koyanagi Y, Chen ISY. Interleukin-1 and tumor necrosis factor α can be induced from mononuclear phagocytes by human immunodeficiency virus type 1 binding to the CD4 receptor. J Virol 1989; 63:4404–8.
71. Clouse KA, Robbins PB, Fernie B, Ostrove JM, Fauci AS. Viral antigen stimulation of the production of human monokines capable of regulating HIV-1 expression. J Immunol 1989; 143:470–5.
72. Popik W, Pitha PM. Binding of human immunodeficiency virus type 1 to CD4 induces association of Lck and Raf-1 and activates Raf-1 by a Ras-independent pathway. Mol Cell Biol 1996; 16:6532–41.
73. Popik W, Pitha P.M. Early activation of mitogen-activated protein kinase kinase, extracellular signal-regulated kinase, p38 mitogen-activated protein kinase, and c-Jun N-terminal kinase in response to binding of simian immunodeficiency virus to Jurkat T cells expressing CCR5 receptor. Virology 1998; 252:210–7.
74. Popik W, Hesselgesser JE, Pitha PM. Binding of human immunodeficiency virus type 1 to CD4 and CXCR4 receptors differentially regulates expression of inflammatory genes and activates the MEK/ERK signaling pathway. J Virol 1998; 72:6406–13.
75. Popik W, Pitha PM. Inhibition of CD3/CD28-mediated activation of the MEK/ERK signaling pathway represses replication of X4 but not R5 human immunodeficiency virus type 1 in peripheral blood CD4(+) T lymphocytes. J Virol 2000; 74:2558–66.
76. Clouse KA, Cosentino LM, Weih KA, Pyle SW, Robbins PB, Hochstein HD, et al. The HIV-1 gp120 envelope protein has the intrinsic capacity to stimulate monokine secretion. J Immunol 1991; 147:2892–901.
77. Pericle F, Pinto LA, Hicks S, Kirken RA, Sconocchia G, Rusnak J, et al. HIV-1 infection induces a selective reduction in STAT5 protein expression. J Immunol 1998; 160:28–31.
78. Bovolenta C, Camorali L, Lorini AL, Ghezzi S, Vicenzi E, Lazzarin A, Poli G. Constitutive activation of STATs upon in vivo human immunodeficiency virus infection. Blood 1999; 94:4202–9.
79. Leonard WJ, O'Shea JJ. Jaks and STATs: biological implications. Annu Rev Immunol 1998; 16:293–322.
80. Collette Y, Dutartre H, Benziane A, Ramos M, Benarous R, Harris M, Olive D. Physical and functional interaction of Nef with Lck. HIV-1 Nef-induced T-cell signaling defects. J Biol Chem 1996; 271:6333–41.
81. De SK, Venkateshan CN, Seth P, Gajdusek DC, Gibbs CJ. Adenovirus-mediated human immunodeficiency virus-1 Nef expression in human monocytes/macrophages and effect of Nef on downmodulation of Fcgamma receptors and expression of monokines. Blood 1998; 91:2108–17.
82. Scala G, Ruocco MR, Ambrosino C, Mallardo M, Giordano V, Baldassarre F, et al. The expression of the interleukin 6 gene is induced by the human immunodeficiency virus 1 TAT protein. J Exp Med 1994; 179:961–71.

83. Buonaguro L, Buonaguro FM, Giraldo G, Ensoli B. The human immunodeficiency virus type 1 Tat protein transactivates tumor necrosis factor beta gene expression through a TAR-like structure. J Virol 1994; 68:2677–82.
84. Zauli G, Davis BR, Re MC, Visani G, Furlini G, La Placa M. tat protein stimulates production of transforming growth factor-beta 1 by marrow macrophages: a potential mechanism for human immunodeficiency virus-1-induced hematopoietic suppression. Blood 1992; 80:3036–43.
85. Conant K, Garzino-Demo A, Nath A, McArthur JC, Halliday W, Power C, et al. Induction of monocyte chemoattractant protein-1 in HIV-1 Tat-stimulated astrocytes and elevation in AIDS dementia. Proc Natl Acad Sci USA 1998; 95:3117–21.
86. Mengozzi M, De Filippi C, Transidico P, Biswas P, Cota M, Ghezzi S, et al. Human immunodeficiency virus replication induces monocyte chemotactic protein-1 in human macrophages and U937 promonocytic cells. Blood 1999; 93:1851–7.
87. Ghezzi S, Noonan DM, Aluigi MG, Vallanti G, Cota M, Benelli R, et al. Inhibition of CXCR4-dependent HIV-1 infection by extracellular HIV-1 Tat. Biochem Biophys Res Commun 2000; 270:992–6.
88. Xiao H, Neuveut C, Tiffany HL, Benkirane M, Rich EA, Murphy PM, Jeang KT. Selective CXCR4 antagonism by Tat: implications for in vivo expansion of coreceptor use by HIV-1. Proc Natl Acad Sci USA 2000; 97:11466-71.
89. Welker R, Harris M, Cardel B, Krausslich HG. Virion incorporation of human immunodeficiency virus type 1 nef is mediated by a bipartite membrane-targeting signal: analysis of its role in enhancement of viral infectivity. J Virol 1998; 72:8833–40.
90. Wong GH, Krowka JF, Stites DP, Goeddel DV. In vitro anti-human immunodeficiency virus activities of tumor necrosis factor-alpha and interferon-gamma. J Immunol 1988; 140:120–4.
91. Wong GH, Goeddel DV. Tumour necrosis factors alpha and beta inhibit virus replication and synergize with interferons. Nature 1986; 323:819–22.
92. Folks TM, Clouse KA, Justement J, Rabson A, Duh E, Kehrl JH, Fauci AS. Tumor necrosis factor alpha induces expression of human immunodeficiency virus in a chronically infected T-cell clone. Proc Natl Acad Sci USA 1989; 86:2365–8.
93. Duh EJ, Maury WJ, Folks TM, Fauci AS, Rabson AB. Tumor necrosis factor alpha activates human immunodeficiency virus type 1 through induction of nuclear factor binding to the NF-kappa B sites in the long terminal repeat. Proc Natl Acad Sci USA 1989; 86:5974–8.
94. Griffin GE, Leung K, Folks TM, Kunkel S, Nabel GJ. Activation of HIV gene expression during monocyte differentiation by induction of NF-kappa B. Nature 1989; 339:70–3.
95. Osborn L, Kunkel S, Nabel GJ. Tumor necrosis factor alpha and interleukin 1 stimulate the human immunodeficiency virus enhancer by activation of the nuclear factor kappa B. Proc Natl Acad Sci USA 1989; 86:2336–40.
96. Siebenlist U, Franzoso G, Brown K. Structure, regulation and function of NF-κB. Annu Rev Cell Biol 1994; 10:405–55.
97. Antoni BA, Rabson AB, Kinter A, Bodkin M, Poli G. NF-kappa B-dependent and -independent pathways of HIV activation in a chronically infected T cell line. Virology 1994; 202:684–94.
98. Poli G, Kinter AL, Fauci AS. Interleukin 1 induces expression of the human immunodeficiency virus alone and in synergy with interleukin 6 in chronically infected U1 cells: inhibition of inductive effects by the interleukin 1 receptor antagonist. Proc Natl Acad Sci USA 1994; 91:108–12.
99. Vicenzi E, Biswas P, Mengozzi M, Poli G. Role of pro-inflammatory cytokines and beta-chemokines in controlling HIV replication. J Leukoc Biol 1997; 62:34–40.
100. Yang X, Chen Y, Gabuzda D. ERK MAP kinase links cytokine signals to activation of latent HIV-1 infection by stimulating a cooperative interaction of AP-1 and NF- kappaB. J Biol Chem 1999; 274:27981–8.

101. Shapiro L, Puren AJ, Barton HA, Novick D, Peskind RL, Shenkar R, et al. Interleukin 18 stimulates HIV type 1 in monocytic cells. Proc Natl Acad Sci USA 1998; 95:12550–5.
102. Poli G, Bressler P, Kinter A, Duh E, Timmer WC, Rabson A, et al. Interleukin 6 induces human immunodeficiency virus expression in infected monocytic cells alone and in synergy with tumor necrosis factor alpha by transcriptional and posttranscriptional mechanisms. J Exp Med 1990; 172:151–8.
103. Biswas P, Poli G, Kinter AL, Justement JS, Stanley SK, Maury WJ, et al. Interferon gamma induces the expression of human immunodeficiency virus in persistently infected promonocytic cells (U1) and redirects the production of virions to intracytoplasmic vacuoles in phorbol myristate acetate-differentiated U1 cells. J Exp Med 1992; 176:739–50.
104. Poli G, Kinter A, Justement JS, Kehrl JH, Bressler P, Stanley S, Fauci AS. Tumor necrosis factor alpha functions in an autocrine manner in the induction of human immunodeficiency virus expression. Proc Natl Acad Sci USA 1990; 87:782–5.
105. Vyakarnam A, McKeating J, Meager A, Beverley PC. Tumour necrosis factors (α, β) induced by HIV-1 in peripheral blood mononuclear cells potentiate virus replication. AIDS 1990; 4:21–7.
106. Weissman D, Poli G, Fauci AS. Interleukin 10 blocks HIV replication in macrophages by inhibiting the autocrine loop of tumor necrosis factor alpha and interleukin 6 induction of virus. AIDS Res Hum Retrovir 1994; 10:1199–206.
107. Kinter AL, Poli G, Fox L, Hardy E, Fauci AS. HIV replication in IL-2-stimulated peripheral blood mononuclear cells is driven in an autocrine/paracrine manner by endogenous cytokines. J Immunol 1995; 154:2448–59.
108. Ruocco MR, Chen X, Ambrosino C, Dragonetti E, Liu W, Mallardo M, et al. Regulation of HIV-1 long terminal repeats by interaction of C/EBP(NF-IL6) and NF-kappaB/Rel transcription factors. J Biol Chem 1996; 271:22479–86.
109. Hottiger MO, Nabel GJ. Interaction of human immunodeficiency virus type 1 Tat with the transcriptional coactivators p300 and CREB binding protein. J Virol 1998; 72:8252–6.
110. Hottiger MO, Felzien LK, Nabel GJ. Modulation of cytokine-induced HIV gene expression by competitive binding of transcription factors to the coactivator p300. Embo J 1998; 17:3124–34.
111. Poli G, Kinter AL, Justement JS, Bressler P, Kehrl JH, Fauci AS. Retinoic acid mimics transforming growth factor beta in the regulation of human immunodeficiency virus expression in monocytic cells. Proc Natl Acad Sci USA 1992; 89:2689–93.
112. Weissman D, Poli G, Fauci AS. IL-10 synergizes with multiple cytokines in enhancing HIV production in cells of monocytic lineage. J Acquir Immune Defic Syndr Hum Retrovirol 1995; 9:442–9.
113. Barcellini W, Rizzardi GP, Marriott JB, Fain C, Shattock RJ, Meroni PL, et al. Interleukin-10-induced HIV-1 expression is mediated by induction of both membrane-bound tumour necrosis factor (TNF)-alpha and TNF receptor type 1 in a promonocytic cell line. AIDS 1996; 10:835–42.
114. Lazdins JK, Klimkait T, Woods-Cook K, Walker M, Alteri E, Cox D, et al. In vitro effect of transforming growth factor-β on progression of HIV-1 infection in primary mononuclear phagocytes. J Immunol 1991; 147:1201–7.
115. Peterson PK, Molitor TW, Chao CC. The opioid-cytokine connection. J Neuroimmunol 1998; 83:63–9.
116. Kazazi F, Mathijs JM, Chang J, Malafiej P, Lopez A, Dowton D, et al. Recombinant interleukin 4 stimulates human immunodeficiency virus production by infected monocytes and macrophages. J Gen Virol 1992; 73:941–9.
117. Schuitemaker H, Kootstra NA, Koppelman MH, Bruisten SM, Huisman HG, Tersmette M, Miedema F. Proliferation-dependent HIV-1 infection of monocytes occurs during differentiation into macrophages. J Clin Invest 1992; 89:1154–60.

118. Mikovits JA, Meyers AM, Ortaldo JR, Minty A, Caput D, Ferrara P, Ruscetti FW. IL-4 and IL-13 have overlapping but distinct effects on HIV production in monocytes. J Leukoc Biol 1994; 56:340–6.
119. Foli A, Saville MW, Baseler MW, Yarchoan R. Effects of the Th1 and Th2 stimulatory cytokines interleukin-12 and interleukin-4 on human immunodeficiency virus replication. Blood 1995; 85:2114–23.
120. Koyanagi Y, O'Brien WA, Zhao JQ, Golde DW, Gasson JC, Chen IS. Cytokines alter production of HIV-1 from primary mononuclear phagocytes. Science 1988; 241:1673–5.
121. Montaner LJ, Doyle AG, Collin M, Georges H, James W, Minty A et al. Interleukin 13 inhibits human immunodeficiency virus type 1 production in primary blood-derived human macrophages in vitro. J Exp Med 1993; 178:743–7.
122. Herbein G, Montaner LJ, Gordon S. Tumor necrosis factor alpha inhibits entry of human immunodeficiency virus type 1 into primary human macrophages: a selective role for the 75-kilodalton receptor. J Virol 1996; 70:7388–97.
123. Brown CC, Poli G, Lubaki N, St. Louis M, Davachi F, Musey L, et al. Elevated levels of tumor necrosis factor-alpha in Zairian neonate plasmas: implications for perinatal infection with the human immunodeficiency virus. J Infect Dis 1994; 169:975–80.
124. Goletti D, Weissman D, Jackson RW, Graham NM, Vlahov D, Klein RS, et al. Effect of Mycobacterium tuberculosis on HIV replication. Role of immune activation. J Immunol 1996; 157:1271–8.
125. Wahl SM, Greenwell-Wild T, Peng G, Hale-Donze H, Doherty TM, Mizel D, Orenstein JM. Mycobacterium avium complex augments macrophage HIV-1 production and increases CCR5 expression. Proc Natl Acad Sci USA 1998; 95:12574–9.
126. Shapira-Nahor O, Kalinkovich A, Weisman Z, Greenberg Z, Nahmias J, Shapiro M, et al. Increased susceptibility to HIV-1 infection of peripheral blood mononuclear cells from chronically immune-activated individuals. AIDS 1998; 12:1731–3.
127. Ryu SE, Kwong PD, Truneh A, Porter TG, Arthos J, Rosenberg M, et al. Crystal structure of an HIV-binding recombinant fragment of human CD4. Nature 1990; 348:419–26.
128. Lores P, Boucher V, Mackay C, Pla M, Von Boehmer H, Jami J, et al. Expression of human CD4 in transgenic mice does not confer sensitivity to human immunodeficiency virus infection. AIDS Res Hum Retrovir 1992; 8:2063–71.
129. Feng Y, Broder CC, Kennedy PE, Berger EA. HIV-1 entry cofactor: cloning of a seven-transmembrane G protein-coupled receptor. Science 1996; 272:872–7.
130. Walker CM, Moody DJ, Stites DP, Levy JA. $CD8^+$ lymphocytes can control HIV infection in vitro by suppressing virus replication. Science 1986; 234:1563–6.
131. Cocchi F, DeVico AL, Garzino-Demo A, Arya SK, Gallo RC, Lusso P. Identification of RANTES, MIP-1 alpha, and MIP-1 beta as the major HIV-suppressive factors produced by $CD8^+$ T cells. Science 1995; 270:1811–5.
132. Center DM, Kornfeld H, Cruikshank WW. Interleukin 16 and its function as a CD4 ligand. Immunol Today 1996; 17:476–81.
133. Mathy NL, Bannert N, Norley SG, Kurth R. Cutting edge: CD4 is not required for the functional activity of IL-16. J Immunol 2000; 164:4429–32.
134. Baier M, Werner A, Bannert N, Metzner K, Kurth R. HIV suppression by interleukin-16. Nature 1995; 378:563.
135. Zhou P, Goldstein S, Devadas K, Tewari D, Notkins AL. Human $CD4^+$ cells transfected with IL-16 cDNA are resistant to HIV-1 infection: inhibition of mRNA expression. Nat Med 1997; 3:659–64.
136. Maciaszek JW, Parada NA, Cruikshank WW, Center DM, Kornfeld H, Viglianti GA. IL-16 represses HIV-1 promoter activity. J Immunol 1997; 158:5–8.
137. Amiel C, Darcissac E, Truong MJ, Dewulf J, Loyens M, Mouton Y, et al. Interleukin-16 (IL-16) inhibits human immunodeficiency virus replication in cells from infected subjects, and serum IL-16 levels drop with disease progression. J Infect Dis 1999; 179:83–91.

138. Alkhatib G, Combadiere C, Broder CC, Feng Y, Kennedy PE, Murphy PM, Berger EA. CC CKR5: a RANTES, MIP-1α, MIP-1β receptor as a fusion cofactor for macrophage-tropic HIV-1. Science 1996; 272:1955–8.
139. Choe H, Farzan M, Sun Y, Sullivan N, Rollins B, Ponath PD, et al. The beta-chemokine receptors CCR3 and CCR5 facilitate infection by primary HIV-1 isolates. Cell 1996; 85:1135–48.
140. Oberlin E, Amara A, Bachelerie F, Bessia C, Virelizier JL, Arenzana-Seisdedos F, et al. The CXC chemokine SDF-1 is the ligand for LESTR/fusin and prevents infection by T-cell-line-adapted HIV-1. Nature 1996; 382:833–5.
141. Nagasawa T, Nakajima T, Tachibana K, Iizasa H, Bleul CC, Yoshie O, et al. Molecular cloning and characterization of a murine pre-B-cell growth-stimulating factor/stromal cell-derived factor 1 receptor, a murine homolog of the human immunodeficiency virus 1 entry coreceptor fusin. Proc Natl Acad Sci USA 1996; 93:14726–9.
142. Premack BA, Schall TJ. Chemokine receptors: gateways to inflammation and infection. Nat Med 1996; 2:1174–8.
143. Littman DR. Chemokine receptors—keys to AIDS pathogenesis. Cell 1998; 93:677–80.
144. Murakami T, Nakajima T, Koyanagi Y, Tachibana K, Fujii N, Tamamura H, et al. A small molecule CXCR4 inhibitor that blocks T cell line-tropic HIV-1 infection. J Exp Med 1997; 186:1389–93.
145. Mack M, Luckow B, Nelson PJ, Cihak J, Simmons G, Clapham PR, et al. Aminooxypentane-RANTES induces CCR5 internalization but inhibits recycling: a novel inhibitory mechanism of HIV infectivity. J Exp Med 1998; 187:1215–24.
146. Sozzani S, Ghezzi S, Iannolo G, Luini W, Borsatti A, Polentarutti N, et al. Interleukin 10 increases CCR5 expression and HIV infection in human monocytes. J Exp Med 1998; 187:439–44.
147. Donzella GA, Schols D, Lin SW, Este JA, Nagashima KA, Maddon PJ, et al. AMD3100, a small molecule inhibitor of HIV-1 entry via the CXCR4 co-receptor. Nat Med 1998; 4:72–7.
148. Hwang SS, Boyle TJ, Lyerly HK, Cullen BR. Identification of the envelope V3 loop as the primary determinant of cell tropism in HIV-1. Science 1991; 253:71–3.
149. Cocchi F, DeVico AL, Garzino-Demo A, Cara A, Gallo RC, Lusso P. The V3 domain of the HIV-1 gp120 envelope glycoprotein is critical for chemokine-mediated blockade of infection. Nat Med 1996; 2:1244–7.
150. Scarlatti G, Tresoldi E, Bjorndal A, Fredriksson R, Colognesi C, Deng HK, et al. In vivo evolution of HIV-1 co-receptor usage and sensitivity to chemokine-mediated suppression. Nat Med 1997; 3:1259–65.
151. Menzo S, Sampaolesi R, Vicenzi E, Santagostino E, Liuzzi G, Chirianni A, et al. Rare mutations in a domain crucial for V3-loop structure prevail in replicating HIV from long-term non-progressors. AIDS 1998; 12:985–97.
152. Michael NL, Moore JP. HIV-1 entry inhibitors: evading the issue. Nat Med 1999; 5:740–2.
153. Michael NL, Moore JP. Viral phenotype and CCR5 genotype. Nat Med 1999; 5:1330.
154. Zhang YJ, Moore JP. Will multiple coreceptors need to be targeted by inhibitors of human immunodeficiency virus type 1 entry? J Virol 1999; 73:3443–8.
155. He J, Chen Y, Farzan M, Choe H, Ohagen A, Gartner S, et al. CCR3 and CCR5 are co-receptors for HIV-1 infection of microglia. Nature 1997; 385:645–9.
156. Rowland-Jones SL, McMichael A. Immune responses in HIV-exposed seronegatives: have they repelled the virus? Curr Opin Immunol 1995; 7:448–55.
157. Paxton WA, Dragic T, Koup RA, Moore JP. The beta-chemokines, HIV type 1 second receptors, and exposed uninfected persons. AIDS Res Hum Retrovir 1996; 12:1203–7.
158. Dean M, Carrington M, Winkler C, Huttley GA, Smith MW, Allikmets R, et al. Genetic restriction of HIV-1 infection and progression to AIDS by a deletion allele of the CKR5 structural gene. Hemophilia Growth and Development Study, Multicenter AIDS Cohort Study, Multicenter Hemophilia Cohort Study, San Francisco City Cohort, ALIVE Study. Science 1996; 273:1856–62.

159. Berger EA, Doms RW, Fenyo EM, Korber BT, Littman DR, Moore JP, et al. A new classification for HIV-1. Nature 1998; 391:240.
160. Biti R, Ffrench R, Young J, Bennetts B, Stewart G, Liang T. HIV-1 infection in an individual homozygous for the CCR5 deletion allele. Nat Med 1997; 3:252–3.
161. Michael NL, Nelson JA, KewalRamani VN, Chang G, O'Brien SJ, Mascola JR, et al. Exclusive and persistent use of the entry coreceptor CXCR4 by human immunodeficiency virus type 1 from a subject homozygous for CCR5 delta32. J Virol 1998; 72:6040–7.
162. Zhu T, Wang N, Carr A, Nam DS, Moor-Jankowski R, Cooper DA, Ho DD. Genetic characterization of human immunodeficiency virus type 1 in blood and genital secretions: evidence for viral compartmentalization and selection during sexual transmission. J Virol 1996; 70:3098–107.
163. Zaitseva M, Blauvelt A, Lee S, Lapham CK, Klaus-Kovtun V, Mostowski H, et al. Expression and function of CCR5 and CXCR4 on human Langerhans cells and macrophages: implications for HIV primary infection. Nat Med 1997; 3:1369–75.
164. Patterson BK, Landay A, Andersson J, Brown C, Behbahani H, Jiyamapa D, et al. Repertoire of chemokine receptor expression in the female genital tract: implications for human immunodeficiency virus transmission. Am J Pathol 1998; 153:481–90.
165. Zhang Z, Schuler T, Zupancic M, Wietgrefe S, Staskus KA, Reimann KA, et al. Sexual transmission and propagation of SIV and HIV in resting and activated $CD4^+$ T cells. Science 1999; 286:1353–7.
166. Vicenzi E, Bordignon PP, Biswas P, Brambilla A, Bovolenta C, Cota M, et al. Envelope-dependent restriction of human immunodeficiency virus type 1 spreading in CD4(+) T lymphocytes: R5 but not X4 viruses replicate in the absence of T-cell receptor restimulation. J Virol 1999; 73:7515–23.
167. Rucker J, Samson M, Doranz BJ, Libert F, Berson JF, Yi Y, et al. Regions in beta-chemokine receptors CCR5 and CCR2b that determine HIV-1 cofactor specificity. Cell 1996; 87:437–46.
168. Alfano M, Schmidtmayerova H, Amella CA, Pushkarsky T, Bukrinsky M. The B-oligomer of pertussis toxin deactivates CC chemokine receptor 5 and blocks entry of M-tropic HIV-1 strains. J Exp Med 1999; 190:597–606.
169. Wang JM, Oppenheim JJ. Interference with the signaling capacity of CC chemokine receptor 5 can compromise its role as an HIV-1 entry coreceptor in primary T lymphocytes. J Exp Med 1999; 190:591–5.
170. Alfano M, Pushkarsky T, Poli G, Bukrinsky M. The B-oligomer of pertussis toxin inhibits HIV-1 replication at multiple stages. J Virol 2000; 74:8767–70.
170a. Alfano M, Vallanti G, Biswas P, Bovolenta C, Vicenzi E, Rappuoli R, et al. The B-oligomeric subunit of pertussis toxin inhibits HIV replication in human macrophages and virus expression in chronically infected promonocytic U1 cells. J Immunol 2001; 166:1863–70.
171. Pal R, Garzino-Demo A, Markham PD, Burns J, Brown M, Gallo RC, DeVico AL. Inhibition of HIV-1 infection by the beta-chemokine MDC. Science 1997; 278:695–8.
172. Arenzana-Seisdedos F, Amara A, Thomas D, Virelizier JL. β-Chemokine MDC and HIV-1 infection. Science 1998; 281:487–87a.
173. Lee B, Rucker J, Doms RW, Tsang M, Hu X, Dietz M, et al. β-Chemokine MDC and HIV-1 infection. Science 1998; 281:487–87a.
174. Cota M, Mengozzi M, Vicenzi E, Panina-Bordignon P, Sinigaglia F, Transidico P, et al. Selective inhibition of HIV replication in primary macrophages but not T lymphocytes by macrophage-derived chemokine. Proc Natl Acad Sci USA 2000; 97:9162–7.
175. Struyf S, De Meester I, Scharpe S, Lenaerts JP, Menten P, Wang JM, et al. Natural truncation of RANTES abolishes signaling through the CC chemokine receptors CCR1 and CCR3, impairs its chemotactic potency and generates a CC chemokine inhibitor. Eur J Immunol 1998; 28:1262–71.
176. Struyf S, Proost P, Sozzani S, Mantovani A, Wuyts A, De Clercq E, et al. Enhanced anti-HIV-1 activity and altered chemotactic potency of NH2-terminally processed macrophage-derived chemokine (MDC) imply an additional MDC receptor. J Immunol 1998; 161:2672–5.

177. Schmidtmayerova H, Sherry B, Bukrinsky M. Chemokines and HIV replication. Nature 1996; 382:767.
178. Kelly MD, Naif HM, Adams SL, Cunningham AL, Lloyd AR. Dichotomous effects of beta-chemokines on HIV replication in monocytes and monocyte-derived macrophages. J Immunol 1998; 160:3091–5.
179. Kinter A, Catanzaro A, Monaco J, Ruiz M, Justement J, Moir S, et al. CC-chemokines enhance the replication of T-tropic strains of HIV-1 in CD4(+) T cells: role of signal transduction. Proc Natl Acad Sci USA 1998; 95:11880–5.
180. Dolei A, Biolchini A, Serra C, Curreli S, Gomes E, Dianzani F. Increased replication of T-cell-tropic HIV strains and CXC-chemokine receptor-4 induction in T cells treated with macrophage inflammatory protein (MIP)-1alpha, MIP-1beta and RANTES beta-chemokines. AIDS 1998; 12:183–90.
181. Koot M, Keet IP, Vos AH, de Goede RE, Roos MT, Coutinho RA, et al. Prognostic value of HIV-1 syncytium-inducing phenotype for rate of $CD4^+$ cell depletion and progression to AIDS. Ann Intern Med 1993; 118:681–8.
182. Kutza J, Hayes MP, Clouse KA, Interleukin-2 inhibits HIV-1 replication in human macrophages by modulating expression of CD4 and CC-chemokine receptor-5. AIDS 1998; 12:F59–64.
183. Wang J, Harada A, Matsushita S, Matsumi S, Zhang Y, Shioda T, Nagai Y, Matsushima K. IL-4 and a glucocorticoid up-regulate CXCR4 expression on human $CD4^+$ T lymphocytes and enhance HIV-1 replication. J Leukoc Biol 1998; 64:642–9.
184. Zella D, Barabitskaja O, Burns JM, Romerio F, Dunn DE, Revello MG, et al. Interferon-gamma increases expression of chemokine receptors CCR1, CCR3, and CCR5, but not CXCR4 in monocytoid U937 cells. Blood 1998; 91:4444–50.
185. Biswas P, Mengozzi M, Mantelli B, Delfanti F, Brambilla A, Vicenzi E, Poli G. 1,25-Dihydroxyvitamin D3 upregulates functional CXCR4 human immunodeficiency virus type 1 coreceptors in U937 minus clones: NF- kappaB-independent enhancement of viral replication. J Virol 1998; 72:8380–3.
186. Sallusto F, Mackay CR, Lanzavecchia A. Selective expression of the eotaxin receptor CCR3 by human T helper 2 cells. Science 1997; 277:2005–7.
187. Sallusto F, Lenig D, Mackay CR, Lanzavecchia A. Flexible programs of chemokine receptor expression on human polarized T helper 1 and 2 lymphocytes. J Exp Med 1998; 187:875–83.
188. Bonecchi R, Bianchi G, Bordignon PP, D'Ambrosio D, Lang R, Borsatti A, et al. Differential expression of chemokine receptors and chemotactic responsiveness of type 1 T helper cells (Th1s) and Th2s. J Exp Med 1998; 187:129–34.
189. Mikovits JA, Taub DD, Turcovski-Corrales SM, Ruscetti FW. Similar levels of human immunodeficiency virus type 1 replication in human TH1 and TH2 clones. J Virol 1998; 72:5231–8.
190. Taub DD, Ortaldo JR, Turcovski-Corrales SM, Key ML, Longo DL, Murphy WJ. Beta chemokines costimulate lymphocyte cytolysis, proliferation, and lymphokine production. J Leukoc Biol 1996; 59:81–9.
191. Wagner L, Yang OO, Garcia-Zepeda EA, Ge Y, Kalams SA, Walker BD, et al. Beta-chemokines are released from HIV-1-specific cytolytic T-cell granules complexed to proteoglycans. Nature 1998; 391:908–11.
192. Kim JJ, Nottingham LK, Sin JI, Tsai A, Morrison L, Oh J, et al. CD8 positive T cells influence antigen-specific immune responses through the expression of chemokines. J Clin Invest 1998; 102:1112–24.
193. Hadida F, Vieillard V, Autran B, Clark-Lewis I, Baggiolini M, Debre P. HIV-specific T cell cytotoxicity mediated by RANTES via the chemokine receptor CCR3. J Exp Med 1998; 188:609–14.
194. Pantaleo G. How immune-based interventions can change HIV therapy. Nat Med 1997; 3:483–6.
195. Lori F, Malykh A, Cara A, Sun D, Weinstein JN, Lisziewicz J, Gallo RC. Hydroxyurea as an inhibitor of human immunodeficiency virus-type 1 replication. Science 1994; 266:801–5.

196. Lori F, Malykh AG, Foli A, Maserati R, De Antoni A, Minoli L, et al. Combination of a drug targeting the cell with a drug targeting the virus controls human immunodeficiency virus type 1 resistance. AIDS Res Hum Retrovir 1997; 13:1403–9.
197. Chapuis AG, Paolo Rizzardi G, D'Agostino C, Attinger A, Knabenhans C, Fleury S, et al. Effects of mycophenolic acid on human immunodeficiency virus infection in vitro and in vivo. Nat Med 2000; 6:762–8.
198. Miles S. The use of hematopoietic growth factors in treating HIV infection. Curr Opin Hematol 1995; 2:227–33.
199. Deresinski SC. Granulocyte-macrophage colony-stimulating factor: potential therapeutic, immunological and antiretroviral effects in HIV infection. AIDS 1999; 13:633–43.
200. Coffey MJ, Phare SM, Cinti S, Peters-Golden M, Kazanjian PH. Granulocyte-macrophage colony-stimulating factor upregulates reduced 5-lipoxygenase metabolism in peripheral blood monocytes and neutrophils in acquired immunodeficiency syndrome. Blood 1999; 94:3897–905.
201. Skowron G, Stein D, Drusano G, Melbourne K, Bilello J, Mikolich D, et al. The safety and efficacy of granulocyte-macrophage colony-stimulating factor (Sargramostim) added to indinavir- or ritonavir-based antiretroviral therapy: a randomized double-blind, placebo-controlled trial. J Infect Dis 1999; 180:1064–71.
202. Trinchieri G, Scott P. The role of interleukin 12 in the immune response, disease and therapy. Immunol Today 1994; 15:460–3.
203. Romani L, Puccetti P, Bistoni F. Interleukin-12 in infectious diseases. Clin Microbiol Rev 1997; 10:611–36.
204. Moss RB, Giermakowska WK, Savary JR, Theofan G, Daigle AE, Richieri SP, et al. A primer on HIV type 1-specific immune function and REMUNE. AIDS Res Hum Retrovir 1998; 14:Suppl 2, S167–75.
205. Cafaro A, Caputo A, Fracasso C, Maggiorella MT, Goletti D, Baroncelli S, et al. Control of SHIV-89.6P-infection of cynomolgus monkeys by HIV-1 Tat protein vaccine. Nat Med 1990; 5:643–50.
206. Bernstein ZP, Porter MM, Gould M, Lipman B, Bluman EM, Stewart CC, et al. Prolonged administration of low-dose interleukin-2 in human immunodeficiency virus-associated malignancy results in selective expansion of innate immune effectors without significant clinical toxicity. Blood 1995; 86:3287–94.
207. Jacobson EL, Pilaro F, Smith KA. Rational interleukin 2 therapy for HIV positive individuals: daily low doses enhance immune function without toxicity. Proc Natl Acad Sci USA 1996; 93:10405–10.
208. Teppler H, Kaplan G, Smith KA, Montana AL, Meyn P, Cohn ZA. Prolonged immunostimulatory effect of low-dose polyethylene glycol interleukin 2 in patients with human immunodeficiency virus type 1 infection. J Exp Med 1993; 177:483–92.
209. Khatri VP, Fehniger TA, Baiocchi RA, Yu F, Shah MH, Schiller DS, et al. Ultra low dose interleukin-2 therapy promotes a type 1 cytokine profile in vivo in patients with AIDS and AIDS-associated malignancies. J Clin Invest 1998; 101:1373–8.
210. Kovacs JA, Baseler M, Dewar RJ, Vogel S, Davey RT Jr, Falloon J, et al. Increases in CD4 T lymphocytes with intermittent courses of interleukin- 2 in patients with human immunodeficiency virus infection. A preliminary study. N Engl J Med 1995; 332:567–75.
211. Kovacs JA, Vogel S, Albert JM, Falloon J, Davey RT Jr, Walker RE, et al. Controlled trial of interleukin-2 infusions in patients infected with the human immunodeficiency virus. N Engl J Med 1996; 335:1350–6.
212. Connors M, Kovacs JA, Krevat S, Gea-Banacloche JC, Sneller MC, Flanigan M, et al. HIV infection induces changes in $CD4^+$ T-cell phenotype and depletions within the $CD4^+$ T-cell repertoire that are not immediately restored by antiviral or immune-based therapies. Nat Med 1997; 3:533–40.
213. Walker RE, Carter CS, Muul L, Natarajan V, Herpin BR, Leitman SF, et al. Peripheral expansion of pre-existing mature T cells is an important means of $CD4^+$ T-cell regeneration HIV-infected adults. Nat Med 1998; 4:852–6.

214. Levy Y, Capitant C, Houhou S, Carriere I, Viard JP, Goujard C, et al. Comparison of subcutaneous and intravenous interleukin-2 in asymptomatic HIV-1 infection: a randomised controlled trial. ANRS 048 study group, Lancet 1999; 353:1923–9.
215. Beverley PC, Michie CA, Young JL. Memory and the lifespan of human T lymphocytes. Leukemia 1993; 7:Suppl 2, S50–4.
216. Bell EB, Sparshott SM, Bunce C. CD4+ T-cell memory, CD45R subsets and the persistence of antigen—a unifying concept. Immunol Today 1998; 19:60–4.
217. De Paoli P, Zanussi S, Simonelli C, Bortolin MT, D'Andrea M, Crepaldi C, et al. Effects of subcutaneous interleukin-2 therapy on CD4 subsets and in vitro cytokine production in HIV+ subjects. J Clin Invest 1997; 100:2737–43.
218. Tambussi G, Ghezzi S, Guffanti M, Vallanti G, Nozza S, Magenta L, et al. Low-dose intermittent subcutaneous interleukin-2 in antiviral-experienced HIV-infected individuals. A controlled study, J Inf Dis, 2001, in press.
219. Bovolenta C, Camorali L, Lorini AL, Vallanti G, Ghezzi S, Tambussi G, et al. In vivo administration of recombinant IL-2 to individuals infected by HIV down-modulates the binding and expression of the transcription factors ying-yang-1 and leader binding protein-1/Late simian virus 40 factor. J Immunol 1999; 163:6892–7.
220. Brinkman K, Huysmans F, Galama JM, Boucher CA. In-vivo anti-CD3-induced HIV-1 viraemia. Lancet 1998; 352:1446.
221. Unutmaz D, Pileri P, Abrignani S. Antigen-independent activation of naive and memory resting T cells by a cytokine combination. J Exp Med 1994; 180:1159–64.
222. Chun TW, Engel D, Mizell SB, Ehler LA, Fauci AS. Induction of HIV-1 replication in latently infected CD4+ T cells using a combination of cytokines. J Exp Med 1998; 188:83–91.
223. Chun TW, Davey RT Jr, Ostrowski M, Shawn Justement J, Engel D, Mullins JI, Fauci AS. Relationship between pre-existing viral reservoirs and the re-emergence of plasma viremia after discontinuation of highly active antiretroviral therapy. Nat Med 2000; 6:757–61.
224. Ho DD, Zhang L. HIV-1 rebound after anti-retroviral therapy. Nat Med 2000; 6:736–7.
225. Davey RT Jr, Bhat N, Yoder C, Chun TW, Metcalf JA, Dewar R, et al. HIV-1 and T cell dynamics after interruption of highly active antiretroviral therapy (HAART) in patients with a history of sustained viral suppression. Proc Natl Acad Sci USA 1999; 96:15109–14.
226. Neumann AU, Tubiana R, Calvez V, Robert C, Li TS, Agut H, et al. HIV-1 rebound during interruption of highly active antiretroviral therapy has no deleterious effect on reinitiated treatment. Comet Study Group. AIDS 1999; 13:677–83.
227. Ruiz L, Martinez-Picadol J, Romeu J, Paredes R, Zayat MK, Marfil S, et al. Structured treatment interruption in chronically HIV-1 infected patients after long-term viral suppression. AIDS 2000; 14:397–403.
228. Friedrich MJ. HAART stopping news: experts examine structured therapy interruption for HIV. JAMA 2000; 283:2917–8.
229. Zou W, Foussat A, Houhou S, Durand-Gasselin I, Dulioust A, Bouchet L, et al. Acute upregulation of CCR-5 expression by CD4+ T lymphocytes in HIV-infected patients treated with interleukin-2. ANRS 048 IL-2 Study Group. AIDS 1999; 13:455–63.
230. Weissman D, Dybul M, Daucher MB, Davey RT Jr, Walker RE, Kovacs JA. Interleukin-2 upregulates expression of the human immunodeficiency virus fusion coreceptor CCR5 by CD4+ lymphocytes in vivo. J Infect Dis 2000; 181:933–8.
231. Loetscher P, Seitz M, Baggiolini M, Moser B. Interleukin-2 regulates CC chemokine receptor expression and chemotactic responsiveness in T lymphocytes. J Exp Med 1996; 184:569–77.
232. Patterson BK, Czerniewski M, Andersson J, Sullivan Y, Su F, Jiyamapa D, et al. Regulation of CCR5 and CXCR4 expression by type 1 and type 2 cytokines: CCR5 expression is downregulated by IL-10 in CD4-positive lymphocytes. Clin Immunol 1999; 91:254–62.

4

Development and Reconstitution of T-Lymphoid Immunity

Krishna V. Komanduri and Joseph M. McCune

INTRODUCTION

Remarkable progress has been made in our understanding of the mechanisms by which the immune system responds to challenge by invading pathogens. Driven by urgent clinical problems, including the pandemic caused by human immunodeficiency virus type 1 (HIV-1) *(1,2)*, these basic advances are starting to yield rewards in the treatment of human disease. Despite these gains, many fundamental questions remain unanswered, including many related to the factors that govern reconstitution of the immune system following its destruction in the setting of human disease.

In the United States and other developed countries, the advent of highly active antiretroviral therapy (HAART), consisting of combinations of antiretroviral agents shown to suppress viral replication, has led to a decline in acquired immune deficiency syndrome (AIDS)-related mortality and hospitalizations as well as to decreases in observed rates of secondary opportunistic infections *(3)*. A number of clinical studies have demonstrated quantitative and qualitative improvements in the functional T-cell receptor (TCR) repertoire *(4–8)*. Although defects in the repertoire may persist even after complete suppression of viral load *(9,10)*, it is clear that progress has been made, at least for those patients with access to HAART.

These clinical advances, although significant, have actually preceded our understanding of immune reconstitution, a process that appears to be more complete in some individuals with HIV-1 disease than in others. Understanding this differential response represents an immediate challenge to those investigating mechanisms of immune reconstitution in the laboratory, as well as to those administering antiretroviral therapy in the clinic. This understanding will also benefit the increasingly large group of patients who receive cytoreductive therapies for the treatment of malignant and autoimmune diseases, often with considerable morbidity and mortality due to prolonged immunosuppression.

Given the clinical importance of lymphoid depletion in the setting of AIDS and after cytoreductive chemotherapy, this chapter focuses on the principles governing development and reconstitution of the T-lymphoid repertoire, including discussions of normal lymphocyte ontogeny and of homeostatic mechanisms governing the function of the central and peripheral lymphoid repertoire.

From: *Retroviral Immunology: Immune Response and Restoration*
Edited by: Giuseppe Pantaleo and Bruce D. Walker © Humana Press Inc., Totowa, NJ

LYMPHOID ONTOGENY

Immunocompetence is normally dependent on developmental processes that generate a diverse functional repertoire of lymphocytes. In the setting of immunodeficiency, some or all of these processes are likely to be disrupted or impaired, contributing to the inability to maintain a healthy complement of cellular immune responses against bacterial, fungal, and viral pathogens. A critical organ for the generation of T cell receptor diversity is the thymus.

The Thymus

The "T cell" is so named because the vast majority of these lymphocytes are thought to be derived from the thymus. As uncontroversial as this simple statement now seems, it was not until the early 1960s that the thymus was demonstrated to be an important source of lymphocytes and, therefore, central to the development of effective immune responses. This observation initially arose as the unexpected result of an experiment designed to identify factors central to the development of malignancy in a murine model of virally induced leukemogenesis *(11)*. Neonatally thymectomized mice were found to succumb to diseases that were unrelated to the onset of leukemia. Subsequent experiments demonstrated that lymphocytes produced in the thymus were essential for protection against opportunistic infection and for the rejection of allogeneic skin grafts. In turn, it was hypothesized that, "during embryogenesis, the thymus would produce the originators of immunologically competent cells many of which would have migrated to other sites at about the time of birth" *(11,12)*. Although it was first assumed that a homogeneous population of small lymphocytes was capable of initiating cellular *and* humoral immune responses *(13)*, further work established that these responses were dependent on distinct cellular subsets, with the thymus-derived T-cell subset essential for the production of antibody by cells later termed B cells *(14)*. As discussed in the following sections, other experiments established the importance of positive and negative thymic selection in the production of a diverse functional T-cell repertoire capable of responding to foreign, but not self antigens.

The Hematopoietic Stem Cell

The fetal liver and bone marrow harbor rare hematopoietic stem cells (HSCs) capable of multilineage differentiation and also of long-term self renewal *(15)* (reviewed in *16*). In human embryogenesis, the human thymic rudiment is formed at a gestational age of approx 7 wk and is soon thereafter colonized by progenitor HSCs from the fetal liver *(17)*. Following colonization of the bone marrow by fetal liver HSCs at approx wk 16, seeding of the thymus by fetal liver HSCs continues, but is accompanied by migration of progenitors from the bone marrow as well *(18)*. Following birth, a population of HSCs that originate in the bone marrow and transit through the peripheral blood is thought to continually seed the thymus throughout its functional life span (reviewed in *19–21*).

The most immature HSC population in the human has been characterized by expression of the markers CD34 and Thy-1 and by lack of expression of the markers CD 2, 14, 15, 16, 19, and glycophorin A (Lin^-) (Fig. 1) *(22)*. A larger subpopulation of cells, delineated by expression of CD34 but unfractionated for other markers, is capable of developing into T and B lymphocytes, as well as into the granulocyte-macrophage, ery-

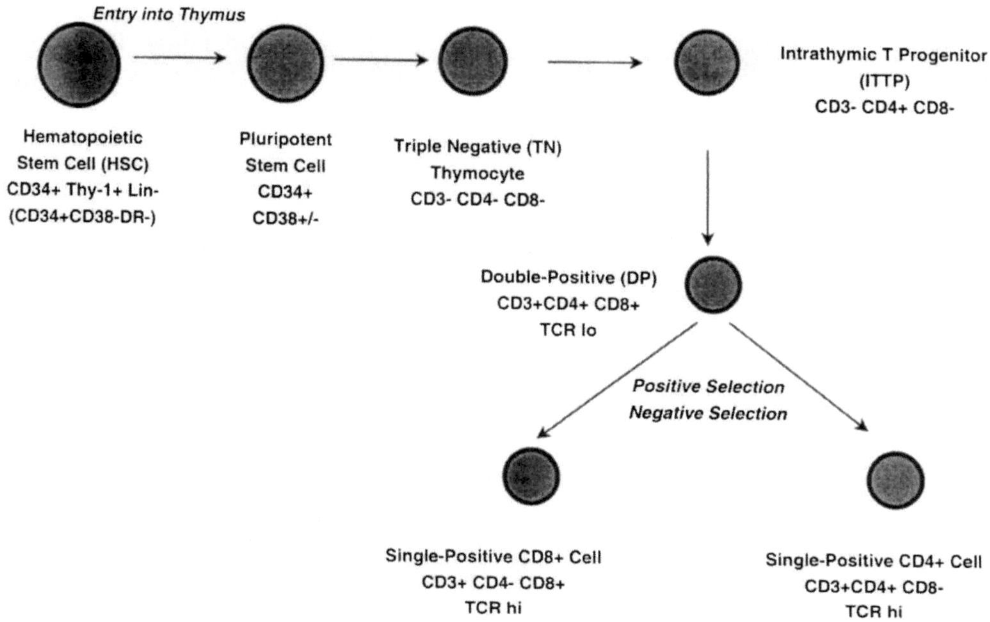

Fig. 1. Defined stages of human thymocyte maturation.

throid, and megakaryocytic lineages. Subsets of the $CD34^+$ population *(23)*, demarcated by site of origin and intensity of expression of the surface marker CD38 ($CD38^-$ or $CD38^+$), have been characterized by their potential to develop into the T-cell lineage *(20,24)*. These studies demonstrated that $CD34^+$ $CD38^-$ cells that originated in the liver had the potential to develop into T cells while the more mature liver-derived $CD34^+$ $CD38^+$ cells could not *(25)*. In contrast, both $CD34^+$ $CD38^-$ and $CD34^+$ $CD38^+$ cells derived from either fetal bone marrow or umbilical cord blood could differentiate into the T-cell lineage *(26)*. Despite the potential of cord blood progenitors to differentiate into the T-cell lineage, it is not clear if they are committed to this lineage prior to entry into the thymus. In some *(19,27)* but not other studies *(26)*, rearrangements of the T-cell receptor (TCR) β chain locus have been noted in prethymic $CD34^+$ cells. These results suggest that pluripotent progenitor cells (expressing CD34 but heterogeneous in their expression of CD38) originating in fetal liver, cord blood, and bone marrow are the immediate predecessors of the most immature thymocytes. Furthermore, it appears likely that these cells do not become fully committed to T-cell differentiation prior to their entry into the thymus.

Intrathymic T-Cell Maturation

The intrathymic maturation of hematopoietic progenitor cells into lymphoid effector cells has been extensively studied in the mouse *(28)* and in the chicken (*28a*), and also in models of human thymopoiesis, such as the SCID-hu Thy/Liv mouse *(29)*. As early as the 1970s, the movement of developing thymocytes from cortical to medullary regions of the thymus was noted to precede export of mature lymphocytes into the peripheral blood *(30,31)*. The identification of cell surface markers and the application

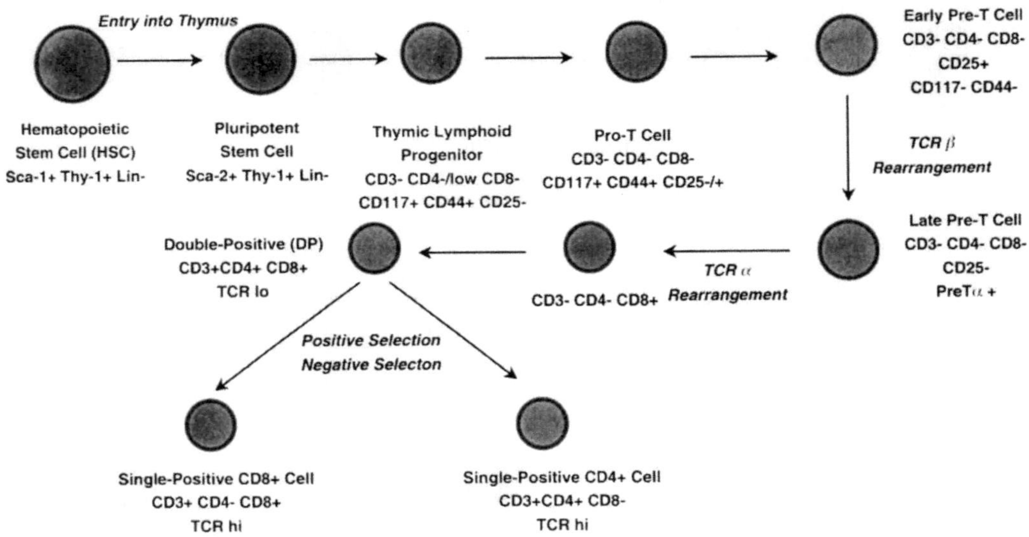

Fig. 2. Defined stages of mouse thymocyte maturation.

of flow cytometry to the study of thymopoiesis has allowed classification of relatively discrete stages of maturation.

Following homing of multilineage progenitor cells to the murine thymus *(32)*, CD34$^+$ cells lacking expression of CD3, CD4, and CD8 downregulate CD34, and in successive stages lose the ability to differentiate into myeloid cells and thymic dendritic cells (DCs) (Fig. 2) *(33)*. Studies in the SCID-hu Thy/Liv mouse have demonstrated that cells with the phenotypes of CD34$^+$ Lin$^-$ CD45RA$^-$, CD34$^+$ Lin$^-$ CD45RA$^+$ CD10$^-$, and CD34$^+$ Lin$^-$ CD45RA$^+$ CD10$^+$ have progressively restricted differentiation potential, with the former consisting of HSC and the latter capable of producing only lymphoid, natural killer (NK) and thymic DC cells *(34,35)*. Studies in human bone marrow *(36)* and fetal thymus *(37)* have demonstrated that downregulation of CD34 represents the point of divergence in the T and NK lineages.

The earliest stages of thymocyte maturation have been best characterized in the mouse (reviewed in *38*), where CD3$^-$ CD4$^-$/low CD8$^-$ or triple-negative (TN) cells have been identified as the most immature thymic lymphoid progenitors *(39)*. These cells, still capable of NK differentiation, are probably capable of limited self-renewal and express CD117 (c-kit, receptor for stem cell factor [SCF]) *(40)* and CD44 (heat-stable antigen [HSA]) while lacking expression of CD25 (the receptor for interleukin-2 [IL-2]) *(41)*. Maturation of the thymic lymphoid progenitor (TLP) cell results in the pro-T cell, characterized by persistent c-kit expression with upregulation of CD25 *(41)*. CD25 upregulation defines a state of activation which, in contrast to that observed in mature peripheral lymphocytes, occurs in a T-cell-receptor–independent fashion, as T-cell receptor β (TCR-β) rearrangement begins only during the transition from the pro-T cell to the pre-T-cell stage *(42)*. Maturation from the pro-T to the pre-T-cell stage is heralded by downregulation of CD44 and CD117, and by the presence of clonotype-independent CD3 complexes (CICs) which appear on the surface of pro-T cells before detectable TCR-β VDJ rearrangement. Recent data suggest that signaling through CIC may be necessary for normal TCR-β rearrangement and thus progression to the pre-T stage *(43)*.

The early pre-T cell ($CD117^-$ $CD44^-$ $CD25^+$) represents an important developmental checkpoint, as cells must undergo productive TCR-β rearrangement, downregulate CD25, and stop actively cycling as they mature to the late pre-T cell-stage *(38)*. At this stage, the pre-T α chain (pTα) *(44)* has been found to covalently associate with TCR-β and the CD3 proteins, forming a signaling complex that is necessary for maturation to the late pre-T-cell stage, a process that has been termed "β selection" (reviewed in *45*). The expression of recombinase-activating gene (RAG) products, which mediate the rearrangements at the TCR loci, is switched off as thymocytes mature to the late pre-T-cell stage. In human thymocytes, it has recently been shown that late pre-T cells may rapidly downregulate surface pre-TCR and progress to resting, smaller cells *(46)*. It is at this stage that TCR-α rearrangement begins, mediated by RAG products that are again expressed at increased levels. Following TCR-α rearrangement, maturation occurs through a rapidly cycling intermediate characterized as $CD3^-$ $CD4^-$ $CD8^+$ in the mouse and as $CD3^-$ $CD4^+$ $CD8^-$ (termed the intrathymic T progenitor, or ITTP cell) in the human thymus *(47)*. The next and perhaps best studied thymocyte is an αβ TCR-bearing cell that upregulates the markers CD4 and CD8 ($CD4^+$ $CD8^+$, or double positive [DP] thymocyte) with low/intermediate expression of CD3 on the cell surface. The pairing of a newly synthesized TCR-α chain with the existing TCR-β chain results in the surface expression of a complex comprised of CD3 and TCR-αβ. The diversity of the surface TCR-αβ–CD3 complexes on DP thymocytes is determined by the germline, and is therefore unselected. It is at the DP stage that positive and negative selection shape the developing T-lymphoid repertoire.

Positive and Negative Selection of Thymocytes

In deciding the fate of thymocytes that mature from DP cells present in the thymic cortex to more mature single positive (SP) cells ($CD3^+$ $CD4^+$ $CD8^-$ and $CD3^+$ $CD4^-$ $CD8^+$), the immune system faces a remarkable problem: how is it possible to generate an efficient, diverse population of effector $CD4^+$ and $CD8^+$ T cells that respond to foreign antigens in the context of self-major histocompatibility complex (MHC) molecules, yet remain incapable of generating potentially deadly autoimmune reactions? The clues to this paradox lie in the processes of positive and negative selection, and continue to be a subject of intense investigation hindered by several experimental limitations: (1) As the in vivo precursor frequency of a T cell recognizing a single native antigen/MHC complex is likely to be below the limit of detection in physiologic conditions, it has been necessary to rely on transgenic model systems, such as mice overexpressing a single TCR; (2) it is unknown how peptides are presented in vivo in an intact thymus, leading to experiments in fetal thymic organ culture (FTOC) that may lack elements of the spatial geometry and cellular interactions present in the native thymus; (3) murine systems, while crucial to our understanding of these processes, may incompletely mirror developmental and selective events in the human thymus. Despite these limitations, several salient features of positive and negative selection have been described that will be discussed further.

Phenotypically, the transition from immature DP to mature SP thymocytes involves upregulation of CD3 and TCR and usually involves downregulation of CD4 on $CD3^+$

CD8+ cells with MHC class I TCR-αβ specificity and downregulation of CD8 on CD3+CD4+ cells with class II TCR-αβ specificity. Concomitantly, there is decreased expression of the recombinase-activating genes 1 and 2 (RAG-1 and RAG-2) which previously mediated α- and β-chain rearrangement, and increasing functional maturity and expression of bcl-2, TCR-αβ, and MHC class I (reviewed in *48*). Cells that are at early stages of this transition express CD69 *(49,50)* and CD1a *(51),* while more mature SP cells do not. The vast majority of cells at the DP stage (perhaps >99%) die by apoptosis after failing to be positively selected or through negative selection.

Phenotypic characterization of the cells undergoing and surviving positive and negative selection has proved easier than delineating the criteria that determine whether an individual cell lives or dies during this process (reviewed in *52–54*). On a simplistic level, binding of a TCR-bearing thymocyte to complex of peptide and either MHC class I (for cells destined to become CD3+ CD8+, or cytotoxic T cells) or class II (for CD3+ CD4+ or helper T cells) is thought to facilitate positive selection if this binding proceeds in the appropriate fashion. Experiments in FTOC from TCR-transgenic mice examining the efficiency of positive selection by a single antigenic peptide have produced conflicting results about the relative importance of avidity *(55,56)* (i.e., the number of TCR per cell triggered during an antigenic stimulus during selection) vs affinity *(57)* (i.e., the strength of interaction between a given TCR and its cognate peptide–MHC ligand). These articles did support the model that naturally occurring peptide–MHC complexes expressed during positive selection were likely to mediate recognition of similar complexes in the periphery by T cells surviving such selection, a fact supported by the demonstration of such a ligand on thymic epithelium *(58).*

Others, however, have demonstrated that multiple, structurally divergent peptides (even some incapable of stimulating selected T cells) can select a single TCR in a transgenic FTOC system *(59)*. This observation suggests that positive selection may be more "promiscuous" *(52)* than initially imagined, an hypothesis supported by experiments characterizing positive selection following introduction of neopeptides into mouse thymus via adenoviral delivery to mouse stromal cells *(60)*. Equally remarkable, structural characterization of human TCRs from two individuals lacking contact residue homology, yet binding the same MHC–peptide complex *(61),* have suggested that functionally "synonymous" TCRs, despite disparate binding regions, may be positively selected on a single MHC–peptide complex (as discussed in *62*). It should be clear from this discussion that no simplistic summary of factors governing positive selection is possible, and that explanations for these seeming contradictions await further study.

Similarly, fascinating and unanswered questions surround the process of negative selection, wherein maturing thymocytes bearing potentially autoreactive TCR are eliminated by apoptosis. It has been estimated that one half to two thirds of positively selected thymocytes (which themselves may represent ≤5% of DP thymocytes) undergo death due to negative selection *(63).* Much of the basis for our understanding of negative selection is derived from the study of superantigens encoded by mouse mammary tumor viruses (MTVs) that are present as integrated sequences in the germline of highly inbred laboratory mouse strains (reviewed in *64*). These studies revealed deletions in the peripheral lymphoid repertoire (but not in DP thymocytes) in TCR-β variable region (Vβ)-restricted T cell subsets *(65–69),* suggesting that negative selection occurred following positive selection during the DP to SP transition. It was later demonstrated that effective Vβ-specific deletion by superantigens was mediated by bone marrow derived dendritic cells rather than by cortical epithelial cells *(70)*. Similar results have been observed in human thymic tissue following exogenous administration of superantigens and indicate that human deletional tolerance also occurs at the late DP to early SP stage *(71–73)*. These and other results (reviewed in *74,75*) suggest that dendritic cell mediated deletional selection occurs primarily at the cortico–medullary junction and in the medulla, while medullary epithelial cells are more likely to induce tolerance by induction of anergy *(76)*. Other intruiging data suggest another potential mechanism for tolerance to self-antigens in the medulla. In a study of intrathymic tolerance induction to human C-reactive protein (hCRP), an inducible serum protein normally produced in the liver of transgenic mice, it was demonstrated that hCRP "ectopically" produced by thymic medullary epithelial cells was necessary and sufficient to produce deletional tolerance *(77)*. When considered with the observations that proteins normally of pancreatic (e.g., insulin *78,79*) or retinal origin *(80)* may be expressed in the thymus, these data suggest that endogenous production of self-proteins (rather than presentation of circulating protein antigens by medullary dendritic cells) may represent an important mechanism of negative selection *(81)*.

Stromal Cells and Cytokines

The role of nonlymphoid cells in the maturation of thymocytes is not restricted to the presentation of antigens during positive and negative selection. The defined elements of thymic stroma include a wide variety of epithelial cells developmentally derived from the pharyngeal pouches as well as dendritic cells and macrophages of hematopoietic origin (reviewed in *74,82,83*). In addition, fibroblasts and networks of extracellular matrix proteins are present. Important interactions between stromal cells and thymocytes are thought to occur at several developmental checkpoints. The first of these points is at the TN stage of development, when the pre-TCR signal is known to induce further maturation. While it is possible that spontaneous signaling may occur after formation of the pre-TCR complex, it is more likely that interaction of the pre-TCR with stromal elements (perhaps fibroblasts or epithelial cells (*84*) is important in this interaction. Other important associations are likely to occur between thymocytes and epithelial cells during positive selection and, as discussed previously, during presentation of self-antigens by dendritic cells or epithelial cells in the medulla or the cortico–medullary junction. The importance of phagocytic activity of macrophages in the thymus is evidenced by the ability of the organ to preserve its normal architecture in the face of massive thymocyte death. During HIV-1 infection, these populations are likely to be of special relevance, as they express CD4 and may become infected by macrophage-tropic viral species, providing a target and potential reservoir for viral replication *(85)*.

Several cytokines have been demonstrated to play a role in intrathymic T-cell maturation. Perhaps the best evidence exists to support the influence of interleukin-7 (IL-7) in early thymocyte maturation. Originally described as a B-cell growth factor *(86)*, further work defined diverse roles in regulation of B- and T-cell development and function (reviewed in *87*). Expression of CD127, the IL-7 receptor (IL-7R), occurs on early thymocytes (from the TLP to TN stages) as well as on mature CD4+ and CD8+ SP thymocytes *(88)*. The importance of IL-7 in early T-cell maturation was clearly defined by the creation of IL-7R knockout mice which were found to be severely deficient in lymphoid cells, including thymocytes *(89,90)*. Overexpression of the antiapoptotic *bcl-2* gene product in these mice led to complete rescue from lymphopenia by restoration of positive selection, suggesting that IL-7 has an antiapoptotic role during thymopoiesis, especially during the period of positive selection. In addition to its antiapoptotic role, it has been demonstrated that IL-7 may induce proliferation in a subset of immature, CD34+ early thymocytes *(91)* and lead to increased numbers of thymic dendritic cells in FTOC *(92)*. Proliferation of early thymic progenitors was also demonstrated to be important in a murine bone marrow transplant model, where administration of IL-7 enhanced thymopoiesis and more rapidly restored normal cellularity after myeloablation *(93)*.

Recent clinical studies, performed in HIV-1–infected adults, have suggested that IL-7 may play an important role in the regulation of peripheral lymphoid numbers in human subjects *(94,95)*, consistent with results from murine systems. In one study, analyses performed in a large number of human subjects (n = 168) demonstrated that increased circulating IL-7 levels were associated with decreased total CD4+ and CD8+ T cell counts *(94)*. Increased IL-7 levels were strongly associated with the depletion of naïve and memory T cells in these subjects *(94)*. Furthermore, retrospective longitudinal analyses of a smaller group of subjects (n = 11) demonstrated that IL-7 levels rose in proportion to a decrease in the circulating CD4+ T cell count (*94*). These results, considered with the established antiapoptotic and proliferative effects of IL-7 on murine and human thymocytes, suggest that IL-7 may be an important homeostatic regulator of lymphocyte numbers, perhaps through its effects on thymopoiesis.

Early thymopoiesis has also been shown to be positively regulated by signaling by stem cell factor (SCF) through its receptor (c-kit) and by the ligand for the flt-3/flk-2 receptor (flt-3 ligand, FL). Both the c-kit and flt-3 receptors have tyrosine kinase activity regulated by binding of their respective ligands on target cells *(96,97)* and to have distinct but partially overlapping patterns of expression on primitive hematopoietic tissues (reviewed in *98*). Analysis of knockout mice deficient in c-kit (W/W) and SCF (SI/SI) revealed that the size of the TN thymocyte compartment was significantly reduced in both strains and that expansion of immature thymocytes in SI/SI mice was also impaired *(99)*. Further studies suggested that combined knockout mice lacking both c-kit and the common cytokine receptor γ (γ_c) chain (i.e., common to IL-2, IL-4, IL-7, IL-9, and IL-15) had a complete abrogation of thymopoiesis, far more severe than that seen in either single knockout *(100)*. Other experiments in FTOC have suggested that SCF may induce a differentiation signal in concert with signals from other cytokines (e.g., IL-3, IL-6, and IL-7), in contrast to FL, which may instead serve as a self-renewal signal for the earliest TLP cells *(101)*. It is relevant to note, however, that peripheral plasma levels of SCF, in a group of HIV-1–infected human subjects (n = 18), did not correlate with the degree of lymphopenia seen in these subjects, in contrast to the inverse relationship observed between IL-7 levels and peripheral CD4+ and CD8+ T cell counts *(94)*.

The number and complexity of signaling pathways known to be important to the maintenance and regulation of thymopoiesis will certainly increase substantially in the coming years *(45)*. In addition to those already discussed, a growing number of signaling intermediates, including protein tyrosine phosphatases (e.g., CD45) *(102)*, Src-family protein tyrosine kinases (PTKs) (e.g., Fyn, Lck *45*, and Csk *103*), as well as transcription factors *(104,105)* have been identified. The role of known intermediates in apoptotic pathways, such as the regulators bcl-2 and bax *(106)*, is only now beginning to emerge. These and other arbitrators of life and death in biological systems, such as members of the tumor necrosis factor family of receptors (e.g., CD30 *107*), may play significant regulatory roles in an organ in which continual cell death is an important aspect of its normal function. While identification of these regulators of thymic development will likely come initially from ex vivo and murine models, it will be important to subsequently determine whether they become dysregulated in the setting of human diseases (e.g., AIDS).

Lymphocyte Adolescence

The product of the maturation process from HSC to mature SP thymocyte is a small lymphocyte, expressing either CD4 or CD8 on its surface, which migrates from the thymic medulla to the peripheral blood. Prior to its initial encounter with an antigenic stimulus, this cell is designated as a "naïve" lymphocyte. The expression of various isoforms of the leukocyte common antigen, CD45, a protein tyrosine phosphatase, has been shown to correlate with "naïve" vs "memory" phenotypes of lymphocytes (reviewed in *108*). Resting T cells (with the phenotype $CD45R^{hi}$ or $CD45RB^{+}$ in the mouse) were found to switch to expression of a low molecular weight isoform of CD45 ($CD45^{lo}$, characterized as $CD45RB^{-}$ in the mouse) in which several exons were deleted. In human T cells, analogous naïve subsets were defined by expression of the marker CD45RA, while memory T cells are recognized by an antibody recognizing a novel epitope at the $CD45^{lo}$ splice site ($CD45RO^{+}$). A more restrictive definition of naïve T cells characterizes them on the basis of coexpression of the cell surface adhesion molecule L-selectin (CD62L) *(109)*. This lectin has an affinity for carbohydrate determinants displayed by specialized vascular structures such as high endothelial venules (HEVs) in lymph nodes. Its expression has been postulated to allow divergent recirculation patterns in naïve and memory T cells, with HEVs serving as a gateway to the lymphatic tissues for naïve cells.

The process whereby a naïve lymphocyte first encounters antigen and becomes activated is a complex one, involving the signal provided by the recognition of a cognate peptide–MHC complex *(110)* by the TCR as well as additional signals provided by cytokines and costimulatory molecules (reviewed in *111*). It is now apparent that multiple ligand–receptor interactions (reviewed in *112*) may play a role in determining the fate of TCR-mediated triggering on naïve T cells, including binding of the B7 ligands (B7-1/CD80 and B7-2/CD86) to intercellular the CD28 and CTLA-4 receptors; of LFA-1 to the intercellular adhesion molecules (ICAM); and of LFA-3 to CD2. Quantitative estimates derived from analysis of TCR downregulation in response to varying antigenic ligand densities led to estimates that T cell activation occurred when approx 8000 TCRs were triggered, irrespective of the activation state of the cell studied *(113)*. Costimulation through CD28, which lowered the activation threshold to approx 1500 TCRs, was much more important for resting (putative naïve) cells than for memory T-cell clones. It has been also suggested that costimulation via CD28 may confer resistance to TCR-mediated activation-induced cell death (AICD) mediated by the fas/fas ligand (CD95/CD95L) pathway, which might otherwise induce a form of peripheral tolerance by deletion of responding T cells *(114,115)*. The product of activation of a naïve T cell through TCR-mediated and costimulatory signals is a lymphocyte which downregulates CD45RA and CD62L, and expresses CD45RO. Whether all of these cells function as effector cells, from which a long-term memory population is derived, or whether memory cell differentiation can occur in a divergent pathway of maturation, has been a topic of considerable debate.

The Persistence of Memory

The establishment of immunologic memory is a task of fundamental importance to the immune system. Our understanding of this process is central to our ability to develop active forms of immunization for human diseases. The Greek historian Thucydides, in describing the plague of Athens in 430 BC, observed that "the same man was never attacked twice" (reviewed in *116*). The reason for this protection is that after primary antigenic challenge, a massive expansion of lymphocytes occurs (with the majority later dying via AICD), followed by a period characterized by long-term memory in which repeat challenge with antigen induces a larger and more rapid response than seen initially *(108,116)*. While it is universally agreed that a population of T-lymphoid memory cells mediates this response, divergent models explaining the derivation and maintenance of memory have been proposed *(108, 116–118)*. One such model proposes that the generation of memory cells may occur without progression through an effector cell intermediate (i.e., through "linear" maturation from naïve to effector to memory cell) and that the fate of naïve (into effector vs memory cells) might be determined by events during its primary activation *(117)*. In support of this model are data suggesting that memory and effector T lymphocytes can be discriminated based upon patterns of proximate and downstream signaling events observed after CD3/TCR triggering *(117)*, extending the results of earlier experiments that showed differences in TCR-mediated signaling through PTK proteins such as ZAP-70 in naïve and memory T cells *(119)*.

In contrast, two studies examined populations of cells expanding in primary and secondary immune responses in animal models of infection and support the notion that the memory pool is derived from the pool of effector cells, consistent with a linear maturation model *(120,121)*. The first of these studies used flow-cytometric methods to analyze the TCR Vβ repertoire of defined $CD8^+$ T cell responses in mice infected with *Listeria monocytogenes* and demonstrated that primary and effector responses were remarkably conserved at the Vβ level, with a somewhat narrower repertoire in the memory-responsive pool *(120)*. The second report, using MHC/peptide tetramers (reviewed in *122*) to scrutinize the diversity of responses within responding Vβ subsets of $CD8^+$ cells in mice experimentally infected with lymphocytic choriomeningitis virus (LCMV), confirmed that the memory pool of $CD8^+$ cells responding to secondary challenge was structurally and functionally similar to that of the primary response *(121)*. It should be noted that the methodology used in these studies to examine longitudinal $CD8^+$ T cell responses has not yet been applied to the study of $CD4^+$ responses during primary and secondary infection, and may not be generalizable to that population. Despite this limitation, these data are compelling in their support for a model wherein long-lived memory cells are stochastically derived from the primary effector response to antigenic challenge.

Further evidence for a linear maturation model of memory cell development arises from studies of the expression pattern of the chemokine receptor CCR7, which is present on a subset of $CD45RA^-$ cells that produce IL-2 only following stimulation *(123)*. In contrast, $CCR7^+$ cells within the CD45RA subset produced high levels of IL-4, IL-5, and IFN-γ and moderately reduced levels of IL-2. $CD45RA^-$ $CCR7^+$ memory cells retain expression of the lymph node homing receptor CD62L, whereas $CD45RA^-$ $CCR7^-$ cells express CD62L to a lesser and more variable extent. Furthermore, rapid production of IFN-γ may be detected in most $CCR7^-$ cells, but only in a negligible fraction of $CCR7^+$ memory cells following superantigen stimulation. These data suggest that a subset of memory cells may retain lymph node homing properties ($CD45RA^-$ $CD62L^+$ $CCR7^+$ cells) and may serve as a precursor population to a population of memory T cells with effector functions and a distinct phenotype ($CD45RA^-$ $CD62L^-$ $CCR7^-$) *(123)*.

An important aspect of T-lymphoid memory relates to phenotypic interconversion of putative naïve and memory subsets. As discussed previously, CD45RA and CD45RO isoforms have been used to characterize naïve and memory subsets of human T cells. Several lines of experimental evidence now support the notion that the $CD45RA^+$ (putative naïve) population may harbor divergent cell types with respect to "naïveté." One such piece of evidence derived from the study of $CD45RA^+$ and $CD45RO^+$ cell populations from patients who had previously undergone radiotherapy *(124)*. A rapid loss of unstable chromosomes induced by the prior radiation exposure was noted in the $CD45RO^+$ but not $CD45RA^+$ pool, and modeling of the data best supported a model in which in vivo reversion from the CD45RO to CD45RA had occurred. Other experiments, examining the responses of mouse lymphocytes to dinitrochlorobenzene (DNCB), demonstrated that primed DNCB-specific memory $CD4^+$ cells ($CD45R^{lo}$) reverted to a $CD45R^{hi}$ (putative naïve) phenotype if they were transferred to a secondary recipient in the absence of further antigenic challenge *(125)*. In the presence of even modest antigenic persistence, the $CD45R^{lo}$ phenotype was preserved. Significantly, memory "revertants" with naïve phenotype behaved initially like naïve cells in their response to rechallenge, consistent with an alternative form of long-term memory cell than previously imagined *(108)*. Further evidence supporting the hypothesis that $CD45RA^+$ cells may represent a functionally diverse population comes from phenotypic studies of lymphocytes in HIV-1–infected adults, demonstrating that the fraction of cells expressing CD45RA (but lacking other markers of naïve cells, e.g., CD62L expression) progressively increases with advancing infection, despite the progressive loss of $CD4^+$ and $CD8^+$ $CD45RA^+$ $CD62L^+$ lymphocytes through the course of infection *(126)*. Other evidence comes from functional studies of reactivity to dust mite allergens that have demonstrated a substantially higher response in the $CD4^+$ $CD45RA^+$ subset of atopic vs nonatopic subjects, suggesting that this population contains memory revertants *(127)*. In aggregate, these results suggest that oversimplification in characterizing putative naïve and memory T-cell subsets may be misleading, and that further work will be necessary to understand the relationship between phenotypic distinctions and functional capacity of these subpopulations.

The Effector Lymphocyte

Although a detailed consideration of the functional importance and diversity of $CD4^+$ and $CD8^+$ T lymphocytes is beyond the scope of this chapter, it is important to

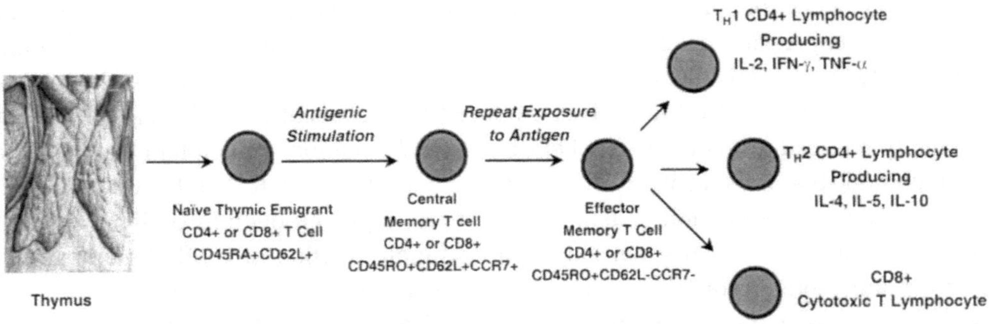

Fig. 3. Phenotypes of peripheral human T cells.

underscore several points. First, the functional breadth of the $CD4^+$ T-cell compartment is likely to be great, with several lines of investigation pointing to divergent functional roles of cells based on their ability to produce subsets of cytokines during effector responses *(128)* (and on their representation in HIV-1–infected individuals *(129,130)* (Fig. 3).

In all likelihood, diverse functional subsets of memory T cells exist, perhaps containing distinct effector functions necessary for protection against the diverse challenges presented by pathogenic organisms. Phenotypic studies have identified surface proteins on T cells that demarcate subsets of memory T cells that exemplify this functional diversity. Among the $CD45RA^-$ population, subsets defined by the phenotypes of $CD62L^+$ $CD11a^{dim}$ and $CD62L^-$ $CD11a^{bright}$ appear to have unique cytokine-secretion profiles *(131)*. The $CD45RA^-$ $CD62L^+$ $CD11a^{dim}$ subset was found to produce cytokines including IL-4 (a T_H2 cytokine) while the CD45RA-CD62L-$CD11a^{bright}$ subset was demonstrated to produce IFN-γ preferentially. While the representation of these two subsets of memory $CD4^+$ T cells was found to be altered in clinical subtypes of mycobacterium-induced leprosy, the individual cytokine-secretion profiles of these subsets within individuals was invariant *(131)*. These data suggest that pathogenic infections (or other disease states including malignancies) *(132)* might be associated with a skewing in the representation of individual effector T-cell subsets. It will be important to determine to what extent such skewing might render an immune response to an infection or a cancer ineffectual, due to the overexpansion of cells with a phenotype incapable of an optimal protective response.

It is becoming clear that complex signaling interactions between $CD4^+$ T cells, so-called "professional" antigen presenting cells (e.g., marrow-derived dendritic cells), and cytotoxic T cells are likely to be important in the development of mature, protective immune responses. The ability of $CD4^+$ T cells to "license" dendritic cells (via CD40/CD40 ligand signaling pathways) to activate $CD8^+$ cytotoxic effector responses is one example of this complexity *(133–136)*. Further evidence lies in the observations that mediators as diverse as leptin *(137)* and regulators of tryptophan catabolism *(138)* may play a role in starvation- and pregnancy-associated immunosuppression, respectively. Dysregulation of such pathways in immunodeficient states may compound the deficits caused by quantitative decreases in effector cells.

LYMPHOID HOMEOSTASIS IN IMMUNODEFICIENCY

In healthy individuals studied longitudinally, hematological parameters such as neutrophil and red blood cell counts, as well as lymphocyte numbers, are maintained with remarkable stability over time. Whereas regulatory proteins such as erythropoietin (in the case of maintenance of red blood cell mass) and myeloid colony-stimulating factors (in the case of neutrophils) have been identified as regulators of such stability in other lineages, similar mechanisms have yet to be elucidated for lymphoid cells. Nonetheless, studies within immunodeficient humans and murine models have provided interesting insights into the general problem of lymphoid homeostasis.

A Hierarchical Regulation of T-Cell Numbers

The concept of "blind T-cell homeostasis," postulating that the size of the total CD3$^+$ T cell compartment is regulated independently of its constituent CD4$^+$ and CD8$^+$ subpopulations, was advanced on the basis of cross-sectional observations of T cell subsets in HIV-1–infected individuals as well as in healthy mice depleted of CD4$^+$ T cells by monoclonal antibodies *(139)*. In the setting of HIV-1 disease, circulating total CD3$^+$ T cell numbers were observed to remain relatively constant despite progressive decline in total circulating CD4$^+$ T cells, a fact that could be explained by a compensatory increase in CD8$^+$ T cell numbers. Supporting data from CD4-depleted mice demonstrated that an initial decrease in the total CD3$^+$ pool size due to CD4$^+$ depletion was followed by an increase in CD8$^+$ numbers in both lymphoid tissues and in the circulation *(139)*. Other investigators have provided supportive data for the principle of blind homeostasis in longitudinal studies of HIV-1–infected subjects (reviewed in *140*) as well as in mathematical models based on FTOC *(141,142)*. Although the blind homeostasis model explains interesting features of intercompartmental regulation of T-cell numbers, it does not directly address the source of the pools from which lymphoid expansion may emanate. Elegant experiments in murine models (reviewed in *143*) have demonstrated that the circulating peripheral lymphocyte compartment does not expand after adoptive transfer of large numbers of lymphocytes or after implantation of multiple thymus grafts. In other experiments, congenitally athymic or thymectomized, irradiated mice injected with relatively small lymphocyte numbers were able to replenish a depleted lymphoid pool *(143)*, albeit to subnormal levels *(144)*. These studies suggest that when athymic hosts are confronted with a deficit in lymphocyte numbers, substantial proliferation of remaining lymphocytes may occur, that this feedback is inhibited when pool size approaches normal levels, and that the CD4$^+$ and CD8$^+$ compartments are interregulated. While these concepts may be sufficient to explain many of the changes observed in athymic hosts, they do not account for the contribution of *de novo* lymphocyte production from the thymus, and its role in homeostatic regulation of the lymphoid compartment.

Thymus-Derived vs Peripheral Expansion

If preservation of total CD3$^+$ T cell numbers is a major determinant of lymphoid homeostasis, it is important to know whether and in what circumstances the system is maintained by thymic and/or extrathymic production. Important experiments utilizing transfer of either bone marrow (BM)-derived or lymph node (LN)-derived inocula into either euthymic or thymectomized murine hosts shed light on this question (reviewed in

145,146). Not surprisingly, BM inocula requiring differentiation in the thymus were unable to reconstitute athymic hosts, where progeny of LN-derived inocula were responsible for $\alpha\beta^+$ T-cell repopulation *(147)*. In contrast, euthymic hosts preferentially reconstituted their lymphoid compartment from BM-derived progeny maturing in the thymus to regenerate a naïve repertoire. Importantly, athymic hosts achieving reconstitution via peripheral expansion were unable to respond to neoantigens, in contrast to euthymic hosts preferentially expanding thymus-derived T cells. This observation suggests that immunodeficiency may persist if a diverse, naïve cell-derived repertoire is not generated, even if $CD3^+$ T-cell numbers are normal. These experiments also demonstrated that extrathymic T cell expansion is antigen driven and that such expansion can lead to a skewed TCR repertoire of limited diversity *(148)*. By analogy, HIV-1–infected subjects have been demonstrated to have dramatic skewing of functional antigen-specific $CD4^+$ T cell responses toward cytomegalovirus (CMV), with >10% of the peripheral $CD4^+$ T cells in some subjects responding to CMV *(7,149)*. In aggregate, these studies in mice and in humans indicate that thymic repopulation is favored and that it is more likely to generate a functionally diverse T-cell repertoire. This conclusion raises questions regarding the persistence of thymic function in human subjects with immunodeficiency states and the role of such function in contributing to immune reconstitution.

Persistence of Thymic Function—Theoretical Considerations

Conventional immunologic wisdom held for decades that the human thymus, while clearly the source of T lymphocyte production in early life, is functionally inert beyond adolescence (reviewed in *150*). Although studies demonstrate that the size and weight of the organ are maintained at relatively constant levels throughout life *(151)*, its adipose content proportionately increases over time, as studied by histology *(151)* and radiographic examination *(152–154)*. Despite the relative increase in fatty tissue, it has been noted that persistent lymphoid islands are present in the gland in individuals as old as 107 yr of age and that the mean lymphoid tissue volume in adults between 20 and 39 yr of age is still approx 45% of that in children in the first decade of life *(151)*. Direct labeling of emigrating thymocytes in mice revealed that the absolute number of thymic emigrants declines in aged mice but that the relative production rate of naïve thymocytes by remaining thymic tissue stays relatively constant. Although these data do not speak to the physiologic role (or importance) of residual thymic function, they suggest that such function may persist beyond adolescence.

Studies of Thymic Function in Children and Adults Treated for Malignancy

Clinical evidence that thymic function may be important in immune reconstitution in children and in some adults has been mounting, initially from the study of immunologic reconstitution in patients treated with chemotherapy for malignant diseases (reviewed in *155–157*). Several investigators have observed "rebound" thymic hypertrophy in the period following such therapy in children and some young adults *(158–161)*. In a study of 15 subjects (varying in age from 1 to 24 yr), naïve $CD4^+$ T-cell counts at 6 mo after therapy (defined by the less restrictive $CD45RA^+$ phenotype) correlated inversely with age. Thymic rebound by CT scan (assessed 3 mo after the completion of therapy) was noted in a majority of children aged <20 yr and in only one subject of age 21 through 24 *(162)*. Those experiencing rebound had higher CD45RA/CD45RO ratios and had more complete and rapid recovery in the 6-mo period following therapy *(162)*. Other studies, examining adults treated with high-dose chemotherapy and autologous transplantation for solid tumors, demonstrated that recovery of normal numbers of $CD4^+$ T cells occurred within 2 yr in only about half of the patients studied, with continued slow increases in the number of circulating ($CD4^+$ $CD45RA^+$) T cells even at intervals greater than 1 yr post-therapy *(146)*.

Further insight into lymphoid recovery patterns comes from studies of patients treated for Hodgkin's disease with mediastinal irradiation, which effectively ablates thymic function *(163,164)*. These studies demonstrated that numbers of naïve ($CD45RA^+$ $CD62L^+$) $CD4^+$ and $CD8^+$ cells never recovered to normal levels, despite recovery of $CD4^+$ and $CD8^+$ memory cells. These data again confirm the importance of intercompartmental regulation, with return of normal total $CD3^+$ T cell numbers by peripheral expansion of memory cells despite the inability to generate cells by a thymic pathway.

Extrathymic T-Cell Maturation

Another consequence of thymic ablation is the appearance of unusual T-cell populations thought to be derived from extrathymic sources (reviewed in *165*). Several of these populations have been noted in patients receiving mediastinal irradiation, including $CD8^+$ T cells with the phenotype of $CD8^{dull}$ and $CD8\alpha\alpha$ (rather than $\alpha\beta$); $CD8^+$ $CD57^+$ $CD28^-$ T cells; $CD3^+$ $CD5^-$ T cells (in contrast to most T cells which express CD5); and $V\delta1^+$ T cells (reviewed in *163*). It is important to note that there is overlap between these cell populations and that their functional capacity (e.g., with respect to their ability to be protective for infection) is not yet known. Although it is thought that these cells are likely to be derived from extrathymic maturation, as described in the mouse *(166,167)*, the significance and mechanisms of extrathymic T-cell maturation in humans remains unclear.

It has been suggested that the pathways for regeneration of $CD4^+$ and $CD8^+$ T cells may not be equally dependent on thymic function. In one study of immunologic reconstitution in a previously thymectomized 15-yr-old child undergoing allogeneic bone marrow transplantation, $CD4^+$ $CD45RA^+$ cells remained depressed even 2 yr after engraftment. In contrast, $CD4^+$ $CD45RO^+$ and $CD8^+$ $CD45RA^+$ cells recovered in a pattern similar to that previously observed for euthymic hosts undergoing transplantation *(168)*. This study is notable, as the presence of allogeneic reconstitution pointed to host-related (and not stem cell dependent) factors in determining the clinical outcome. It is limited, however, by the fact that further subclassification of the $CD4^+$ and $CD8^+$ populations (e.g., by expression of CD62L or other markers of putative extrathymic maturation) was not performed. Therefore, it is unclear whether the rapidly recovering $CD8^+$ $CD45RA^+$ cells (which might have consisted of memory revertants if negative for expression of CD62L) were the result of *de novo* T cell production or of memory T-cell expansion. Others have confirmed that $CD8^+$ $CD45RA^+$ repopulation occurs more rapidly than in the $CD4^+$ $CD45RA^+$ subset, but is associated with cells bearing the $CD28^-$ phenotype. In contrast, repopulation of $CD8^+$ $CD45RA^+$ $CD28^+$ cells occurs at a pace similar to that found for $CD4^+$ $CD45RA^+$ cells, hinting that there are dichotomous routes for $CD8^+$ regeneration that are temporally distinct *(169)*.

Thymic Mass and Function in Healthy and HIV-1–Infected Adults

The lymphopenia that results from HIV-1 disease progression can be viewed as a balance between destruction of lymphocytes (by direct infection and indirect means) and regenerative failure of the thymus and other possible sites of *de novo* lymphocyte production *(170)*. The foregoing sections have highlighted the biological complexity that is likely to underlie regulation of T-cell numbers in healthy and immunocompromised hosts. To evaluate the interplay between extrathymic peripheral expansion and thymic production of new lymphocytes, it is necessary to gather information about thymic mass and function, as well as T cell turnover, in healthy and HIV-1–infected adults.

To examine whether thymic mass and function were likely to be present in healthy adults and in subjects infected with HIV-1, a large group of subjects (n = 131, 99 HIV-1–seropositive and 32 seronegative) was examined by computed tomography (CT) for the presence of thymic tissue. Concomitantly, peripheral blood lymphocyte counts from these individuals were analyzed for absolute number and percentages of naïve (CD45RA$^+$ CD62L$^+$) and memory T cells *(171)*. Results were then stratified by age and HIV-1 serostatus, and in the case of infected subjects, by clinical parameters including circulating CD4$^+$ T cell counts. In HIV-1–seronegative individuals, the presence of abundant thymic tissue correlated with higher absolute number and percentage of circulating CD4$^+$ and CD8$^+$ naïve T cells. Of interest, a surprisingly large fraction of HIV-1–infected adults (47/99) also had abundant thymic tissue by CT. The thymic index (reflective of increased mass by CT) correlated with increases in the absolute number and percentage of naïve cells in the CD4$^+$ (but not CD8$^+$) T-cell compartment in these individuals, a correlation that persisted after controlling for age and duration of infection. In fact, older HIV-1–infected adults (i.e., >40 yr of age) were much more likely to have abundant thymic tissue than control subjects not infected with HIV-1 (5/10 vs 0/10 in the respective groups). These observations suggest that abundant thymic tissue persists in some, but not all, healthy and HIV-1–infected adults. Furthermore, the positive correlation between thymic tissue and circulating naïve CD4$^+$ T cells supports the possibility that persistent thymic function may contribute to lymphoid homeostasis in healthy and HIV-1–infected adults. Consistent with these observations are studies documenting persistent declines in naïve CD4$^+$ and CD8$^+$ populations throughout the course of HIV-1 infection in adults, as well as in children *(126,172)*.

To gather estimates of T-cell turnover in humans, a novel technique has been developed that allows nonradioactive labeling of endogenous lymphocytes in vivo *(173)*. Analysis of T-cell turnover and production rates in a group of HIV-1–infected adults demonstrated that, following initiation of potent antiretroviral therapy, production rates for CD4$^+$ and CD8$^+$ cells increased, even though the half-life of CD4$^+$ populations actually decreased *(174)*. These observations suggested that regenerative failure of lymphocyte production is an important pathogenic mechanism in AIDS, and focus attention on factors that may influence lymphocyte production following HIV-1 infection, including the role of persistent thymic function.

Further analyses of T cell turnover in prospectively studied HIV-1–infected individuals beginning HAART revealed that subjects with abundant thymus (by CT-based radiographic evaluation) had higher levels of naïve-phenotype T cells and lower

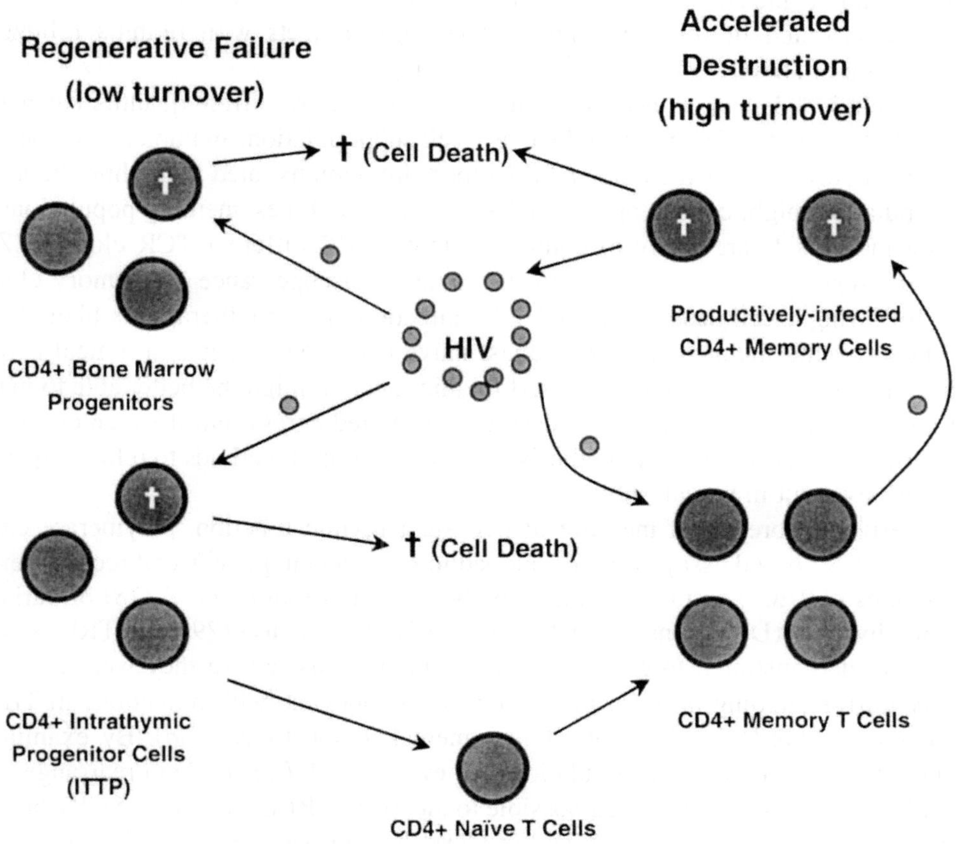

Fig. 4. Kinetics of T-cell dynamics in HIV-1 disease: regenerative failure and accelerated destruction. HIV infection may affect cell subpopulations across the hematopoietic tree, including multilineage $CD4^+$ bone marrow hematopoietic progenitor cells, intrathymic T-cell progenitors in the thymus, and mature $CD4^+$ T cells in the periphery. For discussion, see *170.*

turnover rates for the total $CD4^+$ T cell population *(175)*. These data suggest, in aggregate, that HIV-1–infected subjects may be subdivided into discrete groups with respect to the composition of the peripheral T-cell compartment. One group is typified by abundant thymic tissue, high circulating levels of slowly dividing naïve-phenotype T cells, and low turnover of the total circulating T-cell pool. Another is characterized by nonabundant thymic tissue, lower proportions of naïve-phenotype cells, and higher turnover of the total circulating T-cell pool. Given the presence or absence of thymic tissue and naïve T cells in the peripheral blood, the potential for diversification of the TCR repertoire in lymphopenic individuals may vary (Fig. 4).

The consequence of this distinction, and the long-term clinical sequelae, may have important clinical impact. Individuals in both groups might be able to produce new T cells, but those dependent on extrathymic maturation might remain immunodeficient, by merely expanding clones of T cells with limited diversity. Those with robust thymic output, in contrast, might be better equipped to regenerate a diverse naïve repertoire from a lymphopenic state. By example, increased $CD4^+$ T cell responses to CMV have been demonstrated in some but not all late-stage subjects with retinitis following the initiation of HAART *(7)* (Komanduri et al., in press).

These clinical data are consistent with observations derived from quantitative analyses of TCR diversity of memory and naïve T-cell subpopulations in humans. An elegant study of the diversity of the human TCR repertoire demonstrated that while the naïve cell population might contain approx 10^7 different TCR clones, memory populations of healthy individuals are likely to contain as few as 10^5 different TCR clones *(176)*. Thus, the regeneration of diversity in the event of disappearance of memory clones (e.g., following T-cell destruction by HIV-1 infection or chemotherapy) is likely to be facilitated by the maintenance of a robust naïve cell reservoir. It is a logical consequence that individuals with more robust thymic function might be better able to maintain a diverse naïve TCR repertoire despite accelerated egress into the memory T-cell compartment. Testing of this hypothesis, however, required methods to reliably quantitate thymic output in human subjects.

To derive a more direct measure of persistent thymic function, polymerase chain reaction (PCR)-based assays were developed to take advantage of T cell receptor excision circles (TRECs) formed during recombination and joining *(177,178)* of variable (V) and diversity (D) regions of the TCR-α and TCR-β chains *(179,180)*. TRECs were previously demonstrated to exist in avian lymphoid cells, where they were found to closely mirror ongoing *de novo* production of thymocytes, with reductions in TREC frequency observed as a function of incremental thymectomy *(28a)*. By examining purified human lymphoid subpopulations for evidence of TCR β-chain rearrangement byproducts (βTRECs), it has been possible to identify βTRECs in human SCID-hu thymocytes, in umbilical cord blood, and in $CD4^+$ human peripheral blood lymphocytes *(180)*. βTRECs were most prevalent in $CD45RA^+$ $CD62L^+$ lymphocytes, but were also detectable at reduced frequency in $CD45RO^+$ $CD62L^+$ and $CD45RO^+$ $CD62L^-$ lymphocytes in some individuals, despite the generally accepted notion that these populations should not contain recent thymic emigrants. Consistent with expectations regarding diminished thymic function with aging, βTREC frequency in the $CD45RA^+$ $CD62L^+$ subset of healthy individuals declined logarithmically with age, although persistent function was noted in older adults *(180)*.

Analogous studies examining TRECs formed during the excision of the TCR-δ locus during TCR-α chain rearrangement (δTRECs) also conclusively demonstrated that thymic function persists throughout adulthood, albeit declining with age. Examination of δTREC levels in lymphocytes of HIV-1–infected subjects revealed that δTREC levels were increased following the initiation of antiretroviral therapy *(179)*. It has been suggested that increases in TREC output may be variably detected following antiretroviral therapy and might be insufficient to explain completely the rises in levels of naïve T cells following HAART *(181)*. Despite this, it has been demonstrated that greater TREC production (presumably reflecting an increased level of thymic output into the peripheral T cell pool) is associated with a significant decrease in the risk of progression to AIDS and to death in HIV-1–infected subjects *(182)*. It has also been shown that δTREC levels were significantly increased over baseline levels following myeloablative chemotherapy and autologous stem cell transplantation in subjects with multiple myeloma *(183)*. In those subjects (half of whom were older than 50 yr of age), increased TREC levels following autologous transplantation were associated with improved recovery of increased naïve T-cell numbers as well as broader T-cell repertoires, as studied at the level of TCR Vβ subsets *(183)*.

While recent clinical studies provide tantalizing evidence that the thymus might persist and perhaps increase its level of function in lymphopenic individuals, many questions remain unanswered. Studies of δTRECs and βTRECs performed to date in healthy subjects and in those with cancer and AIDS have demonstrated substantial heterogeneity in levels of *de novo* T cell production even in age-matched individuals. This variation may approach 2–3 log orders of difference *(181,183)*. There also appears to be great heterogeneity on the impact of clinical interventions, such as cytotoxic chemotherapy for cancer, and of HAART, on thymic output. At this time little is known about the impact of individual clinical variables (e.g., effects of antiretroviral drugs, cytotoxic agents, or immunomodulatory therapies) on *de novo* T cell production. More complete studies are needed to establish whether therapeutic regimens for AIDS and cancer might be devised to induce effective control of disease while maximizing the potentially beneficial effects of thymic function. Such studies may also determine to what extent feedback in the setting of lymphoid depletion may influence the persistence (or even augmentation) of thymic function, and what biological variables (e.g., IL-7 levels) *(94)* may control such persistence in some individuals and not in others.

SUMMARY

A complex process underlies the development of a T-cell receptor repertoire that is both functionally diverse and tolerant of self. Regulation of the size, function, and diversity of the peripheral lymphoid pool is equally complicated. More clear is that fact that lymphocyte numbers are maintained by contributions from disparate sources that may provide unequal benefit.

When thymic function is absent (e.g., after thymectomy or radiation-induced ablation), the peripheral T cell repertoire is regulated by antigen-driven expansion. In the setting of peripheral lymphopenia, such expansion may lead to a T-cell compartment that has limited TCR diversity and that is comprised of extrathymically derived cells of uncertain functionality. Even in the presence of adequate numbers of repopulating cells, immunodeficiency may persist (Fig. 5).

Reconstitution of a diverse, functional repertoire will likely require thymic function. Thymopoiesis, as discussed in the preceding sections, requires input of HSC, maturation through a number of defined intermediate stages, and an array of signals from cytokines and stromal cells, many of which may be disrupted by direct or indirect mechanisms in the setting of HIV-1 infection or other pathologic (or iatrogenic) insults. Continued study of thymic function and its dysregulation in animal models *(184–186)* and in healthy and HIV-1–infected individuals *(171)* is likely to help us understand why immune reconstitution is more complete in some individuals than in others. The ultimate result of such understanding may be the development of clinical therapies that can actively influence the process of reconstitution, resulting in improved outcomes for patients suffering from the ravages of immunodeficiency.

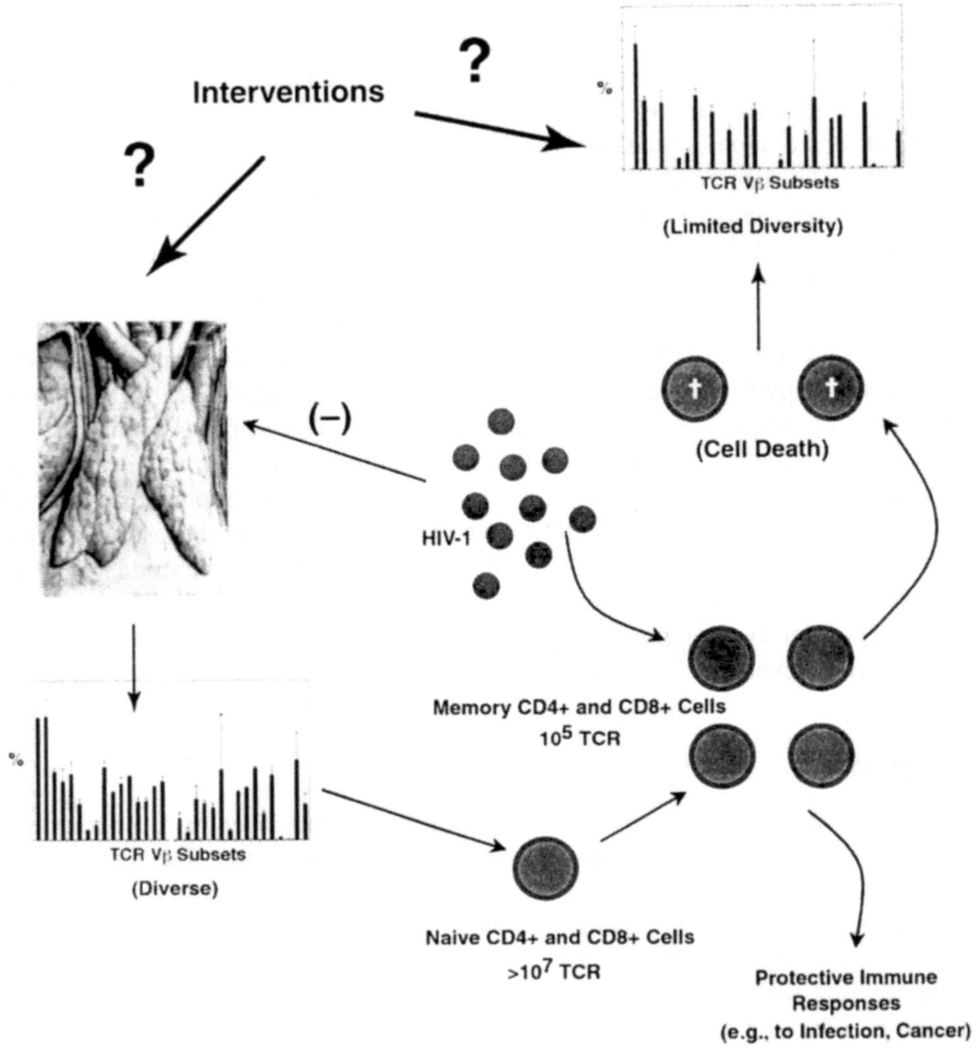

Fig. 5. Overview of lymphoid diversity and reconstitution. Thymic output is diverse (depicted by a normal TCR Vβ profile) and leads to generation of a broad naive T-cell repertoire. The memory T-cell repertoire is less diverse, and prone to attack by HIV-1, leading to cell death and a diminished TCR repertoire. HIV-1 may also directly suppress thymopoiesis. The effects of interventions (e.g., HAART) on thymopoiesis and on the peripheral T cell repertoire need to be studied further.

REFERENCES

1. McCune JM. HIV-1: the infective process in vivo. Cell 1991; 64:351–63.
2. Pantaleo G, Graziosi C, Fauci AS. The immunopathogenesis of human immunodeficiency virus infection. N Engl J Med 1993; 328:327–35.
3. Palella FJ, Delaney KM, Moorman AC, Loveless MO, Fuhrer J, Satten GA, et al. Declining morbidity and mortality among patients with advanced human immunodeficiency virus infection. N Engl J Med 1998; 338:853–60.

4. Autran B, Carcelain G, Li TS, Blanc C, Mathez D, Tubiana R, et al. Positive effects of combined antiretroviral therapy on CD4+ T cell homeostasis and function in advanced HIV disease. Science 1997; 277:112–6.
5. Gorochov G, Neumann AU, Kereveur A, Parizot C, Li T, Katlama C, et al. Perturbation of CD4+ and CD8+ T-cell repertoires during progression to AIDS and regulation of the CD4+ repertoire during antiviral therapy. Nat Med 1998; 4:215–21.
6. Li TS, Tubiana R, Katlama C, Calvez V, Ait Mohand H, Autran B. Long-lasting recovery in CD4 T-cell function and viral-load reduction after highly active antiretroviral therapy in advanced HIV-1 disease. Lancet 1998; 351:1682–6.
7. Komanduri KV, Viswanathan MN, Wieder ED, Schmidt DK, Bredt BM, Jacobson MA, McCune JM. Restoration of cytomegalovirus-specific CD4+ T-lymphocyte responses after ganciclovir and highly active antiretroviral therapy in individuals infected with HIV-1. Nat Med 1998; 4:953–6.
8. Lederman MM, Connick E, Landay A, Kuritzkes DR, Spritzler J, St. Clair M, et al. Immunologic responses associated with 12 weeks of combination antiretroviral therapy consisting of zidovudine, lamivudine, and ritonavir: results of AIDS Clinical Trials Group Protocol 315. J Infect Dis 1998; 178:70–9.
9. Connors M, Kovacs JA, Krevat S, Gea-Banacloche JC, Sneller MC, Flanigan M, et al. HIV infection induces changes in CD4+ T-cell phenotype and depletions within the CD4+ T-cell repertoire that are not immediately restored by antiviral or immune-based therapies. Nat Med 1997; 3:533–40.
10. Jacobson MA, Zegans M, Pavan PR, O'Donnell JJ, Sattler F, Rao N, et al. Cytomegalovirus retinitis after initiation of highly active antiretroviral therapy. Lancet 1997; 349:1443–5.
11. Miller JFAP. Immunological function of the thymus. Lancet 1961; ii:748–9.
12. Miller JFAP. Immunological significance of the thymus of the adult mouse. Nature 1962; 195:1318–9.
13. Gowans JL, McGregor DD, Cowen DM, Ford CE. Initiation of immune responses by small lymphocytes. Nature 1962; 196:651–5.
14. Miller JF, Mitchell GF. The thymus and the precursors of antigen reactive cells. Nature 1967; 216:659–63.
15. Brummendorf TH, Dragowska W, Zijlmans J, Thornbury G, Lansdorp PM. Asymmetric cell divisions sustain long-term hematopoiesis from single-sorted human fetal liver cells. J Exp Med 1998; 188:1117–24.
16. Morrison SJ, Wright DE, Cheshier SH, Weissman IL. Hematopoietic stem cells: challenges to expectations. Curr Opin Immunol 1997; 9:216–21.
17. Haynes BF, Heinly CS. Early human T cell development: analysis of the human thymus at the time of initial entry of hematopoietic stem cells into the fetal thymic microenvironment. J Exp Med 1995; 181:1445–58.
18. Gale RP. Development of the immune system in the human fetal liver. Thymus 1987; 10:45–52.
19. Schmitt C, Ktorza S, Sarun S, Verpilleux MP, Blanc C, Deugnier MA, et al. CD34-positive early stages of human T-cell differentiation. Leuk Lymph 1995; 17:43–50.
20. Spits H. Early stages in human and mouse T-cell development. Curr Opin Immunol 1994; 6:212–21.
21. Scollay R, Smith J, Stauffer V. Dynamics of early T cells: prothymocyte migration and proliferation in the adult mouse thymus. Immunol Rev 1986; 91:129–57.
22. Baum CM, Weissman IL, Tsukamoto AS, Buckle AM, Peault B. Isolation of a candidate human hematopoietic stem cell population. Proc Natl Acad Sci USA 1992; 89:2804–8.
23. Galy A, Verma S, Bárcena A, Spits H. Precursors of CD3+ CD4+ CD8+ cells in the human thymus are defined by expression of CD34. Delineation of early events in human thymic development. J Exp Med 1993; 178:391–401.

24. Res P, Martínez-Cáceres E, Cristina Jaleco A, Staal F, Noteboom E, Weijer K, Spits H. CD34+ CD38dim cells in the human thymus can differentiate into T, natural killer, and dendritic cells but are distinct from pluripotent stem cells. Blood 1996; 87:5196–206.
25. Barcena A, Galy AH, Punnonen J, Muench MO, Schols D, Roncarolo MG, et al. Lymphoid and myeloid differentiation of fetal liver CD34+-lineage cells in human thymic organ culture. J Exp Med 1994; 180:123–32.
26. Blom B, Res P, Noteboom E, Weijer K, Spits H. Prethymic CD34+ progenitors capable of developing into T cells are not committed to the T cell lineage. J Immunol 1997; 158:3571–7.
27. Ramiro AR, Trigueros C, Márquez C, San Millán JL, Toribio ML. Regulation of pre-T cell receptor (pT alpha-TCR beta) gene expression during human thymic development. J Exp Med 1996; 184:519–30.
28. Fehling HJ, von Boehmer H. Early alpha beta T cell development in the thymus of normal and genetically altered mice. Curr Opin Immunol 1997; 9:263–75.
28a. Kong F, Chen CH, Cooper MD. Thymic function can be accurately monitored by the level of recent T cell emigrants in the circulation. Immunity 1998; 8:97–104.
29. McCune JM. Development and applications of the SCID-hu mouse model. Semin Immunol 1996; 8:187–96.
30. Weissman IL. Thymus cell maturation. Studies on the origin of cortisone-resistant thymic lymphocytes. J Exp Med 1973; 137:504–10.
31. Fathman CG, Small M, Herzenberg LA, Weissman IL. Thymus cell maturation. II. Differentiation of three "mature" subclasses in vivo. Cell Immunol 1975; 15:109–28.
32. Dunon D, Imhof BA. Mechanisms of thymus homing. Blood 1993; 81:1–8.
33. Wu L, Li C, Shortman K. Thymic dendritic cell precursors: relationship to the T lymphocyte lineage and phenotype of the dendritic cell progeny. J Exp Med 1996; 184:903–11.
34. Galy AHM, Cen D, Travis M, Chen S, Chen BP. Delination of T-progenitor activity within the CD34+ compartment of adult bone marrow. Blood 1995; 85:2770–78.
35. Galy A, Travis M, Cen D, Chen B. Human T, B, natural killer, and dendritic cells arise from a common bone marrow progenitor cell subset. Immunity 1995; 3:459–73.
36. Miller JS, Verfaillie C, McGlave P. The generation of human natural killer cells from CD34+/DR− primitive progenitors in long-term bone marrow culture. Blood 1992; 69:2182–7.
37. Sánchez MJ, Muench MO, Roncarolo MG, Lanier LL, Phillips JH. Identification of a common T/natural killer cell progenitor in human fetal thymus. J Exp Med 1994; 180:569–76.
38. Zúñiga-Pflücker JC, Lenardo MJ. Regulation of thymocyte development from immature progenitors. Curr Opin Immunol 1996; 8:215–24.
39. Wu L, Scollay R, Egerton M, Pearse M, Spangrude GJ, Shortman K. CD4 expressed on earliest T-lineage precursor cells in the adult murine thymus. Nature 1991; 349:71–4.
40. Godfrey DI, Zlotnik A, Suda T. Phenotypic and functional characterization of c-*kit* expression during intrathymic T cell development. J Immunol 1992; 149:2281–5.
41. Godfrey DI, Kennedy J, Suda T, Zlotnik A. A developmental pathway involving four phenotypically and functionally distinct sets of CD3− CD4− CD8− triple-negative adult mouse thymocytes defined by CD44 and CD25 expression. J Immunol 1993; 150:4244–52.
42. Godfrey DI, Kennedy J, Mombaerts P, Tonegawa S, Zlotnik A. Onset of TCR beta gene rearrangement and role of TCR beta expression during CD3− CD4− CD8− thymocyte differentiation. J Immunol 1994; 152:4783–92.
43. Wurch A, Biro J, Potocnik A, Falk I, Mossmann H, Eichmann K. Requirement of CD3 complex-associated signaling functions for expression of rearranged T cell recepter beta VDJ genes in early thymic development. J Exp Med 1998; 188:1669–78.
44. Saint-Ruf C, Ungewiss K, Groettrup M, Bruno L, Fehling HJ, von Boehmer H. Analysis and expression of a cloned pre-T cell receptor gene. Science 1994; 266:1208–12.

45. Owen MJ, Venkitaraman AR. Signalling in lymphocyte development. Curr Opin Immunol 1996; 8:191–8.
46. Trigueros C, Ramiro AR, Carrasco YR, de Yebenes VG, Albar JP, Tiribio ML. Identification of a late stage of small noncycling pT-alpha negative T cells as immediate precursors of T cell receptor alpha/beta thymocytes. J Exp Med 1998; 188:1401–12.
47. Kraft DL, Weissman IL, Waller EK. Differentiation of $CD3^- 4^- 8^-$ human fetal thymocytes in vivo: characterization of a $CD3^- 4^+ 8^-$ intermediate. J Exp Med 1993; 178:265–77.
48. Guidos CJ. Positive selection of $CD4^+$ and $CD8^+$ T cells. Curr Opin Immunol 1996; 8:225–32.
49. Vanhecke D, Leclercq G, Plum J, Vandekerckhove B. Characterization of distinct stages during the differentiation of human $CD69^+$ $CD3^+$ thymocytes and identification of thymic emigrants. J Immunol 1995; 155:1862–72.
50. Vanhecke D, Verhasselt B, Debacker V, Leclercq G, Plum J, Vandekerckhove B. Differentiation to T helper cells in the thymus. Gradual acquisition of T helper cell function by $CD3^+$ $CD4^+$ cells. J Immunol 1995; 155:4711–8.
51. Res P, Blom B, Hori T, Weijer K, Spits H. Downregulation of CD1 marks acquisition of functional maturation of human thymocytes and defines a control point in late stages of human T cell development. Journal of Exp Med 1997; 185:141–51.
52. Benoist C, Mathis D. Positive selection of T cells: fastidious or promiscuous? Curr Opin Immunol 1997; 9:245–9.
53. Marrack P, Kappler J. Positive selection of thymocytes bearing alpha beta T cell receptors. Curr Opin Immunol 1997; 9:250–5.
54. Lucas B, Germain RN. T-cell repertoire: political correctness in the immune system. Curr Biol 1996; 6:783–7.
55. Ashton-Rickardt PG, Bandeira A, Delaney JR, Van Kaer L, Pircher HP, Zinkernagel RM, Tonegawa S. Evidence for a differential avidity model of T cell selection in the thymus. Cell 1994; 76:651–63.
56. Sebzda E, Wallace VA, Mayer J, Yeung RS, Mak TW, Ohashi PS. Positive and negative thymocyte selection induced by different concentrations of a single peptide. Science 1994; 263:1615–8.
57. Hogquist KA, Jameson CS, Heath WR, Howard JL, Bevan MJ, Carbone FR. T cell receptor antagonist peptides induce positive selection. Cell 1994; 76:17–27.
58. Hogquist KA, Tomlinson AJ, Kieper WC, McGargill MA, Hart MC, Naylor S, Jameson SC. Identification of a naturally occurring ligand for thymic positive selection. Immunity 1997; 6:389–99.
59. Pawlowski TJ, Singleton MD, Loh DY, Berg R, Staerz UD. Permissive recognition during positive selection. Eur J Immunol 1996; 26:851–7.
60. Nakano N, Rooke R, Benoist C, Mathis D. Positive selection of T cells induced by viral delivery of neopeptides to the thymus. Science 1997; 275:678–83.
61. Ding YH, Smith KJ, Garboczi DN, Utz U, Biddison WE, Wiley DC. Two human T cell receptors bind in a similar diagonal mode to the HLA-A2/Tax peptide complex using different TCR amino acids. Immunity 1998; 8:403–11.
62. Janeway CA, Jr. A tale of two T cells. Immunity 1998; 8:391–4.
63. van Meerwijk JPM, Marguerat S, Lees RK, Germain RN, Fowlkes BJ, MacDonald HR. Quantitative impact of thymic clonal deletion on the T cell repertoire. J Exp Med 1997; 185:377–84.
64. Simpson E, Takacs K, Altmann DM. Thymic repertoire selection by superantigens: presentation by human and mouse MHC molecules. Thymus 1994; 23:1–13.
65. Abe R, Vacchio MS, Fox B, Hodes RJ. Preferential expression of the T-cell receptor V beta 3 gene by Mlsc reactive T cells. Nature 1988; 335:827–30.
66. Choi YW, Herman A, DiGiusto D, Wade T, Marrack P, Kappler J. Residues of the variable region of the T-cell-receptor beta-chain that interact with S. aureus toxin superantigens. Nature 1990; 346:471–3.

67. Choi Y, Kappler JW, Marrack P. A superantigen encoded in the open reading frame of the 3′ long terminal repeat of mouse mammary tumour virus. Nature 1991; 350:203–7.
68. Kappler JW, Staerz U, White J, Marrack PC. Self-tolerance eliminates T cells specific for Mls-modified products of the major histocompatibility complex. Nature 1988; 332:35–40.
69. Pullen AM, Marrack P, Kappler JW. The T-cell repertoire is heavily influenced by tolerance to polymorphic self-antigens. Nature 1988; 335:796–801.
70. Jenkinson EJ, Anderson G, Owen JJT. Studies on T-cell maturation on defined thymic stromal cells *in vitro.* J Exp Med 1992; 176:845–53.
71. Baccala R, Vandekerckhove BA, Jones D, Kono DH, Roncarolo MG, Theofilopoulos AN. Bacterial superantigens mediate T cell deletions in the mouse severe combined immunodeficiency-human liver/thymus model. J Exp Med 1993; 177:1481–5.
72. Waller EK, Sen-Majumdar A, Kamel OW, Hansteen GA, Schick MR, Weissman IL. Human T-cell development in SCID-hu mice: staphylococcal enterotoxins induce specific clonal deletions, proliferation, and anergy. Blood 1992; 80:3144–56.
73. Komanduri KV, Salha MD, Sékaly RP, McCune JM. Superantigen-mediated deletion of specific T cell receptor V beta subsets in the SCID-hu Thy/Liv mouse is induced by staphylococcal enterotoxin B, but not HIV-1. J Immunol 1997; 158:544–9.
74. Owen JJ, Moore NC. Thymocyte-stromal-cell interactions and T-cell selection. Immunol Today 1995; 16:336–8.
75. Sprent J, Webb SR. Intrathymic and extrathymic clonal deletion of T cells. Curr Opin Immunol 1995; 7:196–205.
76. Vandekerckhove BA, Namikawa R, Bacchetta R, Roncarolo MG. Human hematopoietic cells and thymic epithelial cells induce tolerance via different mechanisms in the SCID-hu mouse thymus. J Exp Med 1992; 175:1033–43.
77. Klein L, Klein T, Rüther U, Kyewski B. CD4 T cell tolerance to human C-reactive protein, an inducible serum protein, is mediated by medullary thymic epithelium. J Exp Med 1998; 188:5–16.
78. Pugliese A, Zeller M, Fernandez JA, Zalcberg LJ, Bartlett RJ, Ricordi C, et al. The insulin gene is transcribed in the human thymus and transcription levels correlate with allelic variation at the *INS* VNTR-*IDDM2* susceptibility locus for type 1 diabetes. Nat Genet 1997; 15:293–7.
79. Vafiadis P, Bennet ST, Todd JA, Nadeau J, Grabs R, Goodyer CG, et al. Insulin expression in human thymus is modulated by *INS* VNTR alleles at the *IDDM2* locus. Nat Genet 1997; 15:289–92.
80. Egwuagu CE, Charukamnoetkanok P, Gery I. Thymic expression of autoantigens correlates with resistance to autoimmune disease. J Immunol 1997; 159:3109–12.
81. Heath V, Mason D, Ramirez F, Seddon B. Homeostatic mechanisms in the control of autoimmunity. Semin Immunol 1997; 9:375–80.
82. Anderson G, Moore NC, Owen JJ, Jenkinson EJ. Cellular interactions in thymocyte development. Annu Rev Immunol 1996; 14:73–99.
83. Boyd RL, Tucek CL, Godfrey DI, Izon DJ, Wilson TJ, Davidson NJ, et al. The thymic microenvironment. Immunol Today 1993; 14:445–59.
84. Denning SM, Kurtzberg J, Le PT, Tuck DT, Singer KH, Haynes BF. Human thymic epithelial cells directly induce activation of autologous immature thymocytes. Proc Natl Acad Sci USA 1988; 85:3125–9.
85. Berkowitz RD, Alexander S, Bare C, Linquist-Stepps V, Bogan M, Moreno ME, et al. CCR5 and CXCR4-utilizing strains of human immunodeficiency virus type 1 exhibit differential tropism and pathogenesis *in vivo.* J Virol 1998; 72:10108–17.
86. Namen AE, Lupton S, Hjerrild K, Wignall J, Mochizuki DY, Schmierer A, et al. Stimulation of B-cell progenitors by cloned murine interleukin-7. Nature 1988; 333:571–3.
87. Komschlies KL, Grzegorzewski KJ, Wiltrout RH. Diverse immunological and hematological effects of interleukin 7: implications for clinical application. J Leuk Biol 1995; 58:623–33.

88. Sudo T, Nishikawa S, Ohno N, Akiyama N, Tamakoshi M, Yoshida H. Expression and function of the interleukin 7 receptor in murine lymphocytes. Proc Natl Acad Sci USA 1993; 90:9125–9.
89. Maraskovsky E, O'Reilly LA, Teepe M, Corcoran LM, Peschon JJ, Strasser A. Bcl-2 can rescue T lymphocyte development in interleukin-7 receptor-deficient mice but not in mutant rag-$1^{-/-}$ mice. Cell 1997; 89:1011–9.
90. Akashi K, Kondo M, von Freeden-Jeffry U, Murray R, Weissman IL. Bcl-2 rescues T lymphopoiesis in interleukin-7 receptor-deficient mice. Cell 1997; 89:1033–41.
91. Schmitt C, Ktorza S, Sarun S, Blanc C, De Jong R, Debre P. CD34-expressing human thymocyte precursors proliferate in response to interleukin-7 but have lost myeloid differentiation potential. Blood 1993; 82:3675–85.
92. Varas A, Vicente A, Sacedón R, Zapata AG. Interleukin-7 influences the development of thymic dendritic cells. Blood 1998; 92:93–100.
93. Bolotin E, Smogorzewska M, Smith S, Widmer M, Weinberg K. Enhancement of thymopoiesis after bone marrow transplant by in vivo interleukin-7. Blood 1996; 88:1887–94.
94. Napolitano LA, Grant RM, Schmidt DK, De Rosa SC, Herzenberg LA, Deeks SG et al. Circulating interleukin-7 levels are correlated with CD4+ lymphopenia and viral load in HIV-1 infected individuals: implications for disease progression. Nature Med 2001; 7: 73–9.
95. Fry TJ, Connick E, Landay A, Lederman MM, Wood LV, Yarchoan R, Mackall CL. A potential role for IL-7 in T-cell homeostasis in HIV-infected patients. 7th Conf on Retrovirus & Opportunistic Infections presented at San Francisco, 2000.
96. Lyman SD. Biology of flt3 ligand and receptor. Int J Hematol 1995; 62:63–73.
97. Lyman SD, James L, Vanden Bos T, de Vries P, Brasel K, Gliniak B, et al. Molecular cloning of a ligand for the flt3/flk-2 tyrosine kinase receptor: a proliferative factor for primitive hematopoietic cells. Cell 1993; 75:1157–67.
98. Lyman SD, Jacobsen SE. c-kit ligand and Flt3 ligand: stem/progenitor cell factors with overlapping yet distinct activities. Blood 1998; 91:1101–34.
99. Rodewald HR, Kretzschmar K, Swat W, Takeda S. Intrathymically expressed c-kit ligand (stem cell factor) is a major factor driving expansion of very immature thymocytes in vivo. Immunity 1995; 3:313–9.
100. Rodewald HR, Ogawa M, Haller C, Waskow C, DiSanto JP. Pro-thymocyte expansion by c-kit and the common cytokine receptor gamma chain is essential for repertoire formation. Immunity 1997; 6:265–72.
101. Moore TA, Zlotnik A. Differential effects of Flk-2/Flt-3 ligand and stem cell factor on murine thymic progenitor cells. J Immunol 1997; 158:4187–92.
102. Frearson JA, Alexander DR. Protein tyrosine phosphatases in T-cell development, apoptosis and signalling. Immunol Today 1996; 17:385–91.
103. Schmedt C, Saijo K, Niidome T, Kuhn R, Aizawa S, Tarakhovsky A. Csk controls antigen receptor-mediated development and selection of T-lineage cells. Nature 1998; 394:901–4.
104. Shao H, Kono DH, Chen L-Y, Rubin EM, Kaye J. Induction of the early growth response (Egr) family of transcription factors during thymic selection. J Exp Med 1997; 185:731–44.
105. Ting C-N, Olson MC, Barton KP, Leiden JM. Transcription factor GATA-3 is required for development of the T-cell lineage. Nature 1996; 384:474–8.
106. Williams O, Norton T, Halligey M, Kioussis D, Brady HJM. The action of bax and bcl-2 on T cell selection. J Exp Med 1998; 188:1125–33.
107. Amakawa R, Hakem A, Kundig TM, Matsuyama T, Simard JJ, Timms E, et al. Impaired negative selection of T cells in Hodgkin's disease antigen CD30-deficient mice. Cell 1996; 84:551–62.
108. Bell EB, Sparshott SM, Bunce C. $CD4^+$ T cell memory, CD45R subsets and the persistence of antigen—a unifying concept. Immunol Today 1998; 19:60–4.
109. Butcher EC, Picker LJ. Lymphocyte homing and homeostasis. Science 1996; 272:60–6.

110. Rothbard JB, Gefter ML. Interactions between immunogenic peptides and MHC proteins. Annu Rev Immunol 1991; 9:527–65.
111. Bretscher P. The two-signal model of lymphocyte activation twenty-one years later. Immunol Today 1992; 13:74–9.
112. Croft M, Dubey C. Accessory molecule and costimulation requirements for CD4 T cell response. Crit Rev Immunol 1997; 17:89–118.
113. Viola A, Lanzavecchia A. T cell activation determined by T cell receptor number and tunable thresholds. Science 1996; 273:104–6.
114. Lu L, Qian S, Hershberger PA, Rudert WA, Lynch DH, Thomson AW. Fas ligand (CD95L) and B7 expression on dendritic cells provide counter-regulatory signals for T cell survival and proliferation. J Immunol 1997; 158:5676.
115. McLeod JD, Walker LSK, Patel YI, Boulougouris G, Sansom DM. Activation of human T cells with superantigen (staphylococcal enterotoxin B) and CD28 confers resistance to apoptosis via CD95. J Immunol 1998; 160:2072–79.
116. Ahmed R, Gray D. Immunological memory and protective immunity: understanding their relation. Science 1996; 272:54–60.
117. Farber DL. Differential TCR signaling and the generation of memory T cells. J Immunol 1998; 160:535–9.
118. Sprent J, Tough DF. Lymphocyte life-span and memory. Science 1994; 265:1395–400.
119. Farber DL, Acuto O, Bottomly K. Differential T cell receptor-mediated signaling in naive and memory CD4 T cells. Eur J Immunol 1997; 27:2094–101.
120. Busch DH, Pilip I, Pamer EG. Evolution of a complex T cell receptor repertoire during primary and recall bacterial infection. J Exp Med 1998; 188:61–70.
121. Sourdive DJ, Murali-Krishna K, Altman JD, Zajac AJ, Whitmire JK, Pannetier C, et al. Conserved T cell receptor repertoire in primary and memory CD8 T cell responses to an acute viral infection. J Exp Med 1998; 188:71–82.
122. Ogg GS, McMichael AJ. HLA-peptide tetrameric complexes. Curr Opin Immunol 1998; 10:393–6.
123. Sallusto F, Lenig D, Forster R, Lipp M, Lanzavecchia A. Two subsets of memory T lymphocytes with distinct homing potentials and effector functions. Nature 1999; 401:708–12.
124. Michie CA, McLean A, Alcock C, Beverley PC. Lifespan of human lymphocyte subsets defined by CD45 isoforms. Nature 1992; 360:264–5.
125. Bunce C, Bell EB. CD45RC isoforms define two types of CD4 memory T cells, one of which depends on persisting antigen. J Exp Med 1997; 185:767–76.
126. Roederer M, Dubs JG, Anderson MT, Raju PA, Herzenberg LA. CD8 naive T cell counts decrease progressively in HIV-infected adults. J Clin Invest 1995; 95:2061–6.
127. Richards D, Chapman MD, Sasama J, Lee TH, Kemeny DM. Immune memory in $CD4^+$ $CD45RA^+$ T cells. Immunology 1997; 91:331–9.
128. Abbas A, Murphy KM, Sher A. Functional diversity of helper T lymphocytes. Nature 1996; 383:787–93.
129. Romagnani S. The Th1/Th2 paradigm. Immunol Today 1997; 18:263–6.
130. Clerici M, Shearer G. The Th1-Th2 hypothesis of HIV infection: new insights. Immunol Today 1994; 15:575–81.
131. Mitra DK, De Rosa SC, Luke A, Balamurugan A, Khaitan BK, Tung J, et al. Differential representations of memory T cell subsets are characteristic of polarized immunity in leprosy and atopic diseases. Int Immunol 1999; 11:1801–10.
132. Lee PP, Yee C, Savage PA, Fong L, Brockstedt D, Weber JS, et al. Characterization of circulating T cells specific for tumor-associated antigens in melanoma patients. Nat Med 1999; 5:677–85.
133. Ridge JP, Di Rosa F, Matzinger P. A conditioned dendritic cell can be a temporal bridge between a $CD4^+$ T-helper and a T-killer cell. Nature 1998; 393:474–8.

134. Bennett SR, Carbone FR, Karamalis F, Flavell RA, Miller JF, Heath WR. Help for cytotoxic-T-cell responses is mediated by CD40 signalling. Nature 1998; 393:478–80.
135. Schoenberger SP, Toes RE, van der Voort EI, Offringa R, Melief CJ. T-cell help for cytotoxic T lymphocytes is mediated by CD40-CD40L interactions. Nature 1998; 393:480–3.
136. Mackey MF, Gunn JR, Maliszewsky C, Kikutani H, Noelle RJ, Barth RJ Jr. Dendritic cells require maturation via CD40 to generate protective antitumor immunity. J Immunol 1998; 161:2094–8.
137. Lord GM, Matarese G, Howard LK, Baker RJ, Bloom SR, Lechler RI. Leptin modulates the T-cell immune response and reverses starvation-induced immunosuppression. Nature 1998; 394:897–901.
138. Munn DH, Zhou M, Attwood JT, Bondarev I, Conway SJ, Marshall B, et al. Prevention of allogeneic fetal rejection by tryptophan catabolism. Science 1998; 281:1191–3.
139. Adleman LM, Wofsy D. T cell homeostasis: implications in HIV infection. J AIDS 1993; 6:144–52.
140. Margolick JB, Donnenberg AD. T-cell homeostasis in HIV-1 infection. Semin Immunol 1997; 9:381–8.
141. Mehr R, Perelson AS, Fridkis-Hareli M, Globerson A. Regulatory feedback pathways in the thymus. Immunol Today 1997; 18:581–5.
142. Mehr R, Perelson AS. Blind T-cell homeostasis and the CD4/CD8 ratio in the thymus and peripheral blood. J AIDS Hum Retrovirol 1997; 14:387–98.
143. Bell EB, Sparshott SM. The peripheral T-cell pool: regulation by non-antigen induced proliferation? Semin Immunol 1997; 9:347–53.
144. Tanchot C, Rocha B. The peripheral T cell repertoire: independent homeostatic regulation of virgin and activated $CD8^+$ T cell pools. Eur J Immunol 1995; 25:2127–36.
145. Mackall CL, Gress RE. Pathways of T-cell regeneration in mice and humans: implications for bone marrow transplantation and immunotherapy. Immunol Rev 1997; 157:61–72.
146. Mackall CL, Hakim FT, Gress RE. Restoration of T-cell homeostasis after T-cell depletion. Semin Immunol 1997; 9:339–46.
147. Mackall CL, Granger L, Sheard MA, Cepeda R, Gress RE. T-cell regeneration after bone marrow transplantation: differential CD45 isoform expression on thymic-derived versus thymic-independent progeny. Blood 1993; 82:2585–94.
148. Mackall CL, Bare CV, Granger LA, Sharrow SO, Titus JA, Gress RE. Thymic-independent T cell regeneration occurs via antigen-driven expansion of peripheral T cells resulting in a repertoire that is limited in diversity and prone to skewing. J Immunol 1996; 156:4609–16.
149. Waldrop SL, Pitcher CJ, Peterson DM, Maino VC, Picker LJ. Determination of antigen-specific memory/effector $CD4^+$T cell frequencies by flow cytometry: evidence for a novel, antigen-specific homeostatic mechanism in HIV-associated immunodeficiency. J Clin Invest 1997; 99:1739–50.
150. McCune JM. Thymic function in HIV-1 disease. Semin Immunol 1997; 9(6):397–404.
151. Steinmann GG. Changes in the human thymus during aging. Curr Top Pathol 1986; 75:43–88.
152. Moore AV, Korobkin M, Olanow W, Heaston DK, Ram PC, Dunnick NR, Silverman PM. Age-related changes in the thymus gland: CT-pathologic correlation. AJR 1983; 141:241–6.
153. Francis IR, Glazer GM, Brookstein FL, Gross BH. The thymus: reexamination of age-related changes in size and shape. Am J Roentgenol 1985; 145:249–54.
154. Dixon AK, Hilton CJ, Williams GT. Computed tomography and histological correlation of the thymic remnant. Clin Radiol 1981; 32:255–7.
155. Lum LG. The kinetics of immune reconstitution after human marrow transplantation. Blood 1987; 69:369–80.
156. Parkman R, Weinberg KI. Immunological reconstitution following bone marrow transplantation. Immunol Rev 1997; 157:73–8.
157. Guillaume T, Rubinstein DB, Symann M. Immune reconstitution and immunotherapy after autologous hematopoietic stem cell transplantation. Blood 1998; 92:1471–90.

158. Choyke PL, Zeman RK, Gootenberg JE, Greenberg JN, Hoffer F, Frank JA. Thymic atrophy and regrowth in response to chemotherapy: CT evaluation. Am J Roentgenol 1987; 149:269–72.
159. Small EJ, Venook AP, Damon LE. Gallium-avid thymic hyperplasia in an adult after chemotherapy for Hodgkin disease. Cancer 1993; 72:905–8.
160. Miniero R, Busca A, Leonardo E, Mossetti C, Machado D, Vassallo E, Madon E. Rebound thymic hyperplasia following high dose chemotherapy and allogeneic BMT. Bone Marrow Transplant 1993; 11:67–70.
161. Chertoff J, Barth RA, Dickerman JD. Rebound thymic hyperplasia five years after chemotherapy for Wilms' tumor. Pediatr Radiol 1991; 21:596–7.
162. Mackall CL, Fleisher TA, Brown MR, Andrich MP, Chen CC, Feuerstein IM, et al. Age, thymopoiesis, and $CD4^+$ T-lymphocyte regeneration after intensive chemotherapy. N Engl J Med 1995; 332:143–9.
163. Roederer M, De Rosa SC, Watanabe N, Herzenberg LA. Dynamics of fine T-cell subsets during HIV disease and after thymic ablation by mediastinal irradiation. Semin Immunol 1997; 9:389–96.
164. Watanabe N, De Rosa SC, Cmelak A, Hoppe R, Herzenberg LA, Roederer M. Long-term depletion of naive T cells in patients treated for Hodgkin's disease. Blood 1997; 90:3662–72.
165. Beagley KW, Husband AJ. Intraepithelial lymphocytes: origins, distribution, and function. Crit Rev Immunol 1998; 18:237–54.
166. Clegg CH, Rulffes JT, Wallace PM, Haugen HS. Regulation of an extrathymic T-cell development pathway by oncostatin M. Nature 1996; 384:261–3.
167. García-Ojeda ME, Dejbakhsh-Jones S, Weissman IL, Strober S. An alternate pathway for T cell development supported by the bone marrow microenvironment: recapitulation of thymic maturation. J Exp Med 1998; 187:1813–23.
168. Heitger A, Neu N, Kern H, Panzer-Grümayer ER, Greinix H, Nachbaur D, et al. Essential role of the thymus to reconstitute naive ($CD45RA^+$) T-helper cells after human allogeneic bone marrow transplantation. Blood 1997; 90:850–7.
169. Mackall CL, Fleisher TA, Brown MR, Andrich MP, Chen CC, Feuerstein IM, et al. Distinctions between $CD8^+$ and $CD4^+$ T-cell regenerative pathways result in prolonged T-cell subset imbalance after intensive chemotherapy. Blood 1997; 89:3700–7.
170. Hellerstein MK, McCune JM. T cell turnover in HIV-1 disease. Immunity 1997; 7:583–9.
171. McCune JM, Loftus R, Schmidt DK, Carroll P, Webster D, Swor-Yim LB, et al. High prevalence of thymic tissue in adults with human immunodeficiency virus-1 infection. J Clin Invest 1998; 101:2301–8.
172. Rabin RL, Roederer M, Maldonado Y, Petru A, Herzenberg LA. Altered representation of naive and memory CD8 T cell subsets in HIV-infected children. J Clin Invest 1995; 95:2054–60.
173. Macallan DC, Fullerton CA, Neese RA, Haddock K, Park SS, Hellerstein MK. Measurement of cell proliferation by labeling of DNA with stable isotope-labeled glucose: studies *in vitro,* in animals, and in humans. Proc Natl Acad Sci USA 1998; 95:708–13.
174. Hellerstein M, Hanley MB, Cesar D, Siler S, Papageorgopoulos C, Wieder E, et al. Directly measured kinetics of circulating T lymphocytes in normal and HIV-1–infected humans. Nat Med 1999; 5:83–9.
175. McCune JM, Hanley MB, Cesar D, Halvorsen R, Hoh R, Schmidt D, et al. Factors influencing T-cell turnover in HIV-1–seropositive patients. J Clin Invest 2000; 105:R1–8.
176. Arstila TP, Casrouge A, Baron V, Even J, Kanellopoulos J, Kourilsky P. A direct estimate of the human alphabeta T cell receptor diversity. Science 1999; 286:958–61.
177. Lewis SM. The mechanism of V(D)J joining: lessons from molecular, immunological, and comparative analyses. Adv Immunol 1994; 56:27–150.
178. Lewis SM, Wu GE. The origins of V(D)J recombination. Cell 1997; 88:159–62.
179. Douek DC, McFarland RD, Keiser PH, Gage EA, Massey JM, Haynes BF, et al. Changes in thymic function with age and during the treatment of HIV infection. Nature 1998; 396:690–5.

180. Poulin JF, Viswanathan MN, Harris JM, Komanduri KV, Wieder E, Ringuette N, et al. Direct evidence for thymic function in adult humans. J Exp Med 1999; 190:479–86.
181. Zhang L, Lewin SR, Markowitz M, Lin HH, Skulsky E, Karanicolas R, et al. Measuring recent thymic emigrants in blood of normal and HIV-1–infected individuals before and after effective therapy. J Exp Med 1999; 190:725–32.
182. Hatzakis A, Touloumi G, Karanicolas R, Karafoulidou A, Mandalaki T, Anastassopopoulou C, et al. Effect of recent thymic emigrants on progression of HIV-1 disease. Lancet 2000; 355:599–604.
183. Douek DC, Vescio RA, Betts MR, Brenchley JM, Hill BJ, Zhang L, et al. Assessment of thymic output in adults after haematopoietic stem–cell transplant and prediction of T cell reconstitution. Lancet 2000; 355:1875–81.
184. Su L, Kaneshima H, Bonyhadi M, Salimi S, Kraft D, Rabin L, McCune JM. HIV-1–induced thymocyte depletion is associated with indirect cytopathogenicity and infection of progenitor cells in vivo. Immunity 1995; 2:25–36.
185. Jenkins M, Hanley MB, Moreno MB, Wieder E, McCune JM. Human immunodeficiency virus-1 infection interrupts thymopoiesis and multilineage hematopoiesis in vivo. Blood 1998; 91:2672–8.
186. McCune JM. Animal models of HIV-1 disease. Science 1997; 278:2141–2.

5
HIV Gene Products as Manipulators of the Immune System

Aram Mangasarian and Didier Trono

The spread of human immunodeficiency virus (HIV) in the body depends on its fitness to replicate and on its ability to escape immune defenses. The viral proteins Nef, Tat, and Env, best known for their direct effects on the viral life cycle, are also crucially engaged in manipulating various components of the immune system, both to prepare the ground for viral propagation and to facilitate immune evasion. This chapter reviews these lesser known functions of the three HIV gene products, which govern fascinating interactions between the virus and its host.

NEF, AN EARLY BIRD WITH MANY FUNCTIONS

The Nef protein, produced very early in the viral life cycle, is an important virulence factor for both HIV and Simian Immunodeficiency Virus (SIV) *(1–3)*. Three functions of Nef have been extensively characterized in vitro: 1) the downregulation of CD4 and MHC-I, 2) the alteration of T-cell activation pathways, and 3) the enhancement of virion infectivity (Fig 1). The first two reflect typical manipulations of the immune system by the virus.

CD4 and MHC-I Downregulation: A Tale of Bad Connections

Cells infected with HIV exhibit a marked downmodulation of two immune receptors, CD4 and class I major histocompatibility complex (MHC-I). In both cases, this primarily reflects the action of Nef. The main purpose of Nef-induced CD4 downregulation seems to be to protect viral infectivity. Indeed, high levels of CD4 on the surface of a virus producer cell result in sequestering the viral envelope, thereby blocking its virion incorporation. Nef-induced CD4 downregulation counteracts this effect, thus ensuring efficient viral spread *(3a)*. MHC-I downmodulation, on the other hand, prevents the efficient recognition and killing of HIV-infected cells by virus-specific cytotoxic T lymphocytes *(4)*. It therefore likely promotes immune escape and the establishment of a chronic infection.

CD4 downregulation is a highly conserved property of Nef proteins from all primate lentiviruses, including primary isolates of HIV and pathogenic clones of SIV *(5,6)*. Nef-induced CD4 downregulation is a two-step process: first, CD4 is rapidly endocytosed from the cell surface; second, it is targeted from early endosomes to lysosomes

From: *Retroviral Immunology: Immune Response and Restoration*
Edited by: Giuseppe Pantaleo and Bruce D. Walker © Humana Press Inc., Totowa, NJ

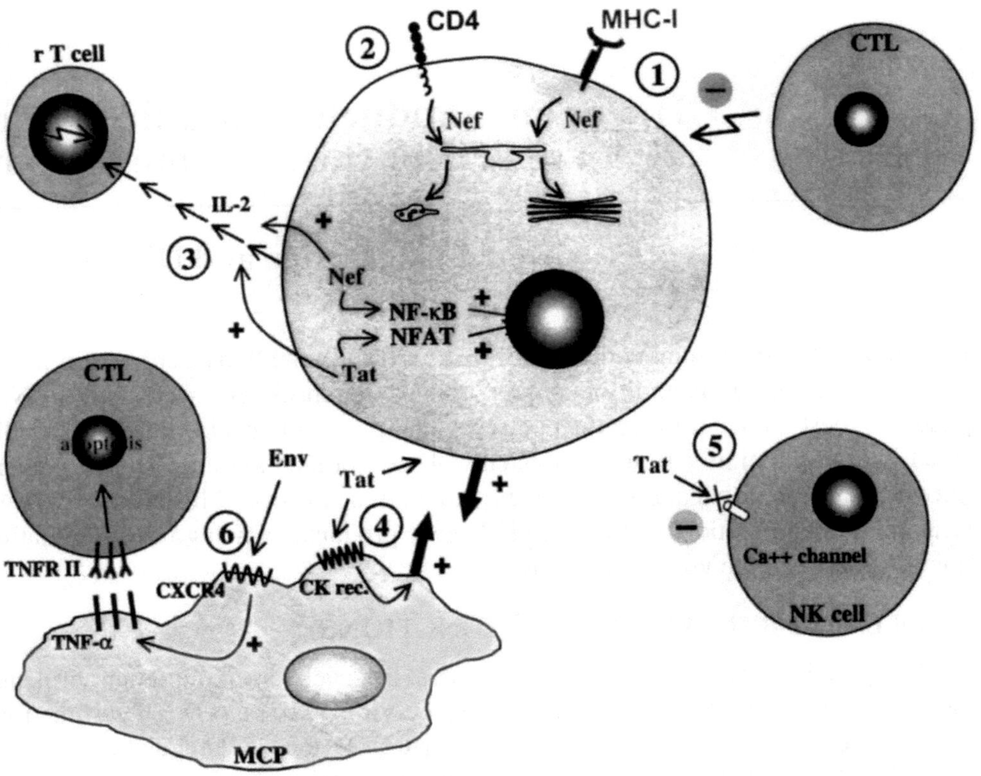

Fig. 1. Immunomodulating effects of HIV-1 proteins. The Nef, Tat, and Env proteins are synthesized in the HIV-infected T cell *(center)*. Nef downregulates the surface expression of MHC-I, thereby protecting this cell against the attacks of virus-specific CTL (1). Nef also downmodulates the immune receptor CD4 (2) and, together with Tat, potentiates the activation of the infected cell. The secretion of IL-2 is promoted, which in turn might render neighboring resting T cells (r T cell) permissive for infection (3). Tat released in the extracellular milieu can act on chemokine receptors (CK rec.) on the surface of macrophages (MCP), thus chemoattracting these targets in the infectious center. Tat also increases the motility of the infected cell itself (4), and inhibits NK cell activity by blocking calcium channels (5). Finally, the Env protein of X4 strains can activate the CXCR4 receptor on macrophages, triggering the TNF-mediated apoptosis of CTL (6).

(7–9). At both of these stages, Nef acts as a connector between CD4 and key components of the protein trafficking machinery. Nef binds to the cytoplasmic tail of CD4, recognizing a critical dileucine-based motif *(7,10,11)*. Chimeric integral membrane proteins harboring Nef as their cytoplasmic domain undergo accelerated internalization via clathrin coated pits at the plasma membrane and are subsequently targeted to lysosomes *(8)*. In addition, in the presence of CD4 or when tethered to the cellular membrane as part of an integral membrane protein, Nef can stimulate the *de novo* formation of clathrin coated pits *(12)*. Together, these results indicate that Nef harbors determinants that can interact with components of the endocytic machinery, and acts by recruiting these molecules beneath CD4.

The first downstream partner of Nef in this process is the adaptor protein (AP) complex of clathrin-coated pits *(9,13)*. Nef associates with APs, and this interaction is essential for efficient CD4 downregulation *(14–17)*. APs are heterotetrameric protein complexes that normally connect receptor cytoplasmic tails with clathrin, and exist in at least three varieties: AP-1 and AP-2, which mediate transport from the Golgi and plasma membrane, respectively *(18)*, and AP-3 which has recently been implicated in cargo-selective transport between the Golgi and the lysosome *(19)*. The Nef proteins of HIV and SIV can interact with all three subsets (*9*). Interestingly, a Carboxy (C)-terminal dileucine motif in HIV-1 Nef is important for AP recruitment *(14–16)*, while in HIV-2 and SIV an amino (N)-proximal tyrosine based signal plays an equivalent role *(9)*. Such convergent evolution emphasizes the biological importance of the Nef–AP interaction. That Nef connects CD4 with both AP-2 and AP-1 probably explains why, in the presence of the viral protein, the receptor is routed to endosomes both from the cell surface and from the *trans* Golgi network (TGN) *(8)*.

After internalization from the cell surface, CD4 reaches the early endosomes, from where it can either recycle to the plasma membrane or move to the late endosomes and lysosomes *(20)*. Nef influences this decision by connecting CD4 to another component of the endocytic machinery, β-COP, a component of COP-I coatomers *(21,22)*. The association of Nef with β-COP is essential for the lysosomal targeting of CD4 *(22)*.

Although it had been noted early on that HIV infection results in MHC-I downmodulation *(17,23)*. Nef was only recently identified as the factor responsible for this effect *(24)*. Like for CD4, Nef triggers the rapid endocytosis of MHC-I and its accelerated degradation *(24)*. However, the two receptors do not appear to be regulated through identical mechanisms. For instance, an interaction between Nef and adaptor complexes is not necessary for efficient MHC-I downmodulation *(14,25,26)*. Furthermore, distinct domains of Nef are necessary for either CD4 or MHC-I downmodulation *(16,26)*. Finally, an interaction between MHC-I and Nef has yet to be demonstrated.

Nef-induced MHC-I downregulation could in theory expose HIV-infected cells to the attacks of natural killer (NK) lymphocytes. However, Nef selectively modulates HLA-A and -B, but not HLA-C, because sensitivity to Nef requires a critical tyrosine residue found in the cytoplasmic tail of the first two, but not the third, groups of MHC-I molecules *(13)*. This stratagem is most astute, because HLA-C is a dominant negative inhibitor of NK recognition. A Tat-mediated inhibition of NK function may complete this effect (*see* p. 114).

Playing with T-Cell Activation Pathways

Abundant evidence points to an effect of Nef on cellular activation pathways. Transgenic mice (Tg) expressing the complete coding sequences of HIV-1 in $CD4^+$ T cells and in cells of the macrophage/dendritic lineages developed several AIDS-like pathologies *(27)*. This phenotype was recapitulated in Tg mice expressing only *nef*, whose thymocytes exhibited a state of hyperactivation and of α-CD3 hyperresponsiveness with increased tyrosine phosphorylation of several substrates, including linker for activation of T cells (LAT) and Erk1/Erk2 mitogen-activated protein (MAP) kinase. In an independent set of experiments, Tg mice that expressed HIV-1 *nef* in T lymphocytes displayed a state of T-cell hyperactivation in the thymus, with CD4 depletion and increased expression of activation markers in the rare mature CD4+ cells found in peripheral lymphoid tissues *(28–30).* In Jurkat human T-lymphoid cells, the surface expression of a CD8–Nef chimera resulted in the appearance of T cell activation markers, in the accumulation of tyrosine phosphorylated proteins, in the induction of NFκB activity and, ultimately, in cell death by apoptosis *(31).* In contrast, the intracytoplasmic accumulation of the CD8–Nef chimera was accompanied by an inhibition of TCR signaling *(31).* Studies in an IL-2–dependent rhesus monkey T-lymphoid cell line infected with herpesvirus saimiri further pointed to a role for Nef in T-cell activation: in the absence of IL-2, SIV strains containing the *nef* gene from either SIV or HIV-1 grew 8–100 times more efficiently in these cells than the same virus without *nef.* Furthermore, *nef*-positive viruses could induce IL-2 production *(32).* Finally, particular SIV Nef variants harboring amino acid sequences which resemble immunoreceptor tyrosine-based activation motifs (ITAMs) could replicate to high levels in peripheral blood mononuclear cells without a need for exogenous stimulation *(33).*

Although several reports have suggested that Nef inhibits lymphocyte activation *(34–42),* this may have reflected the inherent toxicity of Nef in cells functional for activation. Our recent results utilizing Jurkat cells that express Nef in an inducible manner indeed suggest that the viral protein primes T cells for activation *(43).* Moreover, we find that Nef associates with and modifies the content of so-called rafts, which are glycolipid-enriched subdomains of the plasma membrane in which the early events of T cell activation take place *(43).* Further biochemical characterization of the effect of Nef on these structures should shed light on these events.

Several molecular interactions constitute putative links between Nef and signal transduction pathways. Nef recognizes the SH3 domain of the Hck and Lyn nonreceptor protein tyrosine kinases via a conserved proline-rich motif in its core domain *(44–46).* Another interaction was detected between Nef and the T–cell-specific Lck tyrosine kinase, involving apparently both the N-terminus and the central region of the viral protein *(38,39,47).* Also, Nef liberates Lck from the cytoplasmic domain of CD4 when it triggers the accelerated endocytosis of this receptor, thereby increasing levels of free Lck in the cell *(7,48).* Finally, Nef can recruit a member of the p-21 activated kinase (PAK) family *(49–52)* as well as another yet unidentified serine/threonine kinase *(47),* and was found to associate with the theta isoform of protein kinase C (θPKC) *(53).* Members of the PAK family bind to GTPases including cdc42 and RAC1, and as such are the upstream components of a signaling cascade that leads to mitogen-activated protein kinases (MAPK) activation and IL-2 production.

The priming of T cells for activation likely promotes an environment supportive of virus production and propagation. Increased levels of IL-2, which have been observed in the lymph nodes of HIV-infected individuals *(54),* can indeed prime resting cells for infection by HIV-1 in an antigen-independent manner. IL-2 treatment alone of peripheral mononuclear cells is sufficient to render these targets susceptible to infection *(55).*

TAT: BEYOND TRANSACTIVATION

The HIV-1 Tat protein is best known as a potent transcriptional activator of the viral long-terminal repeat (LTR) required for efficient viral replication *(56,57).* An early viral gene product translated from multiply spliced mRNAs, Tat binds an RNA stem-loop structure (TAR) located at the 5′ end of the viral transcript to promote transcriptional elongation. The interaction between the transactivator and its RNA target is mediated by an arginine rich motif (ARM) in Tat, mapping between amino acids 49 and 58. The more N-terminal region of Tat functions as a transcriptional activation domain by recruiting cyclin T, which is bound in vivo to CDK9 *(58)*. CDK9 is a kinase is responsible for phosphorylating the C-terminal domain (CTD) of the RNA–Pol II transcription complex, a modification that augments the processivity of transcription *(58)*. Interestingly, the affinity of Tat for TAR is increased after the viral protein binds cyclin T, ensuring that the target RNA preferentially recruits forms of Tat that are competent for transactivation.

New evidence indicates that Tat plays other roles in HIV-induced pathogenesis, in addition to permitting viral gene expression *(59–63)*. Secreted from infected cells, Tat can indeed recruit new viral targets and can increase their ability to support viral replication. Furthermore, Tat contributes to shielding virus producer cells from some effectors of the innate immune response.

Tat as a Trans-attractant

Leukocytes migrate in response to gradients of chemokines, small cytokines often upregulated as part of the inflammation response. These soluble proteins can be divided into two families distinguished by the spacing of two prototypic cysteines: CC chemokines have two consecutive cysteine residues, while in CXC chemokines there is an intervening amino acid *(64)*. The chemokines trigger their effects through seven-transmembrane receptors coupled to pertussis toxin sensitive, cholera toxin insensitive G-proteins *(64)*. Within each family of chemokines, but not between families, there is considerable sharing of receptor usage. Thus one chemokine may signal to different cell through distinct receptors. In the CC family of receptors, for example, the chemokine MCP-1 (monocyte chemotactic protein-1) binds to CCR2 (CC chemokine receptor-2), and CCR4, while MCP-3 binds CCR1, CCR2, and CCR3. Eotaxin stands out in the CC-chemokine family as it only binds to one receptor, CCR3 *(64)*.

Extracellular Tat has can induce the chemotaxis of both monocytes and neutrophils, and progress has recently been made in understanding the molecular basis of this property *(61,65–67)*. Alignment of Tat with the MCP chemokines reveals a striking homology at the N-terminus *(66)*. Notably, the class-defining CCY sequence as well as an SYXR motif are found both in MCP chemokines and in Tat, with an intervening isoleucine residue at a position that is also conserved. Furthermore, these sequences are present in both HIV-1 and HIV-2 Tat, in spite of being dispensable for the transcriptional activation function of either protein. Conditioned medium from cell lines expressing Tat from the HIV-1 LTR promoter, containing approx 4 ng/mL of Tat, induced the chemotaxis of monocytes *(66)*. Similar levels of Tat have been found in the supernatants of HIV-1 III-B infected H9 cells and in patient serum, indicating that release of Tat is a normal byproduct of the viral life cycle *(62)*. Treating monocytes with 100 ng/mL (6.6 n*M*) of recombinant Tat resulted in significant calcium fluxes across the membrane, reminiscent of those seen following treatment with chemokines such as MCP-3 *(65)*. The calcium signaling correlated with increased migration, and both events could be abrogated by the addition of Tat-specific antibodies or by treating the recombinant Tat with heat or trypsin before use *(65)*. A further proof that Tat signals through the seven-transmembrane chemokine receptors was that pertussis toxin inhibited roughly 80% of the calcium signal generated by Tat, as would be predicted if the signals were generated through chemokine receptors *(65,66)*. The remaining signal is hypothesized to result from the interaction of Tat with other cell surface proteins, such as the integrin receptors *(68,69)*.

The chemotactic activity of Tat stems from its ability to bind chemokine receptors. This was demonstrated through desensitization analyses, which assess whether two agonists share receptors. Tat not only induced the partial desensitization of monocytes to MCP-1, MCP-3, and eotaxin, but also competed with MCP-1 and MCP-3 for binding sites on the plasma membrane of these cells *(65,66)*. Interestingly, when chemokines were used to desensitize monocytes against Tat, their efficiency was only partial, suggesting that the viral protein may interact with a broad range of chemokine receptors, some of which may yet be unidentified. Of note, all members of the MCP family with which Tat shares receptors are potent attractants not only for monocytes but also for activated T cells, and are more efficient at attracting cells across endothelial barriers than RANTES, MIP-1α, or MIP-1β *(64)*.

Why Tat has evolved to promote chemotaxis is an interesting question. An obvious advantage is that it confers HIV with the ability to attract new targets to sites of virus production. However, it was also noted that pretreatment of cells with Tat increases their invasiveness, that is, their movement into and through filters in the absence of a chemotactic gradient *(61)*. It may thus be that Tat induces the migration of the infected cell itself to promote the spread the virus throughout the host.

Following the initiation of highly active antiretroviral therapy (HAART), there is in most patients a rapid increase in the number of circulating $CD4^+$ lymphocytes *(70)*. Though part of this phenomenon seems to represent the proliferation of memory T cells, it probably also reflects a redistribution of lymphocytes from the sites of viral replication, the lymphatic tissue, into the circulation *(71–75)*. It may be that the absence of active viral replication combined with the high turnover rate of infected $CD4^+$ cells leads to a situation where the concentration of Tat in the lymph nodes diminishes to a level insufficient to maintain an effective chemotactic gradient. Further support for this model would be gained through experiments performed in the SIV/rhesus macaque model with viruses expressing Tat variants that cannot act as a chemoattractant, yet are fully functional for transactivation.

A Boost to Coreceptor Expression

Another property of Tat complements its ability to attract putative target cells: Tat can make these cells more vulnerable to infection by upregulating the expression of chemokine receptors that serve as viral coreceptors *(76,77)*. Although HIV-1 virions can efficiently bind $CD4^+$ cells, their subsequent fusion with the cell plasma membrane depends on the presence of a coreceptor, usually CCR5 for macrophage-tropic (R5) viruses and CXCR4 for T-cell-tropic (X4) viruses *(78)*. The clinical importance of these molecules was demonstrated by studies showing that individuals homozygous for a mutation in CCR5 or who had high circulating serum levels of chemokines and low levels of chemokine receptors were highly resistant to HIV infection *(79,80)*. In addition, in vitro analyses have revealed that higher levels of coreceptor on the cell surface correlate with an increased susceptibility to HIV-1 infection *(81–83)*. Exogenous Tat protein could trigger an increase in the expression of the viral coreceptors CCR5,

CXCR4, and CCR3 at the cell surface, which resulted in more than quadrupling the percentage of cells expressing high levels of both CXCR4 and CCR5 in the monocytes/macrophage compartment *(76)*. Interestingly, in T lymphocytes, only CXCR4 was upregulated, and to a lesser extent than in the monocytes/macrophage compartment *(76)*. Whether the increase in coreceptor mRNA transcription is initiated within the cell, or triggered through receptors at the cell surface, is as yet unclear.

Stimulating T-Cell Activation

Infection of human peripheral blood lymphocytes with HIV-1 in vitro was observed to result in increased interleukin-2 (IL-2) *(84)*. Tat alone was shown to recapitulate this phenotype, acting at a transcriptional level via the so-called CD28 responsive element of the IL-2 promoter. Interestingly, this effect was strictly dependent upon the second exon of Tat. This finding suggests that Tat participates in the state of immune hyperactivation observed in HIV-infected individuals. As for Nef-induced priming of T cell activation, this effect is likely to promote viral spread.

Niet to NK Cells

Cytolytic T lymphocytes (CTLs) are particularly important for combating intracellular pathogens like HIV *(85–88)*. In general, CTLs are responsible for the direct killing of cells that display foreign antigens on their surface within the context of MHC-I molecules *(89,90)* though they also have potent noncytolytic properties *(91)*. The Nef-induced downmodulation of MHC-I lessens the efficiency of recognition and killing of HIV-infected cells by CTLs *(4,23)*. Likewise, many other viruses downregulate MHC-I to evade $CD8^+$ cytotoxic lymphocytes *(92)*. For example, human cytomegalovirus (HCMV) has at least four proteins that alter cell surface expression of MHC-I: the US2 and US11 gene products induce the rapid export of MHC-I heavy chains out of the endoplasmic reticulum (ER) into the cytosol where they are degraded by the proteasome *(93)*; the US3 gene product retains fully assembled MHC-I heterodimers in the ER *(94,95)*; finally, the US6 glycoprotein inhibits peptide translocation by TAP (transporters associated with antigen processing) which is required for efficient loading and surface expression of native MHC-I *(94,96)*.

MHC-I downregulation normally would not come without a price, because cells that lack the immune receptor become the targets of NK cells *(97)*. Hence various stratagems developed by viruses to overcome this problem. CMV, for instance, displays an MHC-I homolog that interacts with the CD94 receptors of NK cells to compensate for the downregulation of authentic MHC-I molecules *(98,99)*. The tricks used by HIV are no less sophisticated. First, as described previously, Nef-induced MHC-I downregulation is selective and spares HLA-C, a dominant inhibitor of NK cell activation. Second, Tat can block NK activity *in trans (100)*.

One of the key signaling events triggering NK cells killing functions is a rise in free intracellular calcium *(101)*. This increase is primarily due to intake of ions from the extracellular space *(102,103)*, and occurs through voltage insensitive L-type calcium channels *(100)*. Treatment of NK cells with Tat or verapamil, an L-type calcium channel blocker, inhibits NK-mediated killing in a dose-dependent manner *(100)*. Interestingly, in cell surface binding assays, Tat competes with calcium channel binding compounds, suggesting a direct interaction with cell surface components of the calcium intake apparatus. A more detailed analysis reveals that Tat binds the β^1 subunit of these channels, thereby inhibiting inhibiting calcium influx into the cells *(100)*. This block correlates with an almost complete loss of NK activity in the presence of 100 n*M* recombinant Tat. Of note, pretreatment of NK cells with Bay K 8644, an L-channel agonist, prevents Tat-mediated inhibition of NK activity, but only if added before the viral protein, suggesting that the two molecules exert opposite effects on the same channel *(100)*. Similar results with dendritic cells, which also possess L-type calcium channels, show that Tat treatment can block apoptotic body engulfment as well as the secretion of IL-12 *(104)*. This cytokine aids in the differentiation of the Th1 subset of T-helper cells, which can stimulate further the NK response *(105)*.

ENV: ANGEL OF DEATH

HIV infection is characterized not only by the loss of HIV-infected CD4$^+$ lymphocytes, but also by the accelerated killing of uninfected lymphocytes. For example, there is an increased tendency of CD8$^+$ cytotoxic lymphocytes from HIV-infected individuals to undergo apoptosis *(106–108)*. These cells are also abnormally redistributed into the germinal centers of lymph nodes of AIDS patients, an observation that correlates with increased apoptosis of both T and B cells throughout the node *(109,110)*. In addition, roughly 2 yr before progression to AIDS, the total number of CD8$^+$ T lymphocytes begins to drop in HIV-infected individuals *(72)*. Recent studies suggest that the viral envelope is involved in mediating some of these effects by perverting pathways that normally regulate interactions between macrophages and cytotoxic T cells.

The HIV-1 envelope (Env) is translated as a 160-kDa precursor protein (gp160), and subsequently glycosylated and cleaved in the Golgi apparatus into its functional components: a 41-kDa fusogenic transmembrane moiety (gp41), and a 120-kDa surface subunit (gp120) that binds the viral receptors *(111–113)*. Approximately 50% of gp120 is shed into the extracellular space since its association with gp41 is noncovalent, and thus fairly weak *(111)*.

When peripheral blood mononuclear cells (PBMCs) were exposed to recombinant gp120 of X4 viral strains (which use the chemokine receptor CXCR4 as entry coreceptor), a dose dependent apoptotic death of CD8$^+$ cytotoxic T cells was observed *(114)*. This phenomenon was dependent on the presence of a direct contact between macrophages and CD8$^+$ cells, and correlated with an upregulation of membrane-bound tumor necrosis factor-α (TNF-α) on macrophages and of TNFR-II on CD8$^+$ cells *(114)*. The 26-kDa membrane-bound form of TNF-α is particularly effective at inducing cell death *(115)*. TNFR-II is expressed on the cell surface of resting CD8 cells, where it can induce apoptotis following improper stimulation *(116)*. Interestingly, while SDF-1, the natural ligand for CXCR4, could also induce CD8 cell death in a PBMC culture system, gp120 from an R5 virus had little effect *(114)*. A model can thus be proposed, in which gp120 upregulates membrane-bound TNF-α on macrophages via CXCR4 signaling, to trigger the TNFR-II – mediated apoptosis of CD8$^+$ cells. Interestingly, viruses harvested from patients during the first few years of infection are almost exclusively of the R5 type *(117,118)*, while X4 viruses generally appear late in infection. Whether this switch is the cause or a consequence of a weakening immune system is not clear. The X4 Env-triggered apoptosis of CD8$^+$ cells might explain why lymphocyte depletion is accelerated when X4 viruses become predominant in HIV-infected individuals.

CONCLUSION

The Nef, Tat, and Env gene products are typical examples of multifunctional viral proteins that play critical roles at the interface between the virus and its host. Nef promotes viral spread and facilitates immune evasion by altering the surface expression of specific receptors and by inducing a state of immune hyperresponsiveness. Tat creates a chemotactic gradient that attracts or retains target cells in the lymphatic tissue, the site of viral replication. It increases the susceptibility of putative targets to infection by upregulating the viral coreceptors and inducing partial T cell activation. It also blocks signal transduction steps that would lead to the killing of HIV-infected cells by NK lymphocytes. Env, finally, appears to play a critical role in triggering the destruction of cytotoxic lymphocytes, thereby weakening what would otherwise be an important line of defense against the virus. Important questions for future studies include: Can our understanding of the molecular mechanisms of action of these proteins be exploited to create antiviral approaches targeting their functions? Would such agents significantly affect the course of HIV infection, and the body's ability to limit viral spread? For instance, can antibodies to Tat block some of the *trans* effects of this protein and, if so, would the induction of a strong Tat-specific humoral response constitute a valuable complement to conventional antiviral therapies? Would blocking Nef-induced MHC-I downregulation allow the immune-mediated elimination of the long-term viral reservoir that persists in patients successfully treated with HAART? Addressing these points will shed light on the molecular mechanisms of AIDS pathogenesis and might suggest new avenues for the development of therapies and vaccines.

REFERENCES

1. Deacon NJ, Tsykin A, Solomon A, Smith K, Ludford MM, Hooker DJ, et al. Genomic structure of an attenuated quasi species of HIV-1 from a blood transfusion donor and recipients. Science 1995; 270:988–91.
2. Kestler H, Ringler D, Mori K, Panicali D, Desrosiers R. Importance of the nef gene for maintainance of high viral loads and for development of AIDS. Cell 1991; 65:651–62.
3. Kirchhoff F, Greenough TC, Brettler DB, Sullivan JL, Desrosiers RC. Brief report: absence of intact nef sequences in a long-term survivor with nonprogressive HIV-1 infection [see comments]. N Engl J Med 1995; 332:228–32.

3a. Lama J, Mangasavian A, Trono D. Cell surface expression of CD4 reduces HIV-1 infectivity by blocking Env incorporation in a Nef-and V pu-inhibitable manner. Curr Biol 1999; 9: 622–31.

4. Collins KL, Chen BK, Kalams SA, Walker BD, Baltimore D. HIV-1 Nef protein protects infected primary cells against killing by cytotoxic T lymphocytes. Nature 1998; 391:397–401.
5. Benson RE, Sanfridson A, Ottinger JS, Doyle C, Cullen BR. Downregulation of cell-surface CD4 expression by simian immunodeficiency virus Nef prevents viral super infection. J Exp Med 1993; 177:1561–6.
6. Mariani R, Skowronski J. CD4 down-regulation by nef alleles isolated from human immunodeficiency virus type 1-infected individuals. Proc Natl Acad Sci USA 1993; 90:5549–53.
7. Aiken C, Konner J, Landau NR, Lenburg ME, Trono D. Nef induces CD4 endocytosis: requirement for a critical dileucine motif in the membrane-proximal CD4 cytoplasmic domain. Cell 1994; 76:853–64.

8. Mangasarian A, Foti M, Aiken C, Chin D, Carpentier JL, Trono D. The HIV-1 Nef protein acts as a connector with sorting pathways in the Golgi and at the plasma membrane. Immunity 1997; 6:67–77.
9. Piguet V, Chen Y-L, Mangasarian A, Foti M, Carpentier J, Trono D. Mechanism of Nef induced CD4 endocytosis: Nef connects CD4 with the μ chain of adaptor complexes. EMBO J 1998; 17:2472–81.
10. Grzesiek S, Stahl SJ, Wingfield PT, Bax A. The CD4 determinant for downregulation by HIV-1 Nef directly binds to Nef. Mapping of the Nef binding surface by NMR. Biochemistry 1996; 35:10256–61.
11. Rossi F, Gallina A, Milanesi G. Nef-CD4 physical interaction sensed with the yeast two-hybrid system. Virology 1996; 217:397–403.
12. Foti M, Mangasarian A, Piguet V, Lew D, Krause K, Trono D, Carpentier J. Nef-mediated clathrin coated pit formation. J Cell Biol 1997; 139:37–47.
13. Le Gall S, Erdtmann L, Benichou S, Berlioz-Torrent C, Liu L, Benarous R, et al. Nef interacts with the μ subunit of clathrin adaptor complexes and reveals a cryptic sorting signal in MHC I molecules. Immunity 1998; 8:483–95.
14. Bresnahan PA, Yonemoto W, Ferrell S, Williams-Herman D, Geleziunas R, Greene WC. A dileucine motif in HIV-1 Nef acts as an internalization signal for CD4 downregulation and binds the AP-1 clathrin adaptor. Curr Biol 1998; 8:1235–8.
15. Craig HM, Pandori MW, Guatelli JC. Interaction of HIV-1 nef with the cellular dileucine-based sorting pathway is required for CD4 down-regulation and optimal viral infectivity. Proc Natl Acad Sci USA 1998; 95:11229–34.
16. Greenberg M, DeTulleo L, Rapoport I, Skowronski J, Kirchhausen T. A dileucine motif in HIV-1 Nef is essential for sorting into clathrin- coated pits and for downregulation of CD4. Curr Biol 1998a; 8:1239–42.
17. Kerkau T, Schmitt-Landgraf R, Schimpl A, Wecker E. Downregulation of HLA class I antigens in HIV-1 infected cells. AIDS Res Hum Retroviruses 1989; 5:613–20.
18. Pearse B, Robinson M. Clathrin, adaptors, and sorting. Annu Rev Cell Biol 1990; 6:151–71.
19. Cowles C, Odorizzi G, Payne G, Emrd SD. The AP-3 adaptor complex is essential for cargo-selective transport to the yeast vacuole. Cell 1997; 91:109–18.
20. Pelchen-Matthews A, Parsons I, Marsh M. Phorbol ester-induced downregulation of CD4 is a multistep process involving dissociation from p56lck, increased association with clathrin-coated pits and and altered endosomal sorting. J Exp Med 1993; 178:1209–22.
21. Benichou S, Bomsel M, Bodéus M, Durand H, Douté M, Letourneur F, et al. Physical interaction of the HIV-1 Nef protein with beta-COP, a component of non-clathrin-coated vesicles essential for membrane traffic. J Biol Chem 1994; 269:30073–6.
22. Piguet V, Gu F, Foti M, Demaurex M, Gruenberg J, Carpentier J-L, Trono D. Nef-induced CD4 degradation: a diacidic-based motif in Nef functions as a lysosomal targeting signal through the binding of β-COP in endosomes. Cell 1999; 97:63–73.
23. Scheppler J, Nicholson J, Swan D, Ahmed-Ansari A, McDougal J. Downmodulation of MHC-I in a $CD4^+$ cell line, CEM-E5 after HIV-1 infection. J Immunol 1989; 143:2858.
24. Schwartz O, Maréchal V, Le Gall S, Lemonnier F, Heard JM. Endocytosis of major histocompatibility complex class I molecules is induced by the HIV-1 Nef protein. Nat Med 1996; 2:338–42.
25. Greenberg ME, Iafrate AJ, Skowronski J. The SH3 domain-binding surface and an acidic motif in HIV-1 Nef regulate trafficking of class I MHC complexes. EMBO J 1998b; 17:2777–89.
26. Mangasarian A, Piguet V, Wang J-K, Chen Y-L, Trono D. Nef-induced CD4 and MHC-I down-regulation are governed by distinct determinants: N-terminal alpha helix and proline repeat selectively regulate MHC-I Trafficking. J Virol 1999; 73:1964–73.

27. Hanna Z, Kay DG, Rebai N, Guimond A, Jothy S, Jolicoeur P. Nef harbors a major determinant of pathogenicity for an AIDS-like disease induced by HIV-1 in transgenic mice. Cell 1998; 95:163–75.
28. Brady HJ, Pennington DJ, Miles CG, Dzierzak EA. CD4 cell surface downregulation in HIV-1 Nef transgenic mice is a consequence of intracellular sequestration. EMBO J 1993; 12:4923–32.
29. Lindemann D, Wilhelm R, Renard P, Althage A, Zinkernagel R, Mous J. Severe immunodeficiency associated with a human immunodeficiency virus 1 NEF/3′-long terminal repeat transgene. J Exp Med 1994; 179:797–807.
30. Skowronski J, Parks D, Mariani R. Altered T cell activation and development in transgenic mice expressing the HIV-1 nef gene. EMBO J 1993; 12:703–13.
31. Baur AS, Sawai ET, Dazin P, Fantl WJ, Cheng MC, Peterlin BM. HIV-1 Nef leads to inhibition or activation of T cells depending on its intracellular localization. Immunity 1994; 1:373–84.
32. Alexander L, Du Z, Rosenzweig M, Jung JU, Desrosiers RC. A role for natural simian immunodeficiency virus and human immunodeficiency virus type 1 nef alleles in lymphocyte activation. J Virol 1997; 71:6094–9.
33. Du Z, Lang SM, Sasseville VG, Lackner AA, Ilyinskii PO, Daniel MD, et al. Identification of a nef allele that causes lymphocyte activation and acute disease in macaque monkeys. Cell 1995; 82:665–74.
34. Bandres JC, Luria S, Ratner L. Regulation of human immunodeficiency virus Nef protein by phosphorylation. Virology 1994; 201:157–61.
35. Carreer R, Groux H, Ameisen JC, Capron A. Role of HIV-1 Nef expression in activation pathways in CD4+ T cells. AIDS Res Hum Retrovir 1994; 10:523–7.
36. Collette Y. Towards a consensus for a role of Nef in both viral replication and immunomodulation? Res Virol 1997; 148:23–30.
37. Collette Y, Chang HL, Cerdan C, Chambost H, Algarte M, Mawas C, et al. Specific Th1 cytokine down-regulation associated with primary clinically derived human immunodeficiency virus type 1 Nef gene-induced expression. J Immunol 1996; 156:360–70.
38. Collette Y, Dutartre H, Benziane A, Romas M, Benarous R, Harris M, Olive D. Physical and functional interaction of Nef with Lck. HIV-1 Nef-induced T-cell signaling defects. J Biol Chem 1996; 271:6333–41.
39. Greenway A, Azad A, McPhee D. Human immunodeficiency virus type 1 Nef protein inhibits activation pathways in peripheral blood mononuclear cells and T-cell lines. J Virol 1995; 69:1842–50.
40. Iafrate AJ, Bronson S, Skowronski J. Separable functions of Nef disrupt two aspects of T cell receptor machinery: CD4 expression and CD3 signaling. EMBO J 1997; 16:673–84.
41. Niederman TM, Hastings WR, Luria S, Bandres JC, Ratner L. HIV-1 Nef protein inhibits the recruitment of AP-1 DNA-binding activity in human T-cells. Virology 1993; 194:338–44.
42. Niedermann T, Garcia J, Hastings W, Luria S, Ratner L. Human immunodeficiency virus type 1 Nef protein inhibits NF-κB induction in human T-cells. J Virol 1992; 66:6213–9.
43. Wang J-K, Kiyokawa E, Verdin E, Trono D. The Nef protein of HIV-1 associates with rafts and primes T cells for activation. Proc Natl Acad Sci USA 2000; 97:394–9.
44. Lee CH, Leung B, Lemmon MA, Zheng J, Cowburn D, Kuriyan J, Saksela K. A single amino acid in the SH3 domain of Hck determines its high affinity and specificity in binding to HIV-1 Nef protein. EMBO J 1995; 14:5006–15.
45. Lee CH, Saksela K, Mirza UA, Chait BT, Kuriyan J. Crystal structure of the conserved core of HIV-1 Nef complexed with a Src family SH3 domain. Cell 1996; 85:931–42.
46. Saksela K, Cheng G, Baltimore D. Proline-rich (PxxP) motifs in HIV-1 Nef bind to SH3 domains of a subset of Src kinases and are required for the enhanced growth of Nef+ viruses but not for down-regulation of CD4. EMBO J 1995; 14:484–91.

47. Baur AS, Sass G, Laffert B, Willbold D, Cheng-Mayer C, Peterlin BM. The N-terminus of Nef from HIV-1/SIV associates with a protein complex containing Lck and a serine kinase. Immunity 1997; 6:283–91.
48. Rhee SS, Marsh JW. Human immunodeficiency virus type 1 Nef-induced down-modulation of CD4 is due to rapid internalization and degradation of surface CD4. J Virol 1994; 68:5156–63.
49. Lu X, Wu X, Plemenitas A, Yu H, Sawai ET, Abo A, Peterlin BM. CDC42 and Rac1 are implicated in the activation of the Nef-associated kinase and replication of HIV-1. Curr Biol 1996; 6:1677–84.
50. Nunn MF, Marsh JW. Human immunodeficiency virus type 1 Nef associates with a member of the p21-activated kinase family. J Virol 1996; 70:6157–61.
51. Sawai ET, Baur A, Struble H, Peterlin BM, Levy JA, Cheng MC. Human immunodeficiency virus type 1 Nef associates with a cellular serine kinase in T lymphocytes. Proc Natl Acad Sci USA 1994; 91:1539–43.
52. Sawai ET, Baur AS, Peterlin BM, Levy JA, Cheng MC. A conserved domain and membrane targeting of Nef from HIV and SIV are required for association with a cellular serine kinase activity. J Biol Chem 1995; 270:15307–14.
53. Smith BL, Krushelnycky BW, Mochly RD, Berg P. The HIV nef protein associates with protein kinase C theta. J Biol Chem 1996; 271:16753–7.
54. Graziosi C, Pantaleo G, Fauci AS. Comparative analysis of constitutive cytokine expression in peripheral blood and lymph nodes of HIV-infected individuals. Res Immunol 1994; 145:602–5.
55. Kinter AL, Poli G, Fox L, Hardy E, Fauci AS. HIV replication in IL-2-stimulateed peripheral blood mononuclear cells is driven in an autocrine/paracrine manner by endogenous cytokines. J Immunol 1995; 154:2448–59.
56. Cullen BR. HIV-1 auxiliary proteins: making connections in a dying cell. Cell 1998; 93:685–92.
57. Frankel AD, Young JA. HIV-1: fifteen proteins and an RNA. Annu Rev Biochem 1998; 67:1–25.
58. Wei P, Garber ME, Fang SM, Fischer WH, Jones KA. A novel CDK9-associated C-type cyclin interacts directly with HIV-1 Tat and mediates its high-affinity, loop-specific binding to TAR RNA. Cell 1998; 92:451–62.
59. Chang HC, Samaniego F, Nair BC, Buonaguro L, Ensoli B. HIV-1 Tat protein exits from cells via a leaderless secretory pathway and binds to extracellular matrix-associated heparan sulfate proteoglycans through its basic region. AIDS 1997; 11:1421–31.
60. Ensoli B, Buonaguro L, Barillari G, Fiorelli V, Gendelman R, Morgan RA, et al. Release, uptake, and effects of extracellular human immunodeficiency virus type 1 Tat protein on cell growth and viral transactivation. J Virol 1993; 67:277–87.
61. Lafrenie RM, Wahl LM, Epstein JS, Hewlett IK, Yamada KM, Dhawan S. HIV-1-Tat protein promotes chemotaxis and invasive behavior by monocytes. J Immunol 1996; 157:974–7.
62. Westendorp MO, Frank R, Ochsenbauer C, Stricker K, Dhein J, Walczak H, et al. Sensitization of T cells to CD95-mediated apoptosis by HIV-1 Tat and gp120. Nature 1995; 375:497–500.
63. Wu MX, Schlossman SF. Decreased ability of HIV-1 tat protein-treated accessory cells to organize cellular clusters is associated with partial activation of T cells. Proc Natl Acad Sci USA 1997; 94:13832–7.
64. Baggiolini M, Dewald B, Moser B. Human chemokines: an update. Annu Rev Immunol 1997; 15:675–705.
65. Albini A, Benelli R, Giunciuglio D, Cai T, Mariani G, Ferrini S, Noonan DM. Identification of a novel domain of HIV tat involved in monocyte chemotaxis. J Biol Chem 1998; 273:15895–900.
66. Albini A, Ferrini S, Benelli R, Sforzini S, Giunciuglio D, Aluigi MG, et al. HIV-1 tat protein mimicry of chemokines. Proc Natl Acad Sci USA 1998; 95:13153–8.
67. Benelli R, Mortarini R, Anichini A, Giunciuglio D, Noonan DM, Montalti S, et al. Monocyte-derived dendritic cells and monocytes migrate to HIV-Tat RGD and basic peptides. AIDS 1998; 12:261–8.

68. Barillari G, Gendelman R, Gallo RC, Ensoli B. The Tat protein of human immunodeficiency virus type 1, a growth factor for AIDS Kaposi sarcoma and cytokine-activated vascular cells, induces adhesion of the same cell types by using integrin receptors recognizing the RGD amino acid sequence. Proc Natl Acad Sci USA 1993; 90:7941–5.
69. Ensoli B, Gendelman R, Markham P, Fiorelli V, Colombini S, Raffeld M, et al. Synergy between basic fibroblast growth factor and HIV-1 Tat protein in induction of Kaposi's sarcoma. Nature 1994; 371:674–80.
70. Wei X, Ghosh SK, Taylor ME, Johnson VA, Emini EA, Deutsch P et al. Viral dynamics in human immunodeficiency virus type 1 infection [see comments]. Nature 1995; 373:117–22.
71. Dimitrov DS, Martin MA. HIV results in the frame. CD4+ cell turnover. Nature 1995; 375:194–5; discussion 198.
72. Margolick JB, Donnenberg AD. T-cell homeostasis in HIV-1 infection. Semin Immunol 1997; 9:381–8.
73. Mosier DE. HIV results in the frame. CD4+ cell turnover. Nature 1995; 375:193–4.
74. Nowak MA, Bonhoeffer S, Loveday C, Balfe P, Semple M, Kaye S, et al. HIV results in the frame. Results confirmed [letter; comment]. Nature 1995; 375:193.
75. Sprent J, Tough D. HIV results in the frame. CD4+ cell turnover. Nature 1995; 375:194.
76. Huang L, Bosch I, Hofmann W, Sodroski J, Pardee AB. Tat protein induces human immunodeficiency virus type 1 (HIV-1) coreceptors and promotes infection with both macrophage-tropic and T-lymphotropic HIV-1 strains. J Virol 1998; 72:8952–60.
77. Li CJ, Ueda Y, Shi B, Borodyansky L, Huang L, Li YZ, Pardee AB. Tat protein induces self-perpetuating permissivity for productive HIV-1 infection. Proc Natl Acad Sci USA 1997; 94:8116–20.
78. Littman DR. Chemokine receptors: keys to AIDS pathogenesis? Cell 1998; 93:677–80.
79. Liu R, Paxton WA, Choe S, Ceradini D, Martin SR, Horuk R, et al. Homozygous defect in HIV-1 coreceptor accounts for resistance of some multiply-exposed individuals to HIV-1 infection. Cell 1996; 86:367–77.
80. Paxton WA, Liu R, Kang S, Wu L, Gingeras TR, Landau NR, et al. Reduced HIV-1 infectability of CD4+ lymphocytes from exposed-uninfected individuals: association with low expression of CCR5 and high production of beta-chemokines. Virology 1998; 244:66–73.
81. Alkhatib G, Combadiere C, Broder C, Feng Y, Kennedy P, Murphy P, Berger E. CC-CKR5: A RANTES, MIP-1a, MIP-1b receptor as a fusion cofactor for macrophage tropic HIV. Science 1996; 272:1955–8.
82. Deng H, Liu R, Ellmeier W, Choe S, Unutmaz D, Burkhart M, et al. Identification of a major co-receptor for primary isolates of HIV-1. Nature 1996; 381:661–6.
83. Dragic T, Litvin V, Allaway G, Martin S, Huang Y, Nagashima K, et al. HIV-1 entry into CD4+ cells is mediated by the chemokine receptor CC-CKR-5. Nature 1996; 381:667–73.
84. Ott M, Emiliani S, Van Lint C, Herbein G, Lovett J, Chirmule N, et al. Immune hyperactivation of HIV-1-infected T cells mediated by Tat and the CD28 pathway. Science 1997; 275:1481–5.
85. Harrer T, Harrer E, Kalams SA, Barbosa P, Trocha A, Johnson RP, et al. Cytotoxic T lymphocytes in asymptomatic long-term nonprogressing HIV-1 infection. Breadth and specificity of the response and relation to in vivo viral quasispecies in a person with prolonged infection and low viral load. J Immunol 1996; 156:2616–23.
86. Jassoy C, Harrer T, Rosenthal T, Navia BA, Worth J, Johnson RP, Walker BD. Human immunodeficiency virus type 1-specific cytotoxic T lymphocytes release gamma interferon, tumor necrosis factor alpha (TNF-alpha), and TNF-beta when they encounter their target antigens. J Virol 1993; 67:2844–52.
87. Rosenberg ES, Billingsley JM, Caliendo AM, Boswell SL, Sax PE, Kalams SA, Walker BD. Vigorous HIV-1 Specific CD4+ T-cell responses associated with control of viremia. Science 1997; 278:1447–50.

88. Yang OO, Kalams SA, Trocha A, Cao H, Luster A, Johnson RP, Walker BD. Suppression of human immunodeficiency virus type I replication by $CD8^+$ cells: evidence for HLA class I-restricted triggering of cytolytic and noncytolytic mechanisms. J Virol 1997; 71:3120–8.
89. Fowlkes BJ, Pardoll DM. Molecular and cellular events of T cell development. Adv Imunol 1989; 44:207–64.
90. York I, Rock K. Antigen processing and presentation by the class I major histocompatibility complex. Annu Rev Imunol 1996; 14:369–96.
91. Guidotti L, Ishikawa T, Hobbs M, Matzke B, Schreiber R, Chisari F. Intracellular inactivation of the hepatitis B virus by cytotoxic T lymphocytes. Immunity 1996; 4:25–36.
92. Fruh K, Ahn K, Peterson P. Inhibition of MHC class I antigen presentation by viral proteins. J Mol Med 1997; 75:18–27.
93. Wiertz E, Jones T, Son L, Bogyo M, Geuze H, Ploegh H. The human cytomegalovirus US11 gene product dislocates MHC class I heavy chains from the ER to the cytosol. Cell 1996; 84:769–79
94. Ahn K, Angulo A, Ghazal P, Peterson P, Yang Y, Fruh K. Human cytomegalovirus inhibits antigen presentation by a sequential multistep process. Proc Natl Acad Sci USA 1996; 93:10990–5.
95. Jones R, Weirtz E, Sun L, Fish K, Nelson J, Ploegh H. Human cytomegalovirus US3 impairs and maturation of MHC-I heavy chains. Proc Natl Acad Sci USA 1996; 93:11327–33.
96. Oritz-Navarette V, Hammerling G. Surface appearance and instability of empty H-2 class I molecules under physiological conditions. Proc Natl Acad Sci USA 1991; 88:3594.
97. Hoglund P, Sundback J, Olsson-Alheim M, Johansson M, Salcedo M, Ohlen C, et al. Host MHC-class I gene control of NK cell specificity in the mouse. Immunol Rev 1997; 155:11–28.
98. Farrell H, Vally H, Lynch D, Fleming P, Shellam G, Scalzo A, Davis-Poynter N. Inhibition of natural killer cells by a cytomegalovirus MHC class I homolog in vivo. Nature 1997; 386:510–4.
99. Reyburn H, Mandelbiom O, Vales-Gomez M, Davis D, Pazmany L, Strominger J. The class I MHC homologue of human cytomegalovirus inhibits attack by natural killer cells. Nature 1997; 386:514–7.
100. Zocchi MR, Rubartelli A, Morgavi P, Poggi A. HIV-1 Tat inhibits human natural killer cell function by blocking L-type calcium channels. J Immunol 1998; 161:2938–43.
101. Leibson PJ. Signal transduction during natural killer cell activation: inside the mind of a killer. Immunity 1997; 6:655–61.
102. Huwyler T, Hirt A, Felix D, Morell A. Effect of cations and cation channel blockers on human natural killer cells. Int J Immunopharmacol 1985; 7:573–6.
103. Solovera JJ, Alvarez-Mon M, Casas J, Carballido J, Durantez A. Inhibition of human natural killer (NK) activity by calcium channel modulators and a calmodulin antagonist. J Immunol 1987; 139:876–80.
104. Poggi A, Rubartelli A, Zocchi MR. Involvement of dihydropyridine-sensitive calcium channels in human dendritic cell function. Competition by HIV-1 Tat. J Biol Chem 1998; 273:7205–9.
105. Gately MK, Renzetti LM, Magram J, Stern AS, Adorini L, Gubler U, Presky DH. The interleukin-12/interleukin-12-receptor system: role in normal and pathologic immune responses. Annu Rev Immunol 1998; 16:495–521.
106. Bofill M, Gombert W, Borthwick N, Akbar A, McLaughlin J, Lee C, et al. Presence of $CD3^+$ $CD8^+$ Bcl^- 2(low) lymphocytes undergoing apoptosis and activated macrophages in lymph nodes of HIV-1+ patients. Am J Pathol 1995; 146:1542–55.
107. Carbonari M, Cibati M, Pesce A, Sbarigia D, Grossi P, D'Offizi G, et al. Frequency of provirus-bearing $CD4^+$ cells in HIV type 1 infection correlates with extent of in vitro apoptosis of $CD8^+$ but not of $CD4^+$ cells. AIDS Res Hum Retroviruses 1995; 11:789–94.
108. Gougeon M, Lecoeur H, Duliost A, Enouf M, Crouvoiser M, Goujard C, et al. Programmed cell death in peripheral lymphocytes from HIV-infected persons: increases susceptibility to apoptosis of CD4 and CD8 T cells correlates with lymphocyte activation and disease progression. J Immunol 1996; 156:3509–20.

109. Modlin R, Meyer P, Hofman F, Mehlmauer M, Levy N, Lukes R, et al. T-lymphocyte subsets in lymph nodes from homosexual men. JAMA 1983; 250:1302–5.
110. Muro-Cacho C, Pantaleo G, Fauci A. Analysis of apoptosis in lymph nodes of HIV infected persons. Intensity of apoptosis correlates with the general state of activation of the lymphoid tissue and not with the stage of disease or viral burden. J Immunol 1995; 154:5555–66.
111. Earl PL, Moss B, Doms RW. Folding, interaction with GRP78-BiP, assembly, and transport of the human immunodeficiency virus type 1 envelope protein. J Virol 1991; 65:2047–55.
112. Rowell JF, Stanhope PE, Siliciano RF. Endocytosis of endogenously synthesized HIV-1 envelope protein. Mechanism and role in processing for association with class II MHC. J Immunol 1995; 155:473–88.
113. Willey RL, Bonifacino JS, Potts BJ, Martin MA, Klausner RD. Biosynthesis, cleavage, and degradation of the human immunodeficiency virus 1 envelope glycoprotein gp 160. Proc Natl Acad Sci USA 1988; 85:9580–4.
114. Herbein G, Mahlknecht U, Batliwalla F, Gregersen P, Pappas T, Butler J, et al. Apoptosis of $CD8^+$ T cells is mediated by macrophages through interaction of HIV gp120 with chemokine receptor CXCR4. Nature 1998; 395:189–94.
115. Grell M, Douni E, Wajant H, Lohden M, Clauss M, Maxeiner B, et al. The transmembrane form of tumor necrosis factor is the prime activating ligand of the 80 kDa tumor necrosis factor receptor. Cell 1995; 83:793–802.
116. Zheng L, Fisher G, Miller RE, Peschon J, Lynch DH, Lenardo MJ. Induction of apoptosis in mature T cells by tumour necrosis factor. Nature 1995; 377:348–51.
117. Connor RI, Ho DD. Human immunodeficiency virus type 1 variants with increased replicative capacity develop during the asymptomatic stage before disease progression. J Virol 1994; 68:4400–8.
118. Schuitemaker H, Koot M, Kootstra NA, Dercksen MW, de Goede RE, van Steenwijk RP, et al. Biological phenotype of human immunodeficiency virus type 1 clones at different stages of infection: progression of disease is associated with a shift from monocytotropic to T-cell-tropic virus population. J Virol 1992; 66:1354–60.

6
Immune Response to Murine and Feline Retroviruses

Daniela Finke and Hans Acha-Orbea

INTRODUCTION

Many different retroviruses have developed strategies to infect leukocytes including monocytes, dendritic cells, B cells, and T cells. Because classical antigen-presenting cells are infected, one would assume that the immune system could recognize and control retroviral infections. However, this is rarely the case. Even in the presence of a vigorous cytotoxic T lymphocyte (CTL) response some leukocytes can escape elimination. Infected lymphocytes divide and differentiate upon stimulation, and B- and T-cell infection allows a small population of lymphocytes to generate a state of latent infection in long-lived memory cells. The mobility of leukocytes allows the interaction of many different cell types and hence cell-contact facilitated infection of a wide variety of cells. Alternatively, secretion of infectious viral particles by leukocytes or other cell types leads to a chronic leukocyte infection.

Retrovirus transmission is not very efficient when compared to other viral infections. Despite this inefficiency, the continuous exposure to retroviruses can lead to infection of a large proportion of the exposed individuals. In the case of mouse mammary tumor virus (MMTV) which is transmitted neonatally via milk, 100% of mice become infected when naturally exposed to the virus. However, for transmission to occur, mice have to be infected for more than 2 mo until they reach sexual maturity and have their first offspring. Feline immunodeficiency virus (FIV) is transmitted through biting, an event that is rare between cats living in the same household and that does not occur very frequently between cats from different households. Therefore transmission is dependent on the survival of the retrovirus in a chronic infection.

Several of these retroviruses induce tumors or immunodeficiency syndromes. This usually happens long after infection despite the initially very strong antiviral response. For human immunodeficiency virus (HIV) and FIV the symptom free state lasts several years. The different immunodeficiency models are named murine acquired immune deficiency syndrome (MAIDS), simian AIDS (SAIDS), and feline AIDS (FAIDS) owing to the similarities with the human acquired immune deficiency syndrome (AIDS). All these infections cause loss of $CD4^+$ T cells and generalized immunodeficiency after long latencies. As outlined in this chapter, most of the murine retroviruses use pathogenic mechanisms that are distinct from the strategies used by the more com-

From: *Retroviral Immunology: Immune Response and Restoration*
Edited by: Giuseppe Pantaleo and Bruce D. Walker © Humana Press Inc., Totowa, NJ

plex lentiviruses. For this reason FAIDS induced by the lentivirus FIV is the model that comes closest to AIDS. Although the animal models are not identical to AIDS they provide important insights into the mechanisms leading to retrovirally induced immunodeficiencies.

ENDOGENOUS MURINE RETROVIRUSES

All strains of laboratory mice contain endogenous retroviruses. At least nine different endogenous retroviral groups have been characterized in mice. These are *MLV, Mtv, IAP, VL30, MuRRS, GLN, MuRVY, MuERV-L,* and *ETn.* It has been shown that more than 1% of the mouse genome consists of retroviral sequences, illustrating the continuous interaction between retroviruses and their host. Although closely resembling exogenous viruses, endogenous retroviruses have undergone multiple adaptation steps to render their life cycle compatible with the host. Many proviruses are defective. For example, most of the *Mtv* loci have lost the capacity to form infectious particles. Several other endogenous retroviruses fail to replicate in cells from inbred mice, but can replicate in cells from nonmurine species (xenotropic retroviruses). In only a few mouse strains is there clear evidence that endogenous retroviruses are pathogenic and implicated in spontaneous leukemias, as in SJL, AKR, C58, and HRS/J mice. Transformation can be induced by the enhancer function of the retroviral long terminal repeats (LTR) localized next to host proto-oncogenes. Alternatively, overexpression of a superantigen (SAg) is implicated in the development of follicular B cell lymphomas in SJL mice *(1).* In AKR mice, thymomas are caused by a retrovirus designated as AKV/MCF, which is derived from multiple recombinations between several endogenous retroviruses *(2).* AKR mice do not mount an antiviral immune response against AKV/MCF *(3),* presumably as a result of immunomodulation by tolerance induction to self-antigens by clonal deletion and anergy. In AKR mice an essential role of the thymus in lymphomagenesis has been observed. The murine oncogenic retrovirus SL3-3 derived from spontaneous AKR tumor cell lines first replicates in thymic dendritic cells before it spreads to macrophages and thymic lymphoid cells of neonatally infected AKR mice *(4).* It has been shown that the expression of MCF strains in the thymus correlates with pathogenicity as viruses that are not expressed in the thymus are virtually nonpathogenic *(5).* Whether this is a consequence of the antiviral response of T cells that have not been deleted during thymic development is unclear. In addition to tumor induction, endogenous retroviruses correlate with autoimmune disease manifestations or immunological disorders of mouse strains such as NZB, NZW, NOD, MRL/*lpr,* SL/Ni, and HRS/J *hr/hr.* For example, NZ mice develop an autoimmune disease resembling systemic lupus erythematosus in humans whereas NOD mice show a high incidence of insulin-dependent diabetes mellitus. Although the expression of retroviral proteins has been shown to correlate with disease their causal role in autoimmune destruction remains unclear.

Earlier observations in primary mixed lymphocyte cultures showed that the induction of vigorous T cell proliferation between H-2–identical populations was due to recognition of distinct minor lymphocyte stimulation (Mls) antigens. The description of deletion of T cell subsets expressing a particular TCR Vβ domain in inbred mouse strains led to the identification of Mls antigens as endogenous retroviral superantigens (SAgs) of the MMTV *(6,7).* Neonatal expression of the SAg leads to lifelong clonal deletion of the SAg-reactive TCR $\alpha\beta^+$T cells in thymus. Most inbred and wild mouse strains contain 1–8 *Mtvs (8)*. The large majority of *Mtv*-loci still encode a functional SAg indicating the absence of evolutionary pressure that leads to their elimination.

INFECTIOUS MURINE RETROVIRUSES

Murine Leukemia Virus (MuLV)

MuLVs are responsible for immunodeficieny syndromes such as MAIDS and the development of lymphomas, sarcomas, thymomas, and erythroleukemias in mice. Viruses causing these diseases most often contain mixtures of defective and complete retroviruses. Replication competent helper retroviruses are required for packaging of the defective viruses leading to formation of pseudotypes. Defective particles can induce MAIDS, thymomas, or erythroleukemia in the absence of helper viruses. Viruses causing rapid cancer induction often carry an oncogene in their genome whereas viruses causing slowly developing cancers insert close to and thereby activate host proto-oncogenes. Prominent features of the best known MuLVs are summarized in Table 1.

During the course of infection new viruses are often generated by recombination with endogenous MuLVs. These new viruses can then contain proto-oncogenes taken up from the host or from other viruses and therefore cause diseases with more rapid and severe symptoms. Alternatively, these recombinations often lead to changes in *env* genes which result in altered tissue tropism and increased pathogenicity.

Owing to different receptor usage, infectious MuLVs are classified into four subgroups: (1) ecotropic viruses which are restricted to cells of mouse or rat origin; (2) xenotropic viruses which can infect target cells of several species except mice; (3 and 4) amphotropic and polytropic viruses which use receptors expressed by both rodent cells and cells of other species, but their specificities do not completely overlap.

Several different endogenous loci have been mapped that confer partial or total resistance to MuLV infection. Their features are summarized in Table 2. Three major classes of resistance genes have been described: (1) Several of the resistance genes represent endogenous proviruses that either block infection with their envelope proteins or block integration with HERV-L–related gag proteins by still poorly understood mechanisms. This is also reflected in the fact that infected cells often cannot be superinfected with MuLV, a mechanism called receptor interference. Alternatively, mutations in the receptor can lead to protection from infection. (2) Immune based mechanisms lead to increased cytotoxic, helper, or antibody responses, and are found in mice expressing specific major histocompatibility complex (MHC) class I or II loci, or alternatively non-MHC–linked genes affecting antibody responses. These inhibitions of infection are easily observed in adult mice. Infection of neonatal mice often bypasses some of these effects to the absence of an efficient immune response in neonatal mice. (3) Finally, changes in the growth rates or frequencies of target cells strongly affect the susceptibility to disease development.

MuLV infection is often accompanied by the appearance of *env* gene recombinations with endogenous MuLVs called mink cell focus-inducing (MCV) viruses that are thought to play a role in leukemogenesis. In normal mice 25–100 copies of endogenous MuLVs are found. Although little information is available on the role of these endogenous MuLVs in the development of the immune response to exogenous viruses, it is

Table 1
Characteristics of Mouse Retroviruses

	LB BM5	Friend	Moloney	Rauscher	MMTV
Etiologic agent	BM5def	SFFV	MMuLV	Rauscher	MMTV
Helper virus dependent replication	+	+	–	–	–
Genetic resistance	*xid, scid, nu/nu,* H-2^d, H-2^a	*W,SI,Fv1-6, Rfvl-3,* H-2^b	*Rmvl-3, nu/nu*	*Rv3*	*Mtv, scid, nu/nu*
Early target cell	B cells	Erythroblasts	Lymphocytes, thymocytes	Erythroblasts	B cells
Lymphoid and hematopoetic disorders	*MAIDS:* lymphadenopathy, polyclonal B-cell activation, hyper-gammaglobulinemia, T-cell activation, B/T anergy, FDC loss, lack of presentation of immunogenic epitopes, Th2 cytokine pattern	Erythroproliferation, anemia, polycythemia, EPO-independence, immunosuppression of cellular and humoral response	General immuno-suppression in tumor bearing mice	Erythroproliferation, anemia, polycythemia, EPO-independence, immunosuppression of cellular and humoral response	Polyclonal B cell activation, T cell proliferation, Vβ-restricted anergy and T cell deletion
Malignancy	T-cell lymphoma, B-cell lymphoma	Erythroleukemia	T-cell lymphoma, sarcoma	Erythroleukemia	Mammary carcinoma T cell lymphoma
Prerequisite for cellular disorders	*Fv-$1^{b/n}$* genotype, T/B interaction, proliferation of infected B cells	surface expression of defective SFFV env that binds to EPO receptor	Neonate	Neonate	Sag-specific T cells, T/B interaction, proliferation of infected B cells
Antiviral immune response	$CD4^+$ T cells, CTL, neutralizing Ab	$CD4^+$ T cells, CTL, neutralizing Ab	$CD4^+$ T cells, CTL	$CD4^+$ T cells, CTL, neutralizing Ab	Neutralizing Ab, $CD4^+$ T cells

Table 2
MuLV Resistance Genes

	Name	Chromosomal localization	Gene product	Mode of action	Viruses affected
Genes affecting the immune response					
H-2 Linked					
Rmv1, Rmv2, Rmv3	Resistance to Moloney virus-1	17		Antigen presentation, CTL and helper responses	MV
Rfv1	Resistance to Friend virus-1	17	MHC class I gene H-2D	CTL response	FV
Rfv2	Resistance to Friend virus-2	17	Maps to Q/TL region		FV
Rgv1	Resistance to Gross virus-1	17			GV
Non H-2 linked					
Fv3	Friend virus susceptibility-3	*15*			FV
Rfv3	Resistance to Friend virus-3		Mapped close to *Ly6*, *IL-2Rβ*, *IL-3Rβ1* and *IL-3Rβ2*	Reduced neutralizing antibody response	FV
Mtv	Mammary tumor virus	many	Superantigen	Deletion of superantigen-reactive T cells	MMTV
nu	Nude	11	Winged helix-protein member	affects T-cell development	Thymotropic MLVs, MAIDS, MMTV
Scid	Severe combined immunodeficiency	16	DNA protein kinase	Affects B- and T-cell development	MAIDS, MMTV
xid	X-linked immunodeficiency	X	BTK protein kinase	Affects some B-cell responses	MAIDS
Genes affecting infection					
Interaction with receptor					
Rec1	Receptor for ecotropic viruses	5			Ecotropic viruses
Rmc1	Receptor for MCF virus				MCF
Ram1	Receptor for amphotropic virus	8			Amphotropic viruses

(continues)

Table 2
(Continued)

	Name	Chromosomal localization	Gene product	Mode of action	Viruses affected
Genes affecting infection					
Sxv	Susceptibility to xenotropic virus	1	Allele of polytropic receptor Rmc1?		Xenotropic viruses
Fv4/Akvr1	Friend virus susceptibility-4	12	Ecotropic env	Blocks ecotropic virus receptor	Ecotropic MuLV
Rmcf	Resistance to MCF virus	5	Polytropic env	Blocks polytropic virus receptor	MCF viruses
Postreceptor binding					
Fv1	Friend virus susceptibility-1	4	Endogenous gag-related gene	Blocks integration	Ecotropic MuLV
Genes affecting target cells					
Fv2	Friend virus susceptibility-2	9		Affects target cell availability	FV and related SFFV
Fv5	Friend virus susceptibility-5			Affects kinetics of erythroid cell development?	FV
Sl		10	Stem cell factor SCF	Affects generation of FV targets	FV and related SFFVs
W		5	SCF receptor c-kit	Affects generation of FV targets	FV and related SFFVs
Unknown					
Fv6	Friend virus susceptibility-6				FV
Srlv1	Susceptibility to RadlV-1				RadLV-1
Fhe					FV
Rv3	Rauscher-virus susceptibility-3				RV
Av1, Av2	Abelson-virus susceptibility-1				Ab-MuLV

Abbreviations: FV, Friend virus; Ab, Abelson virus; MCF, mink cell focus forming virus; RadLV, radiation leukemia virus; GV, Gross virus; MV, Moloney virus; RV, Rauscher virus.

Source: Updated from *103*.

likely that tolerance induction reduces the immunogenic epitopes. This is reflected by the absence of an efficient cytotoxic immune response to MAIDS virus in most mouse strains. There is a clear correlation between high, intermediate, and low responder strains, and their MHC haplotype. As for other viruses, $CD4^+$, $CD8^+$ T-cell as well as B-cell responses are important in the anti-MuLV response.

LP-BM5 MuLV (MAIDS)

The LP-BM5 MuLV contains a mixture of retroviruses recovered from a radiation-induced thymic lymphoma. The original mixture was called Duplan–Laterjet strain and induced an immunodeficiency syndrome termed MAIDS in susceptible mouse strains *(9)*. The etiologic agent for MAIDS has been shown to be a replication-defective virus (BM5def or Du5H) *(10)*. In the original isolate it was mixed with a B-tropic replication-competent helper virus (ecotropic MuLV) and a MCF virus. Large deletions within the *pol* and *env* regions of the defective virus result in the production of a single gag precursor ($Pr60^{gag}$) protein *(11)*. The defective virus can induce MAIDS in the absence of a helper virus *(10)* while ecotropic MuLVs have only minor effects on the immune system *(12)*.

Among different inbred mouse strains with the $Fv\text{-}1^b$ genotype which is permissive for B-tropic viruses, the susceptibility to develop MAIDS is determined almost entirely by MHC loci *(13)*. Mice that carry the $H\text{-}2^d$ allele of MHC, such as B10.D2 are resistant and can clear the virus from infected tissue whereas C57BL/6 mice are highly sensitive to MAIDS and develop advanced disease within 10 wk of infection. $H2^d$-linked resistance has been mapped to the D^d region *(13)*.

PATHOGENESIS OF MAIDS

Multiple abnormalities in immune responses are characteristic of MAIDS (Fig. 1A). The first targets of infection are B lymphocytes *(14)*, and helper free virus inoculation is followed by a rapid polyclonal B-cell activation in the lymph node draining the site of injection. At later stages virus infected cells are detectable in most lymphoid organs *(15)*. B-cell activation leads to a large increase in the number of immunoglobulin M (IgM) and IgG secreting plasma cells *(9)* which is followed by the expansion of activated $CD4^+$ T cells *(16)*. Whereas LP BM5 infection leads to strong expansion of B cells and $CD4^+$ T cells in peripheral lymphoid organs in the thymus total cell numbers range between 60% and 80% of controls until 6 wk post-infection and strikingly decreases to 30% thereafter. This decrease is mainly caused by depletion of double positive thymocytes *(17)*. Three to four weeks after virus inoculation splenic B cells of infected animals become unresponsive to T-dependent and T-independent antigens. Dependent on the presence of infected B cells in lymphoid tissue T cells become hyporesponsive to different stimuli, although only a few of them are infected. $CD4^+$ T cells fail to proliferate or to produce interleukin-2 (IL-2) in response to mitogens and alloantigens *(9)*. At the molecular level, impairment in the signaling pathways of both the B-cell receptor (BCR) and the T-cell receptor (TCR) is postulated to be responsible for this unresponsiveness *(18,19)*.

Additionally, a high percentage of apoptotic $CD4^+$ T cells is detectable several weeks after infection and T cells are highly susceptible to TCR crosslinking *(20)*. Fas seems to be involved in the induction of cell death *(21,22)*, but other pathways have also been discussed *(20,23)*. $CD8^+$ T cells appear to be normal at early time points but

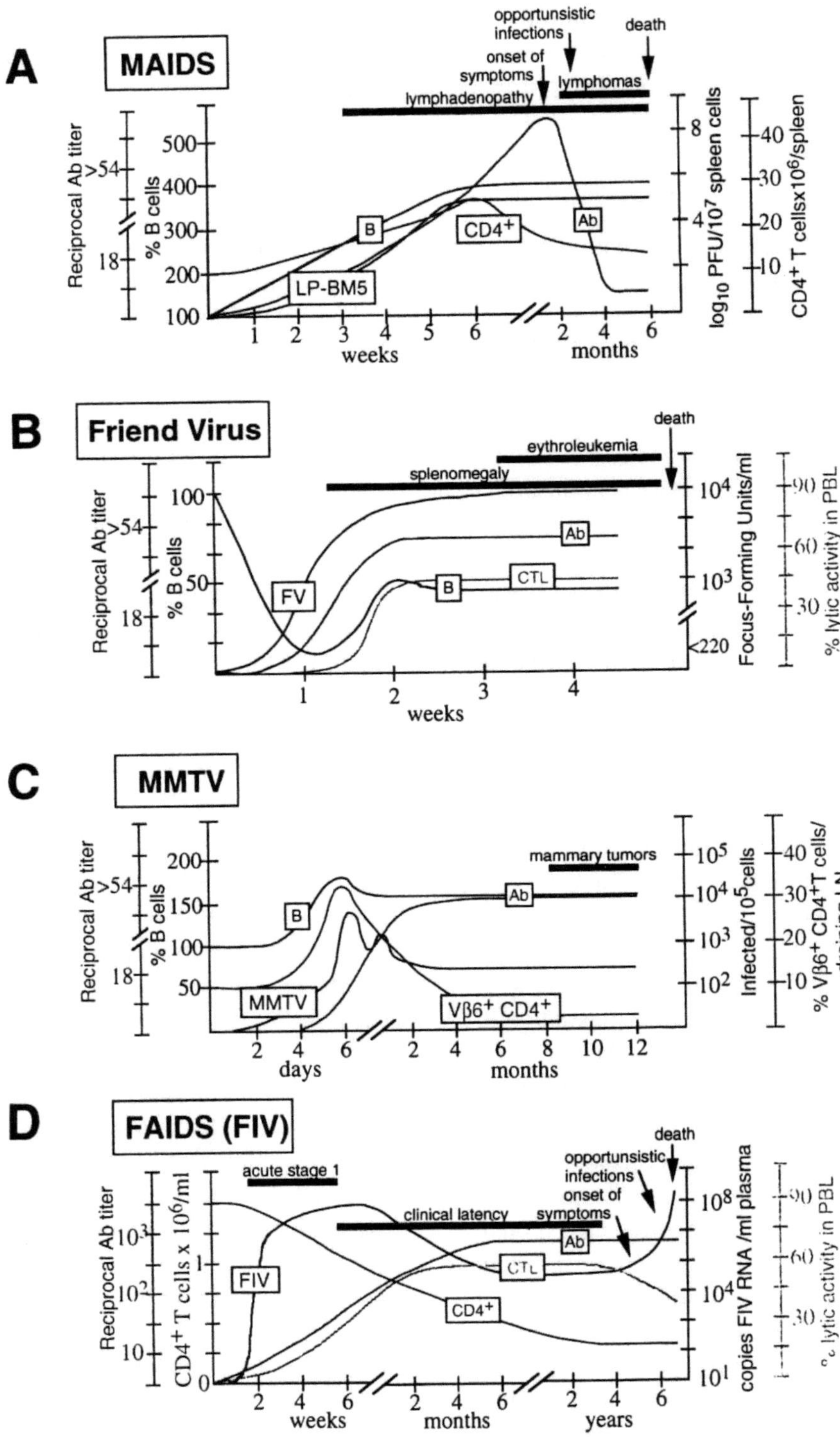

Fig. 1. Kinetics of virus load, immune parameters, and disease development in susceptible mice and cats. **(A)** LP-BM5 infection causing MAIDS; **(B)** Friend virus complex infection inducing erythroleukemia; **(C)** mouse mammary tumor virus infection causing mammary tumors; **(D)** feline immunodeficiency virus infection causing FAIDS. All the values except when indicated were obtained from peripheral blood.

are severely impaired later in infection. This is most probably caused by lack of $CD4^+$ T-cell help *(9,24)*. During later infection, serum antibody levels decrease while B cell proliferation is ongoing with a less diverse repertoire *(25)*. B- and T-cell lymphomas are induced as a consequence of retroviral insertion close to host proto-oncogenes. Death occurs between 16 and 22 wk post-infection due to increased susceptibility to opportunistic infections. Besides the immune disorder, mice infected with BM5def develop an encephalopathy which shares characteristics of AIDS *(26)*.

The induction of MAIDS with helper-free stocks of defective virus suggests that the pathogenesis of disease is determined by clonal expansion of virus-infected cells, rather than virus replication. This explains why the reverse transcriptase inhibitor azidothymidine (AZT) given later in infection cannot prevent the progression to MAIDS. On the other hand, immunosuppressive therapy with cyclophosphamide can prevent MAIDS development and even cure mice when given at later time points *(27)*.

IMPORTANCE OF B CELL/T CELL COLLABORATION FOR MAIDS DEVELOPMENT

Upon infection, B cells proliferate and expand even in the absence of T cells *(28)*, and the viral $Pr60^{gag}$ protein seems to be involved in these early activation events by interacting with signaling molecules *(29)*. On the other hand the full syndrome of lymphadenopathia and immunodeficiency is T cell dependent. For example, athymic C57BL/10 *nu/nu* mice or CD4-deficient mice do not have severe signs of disease after virus inoculation *(28)* (Fig. 2). Most likely, B cells present viral antigens to $CD4^+$ T cells that become activated and provide help for secondary B cell activation and differentiation *(30)*.

There is strong evidence that virus spread, particularly if the virus is replication incompetent, will be favored by direct B-cell/T-cell contact. In B cell deficient mice T cells are not infected with BM5 def whereas in normal mice T cells as well as macrophages contain viral DNA *(14)*. This might be a common viral strategy to exploit the immune system and infect cells expressing insufficient levels of receptor molecules. The importance of T/B collaboration for developing MAIDS is corroborated by the findings that MAIDS is prevented or delayed in mice lacking mature B cells or in *xid* mice that lack T-independent B-cell responses *(31–34)*. Moreover, blocking of the T–B interaction with cyclosporin A or monoclonal antibodies directed against costimulatory molecules can protect from disease *(32,33,35,36)*. Inhibition of intercellular adhesion molecule 1/LFA-1 interaction prevents not only B-cell hyperproliferation, but also replication of BM5def in spleen cells. Taken together, T–B interaction leads to activation of both cell subsets, and seems to be the most cruical step for efficient virus amplification and development of MAIDS.

CYTOKINE PATTERN ON INFECTION

Several reports show that LP-BM5 MuLV alters the cytokine pattern upon infection (for review see *37*). However, the data are conflicting and strongly dependent on mouse strain, time point of observation during infection, and the methods used for restimulation of the cells in vitro before detection of cytokines. An imbalance toward a T helper-2 (Th2) profile observed late in infected susceptible mouse strains is clearly not responsible for MAIDS induction, but the lack of interferon-α and -γ (IFN-α, IFN-γ) in the chronic response might be involved in immune suppression during MAIDS. Consistent with that, interferons induced by infection with other pathogens can delay

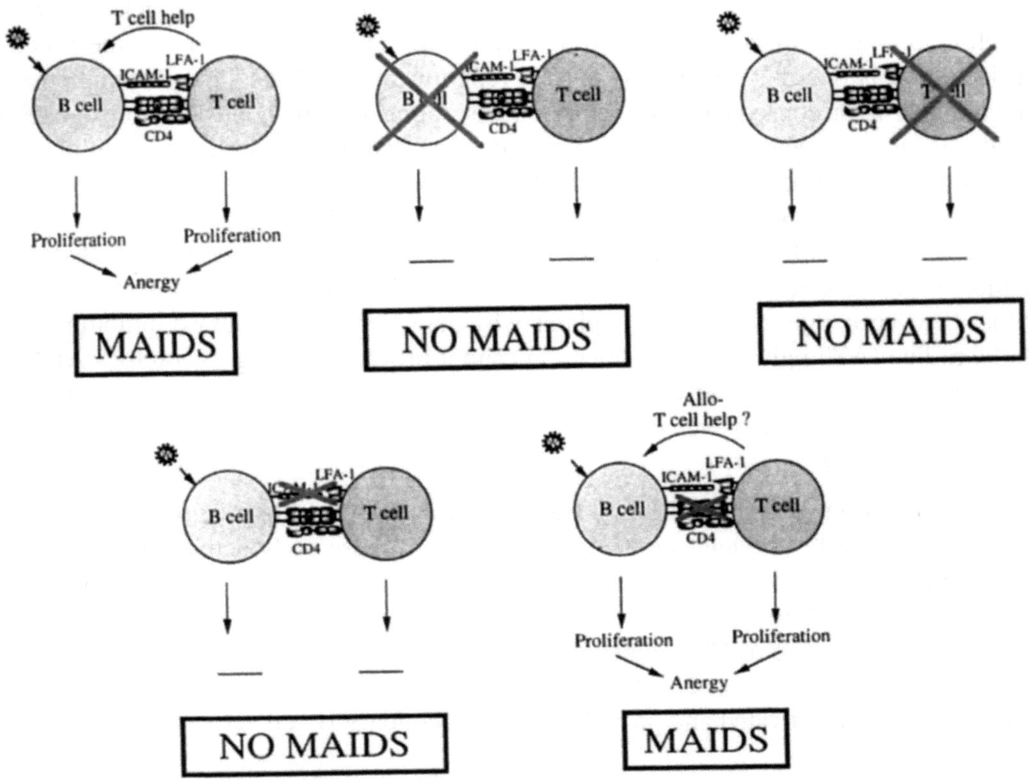

Fig. 2. T cell–B cell interaction is required for MAIDS development. B cell deficient, T cell deficient, or costimulation deficient mice do not develop MAIDS.

MAIDS progression *(38,39)*. In addition, rIL-12 protects susceptible C57BL/6 mice from severe signs of disease most likely via IFN-γ *(40)*. Whether the Pr60^{gag} product of BM5def expressed on the surface of infected cells is responsible for aberrant cytokine expression and clonal expansion of cell subsets is controversial.

TCR Repertoire in Mice Developing MAIDS

Earlier studies concerning the role of gag as a putative T-cell SAg were challenged by the observation that defective MAIDS virus induces only transient alterations in the Vβ T-cell repertoire at d 6 *(41)*, and not at later stages of disease *(16)*. Moreover, a recent paper demonstrates increased expression of endogenous mammary tumor virus *(Mtv)* mRNA encoding the *Mtv* SAg on LP-BM5 infection as an alternative explanation for the described oligoclonal Vβ TCR repertoire in early infected mice *(42)*. However, endogenous *Mtv*-encoded superantigens are not required for the development of MAIDS *(43)*. Gilmore and colleges have used C.B-17 *scid* mice ($H2^d$, IgH^b) reconstituted with B.C-20 ($H2^b$ IgH^a) bone marrow to investigate the stimulatory activity of the B-cell lymphoma line B6-1710 and its impact as a putative SAg. These mice fail to mount an MHC-restricted T–B collaboration and B-cell response to T-dependent antigens, but maintain the capability of their T cells to interact with other syngenic antigen presenting cells (APC) *(44)*. Allochimeric SCID mice are fully susceptible to developing an immunodeficiency disease induced by LP-BM5 (Fig. 2), but T cells from these mice do not respond to a virus-infected B cell lymphoma in vitro. These results appear to be in contradiction to the finding that T–B interaction plays a crucial role in development of disease. But these findings do not exclude the presence of non-MHC–restricted T–B collaboration and/or other APC than B cells, for example, dendritic cells (DC) that participate in MAIDS induction. Taken together these results clearly speak against a role of a SAg in etiology of MAIDS.

Protective Immunity Against MAIDS

The presence of antigen in lymphoid compartments is a prerequisite for stimulation of a protective immune response. Follicular dendritic cells (FDCs) which trap and retain specific Ag can stimulate both T and B cells (for review see *45*). FDCs have the capacity to trap antigen in the form of immune complexes and have been shown to be a major reservoir of HIV early in infection. In MAIDS the ability of follicular dendritic cells to trap antigen and to maintain a specific antibody response is markedly decreased *(46)*. Loss of follicular dendritic cell function and number might contribute to the immunpathology in MAIDS.

LP-BM5 clearance from infected tissues has been shown to be mediated by $CD8^+$T cells, while replication of ecotropic helper virus is controlled by $CD4^+$ T cells, IFN-γ, and IL-2 *(47–49)*. Susceptible mouse strains such as C57BL/6 infected with LP-BM5 are fully capable of generating a specific CTL response *(50)*. However, CTLs from resistant mouse strains are mainly directed against an epitope derived from an additional open reading frame (ORF) of both the bm5def and ecotropic helper *gag* viral coding sequences *(51)*. The failure of susceptible mouse strains to generate this specific CTL response might be a cruical step in their incapacity to clear the virus from infected tissues. Perforin-dependent functions seem to contribute to MAIDS resistance but are not absolutely necessary for virus clearance *(49)*. Instead, an interplay between specific $CD4^+$ T cells, $CD8^+$ T cells, and neutralizing antibodies seems to mediate effective immune control. Indeed, MAIDS infection can be controlled in the presence of MAIDS-resistant immune cells, as shown by infection of allophenic mice containing both a resistant and susceptible genotype as long as at least half of the immune system is derived from the resistant mice *(52)*.

Exogenous Friend/Moloney/Rauscher (FMR)-Type MuLV

Friend Virus Complex (FV)

Until the discovery of Friend virus (FV)-induced leukemia in adult mice *(53–55)* it was believed that the MuLV could cause leukemia only in newborn mice. The subsequent discovery of helper virus RNA in FV-infected cells led to the description of FV as a virus complex composed of a replication competent Friend murine leukemia virus (FMuLV) and a replication defective spleen focus forming virus (SFFV). SFFV is a virus with large deletions in the *gag* and *pol* genes, and a mutant *env* gene. In susceptible mice erythroleukemia develops 1–3 wk after injection of either F-SFFV-A, which induces anemia, or F-SFFV-P, which induces polycythemia. Helper-free SFFVs are pathogenic and induce erythroproliferation which leads to the production of characteristic foci at low virus dose, and to splenomegaly or malignant erythroblast transformation at higher virus doses. FMuLV alone does not induce erythroleukemia in adult mice but causes splenomegaly, anemia, and erythroleukemia when inoculated into newborn mice.

Role of Envelope Glycoprotein in Pathogenesis

The cellular receptor for FMuLV and other ecotropic MuLVs is the 14-transmembrane-pass cationic amino acid transporter MCAT-1 (mouse cationic aminoacid transporter). Lymphocytes and erythroid precursor cells are the preferential targets of infection *(56)*. After infection, the defective SFFV env binds to the eythropoietin (EPO) receptor on erythroid cells via the altered env glycoprotein of SFFV, gp55. Several studies provide conclusive evidence that gp55 acts as a mitogen for erythroid cells (for review see *54*). Mutations of SFFV *env* gene or introduction of SFFV *env* into an M-MuLV-based retroviral vector showed that erythroblastosis is mediated by *env*. Activation of the EPO receptor via gp55 is most probably the reason for polyclonal proliferation of erythroblasts with pronounced splenomegaly shortly after infection *(57)*. Erythroleukemia induced by FMuLV helper virus in newborn mice has been suggested to be initiated by gp-55–like glycoproteins formed by recombination events between exogenous FMuLV and endogenous proviral sequences *(58)*. The various pathogenic aspects of env in FV infection have been supplemented by studies in rats indicating that env protein suppresses hematopoiesis in bone marrow *(59)*. Furthermore, differences in neuropathogenicity between F-MuLV strains have been clearly localized to mutations in the *env* gene *(60)*.

Several weeks after the initial phase of infection and erythroproliferation a few immortalized clones emerge, expand, and finally cause lethal erythroleukemia in most strains of mice (Fig. 1B). Malignancies have two properties in common: first, the provirus activates two cellular oncogenes of the *Ets* family of transcription factors upon integration; second, many leukemic clones transformed by FV have an inactivated p53 gene as a result of internal deletions or SFFV proviral insertions.

Depending on the genetic background some mice can recover from FV leukemia. Various host genes *(W, SI, Fv1-Fv6, rFv1-3, Rmcf)* have been described as conferring resistance to disease (Table 2). Transgenic mice, which express Fv4, a protein with 80% homology to ecotropic MuLV env, were produced. In these mice, the presence of antiviral CTLs, lack of immunosuppression and secretion of soluble env protein have been found to contribute to resistance toward infection *(61,62)*. The *Rfv1* and *Rfv2* genes map to the MHC complex. In addition, four MHC genes (H-2 I-A, I-E, D, and Qa/Tla) are associated with protection against FV leukemia. The H-2^b haplotype carried by C57BL/6 is associated with resistance, whereas H-2^d (BALB/c), H-2^q (FVB/N), H-2^a and H-2^k (C3H) are associated with susceptibility. The contribution of certain MHC alleles to resistance is mediated by the corresponding virus-specific immune response. The b MHC haplotype is important for presentation of viral CTL epitopes and generation of specific $CD4^+$ T cells (for review see *63*). Similarly, viral epitopes presented by H-2 I-A^b induce a strong, specific $CD4^+$ T cell response and protection from disease. H-2 I-E seems to have both positive and negative effects on FV immunity. Inhibition of I-E molecules with monoclonal antibodies reduces the immune response to infection but thymic deletion enhances susceptibility depending on whether or not H-2 I-E recognizing T cells become deleted during thymic maturation.

Protective Immune Response Against FV

A protective immune response against FV in adult mice consists of several parameters including virus-specific CTLs, $CD4^+$ T cells and the production of virus-neutralizing antibodies. CTLs from FV-infected mice have been shown to be H-$2D^b$ and H-$2D^d$

restricted and mainly recognize FMuLV env derived peptides. In contrast to infection with live virus, CTL responses against Friend tumor lines are predominantly specific for gag viral protein. The importance of CTLs has been demonstrated in resistant H-$2^{b/b}$ mice that become susceptible to FV infection after depletion of $CD8^+$ T cells in vivo. On the other hand CTLs seem to be dispensable in the presence of a strong $CD4^+$ T cell and neutralizing B-cell response. Mice immunized with recombinant vaccinia virus expressing env protein mount a $CD4^+$ T-cell response and are protected against leukemia. However, CTLs and neutralizing antibodies are detectable only after virus challenge *(64)*. The lack of CTL induction can be explained by the absence of immunodominant gag-epitopes in the vaccine. Nevertheless it cannot be excluded that the protection observed in vaccinia env-immunized mice is the result of a neutralizing B-cell response and $CD8^+$ T cells that become primed by the live virus challenge, and receive rapid help from preexisting specific $CD4^+$ T cells. However, vaccination with full length FMuLV env protein induces a protective immune response even when mice are $CD8^+$ T cell depleted before virus challenge. These mice mount a rapid and strong neutralizing antibody (Ab) response which efficiently blocks viremia. By contrast env peptide vaccines that do not induce a strong neutralizing Ab response are protective only in the presence of CTLs. These data indicate that CTLs are dispensable only when the virus load is limited. Therefore, compromised recovery from FV infection in $CD4^+$ T cell depleted mice is most likely a consequence of lack of T helper function for CTL and B-cell responses. It was recently published that the protective effect of $CD4^+$ T cells is not only determined by helper function but also by controlling virus replication in persistent FV infection *(65)*. In (C57BL/10 × A.BX)F_1 mice which clear FV from all infected cells except B cells, depletion of $CD4^+$ T cells leads to reactivation of disease in 50% of cases. Hence, virus from persistently FMuLV-infected B cells spreads to erythroid cells, causes splenomegaly and in several cases even leukemia. It remains unclear why a relapse of disease can develop despite the presence of CTLs, and in several cases, highly neutralizing Ab titers. The existence of residual FV-infected spleen cells in recovered mice has already been described. The mechanisms for persistence have not been clarified but it would appear that several virus immune escape strategies might play a role such as impaired presentation of immunodominant viral epitopes. In B cell depleted mice, both $CD4^+$ and $CD8^+$ T-cell responses to FV-induced tumors are reduced, indicating the role of B cells in antigen presentation. Clearly maintenance of virus-neutralizing Ab response by memory $CD4^+$ T cells is important in preventing reinfection and controlling viremia. If mice are not able to mount a neutralizing antibody response to acute FV infection mortality is markedly increased. Treatment of susceptible mice with highly potent virus-neutralizing anti-env MAb, even 10 d after FV-injection, can prevent the outbreak of disease as long as both $CD4^+$ and $CD8^+$ T-cell compartments are functionally intact. The inhibition of virus spread by neutralizing Ab might enable the antiviral T cell response to clear the virus from infected tissue before becoming overrun by the viral load.

IMMUNOSUPPRESSION BY FV

Production of virus-neutralizing antibodies is strongly dependent on *Rfv3 (66)*, a host resistance gene recently mapped to the vicinity of *Ly6*, and three cytokine receptor genes, *IL2rb, IL3rb1,* and *IL3rb2 (67)*. *Rfv3*$^{s/s}$ mice have a compromised FV-specific Ab response, even in the presence of a protective cellular immune response because they have H-2D$^{b/b}$ alleles. However, they can mount a normal humoral immune response to other antigens. A second type of immunosuppression that comprises a general impairment of both humoral and cellular response to common antigens exists after FV infection. The H-2D region is involved in this type of immunosuppression because H-2D$^{b/b}$ mice are resistant to FV-induced immunosuppression, whereas H-2D$^{d/d}$ mice are not. Whether downmodulation of NK cell function by binding of H-2 D^{d} via the Ly-49A receptor on natural killer (NK) cells plays a role in pathogenesis, is unclear. However, FV infection is associated with decreased NK function in several mouse strains *(68)*.

MOLONEY-MULV

Moloney murine leukemia virus (MMuLV) was first isolated in a complex with a murine sarcoma virus (MSV) *(69,70)*. After a latency period of several months MMuLV causes lymphoid tumors by insertion and/or recombination events leading to activation of proto-oncogenes, while MSV contains an oncogene and therefore belongs to the group of rapid transforming viruses. Its replication defect can be overcome through the helper activity of MMuLV. When the MSV–MMuLV complex is injected into susceptible adult mice, T-cell lymphomas develop at the site of injection within 1 week, but undergo spontaneous regression. Conversely, in neonatal mice, regression does not occur, and the consequence is fatal tumor growth. Several mouse strains, for example AKR, SJL/J(v^{+}) and C58, are resistant to infection due to the presence of endogenous ecotropic MuLV and hence receptor interference.

CTL RESPONSE TO M-MULV

Analysis of CTL precursor frequency in C57BL/6 mice that have rejected tumors has identified two distinct populations of CTL. Whereas 40% were specific for viral antigens, 60% were specific for nonviral tumor-antigens. However, tumor specific CTLs have been shown to play no role in in vivo rejection of tumor cells *(71)*. In susceptible adult mice the regression of tumors is dependent on virus-specific cytotoxic T cells and CD4^{+} T cells *(72)* the virus cannot be cleared from the thymus and peripheral T lymphocytes. Neonatal mice fail to generate a tumor-specific CTL response, nor do they produce neutralizing antibodies. However, they respond normally to conventional antigens. The protective CTL response is restricted by H-2K^{d} and H-2D^{b}. H-2D^{b} mutant bm 14 mice have a defect in generating MMuLV-specific CTLs, but normally reject MSV-induced tumors. In these mice an H-2K^{b} restricted CTL response, which is usually not detectable in normal mice, seems to compensate for the lack of H-2D^{b} restricted CTLs. Moreover, priming by dendritic cells plays a role in the generation of CTLs in the absence of functional D^{b} molecules *(73)*. A K^{b} allele-specific epitope of MMuLV (recognized in bm 13 mice) is located in the gp70 env protein *(74)*. The cytotoxicity towards tumors is perforin mediated *(75)*. In vitro studies showed that MMuLV infection of target cells enhances expression of MHC class I molecules and therefore increases susceptibility to lysis by CTLs whereas MSV counteracts this effect. Common cross-reactive CTL epitopes exist between Friend, Molony, and Rauscher types of MuLV referred to as "FMR" antigen complex. CTLs are either specific for the FMR type of MuLV or for the AKV/MCF type (see also *75* Chapter). The immunodominant CTL epitope in endogenous AKV/MCV type MuLV infection differs by a single amino acid from the FMR type CTL epitope *(76)*. This explains why CTLs from H-2^{b} mice primed with endogenous AKV/MCF type MuLV do not recognize tumor cells expressing the FMR type of MuLV. The major CTL epitope of all FMR viruses is located in the leader sequence of the gPr80^{gag} protein *(77)*. It has been shown that the CD8+ T-cell response to Rauscher MuLV and MMuLV is dominated by a highly restricted TCR repertoire to immunodominant epitopes derived from env and gag virus *(78,79)*. Defective processing of the immunodominant epitope KSPWFTTL in tumor cells is one possible mechanism of viral immune escape *(80)*. In the past few years studies on MMuLV have been extended to its application as a retroviral vector since the MMuLV LTR drives gene expression in most hematopoietic cell types. However, only proliferating cells become efficiently transfected by MuLV vectors, whereas lentivirus vectors can also enter nondividing cells *(81,82)*.

NEUROPATHOGENESIS OF MMULV VARIANTS

A temperature-sensitive mutant, *ts*1 of MMuLV in neonatal FVB/N mice, causes hypergammaglobulinemia as well as rapid loss of T cells and neurons without any signs of inflammation (for review see *83*). During the early phase of infection there is a marked increase in mitosis of double-positive thymocytes followed by activation induced apoptosis. Similar to the thymus all cell types of the central nervous system (CNS) become infected but cells that show the most morphological damage are neurons; however, they rarely contain detectable virus or viral antigen *(84)*. In contrast to the beneficial effect of the cellular immune response in MMuLV infection, in *ts*1 infection neuroimmunodeficiency seems to be dependent on T cells and the thymic microenvironment. Whereas athymic BALB/c nude mice are resistant to *ts*1, newborn severe combined immuno-deficiency (SCID) mice are sensitive to infection with *ts* 1 and develop disease after transfer of thymocytes or CD4+ T cells from infected mice, However, neither B cells nor CD8+ T cells induce disease *(85,86)*. Lower virus titers in CD8+ T-cell reconstituted SCID mice leave open the question whether differences in numbers, cell cycle, migration, or survival of transferred *ts* 1-infected lymphocyte subsets are responsible for the lack of neuropathology. Alternatively, an autoimmune response of infected cells rather than the direct consequences of virus replication could participate in *ts* 1-mediated pathology. For example, oxidative stress as a result of excessive cell cycle and cytokine production of accessory cell types has been hypothesized to cause cell death and neurodegeneration.

RAUSCHER-MULV

Rauscher MuLV (RMuLV), a member of the exogenous FMR virus group infects erythropoetic precursors, causes abnormal splenic colony formation within 8 d, marked splenomegaly in 3 wk, and kills infected mice in 4–5 wk *(87)*. The sequence homology between RMuLV and FMuLV is >97% *(88)*. Consistent with that, immunosuppression of both cellular and humoral immune response has been reported. Impaired immune function of dendritic cells and downregultation of costimulatory molecules by RMuLV have been postulated to play a role in immunosuppression *(89,90)*. RMuLV infection has been used as an animal model for studying the ability of antiviral agents to suppress viremia and retroviral disease. Ruprecht and collegues discovered more than 20 yr ago that continuous AZT treatment exerts an antiretroviral effect and prevents infection and development of splenomegaly in mice injected with RMuLV *(91)*. The success of therapy is critically dependent on the virus dose and the presence of a functional cellular immune compartment *(92)*. As for most other exogenous FMR viruses specific

$CD4^+$ and $CD8^+$ T cells transferred into naive mice prevent the outbreak of disease after virus challenge *(93,94)*.

Mouse Mammary Tumor Virus (MMTV)

MMTV is a B-type retrovirus which received its name from its capacity of inducing mammary tumors in infected female mice by insertion close to host proto-oncogenes. Moreover, several of these proto-oncogenes have been defined using MMTV. The discovery of a SAg in the MMTV genome offered an important tool that could be used to study virus–host interactions and antiviral immune responses. Most of the early literature is covered in a recent review *(8)*. Therefore owing to space limitations we will only cite some of the more recent key references.

One characteristics of MMTV is the induction of unresponsiveness (anergy) in a T-cell subpopulation but a lack of a general immunodeficiency.

MMTV Infection (Phase I)

After natural infection of newborn mice, reverse transcribed viral DNA is initially detected in Peyer's patches. The targets of infection are B cells, and dendritic cells have been shown to prime the Sag response. Injection of MMTV into adult mice leads to an immune response localized to the lymph node draining the site of injection, which is undistinguishable from the neonatal infection via milk.

Retroviruses require activated lymphocytes to achieve productive infection. Most retroviruses with the exception of lentiviruses, require cells to be in cycle because the preintegration complex cannot enter into the nucleus without dissolution of the membrane which occurs during mitosis. Despite the fact that lentiviruses can infect cells which are not cycling, infection of lymphocytes requires activation. Most likely, insufficient levels of nucleotides in small resting lymphocytes does not allow reverse transcription. Within hours of injection, MMTV activates a large proportion of B cells but not T cells, as measured by induction of activation markers such as CD69 and CD86. Among these activated B cells only few become infected. Possibly, only the few B cells that enter cell cycle after virus binding can be productively infected. Alternatively, only a small proportion of viral particles are infectious. Since preactivation of B cells prior to virus injection does not increase but rather decreases infection efficiency, it seems likely that MMTV synchronizes the activation state of the target cell to achieve optimal conditions for infection *(95)*. After integration of the reverse transcribed viral genome SAgs are expressed on the cell surface of the infected antigen-presenting cells. This expression leads to concomitant activation of both antigen presenting B cells and SAg-reactive T cells, which becomes detectable between d 2 and 3 after MMTV injection or uptake.

MMTV SAg Response (Phase 2)

Once viral gene products are expressed after integration, the infected antigen presenting cells present an MMTV SAg on the cell surface in the context of MHC class II molecules. It is this step which is cruical for the establishment of a productive infection with MMTV. SAgs are proteins that bind to most MHC class II molecules and stimulate vigorous T-cell responses. Some MMTV isolates such as MMTV(C3H) and MMTV(SIM) require expression of MHC class II I-E molecules to trigger a strong SAg response. For all the described viruses, I-A^q is unable to present SAgs and I-A^s is weak in SAg presentation. SAgs interact with the lateral side of the T cell receptor complex specifically with the HV4 region of the T-cell receptor Vβ chain. Therefore SAgs can interact with 5–35% of the T-cell repertoire which leads to a strong amplification of SAg-reactive T cells (Fig. 1C). The reason for this strong response is the high precursor frequency of SAg-reactive T cells, which is in the order of 10^4 times higher than for classical MHC-restricted peptides. This is due to the recognition of T-cell receptor sequences which are much less polymorphic than the ones important for peptide–MHC recognition. SAg-reactive T cells are primed by dendritic cells and interact with the SAg-presenting infected B cells inducing them to divide, increasing their numbers at least 1000-fold within 6 d of infection, after which they differentiate and become long lived B cells. This classical T–B interaction induced by SAg results in a strong increase in the numbers of infected cells, their differentiation into follicular and extrafollicular B cells, and their involvement in a chronic immune response. This SAg-induced immune response is nearly indistinguishable from classical immune responses. One small difference is the slightly delayed appearance of germinal centers after MMTV injection. Each division of an infected B cell which is induced by SAg-mediated T cell–B cell interaction will increase the number of infected cells. In turn, differentiation of an infected B cell into a long-lived B cell will increase the chances of the virus fulfilling its life cycle. During this early phase of the immune response neutralizing antibodies are detected but no evidence for induction of a CTL response has been reported.

Chronic Infection, Virus Neutralization, and Mammary Gland Infection (Phase 3)

Infection of neonatal or adult mice with MMTV leads to life long infection with an efficiency of 100% in susceptible mouse strains. Shortly after infection, an efficient neutralizing antibody response becomes detectable and high neutralizing titers are observed life long. This efficient response, however, is incapable of controlling the infection. For the moment it is not clear whether this immune response just occurs too late, whether it helps the host to reduce viral spread, or whether it helps the retrovirus to better survive. Interestingly, this neutralizing antibody response is SAg dependent as in the presence of a SAg response neutralization is much stronger than in its absence. It is not clear whether there is preferential infection of MMTV-specific B cells which then are amplified by the SAg response, or whether viral amplification due to the SAg response leads to higher levels of viral protein and hence to induction of a neutralizing response. This SAg-mediated T–B cell collaboration leads to a lifelong chronic neutralizing antibody response in the germinal centers of the lymph node draining the site of injection. A large proportion of SAg-reactive T cells is lost from the repertoire by unknown mechanisms later in the response. Interestingly, the numbers of SAg-reactive T cells remain high in the lymph node draining the site of injection for more than a year. T cells localized in germinal centers are mostly SAg-reactive and are implicated in the chronic immune response. After the initial infection of antigen-presenting cells, the virus spreads to both CD4 and CD8 T cells and is finally brought to the mammary gland by these infected lymphocytes. Since the virus spreads between these lymphocyte subsets it has been difficult to establish which cell is responsible for infection of the mammary gland. Initially, MMTV induces a weak IgM secretion (d 3–4) followed by a strong IgG2a secretion (d 5–7) during the extrafollicular B-cell differentiation and finally IgG_1 during the chronic response in the germinal centers.

Cytokine Induction in MMTV Infection

Little information on cytokine secretion patterns are available but the antibody isotypes produced suggest a response which is initially dominated by Th1 cytokines followed by a chronic Th2 response. Comparable to the response to haptenated protein there is a minimal delay in the cytokine response following T-cell priming with MMTV. Whereas IL-4 mRNA appears later and to a lesser extent in the LN draining the site of MMTV injection, there is a significant elevation of IFN-γ message following infection *(96)*. IFN-γ is involved in the early antiviral IgG_{2a} secretion but studies in IFN-γ-R deficient mice clearly demonstrate that interferons do not play an essential role in antiviral defense during MMTV infection *(97)*.

Antiviral Cellular Immune Response

Cytotoxic immune responses directed against MMTV env and gag peptides have been observed in vitro and in vivo. They were usually directed against mammary carcinoma cells and so far there is no evidence of a role for cytotoxic T cells in the control of MMTV infection (for review see *98*).

Importance of the SAg Response for Infection

Several studies have shown that the SAg presentation step is cruical in the life cycle of MMTV. The absence of SAg-reactive T cells leads to lack of a SAg response and a highly decreased probability of infection of the mammary gland. After one to five generations the virus is lost from the mouse strain it originally infected. Similar results were obtained in mouse strains expressing an MHC class II molecule that cannot present MMTV SAgs (I-A^q) or in mice lacking B cells or MHC class II molecules. In additional experiments it was shown that recombinant MMTVs that express a SAg with a point mutation rendering it non functional select rare mutants reexpressing a functional SAg. Taken together, these data clearly indicate a crucial role for the SAg response in the maintenance of MMTV infection in the mouse population.

Exploitation Instead of Evasion from the Immune System

Many viruses have found strategies to evade the immune response. For example, the pox viruses use a large portion of their genome to evade the host immune response. MMTV is the first well described virus which uses a more offensive strategy to guarantee its survival. It induces a very strong immune response which has as its main purpose an increase in both the number and the survival time of infected B cells. Without the action of its SAg the virus cannot survive in the mouse population.

The Life Cycle of MMTV

A summary of the different stages of the MMTV-induced immune response is given in Fig. 3. High titers of MMTV are produced in the milk of infected female mice, so the babies are infected via their intestines after drinking milk. Infection through this route is only possible during the first 2 wk of life before the stomach acidifies. The virus enters through the dome region that covers the Peyer's patches and infects B cells in the Peyer's patches within days of birth. So far it is unclear whether dendritic cells are infected before B cell infection occurs. Peak SAg responses are found in the Peyer's patches within 8–9 d after birth, and B cells already produce large amounts of antibodies at this stage. After MMTV infection both extrafollicular and follicular B-cell maturation is observed. Several days later the virus-infected cells become detectable in other lymphoid organs. B cells are

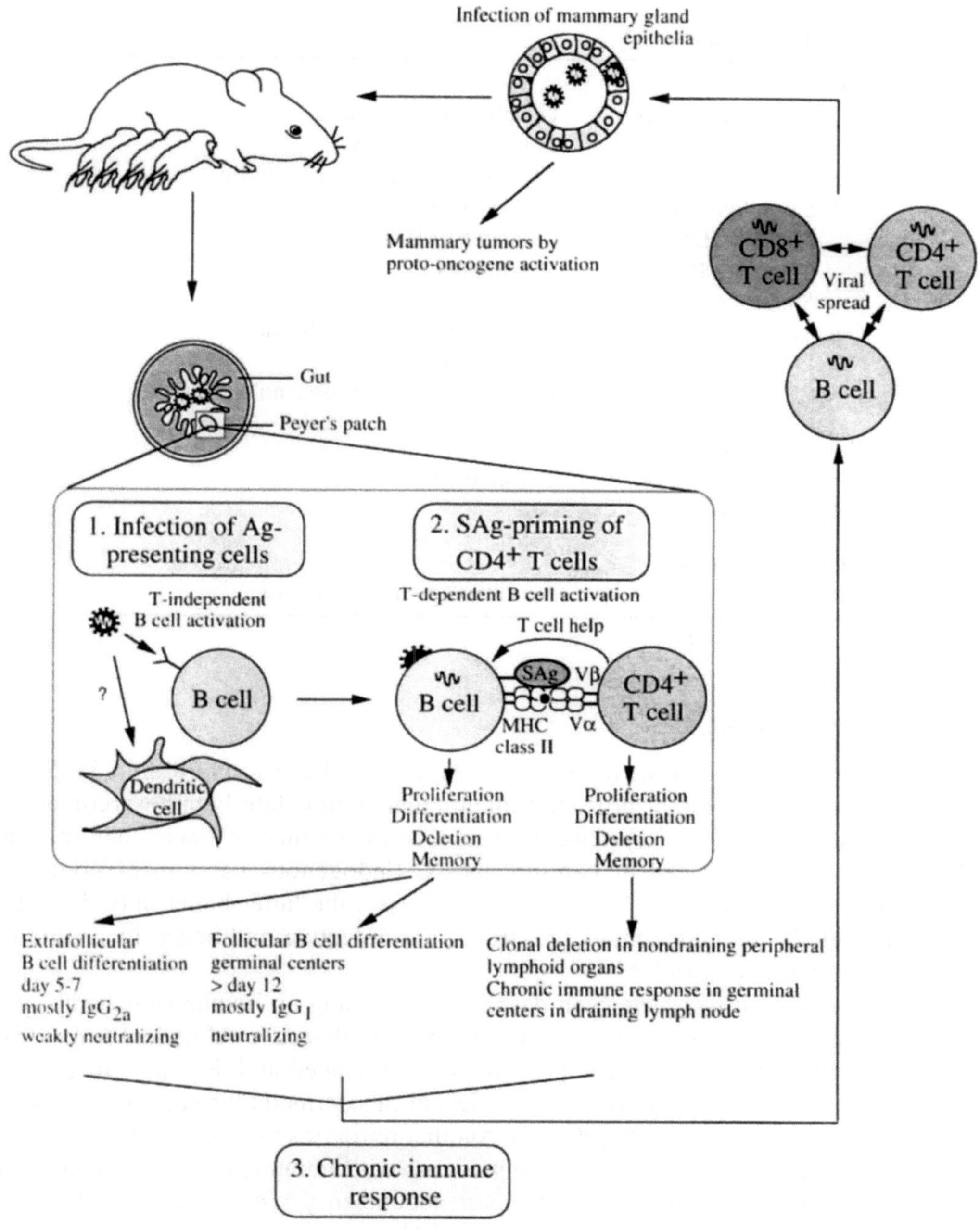

Fig. 3. Life cycle of MMTV infection.

the main infected lymphocyte population within the first week of infection. Thereafter, other lymphoid tissues are infected by unknown mechanism. Throughout the life of the mouse a small fraction of B, CD4+ as well as CD8+ T cells are infected with MMTV and they are found in all lymphoid and in several nonlymphoid organs. Mammary gland infection has been detected around puberty but at which exact time point infection occurs has not been carefully looked at yet.

Table 3
Cat Retroviruses

I. Oncoviruses	
1. Endogenous viruses	Genetically transmitted
2. Exogenous viruses	Spread contagiously
Oncogene-free	Chronic malignancy by insertion
FeLV Subgroup A	Ecotropic
FeLV FAIDS	Induce FAIDS
Subgroup B	Polytropic
Subgroup C	Polytropic
Oncogene positive	Acute transforming malignancy
FeLV	Lymphosarcoma
FeSV	*De novo* sarcoma viruses, no contagiosity
II. Lentiviruses	
FIV	Induce FAIDS
Subgroup A–C	
III. Spumaviruses	
FeSFV	No pathology in natural host

Adapted from *107.*

FELINE RETROVIRUSES

In domestic cats several different retroviruses have been found (Table 3). Some of these viruses cause either profound immunodeficiency, late lymphosarcomas, or sarcomas. As in the MuLV system, the presence or absence of oncogenes in viral RNA determines the speed of carcinogenesis. Endogenous cat viruses comprise 8–12 FeLV and about 20 RD114 xenotropic viruses, the latter being only distantly related to FeLV. The endogenous proviruses are defective and hence incapable of producing infectious particles.

Two feline retroviruses have been described as causing an immunodeficiency syndrome similar to AIDS in humans. First, a replication defective feline leukemia virus (FeLV-FAIDS) with a mutated env protein has been cloned and described to cause a range of neoplastic and hematopoietic disorders in cats, termed feline acquired immunodeficiency syndrome or FAIDS *(99,100).* Another retrovirus that belongs to the family of lentiviruses was discovered in a colony of cats with immunodeficiency syndromes and therefore was referred to as feline immunodeficiency virus (FIV) (*see* Table 4) *(101).* These animals were all negative for FeLV. However, many cats that are naturally infected with FIV, contain also other feline retroviruses, especially FeLV. Coinfection with FeLV may accelerate the development of FIV-induced disease but there is no evidence for direct interaction between FIV and FeLV *(102).* In addition to the immunodeficiency viruses, many cats become infected by FeLV-C strains that induce severe aplastic anemia. These strains originally derive from recombinations between endogenous proviruses and exogenous FeLV-A strains (*see also 103*).

In this section we will focus on FeLV-FAIDS and FIV which are responsible for immunodeficiency in cats, and emphasize their common properties and differences with respect to pathogenesis and immune response.

Table 4
Retroviral Diseases in Cats and Humans

	FAIDS	AIDS
Etiologic agent	FIV	HIV
Receptor	?+fCXCR4	CD4+ CXCR4/CCR5/other chemokine receptors
Tropism	CD4+, CD8+ T cells, B cells, monocytes/macrophages, microglia, astrocytes	CD4+ T cells, monocytes/ macrophages, microglia, infrequent in astrocytes and other cell types
Viral determinants for tropism	V3 loop of env	V3 loop of env
Clinical staging	1–5	1–5
Cellular immune dysfunction	Reduction of CD4+ T cells, anergy of T cells, lymphopenia, reduced lymphoblastogenesis, cutaneous anergy, disappearance of FDC	Reduction of CD4+ T cells, anergy of T cells, lymphopenia, reduced lymphoblastogenesis, cutaneous anergy, NK cell dysfunction, monocyte/ macrophage dysfunction, disappearance of FDC
Humoral immune dysfunction	Early hyperglobulinemia, impaired T-dependent antibody response in chronic infection	Impaired antibody response
Organ manifestation	Thymic and myeloic hyperplasia and atrophy; inflammation of eye, kidney, skin, gastrointestinal tract, respiratory system	Thymic and myeloic hyperplasia and atrophy; inflammation of eye, kidney, skin, gastro-intestinal tract, respiratory system
Neuropathogenesis	Encephalopathy	encephalopathy
tumors	B-cell lymphoma	B-cell lymphoma, cervical carcinoma, Karposi sarcoma

Feline Leukemia Virus (FAIDS)

About 2% of cats are infected with FeLV, and most of them are healthy carriers. FeLVs belong to the family of oncoretroviridae. Exogenous replication competent FeLV can recombine with endogenous FeLV or cellular genes to give rise to highly pathogenic or acute transforming viruses. Subgroups A (ecotropic), B (polytropic), and C (polytropic) are classified according to the species that express the viral receptors recognized by the viral env-glycoprotein. B- and C-type infectious viruses are generated by recombination with endogenous sequences after infection with subgroup A viruses. The subgroup A virus FeLV FAIDS does not contain an oncogene but induces a lymphoproliferative and/or lymphodegenerative disease in cats. Mutations in the env gene have been found which lead to highly pathogenic FAIDS-inducing viruses *(99)*. Some of these mutated viruses have been shown to lack superinfection interference in infected T cells. The clones 61C and 61E represent two closely related FeLV variants with different pathogenicities. Clone 61C is replication defective and capable of inducing fatal immunosuppression whereas 61E is replication competent but poorly pathogenic. The two isolates most likely use distinct receptors *(104)*. The genetic determinant influencing disease manifestation has been mapped to the *env* glycoprotein (env-SU) gene. A 12 nucleotide insertion in the *env* gene is critical in FAIDS-induction. Moreover, 61E chimeras encoding the 12 base pair insertion evolve to T cell cytopathic virus variants and induce FAIDS *(105)*. Lymphopenia, neutropenia, and blastopenia may be the result of extensive replication of FeLV-FAIDS in lymphocytes and myeloid cells. As a consequence, thymic atrophy occurs in young cats after infection, whereas T-cell depletion is found only in peripheral lymphoid organs after infection of adult cats. In particular, $CD4^+$ T cells are the most severely affected as their numbers progressively decline. Virus infection can render animals susceptible to opportunistic infections due to a depressed or deficient cellular immune response. B-cell dysfunction also occurs in FeLV-infected cats *(106)*. High virus levels are found in saliva. Initially, lymphocytes of the head and the neck become infected after licking. On FeLV exposure in cats living in the same houshold, 72% become infected, of which 40% develop chronic infection. The 60% of cats that do not develop a chronic infection become immune to FeLV, and it is thought that both cellular and humoral immunity are required to control infection. In cats that do not become immune at this stage the virus becomes detectable in bone marrow where it replicates. Within 6–8 wk of infection the virus spreads to the salivary glands and oral mucosa *(107)*. Of the chronically infected cats 83% develop the following diseases within 3.5 yr: FAIDS (60%), anemia (25%), lymphosarcoma (5%), and other diseases (10%). Latent, nonreplicating FeLV have been described as persisting in small numbers in mononuclear cells that can become reactivated *(108)*. Moreover, depending on the immune status FeLV can become compartimentalized and persist in a few mammary gland cells (H. Lutz, personal communication). Several months after the infection is controlled, cats are considered virus free if the virus cannot be reactivated in bone marrow cultures.

There exist several vaccines against FeLV infection. Immunization with recombinant env glycoprotein has been shown to mediate protection most efficiently *(109)*. Vaccinated cats produce neutralizing antibodies to FeLV-A and are protected from challenge with FeLV-A, FeLV-B, and FeLV-C. However, the mechanism of protection has not been clarified, and even in the absence of FeLV-specific antibodies cats can become immune against reinfection. Probably induction of a specific cellular immune response plays a major role in the protective effect of vaccines, but to date specific T cell responses in cats remain difficult to analyze.

Feline Immunodeficiency Virus (FIV, FAIDS)

FIV is a lentivirus which can be subdivided into three groups (A–C) dependent on envelope gene sequence and host range *(110)*. The infection, which is transmitted by biting, is distributed worldwide among domestic cats and infected animals carry the virus for life. Transmission between cats living in the same household is rare. Despite phylogenetic divergence, FIV induces immunopathology in cats quite similar to the acquired immunodeficiency syndrome caused by lentiviruses in man *(101)*. FIV isolates from infected cats cause disease with an incidence of close to 100%, leading to death after a mean period of four to five years. On the contrary, a FIV virus variant has been isolated from lions in East Africa for which approx 90% of lions are positive without any clinical signs of immunodeficiency *(111)*. This virus failed to be transferable to cats *(112)*.

Tropism of FIV

FIV can efficiently infect and replicate in activated CD4$^+$ and CD8$^+$ T lymphocytes, B lymphocytes, primary monocytes/macrophages, as well as astrocytes and microglia. In vivo, infected cells are predominantly found in lymph nodes, bone marrow, spleen, and brain *(113)*. As for murine leukemia viruses, alterations in the env SU protein are responsible for tropism *(114)*. A single amino acid substitution in the V3 region of env is sufficient to alter the tropism as has been demonstrated for HIV and SIV infection *(115)*. Depending on the virus clone, FIV replicates preferentially in lymphocytes or macrophages. Primary targets of infection are lymphocytes but a shift to macrophagotropic viruses is already observed in the acute phase of infection *(102)*. A feline homolog of CD9, which is expressed on a wide range of human hematopoetic cells, has been identified as being important for virus release *(116)*. Whereas most retroviruses need lymphocytes in cycle for efficient infection, lentiviruses can replicate in nondividing cells. This was confirmed for FIV in a recent study *(82)*.

Although FIV infection is followed by a marked decrease in CD4$^+$ T cells and reduced expression of CD4 molecules, feline CD4 is not a prerequisite for FIV infection *(117)*. Recently it has been shown that CXCR4 mediates fusion of FIV env SU with cellular membranes. These findings corroborate a cross-species function of seven-transmembrane domain (7TM) molecules as common coreceptors for lentiviruses *(118)*. Feline CXCR4 displays 95% homology at the amino acid level to the human homologue. This homology is reflected by the finding that human stromal cell-derived factor (SDF-1) specifically binds to feline CXCR4 and inhibits FIV infection *(119)*. Infection of IL-2-dependent T cells with FIV can not be inhibited by SDF-1, suggesting a CXCR4-independent mechanism of infection in T cells. At this point it is important to note that under certain conditions chemokines can enhance rather than inhibit infection either by upregulation of cellular chemokine receptors or enhancement of viral replication *(119,120)*.

Pathogenesis of FAIDS

Kinetic studies on the infection levels of different lymphocyte subpopulations reveal that during acute infection, CD4$^+$ T cells represent the main population of infected cells (2–4 wk after infection), followed by B cells, whereas CD8$^+$ T cell are 10 times less infected than CD4$^+$ T cells *(121)*. The primary phase of infection is characterized by an initial burst of viremia which results in widespread dissemination of the virus to other lymphoid organs *(122)* (Fig. ID). At the same time a generalized lymphadenopathy appears with leukopenia, neutropenia, fever and diarrhea. (clinical stage 1). T cell dependent functions are depressed whereas B cells undergo polyclonal B cell activation with hypergammaglobulinemia and normal antibody responses to T-independent antigens (for review see *107,123*). The course of disease is age dependent, as newborn kittens develop severe and persisting lymphadenopathy whereas geriatric cats develop a less severe and shorter clinical stage 1, but proceed faster to the later stages of disease. Moreover, acute FIV infection induces both thymic B cell follicular hyperplasia and atrophy in juvenile cats which might result in the inability of the thymus to replenish the peripheral T-cell pool *(124)*. Stage 1 is followed by an asymptomatic phase where virus can still be isolated from the blood. Decreased numbers of CD4$^+$ T cells as well as inversion of the normal CD4$^+$/CD8$^+$ ratio are observed in this asymptomatic stage 2 (for review see *103*). In chronically infected cats a high percentage of apoptotic lymphocytes has been observed, and is most likely a result of chronic activation. There is a direct inverse correlation between the relative and absolute numbers of CD4$^+$ and CD8$^+$ T cells, and the percentage of apoptosis in PBLs *(125)*.

If cats are kept under pathogen-free conditions, clinical stage 2 can last up to 5 yr or longer. During this chronic phase of infection the B cells represent the major infected lymphocyte subset, with only low levels of infection in CD4$^+$ T cells *(110,126)*. The asymptomatic stage is followed by a third phase with unspecific signs of illness, such as recurrent fever, anemia, anorexia, and lymphadenopathia. This stage is referred to as AIDS-related complex (ACR) with lymphadenopathy syndrome. In the terminal stage cats have symptoms analogous to human AIDS, namely opportunistic infections due to leukopenia, as well as neoplasia, neurological pathology, and hematopoetic disorders. In the ARC stage a variable combination of follicular hyperplasia and involution can be detected in lymphoid tissue, whereas in the terminal stage the lymph node architecture is often abrogated as seen in AIDS patients. In the bone marrow abnormalities consisting either of hyperplasia or myeloid dysplasia are frequently found, both in the ACR and AIDS-like stage (for review see *113*). Maturation arrests, particularly in erythropoiesis are common. Despite the fact that the bone marrow is affected by FIV, infection levels determined by *in situ* hybridization are relatively low. However the numbers of infected cells in the bone marrow and periphery increase during the course of disease. The cats die as a result of severe viral, bacterial, or fungal infections.

Symptomatic FIV-infected animals frequently have FIV-related diseases of other organs. This is relevant for inflammatory and autoimmune diseases of the eye, kidney, skin, gastrointestinal tract, respiratory system, and CNS (for review see *113*). As for HIV infection the most common form of neurological syndromes, FIV encephalopathy, occurs in cats developing AIDS. Neurologic diseases can be a direct consequence of FIV replication in microglia and astrocytes *(127)*, a tropism also displayed by HIV-1 and SIV. Alternatively neuropathogenic effects are indirectly mediated by induction of TNF-α or reactive oxygen derivates. Increased production of TNFα has been reported to induce apoptosis in chronically FIV-infected cells in vitro. Both FIV strain specificity and status of immunosuppression determines the outcome of encephalopathy in cats *(128)*.

FIV also plays a role in tumor development. B cell lymphomas occur late in infection and are more frequent than myeloid tumors or miscellaneous carcinomas and sarcomas (for review see *113*). Another study describes the predominance of miscellaneous forms of B cell lymphosarcomas with uncommon extranodal localization in the heart, eye, spinal cord, and brain *(129)*. Integrated FIV sequences have never been identified in such tumors; therefore tumor development has been hypothesized to be caused by an indirect mechanism during polyclonal B cell activation. However, a recent study strongly indicates that FIV can directly transform B cells after integration into the target cell genome *(130)*.

Antiviral Immune Response

The cellular and humoral immune system seems to be incapable of controlling and clearing FIV from infected tissues, and virtually all cats remain persistently infected for life. Virus-specific antibodies in animals experimentally infected with FIV appear 2–4 wk after infection and mostly stay high for the rest of their life (for review see *131*). The humoral immune response is mainly directed against env followed by a response against gag protein. Nine antibody domains have been identified in the env protein *(132)*. The V3 domain is an important target for virus neutralizing *(133,134)*. This domain also contains determinants for target cell tropism *(114)*. Similar to HIV, infection with primary FIV isolates generates only a poor neutralizing antibody response *(135,136)*. Cellular molecules incorporated into the viral envelope have been suggested to contribute to induction of neutralizing Ab against HIV and SIV. Sera derived from cats infected with FIV-Pet, -A6, or -M2 isolates are efficiently neutralizing, and crossreactive when assayed on a fibroblast cell line. Passive transfer of such antibodies can protect cats from disease *(137)*. However, after a single passage on lymphoid cells in vitro or one passage in vivo they strongly loose neutralizing capacity *(135)*. As for HIV, EIAV and CAEV infection, env-specific Abs have been described even to enhance rather than inhibit FIV infection as well as HIV infection, and therefore may represent a risk in vaccine strategies based on Ab-induction *(138–140)*. Due to protection of cats after vaccination in the absence of detectable neutralizing antibodies, the protective effect of FIV vaccines is likely to be dependent on efficient priming of the cellular immune response (for review see *131*). FIV-specific CTLs in infected cats become detectable either 2 or 9 wk after inoculation in two independent studies *(141,142)*. Functional $CD8^+$ T cells seem to contribute partially to inhibition of virus replication in peripheral blood mononuclear cells *(143)*. Cats vaccinated with inactivated FIV are protected against FAIDS and develop a detectable CTL response against env, and in two of four cats, also against gag *(144,145)*. Cats injected with a FIV DNA vaccine generate env and gag-specific CTLs but this response is only short-lived in the absence of rechallenge *(146)*. Since no antiviral antibodies were detectable in immunized cats, reduced virus levels after FIV challenge were interpreted to be the result of a protective virus specific CTL response. On the other hand, an earlier study demonstrates that a DNA vaccine containing FIV env accelerates viral infection without induction of specific antibodies *(139)*. Therefore, an efficient vaccine against FIV infection is still missing.

CONCLUSIONS

Retroviruses that cause general immunodeficiency syndromes such as FIV, FeLV, and MuLV may use distinct mechanisms leading to progressive destruction of the responding immune system as well as persistence. However, in different species several viruses have common features of disease development. In feline as well as in human immunodeficiency diseases it is generally assumed that the primary phase of immunodeficiency virus infections is critical in determining the overall disease course, that is, whether it proceeds to AIDS over a shorter or longer latency period. A strong cellular immune response seems to be crucial in maintaining the asymptomatic phase in long term nonprogressors in both HIV and FIV infections. On the contrary, the early cellular immune response in MAIDS and MMTV infection is responsible for amplifying infected cells and establishing an efficient infection. Virus replication in the thymus plays a cruical role in the pathogenesis of both murine leukemia virus and lentivirus infections when infections occur early in life. In children or young cats AIDS development progresses more rapidly as a result of thymic atrophy and most likely lack of replenishing the peripheral lymphocyte pool.

The role of the humoral immune response is distinct from one retrovirus to the other. In murine retrovirus infections such as MMTV, neutralizing antibodies clearly can protect the host from reinfection and maintain systemic infection at a low level but the antibody response is not capable of preventing infection of the mammary gland or eradicating the infection. However, in lentivirus infection several observations speak against a major role of the humoral immune response in protection from disease: (1) primary virus isolates poorly induce a neutralizing humoral immune response; (2) vaccination strategies are protective in the absence of neutralizing antibodies; (3) sera that neutralize virus isolates derived from cell lines strongly lose neutralizing capacity after a single passage of the virus in vivo.

Studies in animal models contribute to the molecular understanding of mechanisms leading to immunodeficiency, and it will be highly interesting to see where the different retrovirally induced diseases converge to come to the same effects.

REFERENCES

1. Tsiagbe VK, Asakawa J, Miranda A, Sutherland RM, Paterson Y, Thorbecke GJ. Syngeneic response to SJL follicular center B cell lymphoma (reticular cell sarcoma) cells is primarily in V β 16$^+$ CD4$^+$ T cells. J Immunol 1993; 150:5519–28.
2. Stoye JP, Moroni C, Coffin JM. Virological events leading to spontaneous AKR thymomas. J Virol 1991; 65:1273–85.
3. Green WR. Genetic control of the induction of cytolytic T lymphocyte responses to AKR/Gross viral leukemias. II. Negative control by the Fv-1 locus in AKR mice of responder H-2^b haplotype. J Immunol 1984; 132:2665–71.
4. Uittenbogaart CH, Law W, Leenen P, Bristol G, van Ewijk W, Hays E. Thymic dendritic cells are primary targets for the oncogenic virus SL3–3. J Virol 1998; 72:10118.
5. Cloyd MW. Characterization of target cells for MCF viruses in AKR mice. Cell 1983; 32:217–225.
6. Acha-Orbea H, Shakhov A, Scarpellino L, Kolb E, Müller V, Vessaz-Shaw A, et al. Clonal deletion of Vβ14 positive T cells in mammary tumor virus transgenic mice. Nature 1991; 350:207–11.
7. Choi Y, Kappler J, Marrack P. A superantigen encoded in the open reading frame of the 3′ long terminal repeat of mouse mammary tumor virus. Nature 1991; 350:203–7.
8. Luther SA, Acha-Orbea H. Mouse mammary tumor virus: immunological interplays between virus and host. Adv Immunol 1997; 65:139–243.
9. Mosier DE, Yetter RA, Morse HCL. Retroviral induction of acute lymphoproliferative disease and profound immunosuppression in adult C57BL/6 mice. J Exp Med 1985; 161:766–84.
10. Huang M, Simard C, Jolicoeur P. Immunodeficiency and clonal growth of target cells induced by helper-free defective retrovirus. Science 1989; 246:1614–7.
11. Aziz DC, Hanna Z, Jolicoeur P. Severe immunodeficiency disease induced by a defective murine leukaemia virus. Nature 1989; 338:505–8.
12. Lee JS, Giese NA, Elkins KL, Yetter RA, Holmes KL, Hartley JW, Morse HCR. Effects of exogenous, nonleukemogenic, ecotropic murine leukemia virus infections on the immune systems of adult C57BL/6 mice. J Virol 1995; 69:4182–8.
13. Makino M, Morse HC III, Fredrickson TN, Hartley JW. H-2-associated and background genes influence the development of a murine retrovirus-induced immunodeficiency syndrome. J Immunol 1990; 144:4347–55.
14. Kim WK, Tang Y, Kenny JJ, Longo DL, Morse HCR. In murine AIDS, B cells are early targets of defective virus and are required for efficient infection and expression of defective virus in T cells and macrophages. J Virol 1994; 68:6767–9.

15. Simard C, Huang M, Jolicoeur P. Murine AIDS is initiated in the lymph nodes draining the site of inoculation, and the infected B cells influence T cells located at distance, in noninfected organs. J Virol 1994; 68:1903–12.
16. Muralidhar G, Koch S, Haas M, Swain SL. CD4 T cells in murine acquired immunodeficiency syndrome: polyclonal progression to anergy. J Exp Med 1992; 175:1589–99.
17. Colombi S, Deprez M, De Leval L, Humblet C, Greimers R, Defresne MP, et al. Thymus involvement in murine acquired immunodeficiency (MAIDS). Thymus 1994; 23:27–37.
18. Fitzpatrick EA, Bryson JS, Rhoads C, Kaplan AM, Cohen DA. T-deficient transmembrane signaling in $CD4^+$ T cells of retroviral-induced immune-deficient mice. J Immunol 1992; 148:3377–84.
19. Selvey LA, Morse HCR, June CH, Hodes RJ. Analysis of antigen receptor signaling in B cells from mice with a retrovirus-induced acquired immunodeficiency syndrome. J Immunol 1995; 154:171–9.
20. Muralidhar G, Koch S, Broome HE, Swain SL. TCR triggering of anergic CD4 T cells in murine AIDS induces apoptosis rather than cytokine synthesis and proliferation. J Immunol 1996; 157:625–35.
21. Hiromatsu K, Aoki Y, Makino M, Matsumoto Y, Mizuochi T, Gotoh Y, et al. Increased Fas antigen expression in murine retrovirus-induced immunodeficiency syndrome, MAIDS. Eur J Immunol 1994; 24:2446–51.
22. Kanagawa O, Vaupel BA, Korsmeyer SJ, Russell JH. Apoptotic death of lymphocytes in murine acquired immunodeficiency syndrome: involvement of Fas-Fas ligand interaction. Eur J Immunol 1995; 25:2421–7.
23. Usami J, Hiromatsu K, Aoki Y, Kobayashi N, Makino M, Yagita H, et al. Apoptosis by CD95 (Fas)-dependent and -independent mechanisms in Peyer's patch lymphocytes in murine retrovirus-induced immunodeficiency syndrome. J Virol 1996; 70:8917–25.
24. Morse HCD, Yetter RA, Via CS, Hardy RR, Cerny A, Hayakawa K, et al. Functional and phenotypic alterations in T cell subsets during the course of MAIDS, a murine retrovirus-induced immunodeficiency syndrome. J Immunol 1989; 143:844–50.
25. Portnoi D, Viale AC, Colle JH. Abnormal selection of antibody repertoires in retrovirus-induced murine AIDS. J Immunol 1993; 151:5073–80.
26. Sei Y, Arora PK, Skolnick P, Paul IA. Spatial learning impairment in a murine model of AIDS. FASEB J 1992; 6:3008–13.
27. Jolicoeur P. Murine acquired immunodeficiency syndrome (MAIDS): an animal model to study the AIDS pathogenesis. FASEB J 1991; 5:2398–405.
28. Simard C, Klein SJ, Mak T, Jolicoeur P. Studies of the susceptibility of nude, CD4 knockout, and SCID mutant mice to the disease induced by the murine AIDS defective virus. J Virol 1997; 71:3013–22.
29. Dupraz P, Rebai N, Klein SJ, Beaulieu N, Jolicoeur P. The murine AIDS virus Gag precursor protein binds to the SH3 domain of c-Abl. J Virol 1997; 71:2615–20.
30. Morse HCD, Chattopadhyay SK, Makino M, Fredrickson TN, Hugin AW, Hartley JW. Retrovirus-induced immunodeficiency in the mouse: MAIDS as a model for AIDS. AIDS 1992; 6:607–21.
31. Cerny A, Hugin AW, Hardy RR, Hayakawa K, Zinkernagel RM, Makino M, Morse HCD. B cells are required for induction of T cell abnormalities in a murine retrovirus-induced immunodeficiency syndrome. J Exp Med 1990; 171:315–20.
32. Leval L, Colombi S, Debrus S, Demoitie MA, Greimers R, Linsley P, et al. CD28-B7 costimulatory blockade by CTLA4Ig delays the development of retrovirus-induced murine AIDS. J Virol 1998; 72:5285–90.
33. Green KA, Crassi KM, Laman JD, Schoneveld A, Strawbridge RR, Foy TM, et al. Antibody to the ligand for CD40 (gp39) inhibits murine AIDS-associated splenomegaly, hypergammaglobulinemia, and immunodeficiency in disease-susceptible C57BL/6 mice. J Virol 1996; 70:2569–75.

34. Numata F, Hitoshi Y, Uehara S, Takatsu K. The xid mutation plays an important role in delayed development of murine acquired immunodeficiency syndrome. Int Immunol 1997; 9:139–46.
35. Cerny A, Merino R, Makino M, Waldvogel FA, Morse HCD, Izui S. Protective effect of cyclosporin A on immune abnormalities observed in the murine acquired immunodeficiency syndrome. Eur J Immunol 1991; 21:1747–50.
36. Makino M, Yoshimatsu K, Azuma M, Okada Y, Hitoshi Y, Yagita H, et al. Rapid development of murine AIDS is dependent of signals provided by CD54 and CD11a. J Immunol 1995; 155:974–81.
37. Giese N, Gazzinelli R, Morawetz R, Morse H III. Role of IL12 in MAIDS. Res Immunol 1995; 127:600–5.
38. Doherty TM, Giese N, Morse HCR, Coffman RL. Modulation of murine AIDS-related pathology by concurrent antibody treatment and coinfection with Leishmania major. J Virol 1997; 71:3702–9.
39. Heng JK, Price P, Lai CM, Beilharz MW. Alpha/beta interferons increase host resistance to murine AIDS. J Virol 1996; 70:4517.
40. Gazzinelli RT, Giese NA, Morse HCR. In vivo treatment with interleukin 12 protects mice from immune abnormalities observed during murine acquired immunodeficiency syndrome (MAIDS). J Exp Med 1994; 180:2199–208.
41. Doyon L, Simard C, Sekaly RP, Jolicoeur P. Evidence that the murine AIDS defective virus does not encode a superantigen. J Virol 1996; 70:1–9.
42. Gayama S, Doyon L, Vaupel B, Sekaly RP, Kanagawa O. Induction of endogenous mammary tumor virus in lymphocytes infected with murine acquired immunodeficiency syndrome virus. Cell Immunol 1998; 187:124–30.
43. McCarty TC, Chattopadhyay SK, Scherer MT, Fredrickson TN, Hartley JW, Morse HCR. Endogenous Mtv-encoded superantigens are not required for development of murine AIDS. J Virol 1996; 70:8148–50.
44. Gilmore GL, Cowing C, Mosier DE. LP-BM5 murine retrovirus-induced immunodeficiency disease in allogeneic SCID chimeric mice. Inability to recognize a putative viral superantigen does not prevent induction of disease. J Immunol 1993; 150:185–9.
45. Tew JG, Kosco MH, and Szakal AK. The alternative antigen pathway. Immunol Today 1989; 10:229–32.
46. Masuda A, Burton GF, Fuchs BA, Bhogal BS, Rupper R, Szakal AK, Tew JG. Follicular dendritic cell function and murine AIDS. Immunology 1994; 81:41–6.
47. Makino M, Sei Y, Arora PK, Morse HCD, Hartley JW. Impaired calcium mobilization in $CD4^+$ and $CD8^+$ T cells in a retrovirus-induced immunodeficiency syndrome, murine AIDS. J Immunol 1992; 149:1707–13.
48. Pavlovitch JH, Hulier E, Rizk-Rabin M, Marussig M, Mazier D, Joffret ML, et al. Resistance to murine AIDS in offspring of mice infected with LP-BM5. Role of CD8 T cells. J Immunol 1996; 156:4757–63.
49. Tang Y, Hugin AW, Giese NA, Gabriele L, Chattopadhyay SK, Fredrickson TN, et al. Control of immunodeficiency and lymphoproliferation in mouse AIDS: studies of mice deficient in $CD8^+$ T cells or perforin. J Virol 1997; 71:1808–13.
50. Erbe JG, Green KA, Crassi KM, Morse HCD, Green WR. Cytolytic T lymphocytes specific for tumors and infected cells from mice with a retrovirus-induced immunodeficiency syndrome. J Virol 1992; 66:3251–6.
51. Mayrand SM, Schwarz DA, Green WR. An alternative translational reading frame encodes an immunodominant retroviral CTL determinant expressed by an immunodeficiency-causing retrovirus. J Immunol 1998; 160:39–50.
52. Sechler JM, Lawler A, Hartley JW, Morse HCR, McCarty TC, Swofford R, Rosenberg AS. Induction of murine acquired immunodeficiency syndrome (MAIDS) in allophenic mice generated from strains susceptible and resistant to disease. J Exp Med 1996; 184:2101–8.

53. Friend C. Cell-free transmission in adult Swiss mice of a disease having the character of a leukemia. J Exp Med 1957; 105:307.
54. Kabat D. Molecular biology of Friend viral erythroleukemia. Curr Top Microbiol Immunol 1989; 148:1–42.
55. Ben-David Y, Bernstein A. Friend virus-induced erythroleukemia and the multistage nature of cancer. Cell 1991; 66:831–4.
56. Albritton LM, Tseng L, Scadden D, Cunningham JM. A putative murine ecotropic retrovirus receptor gene encodes a multiple membrane-spanning protein and confers susceptibility to virus infection. Cell 1989; 57:659–6.
57. Li JP, D'Andrea AD, Lodish HF, Baltimore D. Activation of cell growth by binding of Friend spleen focus-forming virus gp55 glycoprotein to the erythropoietin receptor. Nature 1990; 343:762–4.
58. Li JP, Baltimore D. Mechanism of leukemogenesis induced by mink cell focus-forming murine leukemia viruses. J Virol 1991; 65:2408.
59. Mazgareanu S, Muller JG, Czub S, Schimmer S, Bredt M, Czub M. Suppression of rat bone marrow cells by Friend murine leukemia virus envelope proteins. Virology 1998; 242:357–65.
60. Tanaka A, Oka K, Tanaka K, Jinno A, Ruscetti SK, Kai K. The entire nucleotide sequence of friend-related and paralysis-inducing PVC-441 murine leukemia virus (MuLV) and its comparison with those of PVC-211 MuLV and Friend MuLV. J Virol 1998; 72:3423.
61. Nihrane A, Fujita K, Willey R, Lyu MS, Silver J. Murine leukemia virus envelope protein in transgenic-mouse serum blocks infection in vitro. J Virol 1996; 70:1882.
62. Nihrane A, Silver J. Spontaneous priming for anti-viral envelope cytotoxic T lymphocytes in mice transgenic for a murine leukaemia virus envelope gene (Fv4). Immunology 1997; 90:219.
63. Hasenkrug KJ, Chesebro B. Immunity to retroviral infection: the Friend virus model. Proc Natl Acad Sci USA 1997; 94:7811–6.
64. Earl PL, Moss B, Morrison RP, Wehrly K, Nishio J, Chesebro B. T-lymphocyte priming and protection against Friend leukemia by vaccinia-retrovirus env gene recombinant. Science 1986; 234:728.
65. Hasenkrug KJ, Brooks DM, Dittmer U. Critical role for CD4(+) T cells in controlling retrovirus replication and spread in persistently infected mice. J Virol 1998; 72:6559–64.
66. Morrison RP, Nishio J, Chesebro B. Influence of the murine MHC (H-2) on Friend leukemia virus-induced immunosuppression. J Exp Med 1986; 163:301–14.
67. Hasenkrug KJ, Valenzuela A, Letts VA, Nishio J, Chesebro B, Frankel WN. Chromosome mapping of Rfv3, a host resistance gene to Friend murine retrovirus. J Virol 1995; 69:2617–20.
68. Lu L, Zhou Z, Wu B, Xiao M, Shen RN, Williams DE, et al. Influence of recombinant human interleukin (IL)-7 on disease progression in mice infected with Friend virus complex. Int J Cancer 1992; 52:261–5.
69. Chieco-Bianchi L, Collavo D, Biasi G. Immunologic unresponsiveness to murine leukemia virus antigens: mechanisms and role in tumor development. Adv Cancer Res 1988; 51:277.
70. Moloney JB. Biological studies on a lymphoid leukemia virus extracted from sarcoma 537 I. Origin and introductory investigations. J Natl Cancer Inst 1960; 24:933.
71. Jiang D, Flyer DC. Immune response to Moloney murine leukemia virus nonviral, tumor-associated antigens fails to provide in vivo tumor protection. J Immunol 1992; 148:974–80.
72. Biasi G, Mazzocchi M, Facchinetti A, Panozzo M, Zanovello P, Collavo D, Chieco-Bianchi L. Induction of Moloney murine sarcoma virus tolerance in adult mice by anti-CD4 monoclonal antibody treatment. Cancer Res 1990; 50:5703S–6S.
73. Kast WM, Boog CJ, Roep BO, Voordouw AC, Melief CJ. Failure or success in the restoration of virus-specific cytotoxic T lymphocyte response defects by dendritic cells. J Immunol 1988; 140:3186–93.
74. Sijts AJ, Ossendorp F, Mengede EA, van den Elsen PJ, Melief CJ. Immunodominant mink cell focus-inducing murine leukemia virus (MuLV)-encoded CTL epitope, identified by its MHC class I-binding motif, explains MuLV-type specificity of MCF-directed cytotoxic T lymphocytes. J Immunol 1994; 152:106–16.

75. van den Broek ME, Kagi D, Ossendorp F, Toes R, Vamvakas S, Lutz WK. et al. Decreased tumor surveillance in perforin-deficient mice. J Exp Med 1996; 184:1781.
76. Sijts AJ, De Bruijn ML, Ressing ME, Nieland JD, Mengede EA, Boog CJ. Identification of an H-2 Kb-presented Moloney murine leukemia virus cytotoxic T-lymphocyte epitope that displays enhanced recognition in H-2 Db mutant bm13 mice. J Virol 1994; 68:6038–46.
77. Chen W, Qin H, Chesebro B, Cheever MA. Identification of a gag-encoded cytotoxic T- lymphocyte epitope from FBL-3 leukemia shared by Friend, Moloney, and Rauscher murine leukemia virus-induced tumors. J Virol 1996; 70:7773–82.
78. Iezzi G, Rivolta L, Ronchetti A, Martin-Fontecha A, Rosato A, Protti MP, et al. The immunogenicity of experimental tumors is strongly biased by the expression of dominant viral cytotoxic T-lymphocyte epitopes. Cancer Res 1997; 57:2564–8.
79. Brawand P, Biasi G, Horvath C, Cerottini JC, MacDonald HR. Flow-microfluorometric monitoring of oligoclonal CD8+ T cell responses to an immunodominant Moloney leukemia virus-encoded epitope in vivo. J Immunol 1998; 160:1659–65.
80. Ossendorp F, Eggers M, Neisig A, Ruppert T, Groettrup M, Sijts A, et al. A single residue exchange within a viral CTL epitope alters proteasome-mediated degradation resulting in lack of antigen presentation. Immunity 1996; 5:115–24.
81. Naldini L, Blomer U, Gallay P, Ory D, Mulligan R, Gage FH, et al. In vivo gene delivery and stable transduction of nondividing cells by a lentiviral vector. Science 1996; 272:263–7.
82. Poeschla EM, Wong-Staal F, Looney DJ. Efficient transduction of nondividing human cells by feline immunodeficiency virus lentiviral vectors. Nat Med 1998; 4:354–7.
83. Lynn WS, Wong PK. Neuroimmunodegeneration: do neurons and T cells use common pathways for cell death? FASEB J 1995; 9:1147–56.
84. Gonzales-Scarano F, Nathanson N, Wong P. Retroviruses and the nervous system. In: Levy JA (ed). The Retroviridae Vol. 4. New York: Plenum Press, 1995; p. 409.
85. Saha K, Wong PK. T, not B, lymphocytes are required for immunodeficiency and paralysis induced by ts1, a mutant of Moloney murine leukemia virus-TB. Virology 1991; 183:815–20.
86. Saha K, Wong PK. Rudimentary thymus of SCID mouse plays an important role in the development of retrovirus-induced neurologic disorders. Virology 1993; 195:211–8.
87. Rauscher F. A virus-induced disease of mice characterized by erythropoiesis and lymphoid leukemia. J Natl Cancer Inst 1962; 29:515–43.
88. Khimani AH, Lim M, Graf TG, Smith TF, Ruprecht RM. Phylogenetic relationship of the complete Rauscher murine leukemia virus genome with other murine leukemia virus genomes. Virology 1997; 238:64–7.
89. Gabrilovich DI, Roberts MS, Harvey JJ, Botcherby M, Bedford PA, Knight SC. Effects of murine leukemia viruses on the function of dendritic cells. Eur J Immunol 1993; 23:2932–8.
90. Gabrilovich DI, Woods GM, Patterson S, Harvey JJ, Knight SC. Retrovirus-induced immunosuppression via blocking of dendritic cell migration and down-regulation of adhesion molecules. Immunology 1994; 82:82–7.
91. Ruprecht RM, O'Brien LG, Rossoni LD, Nusinoff-Lehrman S. Suppression of mouse viraemia and retroviral disease by 3′-azido-3′-deoxythymidine. Nature 1986; 323:467–9.
92. Ruprecht RM, Bronson R. Chemoprevention of retroviral infection: success is determined by virus inoculum strength and cellular immunity. DNA Cell Biol 1994; 13:59–66.
93. Ruprecht RM, Mullaney S, Bernard LD, Gama Sosa MA, Hom RC, Finberg RW. Vaccination with a live retrovirus: the nature of the protective immune response. Proc Natl Acad Sci USA 1990; 87:5558–62.
94. Hom RC, Finberg RW, Mullaney S, Ruprecht RM. Protective cellular retroviral immunity requires both CD4+ and CD8+ immune T cells. J Virol 1991; 65:220–4.
95. Finke D, Mortezavi L, Acha-Orbea H. Preactivation of B lymphocytes does not enhance mouse mammary tumor virus infection. J Virol 1998; 72:7688–91.

96. Toellner KM, Luther SA, Sze DM, Choy RK, Taylor DR, MacLennan ICM, Acha-Orbea H. T helper 1 (Th1) and Th2 characteristics start to develop during T cell priming and are associated with an immediate ability to induce immunoglobulin class switching. J Exp Med 1998; 187:1193–204.
97. Maillard I, Launois P, Xenarios I, Louis JA, Acha-Orbea H, Diggelmann H. Immune response to mouse mammary tumor virus in mice lacking the alpha/beta interferon or the gamma interferon receptor. J Virol 1998; 72:2638–46.
98. Acha-Orbea H, Finke D, Attinger A, Schmid S, Wehrli N, Vacheron S, et al. Interplays between mouse mammary tumor virus and the cellular and humoral immune response. Immunol Rev 1999; 168:287–303.
99. Overbaugh J, Donahue PR, Quackenbush SL, Hoover EA, Mullins JI. Molecular cloning of a feline leukemia virus that induces fatal immunodeficiency disease in cats. Science 1988; 239:906–10.
100. Overbaugh J, Riedel N, Hoover EA, Mullins JI. Transduction of endogenous envelope genes by feline leukaemia virus in vitro. Nature 1988; 332:731–4.
101. Pedersen NC, Ho EW, Brown ML, Yamamoto JK. Isolation of a T-lymphotropic virus from domestic cats with an immunodeficiency-like syndrome. Science 1987; 235:790.
102. Beebe AM, Faith TG, Sparger EE, Torten M, Pedersen NC, Dandekar S. Evaluation of in vivo and in vitro interactions of feline immunodeficiency virus and feline leukemia virus. AIDS 1994; 8:873–8.
103. Rosenberg N and Jolicoeur P. Retroviral pathogenesis In: Coffin JM, Hughes SM, Varmus ME, eds. Retroviruses, 1997, p 475 Cold Spring Harbor Laboratory Press. Cold Spring Harbor, NY.
104. Moser M, Burns CC, Boomer S, Overbaugh J. The host range and interference properties of two closely related feline leukemia variants suggest that they use distinct receptors. Virology 1998; 242:366.
105. Rohn JL, Moser MS, Gwynn SR, Baldwin DN, Overbaugh J. In vivo evolution of a novel, syncytium-inducing and cytopathic feline leukemia virus variant. J Virol 1998; 72:2686–96.
106. Trainin Z, Wernicke D, Ungar-Waron H, Essex M. Suppression of the humoral antibody response in natural retrovirus infections. Science 1983; 220:858–9.
107. Hardy WD. Feline oncoretroviruses. In: Levy JA (ed). The Retroviridae, vol. 2. New York: Plenum, 1993, p. 109.
108. Rojko JL, Hoover EA, Quackenbush SL, Olsen RG. Reactivation of latent feline leukaemia virus infection. Nature 1982; 298:385–8.
109. Lehmann R, Franchini M, Aubert A, Wolfensberger C, Cronier J, Lutz H. Vaccination of cats experimentally infected with feline immunodeficiency virus, using a recombinant feline leukemia virus vaccine. J Am Vet Med Assoc 1991; 199:1446–52.
110. Pedersen NC. The feline immunodeficiency virus. In: Levy JA (ed). New York: The Retroviridae, vol 2. Plenum 1993, p. 181.
111. Roelke-Parker ME, Munson L, Packer C, Kock R, Cleaveland S, Carpenter M, et al. A canine distemper virus epidemic in Serengeti lions (Panthera leo). Nature 1996; 379:441–5.
112. Lutz H, Isenbugel E, Lehmann R, Sabapara RH, Wolfensberger C. Retrovirus infections in non-domestic felids: serological studies and attempts to isolate a lentivirus. Vet Immunol Immunopathol 1992; 35:215–24.
113. Hartmann K. Feline immunodeficiency virus infection: an overview. Vet J 1998; 155:123–37.
114. Verschoor EJ, Boven LA, Blaak H, van Vliet AL, Horzinek MC, de Ronde A. A single mutation within the V3 envelope neutralization domain of feline immunodeficiency virus determines its tropism for CRFK cells. J Virol 1995; 69:4752–7.
115. Vahlenkamp TW, Verschoor EJ, Schuurman NN, van Vliet AL, Horzinek MC, Egberink HF, de Ronde A. A single amino acid substitution in the transmembrane envelope glycoprotein of feline immunodeficiency virus alters cellular tropism. J Virol 1997; 71:7132–5.

116. de Parseval A, Lerner DL, Borrow P, Willett BJ, Elder JH. Blocking of feline immunodeficiency virus infection by a monoclonal antibody to CD9 is via inhibition of virus release rather than interference with receptor binding. J Virol 1997; 71:5742–9.
117. Willett BJ, Hosie MJ, Dunsford TH, Neil JC, Jarrett O. Productive infection of T-helper lymphocytes with feline immunodeficiency virus is accompanied by reduced expression of CD4. AIDS 1991; 5:1469–75.
118. Willett BJ, Adema K, Heveker N, Brelot A, Picard L, Alizon M, et al. The second extracellular loop of CXCR4 determines its function as a receptor for feline immunodeficiency virus. J Virol 1998; 72:6475–81.
119. Hosie MJ, Broere N, Hesselgesser J, Turner JD, Hoxie JA, Neil JC, Willett BJ. Modulation of feline immunodeficiency virus infection by stromal cell-derived factor. J Virol 1998; 72:2097–104.
120. Kinter A, Catanzaro A, Monaco J, Ruiz M, Justement J, Moir S, et al. CC-chemokines enhance the replication of T-tropic strains of HIV-1 in CD4(+) T cells: role of signal transduction. Proc Natl Acad Sci USA 1998; 95:11880–5.
121. Dean GA, Reubel GH, Moore PF, Pedersen NC. Proviral burden and infection kinetics of feline immunodeficiency virus in lymphocyte subsets of blood and lymph node. J Virol 1996; 70:5165–9.
122. Diehl LJ, Mathiason-DuBard CK, O'Neil LL, Hoover EA. Longitudinal assessment of feline immunodeficiency virus kinetics in plasma by use of a quantitative competitive reverse transcriptase PCR. J Virol 1995; 69:2328–32.
123. Flynn JN, Cannon CA, Lawrence CE, Jarrett O. Polyclonal B-cell activation in cats infected with feline immunodeficiency virus. Immunology 1994; 81:626–30.
124. Woo JC, Dean GA, Pedersen NC, Moore PF. Immunopathologic changes in the thymus during the acute stage of experimentally induced feline immunodeficiency virus infection in juvenile cats. J Virol 1997; 71:8632–41.
125. Holznagel E, Hofmann-Lehmann R, Leutenegger C, Allenspach K, Huettner S, Forster U, et al. The role of in vitro-induced lymphocyte apoptosis in feline immunodeficiency virus infection: correltation with different markers of disease progression. J Virol 1998; 72:9025–33.
126. English RV, Johnson CM, Gebhard DH, Tompkins MB. In vivo lymphocyte tropism of feline immunodeficiency virus. J Virol 1998; 67:5175–86.
127. Yu N, Billaud JN, Phillips TR. Effects of feline immunodeficiency virus on astrocyte glutamate uptake: implications for lentivirus-induced central nervous system diseases. Proc Natl Acad Sci USA 1998; 95:2624–9.
128. Power C, Buist R, Johnston JB, Del Bigio MR, Ni W, Dawood MR, Peeling J. Neurovirulence in feline immunodeficiency virus-infected neonatal cats is viral strain specific and dependent on systemic immune suppression. J Virol 1998; 72:9109.
129. Callanan JJ, Jones BA, Irvine J, Willett BJ, McCandlish IA, Jarrett O. Histologic classification and immunophenotype of lymphosarcomas in cats with naturally and experimentally acquired feline immunodeficiency virus infections. Vet Pathol 1996; 33:264–72.
130. Beatty JA, Callanan JJ, Terry A, Jarrett O, Neil JC. Molecular and immunophenotypical characterization of a feline immunodeficiency virus (FIV)-associated lymphoma: a direct role for FIV in B-lymphocyte transformation? J Virol 1998; 72:767–71.
131. Willett BJ, Flynn JN, Hosie MJ. FIV infection of the domestic cat: an animal model for AIDS. Immunol Today 1997; 18:182–9.
132. Pancino G, Chappey C, Saurin W, Sonigo P. B epitopes and selection pressures in feline immunodeficiency virus envelope glycoproteins. J Virol 1993; 67:664–72.
133. de Ronde A, Stam JG, Boers P, Langedijk H, Meloen R, Hesselink W, et al. Antibody response in cats to the envelope proteins of feline immunodeficiency virus: identification of an immunodominant neutralization domain. Virology 1994; 198:257–64.

134. Richardson J, Fossati I, Moraillon A, Castelot S, Sonigo P, Pancino G. Neutralization sensitivity and accessibility of continuous B cell epitopes of the feline immunodeficiency virus envelope. J Gen Virol 1996; 77:759–71.
135. Baldinotti F, Matteucci D, Mazzetti P, Giannelli C, Bandecchi P, Tozzini F, Bendinelli M. Serum neutralization of feline immunodeficiency virus is markedly dependent on passage history of the virus and host system. J Virol 1994; 68:4572–9.
136. Del Mauro D, Matteucci D, Giannecchini S, Maggi F, Pistello M, Bendinelli M. Autologous and heterologous neutralization analyses of primary feline immunodeficiency virus isolates. J Virol 1998; 72:2199–207.
137. Hohdatsu T, Pu R, Torres BA, Trujillo S, Gardner MB, Yamamoto JK. Passive antibody protection of cats against feline immunodeficiency virus infection. J Virol 1993; 67:2344.
138. Lombardi S, Garzelli C, Pistello M, Massi C, Matteucci D, Baldinotti F, et al. A neutralizing antibody-inducing peptide of the V3 domain of feline immunodeficiency virus envelope glycoprotein does not induce protective immunity. J Virol 1994; 68:8374–9.
139. Richardson J, Moraillon A, Baud S, Cuisinier AM, Sonigo P, Pancino G. Enhancement of feline immunodeficiency virus (FIV) infection after DNA vaccination with the FIV envelope. J Virol 1997; 71:9640–9.
140. Siebelink KH, Tijhaar E, Huisman RC, Huisman W, de Ronde A, Darby IH, et al. Enhancement of feline immunodeficiency virus infection after immunization with envelope glycoprotein subunit vaccines. J Virol 1995; 69:3704–11.
141. Beatty JA, Willett BJ, Gault EA, Jarrett O. A longitudinal study of feline immunodeficiency virus-specific cytotoxic T lymphocytes in experimentally infected cats, using antigen-specific induction. J Virol 1996; 70:6199–206.
142. Song W, Collisson EW, Billingsley PM, Brown WC. Induction of feline immunodeficiency virus-specific cytolytic T-cell responses from experimentally infected cats. J Virol 1992; 66:5409–17.
143. Jeng CR, English RV, Childers T, Tompkins MB, Tompkins WA. Evidence for CD8+ antiviral activity in cats infected with feline immunodeficiency virus. J Virol 1996; 70:2474–80.
144. Flynn JN, Beatty JA, Cannon CA, Stephens EB, Hosie MJ, Neil JC, Jarrett O. 1995. Involvement of gag- and env-specific cytotoxic T lymphocytes in protective immunity to feline immunodeficiency virus. AIDS Res Hum Retrovir 1995; 11:1107–13.
145. Flynn JN, Keating P, Hosie MJ, Mackett M, Stephens EB, Beatty JA et al. Env-specific CTL predominate in cats protected from feline immunodeficiency virus infection by vaccination. J Immunol 1996; 157:3658–65.
146. Hosie MJ, Flynn JN, Rigby MA, Cannon C, Dunsford T, Mackay NA, et al. DNA vaccination affords significant protection against feline immunodeficiency virus infection without inducing detectable antiviral antibodies. J Virol 1998; 72:7310–9.

7
Immune Response to HTLV-I and HTLV-II

Samantha S. Soldan and Steven Jacobson

INTRODUCTION

Originally identified from a T-lymphoblastoid cell line (HUT 102) of a patient diagnosed with a cutaneous T-cell lymphoma, the human T-lymphotropic virus type I (HTLV-I) was the first described human retrovirus *(1)*. In 1981, HTLV-I was established as the etiologic agent for adult T-cell leukemia (ATL) *(2)*, a hematological malignancy first characterized in Japan *(3)*. Since the initial description of ATL and the discovery of HTLV-I, the virus has been associated with an inflammatory, chronic, progressive neurologic disease known as HTLV-I associated myelopathy/tropical spastic paraparesis (HAM/TSP) in addition to several other inflammatory diseases *(4–14)*. Although an increasing number of human diseases have been linked to HTLV-I the vast majority of HTLV-I–infected individuals remain clinically asymptomatic.

Shortly after the discovery of HTLV-I, the human T-lymphotropic virus type II (HTLV-II) was identified in a T-cell line established from the splenic tissue of a patient with hairy cell leukemia *(15)*. The association of HTLV-II with hairy cell leukemia was never firmly established and to date HTLV-II has not been demonstrated as the definitive etiologic agent of a well defined human pathology. Therefore, HTLV-II has been considered a harmless infection and has received substantially less attention than HTLV-I. However, the fascinating epidemiology of HTLV-II infection coupled with mounting evidence that suggests that HTLV-II may be associated with a range of neurologic and lymphoproliferative disorders warrants further consideration of this virus.

The study of HTLV-I and HTLV-II has led to advances in the understanding of retrovirology, retroviral associated diseases pathogenesis, the immune system, and human evolution and migration. This chapter concentrates on the epidemiological, pathological, and immunological aspects of HTLV-I and HTLV-II infection. The well studied immune abnormalities of HAM/TSP and the cellular immune response to HTLV-I are given special attention. The elucidation of the immunopathology of HAM/TSP will enhance our understanding of other HTLV-I associated disorders as well as other neurological, hematologic, and inflammatory diseases for which viral etiologies have been suggested.

STRUCTURE AND BIOLOGY OF HTLV-I AND HTLV-II

Genetic Structure

HTLV-I and HTLV-II are members of the *Oncoviridae* subfamily of retroviruses which includes the bovine leukemia virus (BLV) and the simian T-cell leukemia

From: *Retroviral Immunology: Immune Response and Restoration*
Edited by: Giuseppe Pantaleo and Bruce D. Walker © Humana Press Inc., Totowa, NJ

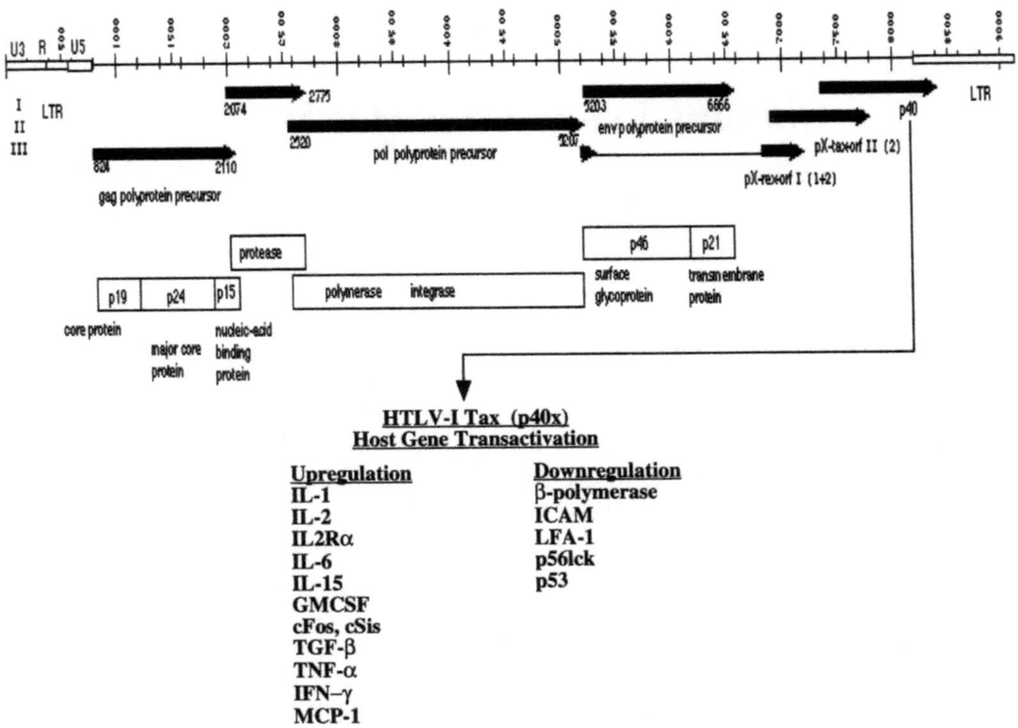

Fig. 1. Structure of HTLV-I with coded proteins. The HTLV-I genome is 9032 bp in length and contains the group antigen (*gag*), polymerase (*pol*), and envelope (*env*) and *pX* genes flanked by long terminal repeats (LTRs). The *pX* gene codes for the regulatory proteins p40 Tax and p27 Rex. The Tax protein transactivates viral transcription through indirect action of the Tax responsive element in the U3 region and is known to upregulate and downregulate several cellular genes, some of which are listed here. This figure was adapted with permission from www.ncbi.nlm.nih.gov/retroviruses/HTLV/index.html.

viruses type I (STLV-I) and type II (STLV-II) *(16)*. HTLV-I and HTLV-II share 65% homology at the nucleotide sequence level. The homology between HTLV-I and HTLV-II is highest in the *tax* and *rex* genes and lowest in the long terminal repeat (LTR). In contrast to infection with lentiviruses such as HIV-1, genetic variability within an individual, known as quasispecies or intrapatient variation is extremely limited in HTLV infection *(17,18)*.

Although HTLV-I and HTLV-II contain the complement of group antigen *(gag)*, polymerase *(pol)*, and envelope *(env)* genes present in other retroviruses, the genetic structure of the *Oncoviridae* is distinct (Fig. 1). Two genes located in the *pX* region of the 3′ end of the *Oncoviridae* genome, known as the *tax* and *rex* genes, are responsible for the transcriptional activation of the LTR and expression of structural proteins respectively. The LTR is comprised of U3, R, and U5 regions. Essential components for viral transcription including the TATA box, Tax responsive elements, poly(A) site, and primer binding site are located in the U3 region *(19,20)*. The majority of the Rex-responsive element is contained in the R region but overlaps the 3′ of the U3 region.

Full-length RNA is utilized for synthesis of HTLV *gag* and *pol* gene products as it is in other retroviruses. $tRNA^{Pro}$ is used for reverse transcription of genomic HTLV RNA. Three messenger RNA (mRNA) species have been identified for HTLV. One single spliced subgenomic mRNA encodes the *env* gene product while a second subgenomic mRNA has two introns removed and encodes the Tax and Rex proteins. Four open reading frames located in the HTLV *pX* region encode the three major regulatory proteins: p40x *tax,* p27 *rex,* and p21 *rex* for HTLV-I and p37 *tax,* p26 *rex,* and p24 *rex* for HTLV-II. In both HTLV-I and HTLV-II, Tax is expressed preferentially over Rex *(20).* The p40/37 *tax* (Tax) protein *trans*-activates viral expression by indirect action upon the Tax-responsive element. In addition, HTLV-I Tax activates several cellular genes through the nuclear transcription factor NF-κB and the bZIP family of transcription activators. These Tax-induced genes include interleukin-2 (IL-2), IL-2 receptor 1-chain (IL-2Rα), IL-15, IL-6, monocyte chemoattractant protein-1, and granulocyte/macrophage colony stimulating factor (GM-CSF) *(21–29).* HTLV-I Tax also activates the transcription of the proto-onocogenes c-*fos* and c-*sis,* and parathyroid hormone related protein *(30–33)* and downregulates the transcription of β-polymerase gene, ICAM, LFA-1, and 56lck *(34–36).* Like HTLV-I Tax, HTLV-II Tax upregulates several cellular genes including the parathyroid hormone related protein and GM-CSF *(37,38)* and downregulates others including IL-10 *(38).* The ability of both HTLV-I and HTLV-II Tax to regulate the transcription of a variety of genes that encode for cytokines, adhesion molecules, proto-oncogenes, and tumor suppressers suggests that Tax has the ability to modulate the host immune response through cytokine expression, cellular proliferation and transformation, and viral replication.

The HTLV-I/HTLV-II p27/26 Rex protein regulates viral gene expression through post-transcriptional regulation of mRNA transport and splicing *(39,40)* and is essential for HTLV replication. Rex increases the expression of the unspliced mRNA coding for Gag, Pol, and Env protein and allows for viral assembly and budding *(39,40).* HTLV-I Rex increases the ratio of nonspliced to completely spliced mRNA *(41).* At increased concentrations, HTLV-II Rex has a negative regulatory effect resulting in decreased levels of viral mRNA and has been suggested to be involved in establishing HTLV-II latency *(42).* The function of the smaller HTLV-I/HTLV-II p21/24 *rex* subunits has not been established *(41).*

Transmission and Transformation

Transmission of HTLV-I requires direct cell-to-cell contact and typically occurs through one of three routes. Mother-to-child transmission may either occur through transplacental passage of infected maternal lymphocytes to the fetus or through infected lymphocytes in breast milk *(43–46).* From 10% to 27% of breast-fed children of HTLV-I–infected mothers become HTLV-I positive compared to fewer than 5% of bottle-fed children of HTLV-I infected mothers *(47).* In addition, polymerase chain reaction (PCR) amplification detected HTLV-I proviral DNA in the breast milk of all HTLV-I–infected mothers but only occasionally from carrier mothers' neonates, which suggests that transplacental infection with HTLV-I is rare and that postpartum infection via breast milk is the major perinatal transmission route *(48).* These observations have led to recommendations that HTLV-I carrier mothers refrain from breast feeding in order to reduce the incidence of HTLV-I transmission to their offspring. Sexual transmission of

HTLV-I may occur from male-to-female during sexual intercourse via HTLV-I–infected cells in semen with infection rates among females increasing with age *(49)*. Female-to-male transmission of HTLV-I also occurs but at a far lower rate *(50)*. The third route of HTLV-I transmission is through infected blood or blood products. Unlike human immunodeficiency virus (HIV), only blood products that involve the passage of whole lymphocytes from donor to recipient can transmit the virus. There is no evidence for the transmission of HTLV-I from cell-free blood products *(51)*. An increased risk for developing HAM/TSP has been suggested to be associated with transfusion *(52,53)*. Therefore, blood bank screening for HTLV-I seropositivity was initiated in Japan (1986), the United States (1988), France (1991), and the Netherlands (1993).

Like HTLV-I, HTLV-II is transmitted sexually, vertically from mother to child, by transfusion of contaminated cellular blood products, and through intravenous drug abuse *(54–58)*. The infection rates following transfusion with HTLV-II contaminated blood products are similar to infection rates following transfusion with HTLV-I–contaminated blood products reported in Japan *(56)*. However, there is an increased prevalence of HTLV-II compared to HTLV-I observed in intravenous drug abusers (IVDAs). The apparent increased efficiency of HTLV-II transmission through intravenous drug abuse is not well understood and may reflect different cellular tropisms or higher viral loads in HTLV-II–infected individuals *(59)*. Sexual transmission is an important route of HTLV-II infection *(60)*. In contrast to HTLV-I, where transmission of HTLV-I from male to female is far more efficient than from female to male *(49)*, HTLV-II sexual transmission rates are high. There appears to be equivalent transmission efficiencies between the sexes with infection rates increasing with age in both males and females *(58,60,61)*.

Although HTLV-I infects a number of cell types in vitro, the virus is detected mainly in $CD4^+$ T cells in vivo with 99% of HTLV-I DNA in the peripheral blood from infected patients found in $CD4^+$ cells *(20,62,63)*. EBV-transformed B-cell lines productively infected with HTLV have been established from patients but there is no direct evidence for HTLV-I infection of B cells in vivo *(64)*. Unlike HIV-1, HTLV-I does not use the CD4 molecule as a binding receptor and the mechanism for the preferred tropism of HTLV-I for $CD4^+$ cells is unknown. Although the cellular receptor for HTLV-I is unclear, one report suggested that the HTLV-I receptor may be encoded on chromosome 17 *(65)*. In contrast to HTLV-I, HTLV-II is reported to have a preferred tropism for $CD8^+$ lymphocytes in vivo *(66,67)*. HTLV-II may also infect $CD4^+$ T cells, B cells, natural killer cells, and monocytes at a lower frequency in vivo *(67)*.

Both HTLV-I and HTLV-II will immortalize primary human peripheral blood T cells in vitro. In addition to human T cells, T lymphocytes from monkeys, rabbits, cats, and rats have been transformed in vitro by HTLV-I *(68–70)*. Initially, the population of transformed cells shows a polyclonal pattern of integration of HTLV proviruses. Over time, dominant clones often predominate resulting in an oligoclonal pattern of integration. This transformation is typically of $CD4^+$ lymphocytes. However, $CD8^+$ and immature $CD4^+$ $CD8^-$ cells from bone marrow can also be transformed. HTLV transformed cells display phenotypes and surface markers associated with T cells functionally activated by specific antigens or lectin. HTLV Tax is essential for transformation of T lymphocytes and it has been demonstrated that specific mutations of *tax* abrogate the transforming ability of the virus *(71)*.

Epidemiology of HTLV-I and HTLV-II

HTLV-I is endemic in several regions throughout the world with clusters of high prevalence in the Caribbean, Japan (Kyushu, Shikoku, Okinawa), equatorial Africa (Ivory Coast, Nigeria, Zaire, Kenya, Tanzania), South America (Columbia), the Middle East (Iran), and Melanesia *(72–78)*. Additional areas of low prevalence have been reported in Taiwan, India, China, Korea, Iraq, Kuwait, and the Soviet Union *(75,78)*. Five main geographic subtypes of HTLV-I have been identified and are known as the Cosmopolitan subtype, Japanese subtype, West African subtype, Central African subtype, and Melanesian subtype *(77,78)*. Sequence homology between various subtypes is highly conserved, with the Melanesian subtype being the most divergent.

While between 15 and 25 million individuals are infected worldwide and seroprevalence rates in endemic areas can exceed 30%, the majority of individuals infected with HTLV-I are clinically asymptomatic *(72)*. It has been reported that the seroprevalence of HTLV-I may be higher than currently estimated based on HTLV-I *tax* sequences detected in HTLV-I/II enzyme immunoassay (EIA)-negative US blood donors *(79)*. Support for this includes the presence of HTLV-I provirus in a large percentage of seronegative individuals with mycosis fungoides and a minority of other seronegative individuals who are HTLV-I/II PCR positive *(79,80)*.

HTLV-II is endemic in several native American Indian populations in North, South, and Central America, geographically distinct Pygmy populations of the Cameroon and Zaire *(80–82)*, and sporadically throughout West, Central, and East Africa *(83–87)*. In the Americas, HTLV-II is endemic among the Navajo and Pueblo Indians of New Mexico *(88–90)*, the seminole Indians of Florida *(91)*, the Guyami Indians of Panama *(92)*, and several populations in South America including the Wayu, Guahibo, and Tunebo of Columbia *(93–95)*, the Kayapo, Mondruku, and Kraho of Brazil *(61,96,97)*, and the Toba and Matacco Indians of Argentina *(98)*. The seroprevalence rates differ substantially among various tribes from a high of >30% among the Kayapo to 2–3% among the Navajo and Pueblo *(97,99)*. High rates of HTLV-II infection are found among (IVDAs) throughout the world *(92,100,101)*, with up to 20% seroprevalance rates among IVDAs in the United States, Spain, Italy, and Scandinavia. Among IVDAs in the United States, HTLV-II is more common in African Americans and Hispanics than in non-Hispanic Caucasians *(102)*. Up to 12.5% of the HIV-infected IVDAs in New York City are concomitantly infected with HTLV-II *(103)*.

Two major subtypes of HTLV-II (HTLV-IIa and HTLV-II b) have been identified *(100,101,103)*. The divergence of nucleotide sequence for HTLV-II subtypes ranges between 4% and 7% *(100,101,103,104)*, with the greatest sequence divergence occurring in the LTR. Subtype divergence found in the *pX* region, however, may cause important differences in different subtypes. Nucleotide substitutions in the 3′ end of HTLV-IIb *tax* would abrogate the stop codon present in the HTLV-IIa subtypes and could result in the synthesis of an elongated Tax protein with 25 additional amino acids at the carboxy (c)-terminus *(105,106)*. HTLV-IIa is the predominant subtype among IVDAs in urban areas of North America and Sweden *(96,100,101)*. However, HTLV-IIb is more prevalent in IVDAs of Spain and Italy. The majority of American Indian groups endemic for HTLV-II carry the HTLV-IIb subtype *(101,103,104)*. An exception is the Kayapo of Brazil, who carry a distinct variant of the HTLV-IIa subtype *(61,107)*.

CLINICAL FEATURES OF HTLV-I– AND HTLV-II–ASSOCIATED DISEASES

Diagnosis of HTLV-I Seropositivity

Many serological procedures are used to detect HTLV-I seropositivity including EIA, particle agglutination, Western blot, radioimmunoprecipitation assay (RIPA), and immunofluorescent assays. In the United States, diagnostic criteria for HTLV-I and HTLV-II seropositivity is based on HTLV-I/II–positive EIA results which are confirmed by RIPA or Western blot. Recombinant proteins specific for HTLV-I and HTLV-II Env glycoproteins are incorporated into Western blot strips to increase sensitivity and distinguish between antibody responses to HTLV-I and HTLV-II. An HTLV-I– or HTLV-II–infected seropositive individual must have an antibody response to all of the core bands and the respective recombinant glycoprotein according to World Health Organization criteria *(72)*. However, anomalous HTLV-I/II Western blot banding patterns have been described from individuals who are HTLV-I/II EIA–positive and show a response to some but not all of the core HTLV-I Western blot bands *(72,108,109)*. These individuals are described as being HTLV-I/II seroindeterminate. HTLV-I/II seroindeterminate Western blot profiles have been reported throughout the world *(72,108,109)*. Although the significance of the HTLV-I/II seroindeterminate Western blot remains unclear, the etiology of the HTLV-I/II seroindeterminate Western blot pattern may be attributable to cross-reactivity with other infectious agents such as *Plasmodium falciparum,* autoantibodies to endogenous retroviruses with homology to HTLV-I, infection with novel or defective HTLV, or infection with HTLV at low copy number *(109–112)*. Recent studies have supported the theory that HTLV-I/II–seroindeterminate individuals may harbor HTLV-I at an extremely low viral load *(113,114)*. These reports have demonstrated periodic detection of HTLV-I *tax* sequence in the peripheral blood mononuclear cells (PBMCs) of individuals with an HTLV-I/II seroindeterminate Western blot pattern by nested PCR and the sequencing of prototypic HTLV-I from a B-cell line generated from an HTLV-I/II seroindeterminate *(113,114)*. An additional study has reported the eventual HTLV-I seroconversion of a small percentage of long-term HTLV-I/II seroindeterminate individuals from the Martinique with strong p19 reactivity, suggesting that continued observation of HTLV-I/II–seroindeterminate individuals may be important in detecting delayed seroconversion *(115)*.

Clinical Features of Adult T-Cell Leukemia

Adult T-cell leukemia (ATL) generally occurs in adulthood at least 20–30 yr following infection. The mean age at ATL onset is 57 yr in Japan and between 40 and 45 yr in the Caribbean, South America, and Africa *(116–119)*, which may indicate that environmental cofactors play an important role in the pathogenesis of this disease. An HTLV-I–infected individual has roughly a 1% chance of developing ATL over a lifetime. Males are 1.4 times as likely to develop ATL as females *(120,121)*. Diagnosis of ATL was once made by the detection of leukocytosis and morphologically abnormal lymphocytes but is now confirmed by the detection of monoclonal integration of HTLV-I in tumor cells from peripheral blood lymphocytes (PBLs) and lymph nodes by Southern blot hybridization *(118,119)*.

ATL patients are usually classified into four subtypes according to clinical and laboratory status. These stages of ATL are termed: acute, chronic, smoldering, and lymphoma *(121–123)*. Approximately 30% of patients diagnosed with ATL are placed in the smoldering ATL stage, which is typically characterized by skin lesions and marrow involvement. Chronic ATL patients generally have elevated numbers of circulating ATL cells with a $CD3^+$ $CD4^+$ $CD25^+$ and $HLADR^+$ surface phenotype and an increased leukocyte count. Characteristic lobulated or flower-shaped nuclei are observed in patients with acute ATL. Chronic or smoldering ATL may progress to acute ATL within a matter of months. The average survival time after diagnosis with acute ATL is 6 mo in spite of clinical intervention. In acute ATL, a dominant clone of malignant cells is present and is marked by a single rearrangement of T-cell antigen receptor genes and one or a few proviruses arranged in an oligoclonal fashion within the population of malignant cells *(124–126)*.

Clinical Features of HAM/TSP

In 1985, Gessain et al. found that a group of patients with a neurologic disease known as tropical spastic paraparesis (HAM) was HTLV-I seropositive *(4)*. One year later, Osame et al. reported a number of Japanese patients with a slowly progressing myelopathy and increased HTLV-I antibody titers *(5)*. Osame et al. termed this disease HTLV-I associated myelopathy (HAM) and it was soon realized that TSP and HAM were clinically identical. Therefore, it was decided that the diseases termed HAM and HTLV-I TSP were both to be called HAM/TSP *(127,128)*.

The clinical hallmark of HAM/TSP is a gradual onset of lower extremity weakness, bowel and bladder dysfunction, fecal incontinence, Babinski sign and variable sensory loss *(129–132)*. Cerebrospinal fluid (CSF) analysis in HAM/TSP is remarkable for a mild lymphocytic pleocytosis, mild protein elevation, increased neopterin, elevated IgG synthesis and IgG index, and oligoclonal bands some of which are directed against HTLV-I *(129,133–136)*. Magnetic resonance imaging has demonstrated lesions in both the white matter and the paraventricular regions of HAM/TSP brains and swelling or atrophy in the spinal cord *(137–139)*. Electrophysiologic and electromyographic abnormalities are often helpful in the diagnosis of HAM/TSP *(140–143)*. ATL cells are found in about 50% of HAM/TSP patients' PBL and CSF at a frequency of about 1% *(129)*. Several other diseases including leukoencephalopathy, abnormal chest X-ray film, Sjögren's syndrome, and arthropathy are frequently observed in HAM/TSP patients *(144)*.

The lifetime risk of an HTLV-I–infected individual developing HAM/TSP over a lifetime is 0.25% *(52)*. More than 2000 HAM/TSP patients have been reported worldwide, with approx 700 of them residing in Japan *(52)*. The average age at onset for HAM/TSP is from 35 to 45 yr but has been reported in individuals as young as 12 yr of age *(52)*. The incubation period from infection to HAM/TSP usually takes years but can be as short as 18 wk posttransfusion with HTLV-I infected blood. Disease progression tends to be more rapid in HAM/TSP patients who were infected by transfusion *(52)*. HTLV-I infected females are three times as likely to develop HAM/TSP as are males *(131)*. The increased prevalence of HAM/TSP among females is a feature of the disease that is consistent with other diseases that have an autoimmune component.

Clinical Features of Other HTLV-I–Associated Disease

HTLV-I has recently been associated in a subset of patients with other inflammatory diseases including HTLV-I–associated arthropathy, myositis, alveolitis, uveitis, Sjögren's syndrome, Behçet disease, systemic lupus erythematosus, and pseudohypoparathyroidism *(6,9,11–13,145–152)*. Of the more recent diseases associated with HTLV-I, HTLV-I–associated uveitis is perhaps the best studied. Infiltrating lymphocytes containing HTLV-I are found in the anterior chamber of patients with HTLV-I–associated uveitis. Furthermore, patients with HTLV-I–associated have an increased proviral load in their PBLs compared to HTLV-I asymptomatic carriers *(150,151)*. In addition, HTLV-I sequences have been detected in PBLs of HTLV-I seronegative patients with mycosis fungoides or neurologic disease *(80,152,153)*. Many of these studies base their associations on limited data making the role of HTLV-I in these various diseases difficult to interpret.

HTLV-II–Associated Disease

The role of HTLV-II as a human pathogen is not as well defined as that of HTLV-I. Given the similarities between HTLV-I and HTLV-II it was anticipated that HTLV-II would be associated with the same spectrum of lymphoproliferative and neurologic diseases as HTLV-I. However, no disorders as yet have been definitively associated with HTLV-II infection. HTLV-II has been associated with a $CD8^+$ lymphoproliferative disorder *(154)*. In addition, a variety of skin disorders with similarities to cutaneous T cell leukemia/lymphomas and smoldering ATL have been described in individuals with HIV and HTLV-II infection *(155,156)*. HTLV-II seropositive IVDUs are reported to have an to have an increased risk for bacterial pneumonia, abscess, and lymphadenopathy *(157)*.

Accumulating evidence suggests that HTLV-II infection may be associated with neurological disease. In 1991, a patient with dual HIV/HTLV-II infection was reported to have a progressive neurologic disease clinically indistinguishable from HAM/TSP *(158)*. This report has been followed by several reports of HTLV-II–infected individuals with HAM/TSP-like disease *(159–161)*. Other individuals with neurologic disease clinically dissimilar to HAM/TSP in conjunction with an HTLV-II infection have also been reported *(162)*. Recently, six patients dually infected with HIV-1 and HTLV-II with predominantly sensory polyneuropathy have been described *(163)*. Of interest, the patients with predominantly sensory polyneuropathy had higher HTLV-II proviral loads than their noneffected dually infected counterparts. This report is reminiscent of higher viral loads observed in HAM/TSP patients compared to HTLV-I–infected asymptomatic controls. Most individuals described with HTLV-II and neurologic disease have been infected with the HTLV-IIa subtype. This may be reflective of the increased prevalence of HTLV-IIa in the United States rather than an increased neuropathology associated with the HTLV-IIa variant.

While dual infection with HIV and HTLV-I has been shown to accelerate the development of acquired immunodeficiency syndrome (AIDS) compared to individuals infected with HIV alone *(164)*, there appears to be no increase in disease progression in individuals concommitantly infected with HTLV-II and HIV *(165)*. The increase in disease progression in HIV/HTLV-I infected individuals may be explained by the shared $CD4^+$ tropism of HTLV-I and HIV. The apparent preferred $CD8^+$ tropism of HTLV-II may account for the lack of influence of HTLV-II on HIV disease progression.

IMMUNOPATHOGENESIS OF HAM/TSP

Host susceptibility to HAM/TSP and Other HTLV-I–Associated Disease

The propensity for certain individuals to develop HAM/TSP, ATL or other HTLV-I associated neurologic disease while others remain clinically asymptomatic is not fully understood. It has been suggested that some individuals may be genetically predisposed to developing HTLV-I–associated disease. In Japan, associations have been made between HAM/TSP and particular human leukocyte antigens (HLAs) *(166,167)*. HAM/TSP patients of Japanese descent have an increased frequency of certain HLA-Cw7, B7, and DR1 alleles represented by the A26CwB16DR9DQ3 and A24Cw7B&DR1DQ1 haplotypes. Japanese ATL patients have an increased frequency HLA-A26, B16, and DR19 and decreased frequency of HLA A24 and Cw1 compared to controls. HLA class II markers in the Japanese population are useful in defining genetic differences between HAM/TSP patients, ATL patients, and asymptomatic HTLV-I carriers *(167)*. The HLA types DRB1*0901, DQB1*0303 and DRB1*1501 in ATL patients and HLA types DRB1*0101, DRB1*0803, DRB1*1403 and DRB1*in HAM/TSP patients were found to be mutually exclusive *(167)*. Recently, a protective effect of HLA-A*02 resulting in a decreased susceptibility to HAM/TSP has been reported *(168)*. It has been suggested that HLA-A*02 reduces the risk of HAM/TSP by reducing HTLV-I provirus load *(168)*. Of interest, HLA-A*02 has also been demonstrated to confer protection against an individual's susceptibility to developing multiple sclerosis, another neurologic disorder with a suspected viral etiology *(169)*. Collectively, these data suggest that HTLV-I disease outcomes may be associated with unique HLA types. More extensive studies in different geographic regions and ethnic groups will be useful in determining whether or not particular HLA types dictate the extent and nature of the immune response to HTLV-I and the likelihood of developing particular HTLV-I–associated disease.

Increased Viral Load in HAM/TSP

Although the idea of disease specific HTLV-I strains has been dismissed as a factor in the determination of disease development, increased viral load has been implicated in the pathogenesis of HAM/TSP. Significantly higher levels of HTLV-I proviral DNA have been consistently detected in the PBLs of HAM/TSP patients *(170–173)*. An estimated 3–15% HAM/TSP PBLs are infected with HTLV-I with 2–20 HTLV-I copies present per 100 PBLs compared to 0.4–8 copies per 100 PBLs in asymptomatic HTLV-I carriers *(172,173)*. A recent study measured HTLV-I proviral load in 202 HAM/TSP patients, 200 nonrelated HTLV-I carriers, and 43 HTLV-I genetically related asymptomatic HTLV-I carriers suggested by TaqMan™ fluorescence energy transfer assay *(170)*. The results of this study indicate that HTLV-I proviral load is increased 16-fold compared to HTLV-I–nonrelated asymptomatic carriers. Of interest, HTLV-I proviral loads were approximately ninefold higher in the HAM/TSP genetically related asymptomatic carriers compared to nonrelated carriers *(170)*. Further studies are needed to determine whether or not increased proviral loads may be predictor for the development of HAM/TSP.

Although there is an increased proviral load in the PBLs of HAM/TSP patients, the detection of HTLV-I mRNA and proteins from PBL has been difficult by conventional

Northern blot analysis and immunofluoresence techniques *(173)*. The surprising absence of HTLV-I viral expression in vivo is not well understood but may be the result of viral latency, or immune elimination of cells expressing viral protein by HTLV-I specific cytotoxic T-lymphocytic (CTL) activity *(174)*. A study using quantitative reverse transcriptase (RT)-PCR technology was able to detect small levels of HTLV-I mRNA and found that the average amount of HTLV-I in asymptomatic HTLV-I carriers and HAM/TSP patients was similar. However, HTLV-I mRNA expression is 50-fold lower in ATL patients *(175)*.

Neuropathology of HAM/TSP

Pathological descriptions of HAM/TSP autopsy material indicate that the disease primarily effects the spinal cord at the thoracic level *(176–182)*. Loss of myelin and axons in the lateral, anterior, and posterior columns occurs frequently in HAM/TSP and is associated with perivascular and parenchymal lymphocytic infiltration, foamy macrophages, proliferation of astrocytes, and fibrillary gliosis *(181,182)*. A symmetrical loss of myelin and axonal dystrophy of the lateral columns within the corticospinal tracts is common with damage being most severe in both the thoracic and lumbar regions *(182)*. Damage to the anterior and posterior columns is variable and less extensive.

The neuropathology of HAM/TSP changes gradually during the progression of the disease. In the initial stages of the disease (up to 5 yr after onset), the leptomeninges and blood vessels are infiltrated with lymphocytes that are thought to penetrate the surrounding parenchyma. Large numbers of inflammatory cells including $CD8^+$ and $CD4^+$ T cells, B cells, and foamy macrophages are present in damaged areas of the spinal cord parenchyma *(181,183)*. HLA class I and β_2-microglobulin are expressed on endothelial cells and infiltrating mononuclear cells *(179,182,184)*. HLA class II expression has also been demonstrated in the endothelial cells, microglia, and infiltrating mononuclear cells of affected lesions *(182,184)*. HLA class II expression is rare in normal central nervous system (CNS) material, and therefore the expression of HLA class II in the affected lesions suggests that resident microglia may be involved in the development of HAM/TSP inflammatory lesions. $CD8^+$ cytotoxic T cells that stain with the monoclonal TIA-1 antibody are thought to represent functionally cytotoxic cells and are observed frequently in active-chronic lesions and occasionally in inactive chronic lesions in HAM/TSP patients *(183)*. The amount of proviral DNA in a HAM/TSP lesion has been shown to correlate with the number of $T1A\text{-}1^+$ cells. The amount of inflammatory cells and HTLV-I proviral DNA decrease with duration of disease.

An increased expression of inflammatory cytokines including IL-1β, interferon-γ (IFN-γ), and tumor necrosis factor-α (TNF-α) is found in the spinal cord of HAM/TSP patients with a short duration of disease *(183)*. In addition, there is elevated expression of several adhesion molecules including vascular cell adhesion molecule-1 (VCAM-1) on endothelial cells, very late antigen-4 (VLA-4) on perivascular molecule-1 (VCAM-1) perivascular infiltrating lymphocytes, and lymphocyte function-associated antigen-1 (LFA-1) in affected areas *(185)*. The chemokine monocyte chemoattractant protein-1 (MCP-1) is also upregulated in the CNS lesions of HAM/TSP *(185)*. As the disease becomes chronic (duration greater than 5 yr), the number of inflammatory cells decreases substantially. The inflammatory cells that persist in the CNS of chronic HAM/TSP are predominantly (>95%) $CD8^+$ *(185,186)*.

The expression of inflammatory cytokines is also reduced over the duration of the disease and, with the exception of IFN-γ, become undetectable.

Infiltrating $CD8^+$ cells are thought to play an important role in the development of HAM/TSP. Therefore, an effort has been made to localize HTLV-I in the CNS of HAM/TSP patients and determine which cells might serve as targets for the $CD8^+$ infiltrates. HTLV-I *gag, pX,* and *pol* sequences have been localized to the thoracic cord areas *(180,181)*. HTLV-I *pX* and *pol* sequences in the thoracic cord were found to be increased in areas of increased $CD4^+$ infiltration. HTLV-I *pX* and *env* sequences have been localized to affected spinal cord *(187,188)*. In addition, HTLV-I RNA has been localized to astrocytes *(180,181)*.

Immune Dysregulation in HAM/TSP

The neuropathology of HAM/TSP suggests that immune-mediated mechanisms are involved in the pathogenesis of this disease. Furthermore, several lines of evidence indicate that the cellular and humoral immune responses of HAM/TSP patients are altered from that of HTLV-I asymptomatic carriers and uninfected controls. The immunologic hallmarks of HAM/TSP include an increase in spontaneous lymphoproliferation *(189)*, the presence of HTLV-I specific, $CD8^+$ CTLs in the PBLs *(190–192)*, and an increase in antibodies to HTLV-I in sera and CSF *(4)*.

Several immune abnormalities occur in the sera and CSF of HAM/TSP patients and may be used in the diagnosis of the disease. Anti-HTLV-I IgM antibodies are present in 83% of HAM/TSP patients and 19% of HTLV-I–infected asymptomatic carriers and are suggestive of continuous HTLV-I antigen production *(193)*. The persistence of an antiviral IgM after initial infection is atypical but has been reported in other systems in which persistent viral infections have been implicated with disease such as chronic type-B Hepatitis. Some HAM/TSP patients develop hypergammaglobulinemia obligoclonal bands in their CSF in addition to elevated levels of neopterin and β_2 microglobulin *(136,139,194,195)*. Increased levels of the cytokines IFN-γ, TNF-α, and IL-6 have been reported in the sera and CSF *(195–197)* and mRNA for IL-1β, IL-2, TNF-α, and IFN-γ are upregulated in HAM/TSP PBL *(198,199)*. In addition, increased levels of soluble VCAM-1 and complement have been identified in the sera and CSF respectively *(200,201)*.

Abnormalities in cellular immune responses of HAM/TSP patients have also been identified. Natural killer cells tend to be diminished in both number and activity in HAM/TSP *(202,203)*. Spontaneous lymphoproliferation, defined as the ability of PBLs to proliferate ex vivo in the absence of antigenic stimulation or IL-2, has been described in HAM/TSP PBL as well as in that of HTLV-I asymptomatic carriers and HTLV-II–infected individuals *(204–206)*. However, the magnitude of spontaneous lymphoproliferation demonstrated ex vivo is typically higher in HAM/TSP PBLs and may be driven by the increased HTLV-I viral load in these patients. The spontaneous lymphoproliferation of HTLV-I–infected PBLs is thought to consist of the proliferation of HTLV-I infected $CD4^+$ cells and the expansion of $CD8^+$ cells based on the demonstration of an increase in virus expressing cells concomitant with an increase in the percentage of $CD8^+$ $CD28^+$ lymphocytes *(207–209)*. Spontaneous lymphoproliferation from the PBLs of HTLV-I infected individuals may be inhibited by antibodies to IL-2, IL-2R, and the costimulatory molecules CD80 and CD86 *(210,211)*. The most striking feature of the cellular immune response of HAM/TSP patients is the highly increased numbers of CD8+ HTLV-I–specific CTLs in the PBL and CNS. This increase in HTLV-I specific CTL in HAM/TSP leaves us with an interesting and largely unexplained paradox: How does an increased HTLV-I viral load persist in patients with extraordinarily high numbers of CD8+ HTLV-I–specific CTLs?

Virus Specific Cytotoxic T-Cell Responses in HAM/TSP

CD8+ and CD4+ subsets of HTLV-I specific CTLs have been described in the PBLs of HAM/TSP patients. CD8+ CTL recognize viral and other foreign antigens in the context of HLA class I molecules while CD4+ CTL recognize larger peptide fragments in association with HLA class II. Although both CTL subtypes are generally important in the elimination of infected cells, the HTLV-I–specific CTLs are thought to be capable of destroying CNS tissue and becoming immunopathogenic in HAM/TSP.

CD4+ T-cell lines that are cytotoxic and HLA class II restricted have been generated by in vitro stimulation with HTLV-I–infected cells from the PBLs of patients with HAM/TSP as well as HTLV-I–infected asymptomatic carriers *(191,212)*. The majority of these CD4+ HTLV-I–specific CTLs recognized the HTLV-I Env between amino acids 196–209 *(191)*. CD4+ CTLs must be expanded by repeated stimulation in vitro to be detected by standard ^{51}Cr release CTL assay which is reflective of the low frequency of CD4+ CTLs in the PBLs. By contrast, CD8+ CTLs may be demonstrated without antigenic stimulation from the PBLs and CSF of HAM/TSP patients *(191,192,212–216)*.

HTLV-I specific CD8+ CTL activity in HAM/TSP PBLs is typically restricted to the p27x and p40x products of the HTLV-I *tax* gene *(191,217)*. However, CD8+ CTL responses to other HTLV-I antigens, particularly the Env proteins, can occur at a lower frequency. HTLV-I CD8+ CTL activity has not typically been demonstrated from the PBLs of HTLV-I positive asymptomatic carriers. However, this observation has been challenged *(215)*. The ability to demonstrate HTLV-I specific CTL directly from the PBLs of HAM/TSP patients without expansion in vitro is thought to reflect an unusually high precursor frequency of virus-specific CTLs in these patients *(213)*. Precursor frequency analysis of the PBLs from five HAM/TSP patients indicates that between 1 in 75 and 1 in 320 PBLs are HTLV-I p40x specific CTLs *(192,213)*. The precursor frequencies of CTLs to more common viruses such as influenza or measles in typically in the range of 1 in 100,000 and 1 in 1,000,000 PBLs *(218)*. Precursor frequencies comparable to that seen in HAM/TSP have been described only in healthy HIV-1 carriers. The high frequency of retrovirus-specific CTLs in these two retroviral systems may reflect persistently high viral load *(219)*.

Class I restricted CTL recognize relatively short peptide fragments that are endogeneously processed and bound to an HLA class I molecule *(220–222)*. It has been demonstrated first by clonal analysis and then by precursor frequency analysis that PBLs from HAM/TSP patients who have the HLA-A201 haplotype preferentially recognize a nine amino acid peptide Tax 11–19 (LLFGYPVYV) (Fig. 2). The recognition of Tax 11–19 by HAM/TSP patients with the HLA-A201 allele is consistent throughout several geographic regions *(192,214,216)*. This peptide conforms to a known HLA-A201 binding motif which has a leucine in the second position and a valine or leucine in position 9 *(223–225)* and has one of the highest affinities known for any peptide–HLA complex *(224)*. HTLV-I Tax-specific CTL in association with other HLA

	Precursor Frequency	
	p40x	**tax peptide**
HAM/TSP Patient #1 **(HLA A201, A28, B18, B44)**	**1/120**	**1/110**
HAM/TSP Patient #2 **(HLA A1, A201, B37, B60)**	**1/250**	**1/290**

Fig. 2. CD8$^+$ CTL activity in HAM/TSP PBL is typically restricted to the p27x and p40x products of the HTLV-I *tax* gene. The precursor frequencies of CTLs to more common viruses such as influenza or measles is usually in the range of 1 in 100,000 and 1 in 1,000,000. PBLs from HAM/TSP patients who have the HLA-A201 haplotype preferentially recognize a nine amino acid peptide Tax 11–19 (LLFGYPVYV). The two HLA-A201 HAM/TSP patients shown here have precursor frequencies of p40x specific CTL between 1 in 120 and 1 in 250. The p40x CD8$^+$ CTLs of these HLA-A201 HAM/TSP patients are overwhelmingly directed to the Tax 11–19 peptide.

class I alleles has been demonstrated. The Tax 90–55 peptide (VPYKRIEEL), for example, has been defined as the sequence preferentially recognized by HLA-B14 *(191,192,213,214)* with equivalent precursor frequencies. It is possible to map the predominant CTL epitopes for each HAM/TSP patient in association with their HLA. Theoretically, this information could lead to immunotherapeutic strategies which would change CTL function and change the immunopathogenic properties of the CTLs. Such strategies have been employed in the treatment and prevention of T cell mediated experimental allergic encephalomyelitis (EAE) *(226,227)*.

The precursor frequency of HTLV-I–specific CTLs is estimated to be between 40- and 100-fold less in asymptomatic HTLV-I carriers than in HAM/TSP patients *(228,229)*. When expanded from the PBLs of HTLV-I asymptomatic carriers in vitro, the predominant CTL response appears to be CD4$^+$ *(192)*. The high precursor frequency of HTLV-I specific CTL in HAM/TSP in comparison to that of HTLV-I–infected asymptomatic carriers and those with other HTLV-I–associated diseases suggests that these CTL may be disease specific and immunopathogenic in HAM/TSP. More recently, HTLV-I–specific CD8$^+$ CTLs have also been demonstrated in HTLV-I–infected patients with other inflammatory disorders including uveitis, arthritis, and Sjögren's syndrome *(212)*, which further suggest that HTLV-I–specific CD8$^+$ CTLs may be immunopathogenic.

The relatively high frequency of HTLV-I–specific CD8$^+$ CTL in HAM/TSP patients has been found to correlate with the production of several cytokines. IFN-γ, TNF-α, and IL-2 were significantly elevated in the HTLV-I–specific CD8$^+$ cells of HAM/TSP patients compared to asymptomatic carriers and HTLV-I–seronegative healthy controls by the use of intracellular cytokine staining coupled with flow cytometry (Fig. 3) *(230)*. INF-γ production from CD8$^+$ cells of an HLA-A201 HAM/TSP patient could be upregulated by the addition of the immunodominant Tax 11–19 peptide. Moreover, anti-HLA class I antibodies were able to inhibit the production of IFN-γ from HAM/TSP CD8$^+$ cells, which suggests that expression of cytokines from CD8$^+$ cells is a result of a

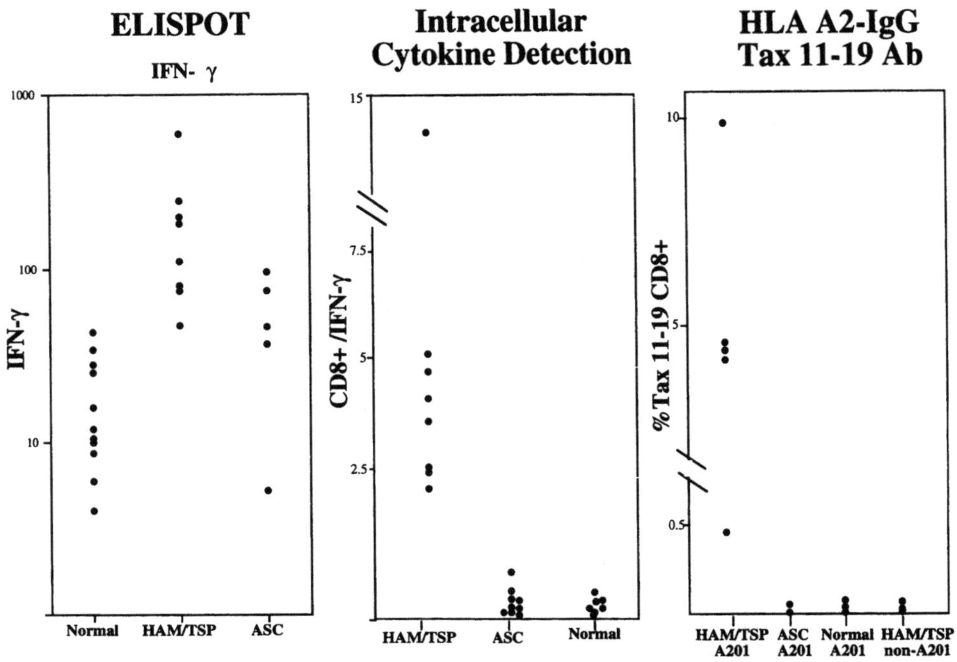

Fig. 3. The high precursor frequency of HTLV-I specific CTL in HAM/TSP correlates with the production of several cytokines. IFN-γ, was significantly elevated in the HTLV-I specific $CD8^+$ cells of HAM/TSP patients compared to asymptomatic carriers HTLV-I seronegative healthy controls by the use of intracellular cytokine staining coupled with flow cytometry and by ELISPOT. In addition, IFN-γ production could be upregulated by the addition of the Tax 11–19 peptide *(230)*. The upregulation of INF-γ reflected the increase in HTLV-I specific CTL observed with an HLA-A2/Ig/Tax 11–19 chimeric antibody. Tricolor analysis ($CD8^+$ vs HLA-A2/Ig/Tax 11–19 vs TNF-α or INF-γ) revealed that approx 28% of $CD8^+$ Tax-A2/Ig^+ cells expressed intracellular INF-γ.

virus-induced inflammatory process rather than *trans*-activation by the HTLV-I *pX* gene. It has been suggested that cytokine expression may be associated with an interaction of the TCR/Ag/HLA trimolecular complex *(231)*. The increased expression of TNF-α observed by intracellular cytokine staining is of particular importance of TNF-α has been demonstrated to be cytotoxic to oligodendrocytes in culture and is capable of inducing demyelination. In a recent study using peptide-loaded divalent HLA-A2/Ig chimeras, HTLV-I Tax 11–19 specific, HLA-A201 restricted $CD8^+$ lymphocytes were visualized directly from the peripheral blood of HAM/TSP patients and found to be present in up to 10% of the $CD8^+$ cells from HLA-A201 HAM/TSP patients *(231)*. Similar frequencies of specific $CD8^+$ lymphocytes were found for HAM/TSP patients in a separate study using MHC class I tetramers loaded with the Tax 11–19 peptide *(232)*. In addition, HTLV-I Tax 11–19 specific $CD8^+$ lymphocytes were found to comprise 23.7% of the $CD8^+$ T cells in the CSF of one patient with a 19-yr disease history *(231)*. The HLA-A2/Ig chimera did not detect HTLV-I Tax 11–19 specific $CD8^+$ lymphocytes from HLA-A201 asyptomatic carriers, HLA-A201 seronegative normal donors, or non-HLA-A201 HAM/TSP patients. These observations support previous data that demonstrated HTLV-I Tax-specific CTL directly from the PBLs of patients with HAM/TSP but not from HTLV-I asymptomatic carriers. Tricolor analysis ($CD8^+$ vs HLA-A2/Ig/Tax 11–19 vs TNF-α or INF-γ) revealed that approximately 28% of $CD8^+$ Tax-A2/Ig^+ cells expressed intracellular INF-γ and TNF-α, suggesting that these circulating Tax-specific $CD8^+$ cells are not uniformly activated *(231)*.

IL-2, IFN-γ, and IL-4, were found to be significantly elevated in PBLs isolated from HAM/TSP patients compared to both asymptomatic carriers and seronegative normal donors by enzyme-linked immunospot (ELISPOT) assay *(233,259,260)* (Fig. 3). IL-4 production was found to be increased 38-fold in HAM/TSP patients compared to seronegative normal donors and 19-fold compared to HTLV-I infected asymptomatic carriers. While IFN-γ and IL-4 were found to be produced by both $CD4^-$ and $CD8^-$ cells, $CD8^-$ cells were the major source of IL-2. Furthermore, when PBLs from two HLA A201 HAM/TSP patients were stimulated with the immunodominant HTLV-I Tax 11–19 peptide, Tax 11–19 responsive cells were estimated to be 1/253 and 1/595 PBLs, respectively by measuring IFN-γ secretion by ELISPOT. The numbers of Tax 11–19-responsive cells obtained by this assay corresponds well with CTL frequencies previously reported on the same individuals *(192)*. In addition, HLA-A201 restricted HTLV-I Tax 11–19-specific $CD8^+$ CTL lines derived from a HAM/TSP patient released IFN-γ, IL-4, and IL-2 with higher magnitude upon stimulation with Tax 11–19. The finding of increased IL-4 secretion in HAM/TSP is unique to this study. IL-4 has been implicated as a helper factor for CTL development and is produced by $CD8^+$ cells in a secondary mixed lymphocyte–tumor cell *(234,235)*.

The high precursor frequency of HTLV-I specific CTL and the subsequent production of IFN-γ, TNF-α, IL-2, and IL-4 in HAM/TSP patients but not in assymptomatic carriers has been demonstrated by conventional CTL assay, HLA specific Ig chimeric antibody detection, intracellular cytokine staining, and ELISPOT. Collectively, these data indicate that is there is a remarkable difference in the magnitude of the HTLV-I specific CTL response of patients with HAM/TSP compared to asymptomatic carriers. Therefore, this body of data suggests that HTLV-I specific CTLs are involved in the pathogenesis of HAM/TSP.

The hypothesis that HTLV-I–specific $CD8^+$ CTL play a role in the development of HAM/TSP is supported by localization of these CTLs in the CNS. Inflammatory $CD8^+$ cells have been demonstrated in the spinal cord lesions of HAM/TSP patients *(179,182,184,236)* and tend to increase with disease progression. As it is not possible to retrieve functionally active T cells from autopsy material, HTLV-I specific CTL activity in the CNS has only been demonstrated through CSF lymphocytes *(213)*. Activated T cells have been reported in HAM/TSP patient CSF and are generally of the $CD8^+$, $CD11^+$, CD45 RO^+, $CD28^-$ phenotype *(237)*. The precursor frequency of HTLV-I–specific CTLs from CSF lymphocytes is extraordinarily high and can represent up to 1 in 60 $CD8^+$ cells *(192)*. In addition, HTLV-I genomic sequences, RNA, and the HTLV-I p19 protein *(238,239)* have been localized to these spinal cord lesions. Therefore, all requirements for CTL recognition, including viral antigen and HLA class I expression, are present in the HAM/TSP lesion, which lends support to the argument that $CD8^+$ CTLs are immunopathogenic in this disease.

Recently, the presence of inflammatory T cells in the parenchyma and leptomininges predominantly of the $CD3^+$, $CD45RO^+$, and $CD8^+$ phenotype were reported in the spinal cord biopsy of a HAM/TSP patient by immunohistochemical analysis *(240)*. In addition, a CD8+ T-cell line established from the cells of this biopsy was able to lyse autologous, CSF derived HTLV-I–infected CD4+ cells as well as an autologous EBV transformed B-cell line which expressed HTLV-I pX proteins. Therefore, this study effectively demonstrated the presence of HTLV-I–specific CTLs in the spinal cord of a HAM/TSP patient. Collectively, these data support the hypothesis that HTLV-I–-specific CD8+ CTLs play a pivotal role in the immunopathogenesis of HAM/TSP.

T-Cell Receptor Usage in HAM/TSP

T-cell recognition of foreign antigens occurs via trimolecular interactions with MHC-bound antigenic peptide with an antigen specific T-cell receptor (TCR). The TCR is a heterodimer comprised of an α- and a β-chain. Somatic rearrangement of the V, D, and J regions generates TCR heterogengeneity with additional diversity conferred by the non germline encoded nucleotides that the VDJ segment junctions. The complementarity-determining region 3 (CDR3) codes for highly variable regions which may bind the antigenic peptide–MHC complex directly. Immunnodirected therapeutic strategies for HAM/TSP must take into consideration whether or not antigen specific immune T cells restricted to an immunodominant peptide–MHC complex are dominated by a single, limited, or heterogeneous set of TCRs. These therapeutic therapies would target specific TCRs of immunopathogenic T cells.

PCR analysis of The TCR Vα and Vβ chains of CD8+ lines cloned from HLA-A201 HAM/TSP patients have demonstrated limited TCR usage *(237,241,242)*. Differences in the TCR repertoires of CTL lines obtained from these HLA-A201 HAM/TSP patients correlated with disease progression. Clones derived from an HLA-A201 HAM/TSP patient with a disease duration of two years with mild disease severity used Vα2. A recent report of limited TCR usage by short-term CD8+ CTL lines from HAM/TSP patients is consistent with these results *(223)*. In CD8+ cell lines derived from HLA-A201 patients with longer duration and increased severity of disease, the TCR usage was more diverse. The TCR usage of lines derived from HAM/TSP patients does not appear to correlate with HLA haplotype. Sequence analysis of the TCR of HAM/TSP patient CTLs suggests that there is oligoclonal expansion of a few founder T cells in these patients *(223)*. A single clone was detected for >3 yr in one HAM/TSP patient.

In one study, TCR Vα/β sequences in the PBLs and CSF were analyzed by reverse transcriptase-polymerase chain reaction/single strand conformation polymorphism (RT-PCR/SSCP) which allows for the detection of single nucleotide changes in TCR mRNA and can be used to detect expansion of clonotypes in the PBLs *(243)*. It was demonstrated by RT-PCR/SSCP that there was oligoclonal expansion of T cells in individuals with HAM/TSP. Identical TCR Vα/β sequences were demonstrated in fresh PBLs and CSF as well as in PBL cultured from HAM/TSP HLA-A201 patients and subsequently found to have Tax 11–19 CTL activity. These data indicated that HTLV-I–specific CD9+ CTLs are subject to oligoclonal expansion in both the CSF and PBLs of patients with HAM/TSP.

It is believed that HTLV-I–specific T cells that are potentially immunopathogenic use a restricted set of V family genes early in disease *(243)*. A more heterogeneous set of V genes may recognize the same HLA–peptide complexes as the disease progresses *(243)*. Heterogeneous V gene usage by potentially immunopathogenic T cells in late stage HAM/TSP has been reported in two autopsy cases where four to seven Vβ family genes were used *(279)*. This theory of increasingly heterogeneous V gene usage with the progression of chronic progressive inflammatory neurologic disease is compatible with the demonstration of restricted TCR gene usage in MBP-reactive T cells in the spinal cord of mice with early stage EAE *(243)*. As disease in these animals progressed, the TCR repertoires of spinal cord infiltrates became increasingly heterogeneous. It has also been demonstrated that TCR usage becomes more heterogeneous with disease progression in multiple sclerosis *(241)*.

X-ray crystal structural analysis of four antigenic viral peptides (influenza A virus matrix M1 58–66, HIV-RTasw 309–317, HIV-1 gp120 197–205, and HTLV-I tax 11–19) presented by HLA-A201 revealed that the structures of the main chains of these peptides are strikingly similar *(223,224)*. The main chains of the peptides sit deep in the cleft near the N-termini and rise toward the surface of the complex due to a kink at residues in positions 3 and 4 and return toward the floor of the cleft at the C-termini. The structures of the main chains at the first three and last two positions of the peptides are highly conserved, which is consistent with the amino acid sequence of the HLA-A2 binding peptides. In contrast, the side chains at the center of the cleft are dramatically different for each of the four viral peptides analyzed. Crystallography of the Tax 11–19/HLA-A201 complex revealed that the tyrosine at position 5 is bound in a deep packet at the center of the CDR3a and CDR3b while the tyrosine at position 8 is bound to both the CDR1b and CDR3b. These data suggest that the tyrosine at position 5 is the primary contact residue of the TCR of a Tax 11–19 specific clone *(244,245)*. The substitution of alanine for tyrosine at position 5 of the Tax 11–19 peptide alters the $CD8^+$ CTL function of CTL clones. These data suggest that altered peptide ligands, which are analog peptides modified at TCR contact residues of a native peptide, may change CTL function. Recently, it has been demonstrated that altered peptide ligands (APL) derived from Tax 11–19 were able to inhibit CTL responses in clones and bulk PBMC of HLA-A*201 HAM/TSP patients when an APL was substituted for tyrosine at position 5 *(246)*. This study suggests that modifications of the antigenic peptide (Tax 11–19) at this central position can modify T-cell responses from bulk PBMCs of individuals with HAM/TSP and provides an ideal system for developing APL-based immunotherapies in humans.

Immunopathogenic Models in HAM/TSP

Several models for the immunopathogenesis of HAM/TSP have been proposed. All of these models are based on an HTLV-I–induced immune-mediated response in the CNS to either specific viral antigens or cross-reactive self peptides, and none of these models are mutually exclusive. One model, known as the cytotoxic hypothesis, suggests that the recognition of HTLV-I gene products in the CNS results in the lysis of glial cells and cytokine release *(247)*. This model is based on the observation that HTLV-I–specific CTLs restricted to immunodominant epitopes of HTLV-I gene products can be demonstrated in the PBLs and CSF of HAM/TSP patients and that the frequency of HTLV-I–specific CTLs is lower or absent in HTLV-I asymptomatic carriers. The presence of viral antigen expressing cells in the CNS could result from hemodynamic forces and anatomical watershed zones in thoracic cord. Lymphocytes may attach to the endothelium and invade the CNS due to decreased blood flow to these areas and interaction with adhesion molecules. The target of the HTLV-I–specific CTLs in the CNS could be either a resident glial cell (oligodendrocytes, astrocytes, or resident microglia) infected with HTLV-I or an infiltrating CD4+ cell. HLA class I and II are not normally expressed in the CNS, which would prevent antigen presentation necessary for CTL activity. However, class I and class II expression are upregulated by several cytokines including IFN-γ and TNF-α which can be induced by HTLV-I and are known to be upregulated in HAM/TSP patients. The release of cytokine and chemokine production by HTLV-I is potentially destructive to cells of the CNS. Furthermore, the induction of inflammatory cytokines alone, such as TNF-α, has been shown to induce demyelination. HLA class I and class II expression has been demonstrated in HTLV-I–infected cells of neuronal origin in vivo. The colocalization of HTLV-I tax RNA in HAM/TSP patient CNS cells which express the glial fibrillary acidic protein (GFAP), a marker of astrocytes, suggests that these cells may be infected in vivo, express HLA class I and become targets for CD8+ CTLs. This cytotoxic hypothesis could potentially be applied to other HTLV-I–associated inflammatory disease including HTLV-I associated arthropathy or HTLV-I associated uveitis.

An alternative immunopathogenic model for HAM/TSP, known as the autoimmune hypothesis, HTLV-I activates autoreactive T cells from the periphery and allows them to migrate into the CNS *(248)*. Autoreactive cells in the CNS would recognize their targets, which could include processed myelin antigens or altered self antigens, and result in cytokine secretion, inflammation, and CNS tissue damage. This model has also been proposed for multiple sclerosis, another inflammatory chronic progressive neurologic disease for which a viral etiology has been proposed.

The study of HTLV-I and HTLV-II has generated a large body of information concerning leukemogenesis, viral induction of inflammatory diseases, host–virus interactions, and virus-induced neuropathogenesis. Immunopathogenic models devised for HAM/TSP may lead to new therapeutic strategies for clinical intervention in these patients and other patients with HTLV-I– or HTLV-II–associated disease. Furthermore, it is hoped that insights into the pathogenesis of HAM/TSP will lead to a better understanding of other neurologic disorders, such as neuro-AIDS and multiple sclerosis in which virus-mediated immunopathogenesis may occur.

REFERENCES

1. Poiesz BJ, Ruscetti FW, Gazdar AF, Bunn PA, Minna JD, Gallo RC. Detection and isolation of type C retrovirus particles from fresh and cultured lymphocytes of a patient with cutaneous T-cell lymphoma. Proc Natl Acad Sci USA 1980; 77:7415–9.
2. Hinuma Y, Nagata K, Hanaoka M, Nakai M, Matsumoto T, Kinoshita KI, et al. Adult T-cell leukemia: antigen in an ATL cell line and detection of antibodies to the antigen in human sera. Proc Natl Acad Sci USA 1981; 78:6476–80.
3. Uchiyama T, Yodoi J, Sagawa K, Takatsuki K, Uchino H. Adult T-cell leukemia: clinical and hematologic features of 16 cases. Blood 1977; 50:481–92.
4. Gessain A, Barin F, Vernant JC, Gout O, Maurs L, Calender A, de The G. Antibodies to human T-lymphotropic virus type-I in patients with tropical spastic paraparesis. Lancet 1985; ii:407–10.
5. Osame M, Usuku K, Izumo S, Ijichi N, Amitani H, Igata A, et al. HTLV-I associated myelopathy, a new clinical entity [letter]. Lancet 1986; i:1031–2.
6. Sasaki K, Morooka I, Inomata H, Kashio N, Akamine T, Osame M. Retinal vasculitis in human T-lymphotropic virus type I associated myelopathy. Br J Ophthalmol 1989; 73:812–5.

7. Ohba N, Matsumoto M, Sameshima M, Kabayama Y, Nakao K, Unoki K, et al. Ocular manifestations in patients infected with human T-lymphotropic virus type I. Jpn J Ophthalmol 1989; 33:1–12.
8. Mochizuki M, Watanabe T, Yamaguchi K, Takatsuki K, Yoshimura K, Shirao M, et al. HTLV-I uveitis: a distinct clinical entity caused by HTLV-I. Jpn J Cancer Res 1992; 83:236–9.
9. Nishioka K, Maruyama I, Sato K, Kitajima I, Nakajima Y, Osame M. Chronic inflammatory arthropathy associated with HTLV-I [letter]. Lancet 1989; 1:441.
10. Sato K, Maruyama I, Maruyama Y, Kitajima I, Nakajima Y, Higaki M, et al. Arthritis in patients infected with human T lymphotropic virus type I. Clinical and immunopathologic features. Arthritis Rheum 1991; 34:714–21.
11. Morgan OS, Rodgers-Johnson P, Mora C, Char G. HTLV-1 and polymyositis in Jamaica. Lancet 1989; ii:1184–7.
12. Sugimoto M, Nakashima H, Watanabe S, Uyama E, Tanaka F, Ando M, et al. T-lymphocyte alveolitis in HTLV-I-associated myelopathy [letter]. Lancet 1987; ii:1220.
13. Vernant JC, Buisson G, Magdeleine J, De Thore J, Jouannelle A, Neisson-Vernant C, Monplaisir N. T-lymphocyte alveolitis, tropical spastic paresis, and Sjogren syndrome [letter]. Lancet 1988; i:177.
14. Terada K, Katamine S, Eguchi K, Moriuchi R, Kita M, Shimada H, et al. Prevalence of serum and salivary antibodies to HTLV-1 in Sjogren's syndrome [see comments]. Lancet 1994; 344:1116–9.
15. Kalyanaraman VS, Sarngadharan MG, Robert-Guroff M, Miyoshi I, Golde D, Gallo RC. A new subtype of human T-cell leukemia virus (HTLV-II) associated with a T-cell variant of hairy cell leukemia. Science 1982; 218:571–3.
16. Coffin J. Retroviridae: the viruses and their replication. In: Fields BN, Knipe DM, et al. (eds). Virology, 3rd edit. Philadelphia: Lippincott-Raven, 1996, pp. 1767–847.
17. Gessain A, Gallo RC, Franchini G. Low degree of human T-cell leukemia/lymphoma virus type I genetic drift in vivo as a means of monitoring viral transmission and movement of ancient human populations. J Virol 1992; 66:2288–95.
18. Ehrlich GD, Andrews J, Sherman MP, Greenberg SJ, Poiesz BJ. DNA sequence analysis of the gene encoding the HTLV-I p21e transmembrane protein reveals inter- and intraisolate genetic heterogeneity. Virology 1992; 186:619–27.
19. Koralnik I. Structure of HTLV-I. In: P Holsberg, Hafler D (eds). Human T-cell Lymphotropic Virus Type I. Chichester, England: John Wiley & Sons, 1996, pp. 79–112.
20. Brady J. Biology of HTLV-I: Host cell interactions. In: Hollsberg P, Hafler D (eds). Human T-Cell Lymphotropic Virus Type I. Chichester, England: John Wiley & Sons, 1996, pp. 79–112.
21. Inoue J, Seiki M, Taniguchi T, Tsuru S, Yoshida M. Induction of interleukin 2 receptor gene expression by p40x encoded by human T-cell leukemia virus type 1. EMBO J 1986; 5:2883–8.
22. Cross SL, Feinberg MB, Wolf JB, Holbrook NJ, Wong-Staal F, Leonard WJ. Regulation of the human interleukin-2 receptor alpha chain promoter: activation of a nonfunctional promoter by the transactivator gene of HTLV-I. Cell 1987; 49:47–56.
23. Leung K, Nabel GJ. HTLV-1 transactivator induces interleukin-2 receptor expression through an NF-kappa B-like factor. Nature 1988; 333:776–8.
24. Hoyos B, Ballard DW, Bohnlein E, Siekevitz M, Greene WC. Kappa B-specific DNA binding proteins: role in the regulation of human interleukin-2 gene expression. Science 1989; 244:457–60.
25. Green JE, Begley CG, Wagner DK, Waldmann TA, Jay G. trans activation of granulocyte-macrophage colony-stimulating factor and the interleukin-2 receptor in transgenic mice carrying the human T-lymphotropic virus type 1 tax gene. Mol Cell Biol 1989; 9:4731–7.
26. Curtiss VE, Smilde R, McGuire KL. Requirements for interleukin 2 promoter transactivation by the Tax protein of human T-cell leukemia virus type 1. Mol Cell Biol 1996; 16:3567–75.

27. Azimi N, Brown K, Bamford RN, Tagaya Y, Siebenlist U, Waldmann TA. Human T cell lymphotropic virus type I Tax protein trans-activates interleukin 15 gene transcription through an NF-kappaB site. Proc Natl Acad Sci USA 1998; 95:2452–7.
28. Yamashita I, Katamine S, Moriuchi R, Nakamura Y, Miyamoto T, Eguchi K, Nagataki S. Transactivation of the human interleukin-6 gene by human T-lymphotropic virus type 1 Tax protein. Blood 1994; 84:1573–8.
29. Mori N, Ueda A, Ikeda S, Yamasaki Y, Yamada Y, Tomonaga M, et al. Human T-cell leukemia virus type I tax activates transcription of the human monocyte chemoattractant protein-1 gene through two nuclear factor-kappaB sites [In Process Citation]. Cancer Res 2000; 60:4939–45.
30. Fujii M, Sassone-Corsi P, Verma IM. c-fos promoter trans-activation by the tax1 protein of human T-cell leukemia virus type I. Proc Natl Acad Sci USA 1988; 85:8526–30.
31. Nagata K, Ohtani K, Nakamura M, Sugamura K. Activation of endogenous c-*fos* proto-oncogene expression by human T-cell leukemia virus type I-encoded p40tax protein in the human T-cell line, Jurkat. J Virol 1989; 63:3220–6.
32. Ratner L. Regulation of expression of the c-*sis* proto-oncogene. Nucleic Acids Res 1989; 17:4101–15.
33. Watanabe T, Yamaguchi K, Takatsuki K, Osame M, Yoshida M. Constitutive expression of parathyroid hormone-related protein gene in human T cell leukemia virus type 1 (HTLV-1) carriers and adult T cell leukemia patients that can be transactivated by HTLV-1 *tax* gene. J Exp Med 1990; 172:759–65.
34. Lemasson I, Robert-Hebmann V, Hamaia S, Duc Dodon M, Gazzolo L, Devaux C. Transrepression of *lck* gene expression by human T-cell leukemia virus type 1-encoded p40tax. J Virol 1997; 71:1975–83.
35. Tanaka Y, Fukudome K, Hayashi M, Takagi S, Yoshie O. Induction of ICAM-1 and LFA-3 by Tax1 of human T-cell leukemia virus type 1 and mechanism of downregulation of ICAM-1 or LFA-1 in adult-T-cell-leukemia cell lines. Int J Cancer 1995; 60:554–61.
36. Jeang KT, Widen SG, Semmes OJt, Wilson SH. HTLV-I trans-activator protein, tax, is a transrepressor of the human beta-polymerase gene. Science 1990; 247:1082–4.
37. Ejima E, Rosenblatt JD, Massari M, Quan E, Stephens D, Rosen CA, Prager D. Cell-type-specific transactivation of the parathyroid hormone-related protein gene promoter by the human T-cell leukemia virus type I (HTLV-I) tax and HTLV-II tax proteins. Blood 1993; 81:1017–24.
38. Nimer SD, Gasson JC, Hu K, Smalberg I, Williams JL, Chen IS, Rosenblatt JD. Activation of the GM-CSF promoter by HTLV-I and -II tax proteins. Oncogene 1989; 4:671–6.
39. Seiki M, Inoue J, Hidaka M, Yoshida M. Two *cis*-acting elements responsible for posttranscriptional trans- regulation of gene expression of human T-cell leukemia virus type I. Proc Natl Acad Sci USA 1988; 85:7124–8.
40. Hidaka M, Inoue J, Yoshida M, Seiki M. Post-transcriptional regulator (rex) of HTLV-1 initiates expression of viral structural proteins but suppresses expression of regulatory proteins. EMBO J 1988; 7:519–23.
41. Inoue J, Itoh M, Akizawa T, Toyoshima H, Yoshida M. HTLV-1 Rex protein accumulates unspliced RNA in the nucleus as well as in cytoplasm. Oncogene 1991; 6:1753–7.
42. Cann AJ, Chen I. Human T-cell leukemia virus types I and II. In: BN Fields, DM Knipe, Howley P (eds). Fields Virology. Philadelphia: Lippincott-Raven, 1996, pp. 1849–50.
43. Kinoshita K, Hino S, Amagaski T, Ikeda S, Yamada Y, Suzuyama J, et al. Demonstration of adult T-cell leukemia virus antigen in milk from three sero-positive mothers. Gann 1984; 75:103–5.
44. Nakano S, Ando Y, Ichijo M, Moriyama I, Saito S, Sugamura K, Hinuma Y. Search for possible routes of vertical and horizontal transmission of adult T-cell leukemia virus. Gann 1984; 75:1044–5.
45. Ando Y, Nakano S, Saito K, Shimamoto I, Ichijo M, Toyama T, Hinuma Y. Transmission of adult T-cell leukemia retrovirus (HTLV-I) from mother to child: comparison of bottle- with breast-fed babies. Jpn J Cancer Res 1987; 78:322–4.

46. Kouro A, Hayami M, Fujii H, et al. Vertical transmission of adult T-cell leukemia virus. Lancet 1983; i:240.
47. Hino S, Yamaguchi K, Katamine S, Sugiyama H, Amagasaki T, Kinoshita K, et al. Mother-to-child transmission of human T-cell leukemia virus type-I. Jpn J Cancer Res 1985; 76:474–80.
48. Nyambi PN, Ville Y, Louwagie J, Bedjabaga I, Glowaczower E, Peeters M, et al. Mother-to-child transmission of human T-cell lymphotropic virus types I and II (HTLV-I/II) in Gabon: a prospective follow-up of 4 years. J Acquir Immune Defic Syndr Hum Retrovirol 1996; 12:187–92.
49. Kajiyama W, Kashiwagi S, Ikematsu H, Hayashi J, Nomura H, Okochi K. Intrafamilial transmission of adult T cell leukemia virus. J Infect Dis 1986; 154:851–7.
50. Brodine SK, Oldfield ECD, Corwin AL, Thomas RJ, Ryan AB, Holmberg J, et al. HTLV-I among U.S. Marines stationed in a hyperendemic area: evidence for female-to-male sexual transmission. J Acquir Immune Defic Syndr 1992; 5:158–62.
51. Canavaggio M, Leckie G, Allain JP, Steaffens JW, Laurian Y, Brettler D, Lee H. The prevalence of antibody to HTLV-I/II in United States plasma donors and in United States and French hemophiliacs. Transfusion 1990; 30:780–2.
52. Osame M, Janssen R, Kubota H, Nishitani H, Igata A, Nagataki S, et al. Nationwide survey of HTLV-I-associated myelopathy in Japan: association with blood transfusion. Ann Neurol 1990; 28:50–6.
53. Osame M, Izumo S, Igata A, Matsumoto M, Matsumoto T, Sonoda S, et al. Blood transfusion and HTLV-I associated myelopathy [letter]. Lancet 1986; 2:104–5.
54. Donegan E, Busch MP, Galleshaw JA, Shaw GM, Mosley JW. Transfusion of blood components from a donor with human T-lymphotropic virus type II (HTLV-II) infection. The Transfusion Safety Study Group. Ann Intern Med 1990; 113:555–6.
55. Sullivan MT, Williams AE, Fang CT, Grandinetti T, Poiesz BJ, Ehrlich GD. Transmission of human T-lymphotropic virus types I and II by blood transfusion. A retrospective study of recipients of blood components (1983 through 1988). The American Red Cross HTLV-I/II Collaborative Study Group. Arch Intern Med 1991; 151:2043–8.
56. Rios M, Khabbaz RF, Kaplan JE, Hall WW, Kessler D, Bianco C. Transmission of human T cell lymphotropic virus (HTLV) type II by transfusion of HTLV-I-screened blood products. J Infect Dis 1994; 170:206–10.
57. Hjelle B, Cyrus S, Swenson SG. Evidence for sexual transmission of human T lymphotropic virus type II [letter]. Ann Intern Med 1992; 116:90–1.
58. Vitek CR, Gracia FI, Giusti R, Fukuda K, Green DB, Castillo LC, et al. Evidence for sexual and mother-to-child transmission of human T lymphotropic virus type II among Guaymi Indians, Panama. J Infect Dis 1995; 171:1022–6.
59. Hall WW, Ishak R, Zhu SW, Novoa P, Eiraku N, Takahashi H, et al. Human T lymphotropic virus type II (HTLV-II): epidemiology, molecular properties, and clinical features of infection. J Acquir Immune Defic Syndr Hum Retrovirol 1996; 13:S204–14.
60. Maloney EM, Armien B, Gracia F, Castillo L, Kruger H, Levin A, et al. Risk factors for human T cell lymphotropic virus type II infection among the Guaymi Indians of Panama. J Infect Dis 1999; 180:876–9.
61. Ishak R, Harrington WJ Jr, Azevedo VN, Eiraku N, Ishak MO, Guerreiro JF, et al. Identification of human T cell lymphotropic virus type IIa infection in the Kayapo, an indigenous population of Brazil. AIDS Res Hum Retrovir 1995; 11:813–21.
62. Yoshikura H, Nishida J, Yoshida M, Kitamura Y, Takaku F, Ikeda S. Isolation of HTLV derived from Japanese adult T-cell leukemia patients in human diploid fibroblast strain IMR90 and the biological characters of the infected cells. Int J Cancer 1984; 33:745–9.
63. Ho DD, Rota TR, Hirsch MS. Infection of human endothelial cells by human T-lymphotropic virus type I. Proc Natl Acad Sci USA 1984; 81:7588–90.

64. Koyanagi Y, Yamamoto N, Kobayashi N, Hirai K, Konishi H, Takeuchi K, et al. Characterization of human B-cell lines harbouring both adult T-cell leukaemia (ATL) virus and Epstein–Barr virus derived from ATL patients. J Gen Virol 1984; 65:1781–9.
65. Sommerfelt MA, Williams BP, Clapham PR, Solomon E, Goodfellow PN, Weiss RA. Human T cell leukemia viruses use a receptor determined by human chromosome 17. Science 1988; 242:1557–9.
66. Ijichi S, Ramundo MB, Takahashi H, Hall WW. In vivo cellular tropism of human T cell leukemia virus type II (HTLV-II). J Exp Med 1992; 176:293–6.
67. Lal RB, Owen SM, Rudolph DL, Dawson C, Prince H. In vivo cellular tropism of human T-lymphotropic virus type II is not restricted to $CD8^+$ cells. Virology 1995; 210:441–7.
68. Inoue H, Yamaoka S, Imamura M, Hatanaka M. Suppression of the transformed phenotype in hybrids of human T-cell leukemia virus type I *tax*-transformed rat fibroblasts and normal human fibroblasts. Exp Cell Res 1994; 215:68–74.
69. Hoshino H, Tanaka H, Shimotohno K, Miwa M, Nagai M, Shimoyama M, Sugimura T. Immortalization of peripheral blood lymphocytes of cats by human T-cell leukemia virus. Int J Cancer 1984; 34:513–7.
70. Collins ND, Newbound GC, Ratner L, Lairmore MD. In vitro $CD4^+$ lymphocyte transformation and infection in a rabbit model with a molecular clone of human T-cell lymphotrophic virus type 1. J Virol 1996; 70:7241–6.
71. Grassmann R, Berchtold S, Radant I, Alt M, Fleckenstein B, Sodroski JG, et al. Role of human T-cell leukemia virus type 1 X region proteins in immortalization of primary human lymphocytes in culture. J Virol 1992; 66:4570–5.
72. Gessain A. Epidemiology of HTLV-I and Associated Diseases. In: Hollsberg P, Hafler D (eds). Human T-Cell Lymphotropic Virus Type I. Chichester, England: John Wiley & Sons, 1996, pp 33–64.
73. Blattner WA, Gallo RC. Epidemiology of HTLV-I and HTLV-II infection. In: Takatsuki K (ed). Adult T-Cell Leukemia. Oxford: Oxford University Press, 1994, pp. 45–90.
74. Mueller N. The epidemiology of HTLV-I infection. Cancer Causes Control 1991; 2:37–52.
75. Kaplan JE, Khabbaz RF. The epidemiology of human T-lymphotropic virus types I and II. Med Virol 1993; 3:137–48.
76. Levine PH, Blattner WA, Clark J, Tarone R, Maloney EM, Murphy EM, et al. Geographic distribution of HTLV-I and identification of a new high-risk population. Int J Cancer 1988; 42:7–12.
77. Tajima K, Hinuma Y. Epidemiological features of adult T cell leukemia. In: Mathe G, Rizenstein P (eds). Pathophysiological Aspects of Cancer Epidemiology. Oxford: Pergamon Press, 1984, pp. 75–87.
78. Tajima K, Inoue H, Takezaki T, Itoh M, Itoh SI. Ethnoepidemiology of ATL in Japan with special reference to the Mongoloid dispersal. In: Takatsuki K (ed). Adult T-Cell Leukemia. Oxford: Oxford University Press, 1994, pp. 91–112.
79. Zucker-Franklin D, Pancake BA, Marmor M, Legler PM. Reexamination of human T cell lymphotropic virus (HTLV-I/II) prevalence. Proc Natl Acad Sci USA 1997; 94:6403–7.
80. Zucker-Franklin D, Coutavas EE, Rush MG, Zouzias DC. Detection of human T-lymphotropic virus-like particles in cultures of peripheral blood lymphocytes from patients with mycosis fungoides. Proc Natl Acad Sci USA 1991; 88:7630–4.
81. Goubau P, Liu HF, De Lange GG, Vandamme AM, Desmyter J. HTLV-II seroprevalence in pygmies across Africa since 1970. AIDS Res Hum Retrovir 1993; 9:709–13.
82. Froment A, Delporte E, Dazza MC, Larouze B. HTLV-II infection in Guinea West Africa. AIDS Res Hum Retrovir 1993; 9:707.
83. Gessain A, Fretz C, Koulibaly M, Boudret ML, Bah A, Raphael M, et al. Evidence of HTLV-II infection in Guinea, West Africa [letter] [see comments]. J Acquir Immune Defic Syndr 1993; 6:324–5.

84. Igarashi T, Yamashita M, Miura T, Osei-Kwasi M, Aysi NK, Shiraki H, et al. Isolation and genomic analysis of human T lymphotropic virus type II from Ghana. AIDS Res Hum Retrovir 1993; 9:1039–42.
85. Bonis J, Verdier M, Dumas M, Denis F. Low human T cell leukemia virus type II seroprevalence in Africa [letter]. J Infect Dis 1994; 169:225–7.
86. Vallejo A, Benito A, Varela JM, Casado C, Roche J, Alvar J, Garcia-Saiz A. Human T-cell leukaemia virus-I/II infection in Equatorial Guinea [letter]. AIDS 1994; 8:1501–3.
87. Buckner C, Roberts CR, Foung SK, Lipka J, Reyes GR, Hadlock K, et al. Immune responsiveness to the immunodominant recombinant envelope epitopes of human T lymphotropic virus types I and II in diverse geographic populations. J Infect Dis 1992; 166:1160–3.
88. Hjelle B, Scalf R, Swenson S. High frequency of human T-cell leukemia-lymphoma virus type II infection in New Mexico blood donors: determination by sequence-specific oligonucleotide hybridization. Blood 1990; 76:450–4.
89. Hjelle B, Mills R, Swenson S, Mertz G, Key C, Allen S. Incidence of hairy cell leukemia, mycosis fungoides, and chronic lymphocytic leukemia in first known HTLV-II-endemic population. J Infect Dis 1991; 163:435–40.
90. Hjelle B. Human T-cell leukemia/lymphoma viruses. Life cycle, pathogenicity, epidemiology, and diagnosis. Arch Pathol Lab Med 1991; 115:440–50.
91. Levine PH, Jacobson S, Elliott R, Cavallero A, Colclough G, Dorry C, et al. HTLV-II infection in Florida Indians. AIDS Res Hum Retrovir 1993; 9:123–7.
92. Lairmore MD, Jacobson S, Gracia F, De BK, Castillo L, Larreategui M, et al. Isolation of human T-cell lymphotropic virus type 2 from Guaymi Indians in Panama. Proc Natl Acad Sci USA 1990; 87:8840–4.
93. Duenas-Barajas E, Bernal JE, Vaught DR, Briceno I, Duran C, Yanagihara R, Gajdusek DC. Coexistence of human T-lymphotropic virus types I and II among the Wayuu Indians from the Guajira Region of Colombia. AIDS Res Hum Retrovir 1992; 8:1851–5.
94. Fujiyama C, Fujiyoshi T, Miura T, Yashiki S, Matsumoto D, Zaninovic V, et al. A new endemic focus of human T lymphotropic virus type II carriers among Orinoco natives in Colombia [letter]. J Infect Dis 1993; 168:1075–7.
95. Duenas-Barajas E, Bernal JE, Vaught DR, Nerurkar VR, Sarmiento P, Yanagihara R, Gajdusek DC. Human retroviruses in Amerindians of Colombia: high prevalence of human T cell lymphotropic virus type II infection among the Tunebo Indians. Am J Trop Med Hyg 1993; 49:657–63.
96. Black FL, Biggar RJ, Neel JV, Maloney EM, Waters DJ. Endemic transmission of HTLV type II among Kayapo Indians of Brazil. AIDS Res Hum Retrovir 1994; 10:1165–71.
97. Maloney EM, Biggar RJ, Neel JV, Taylor ME, Hahn BH, Shaw GM, Blattner WA. Endemic human T cell lymphotropic virus type II infection among isolated Brazilian Amerindians. J Infect Dis 1992; 166:100–7.
98. Ferrer JF, Del Pino N, Esteban E, Sherman MP, Dube S, Dube DK, et al. High rate of infection with the human T-cell leukemia retrovirus type II in four Indian populations of Argentina. Virology 1993; 197:576–84.
99. Hjelle B, Khabbaz RF, Conway GA, North C, Green D, Kaplan JE. Prevalence of human T cell lymphotropic virus type II in American Indian populations of the southwestern United States. Am J Trop Med Hyg 1994; 51:11–5.
100. Hall WW, Takahashi H, Liu C, Kaplan MH, Scheewind O, Ijichi S, et al. Multiple isolates and characteristics of human T-cell leukemia virus type II. J Virol 1992; 66:2456–63.
101. Hjelle B, Zhu SW, Takahashi H, Ijichi S, Hall WW. Endemic human T cell leukemia virus type II infection in southwestern US Indians involves two prototype variants of virus. J Infect Dis 1993; 168:737–40.

102. Khabbaz RF, Onorato IM, Cannon RO, Hartley TM, Roberts B, Hosein B, Kaplan JE. Seroprevalence of HTLV-1 and HTLV-2 among intravenous drug users and persons in clinics for sexually transmitted diseases. N Engl J Med 1992; 326:375–80.
103. Hall WW, Kubo T, Ijichi S, Takahashi H, Zhu SW. Human T-cell leukemia/lymphoma virus type II (HTLV-II): emergence of an important newly recognised pathogen. Semin Virol 1994; 5:165–78.
104. Dube DK, Sherman MP, Saksena NK, Bryz-Gornia V, Mendelson J, Love J, et al. Genetic heterogeneity in human T-cell leukemia/lymphoma virus type II. J Virol 1993; 67:1175–84.
105. Pardi D, Switzer WM, Hadlock KG, Kaplan JE, Lal RB, Folks TM. Complete nucleotide sequence of an Amerindian human T-cell lymphotropic virus type II (HTLV-II) isolate: identification of a variant HTLV-II subtype b from a Guaymi Indian. J Virol 1993; 67:4659–64.
106. Pardi D, Kaplan JE, Coligan JE, Folks TM, Lal RB. Identification and characterization of an extended Tax protein in human T-cell lymphotropic virus type II subtype b isolates. J Virol 1993; 67:7663–7.
107. Eiraku N, Novoa P, da Costa Ferreira M, Monken C, Ishak R, da Costa Ferreira O, et al. Identification and characterization of a new and distinct molecular subtype of human T-cell lymphotropic virus type 2. J Virol 1996; 70:1481–92.
108. Lal RB, Rudolph DL, Coligan JE, Brodine SK, Roberts CR. Failure to detect evidence of human T-lymphotropic virus (HTLV) type I and type II in blood donors with isolated gag antibodies to HTLV-I/II. Blood 1992; 80:544–50.
109. Lal RB, Rudolph D, Alpers MP, Sulzer AJ, Shi YP, Lal AA. Immunologic cross-reactivity between structural proteins of human T-cell lymphotropic virus type I and the blood stage of *Plasmodium falciparum.* Clin Diagn Lab Immunol 1994; 1:5–10.
110. Hayes CG, Burans JP, Oberst RB. Antibodies to human T lymphotropic virus type I in a population from the Philippines: evidence for cross-reactivity with *Plasmodium falciparum.* J Infect Dis 1991; 163:257–62.
111. Mauclere P, Le Hesran JY, Mahieux R, Salla R, Mfoupouendoun J, Abada ET, et al. Demographic, ethnic, and geographic differences between human T cell lymphotropic virus (HTLV) type I-seropositive carriers and persons with HTLV-I Gag-indeterminate Western blots in Central Africa. J Infect Dis 1997; 176:505–9.
112. Busch MP, Switzer WM, Murphy EL, Thomson R, Heneine W. Absence of evidence of infection with divergent primate T-lymphotropic viruses in United States blood donors who have seroindeterminate HTLV test results. Transfusion 2000; 40:443–9.
113. Soldan SS, Graf MD, Waziri A, Flerlage AN, Robinson SM, Kawanishi T, et al. HTLV-I/II seroindeterminate Western blot reactivity in a cohort of patients with neurological disease. J Infect Dis 1999; 180:685–94.
114. Waziri A, Soldan SS, Graf MD, Nagle J, Jacobson S. Characterization and sequencing of prototypic human T-lymphotropic virus type 1 (HTLV-1) from an HTLV-1/2 seroindeterminate patient [In Process Citation]. J Virol 2000; 74:2178–85.
115. Cesaire R, Bera O, Maier H, Lezin A, Martial J, Ouka M, et al. Seroindeterminate patterns and seroconversions to human T-lymphotropic virus type I positivity in blood donors from Martinique, French West Indies. Transfusion 1999; 39:1145–9.
116. Group TaBCMS. The third nation-wide study on adult-T-cell leukemia/lymphoma (ATL) in Japan: characteristic patterns of HLA antigen and HTLV-I infection in ATL patients and their relatives. Int J Cancer 1988; 41:505–12.
117. Tajima K. The 4th nation-wide study of adult T-cell leukemia/lymphoma (ATL) in Japan: estimates of risk of ATL and its geopraphical and clinical features. The T- and B-cell Malignancy Study Group. Int J Cancer 1990; 45:237–43.
118. Takatsuki K, Yamaguchi K, Matsuoka M. Adult T-Cell Leukemia. Human T-Cell Lymphotropic Virus Type I. Chichester, England: John Wiley & Sons, 1996, pp. 219–46.

119. Takatsuki K, Yamaguchi K, Matsuoka M. ATL and HTLV-I related diseases. In: Takatsuki K (ed). Adult T-Cell Leukaemia. Oxford: Oxford University Press, 1994, pp. 1–27.
120. Kondo T, Nonaka H, Miyamoto N. Epidemiology of ATLL and preceding stage in a cluster area. Recent Adv Res 1987; 24:156–61.
121. Kawano F, Yamaguchi K, Nishimura H, Tsuda H, Takatsuki K. Variation in the clinical courses of adult T-cell leukemia. Cancer 1985; 55:851–6.
122. Yamaguchi K, Nishimura H, Kohrogi H, Jono M, Miyamoto Y, Takatsuki K. A proposal for smoldering adult T-cell leukemia: a clinicopathologic study of five cases. Blood 1983; 62:758–66.
123. Shimoyama M. Diagnostic criteria and classification of clinical subtypes of adult T-cell leukaemia-lymphoma. A report from the Lymphoma Study Group (1984–87). Br J Haematol 1991; 79:428–37.
124. Blayney DW, Jaffe ES, Blattner WA, Cossman J, Robert-Guroff M, Longo DL, et al. The human T-cell leukemia/lymphoma virus associated with American adult T-cell leukemia/lymphoma. Blood 1983; 62:401–5.
125. Bunn PA Jr, Schechter GP, Jaffe E, Blayney D, Young RC, Matthews MJ, et al. Clinical course of retrovirus-associated adult T-cell lymphoma in the United States. N Engl J Med 1983; 309:257–64.
126. Hoshino H, Esumi H, Miwa M, Shimoyama M, Minato K, Tobinai K, et al. Establishment and characterization of 10 cell lines derived from patients with adult T-cell leukemia. Proc Natl Acad Sci USA 1983; 80:6061–5.
127. Roman GC, Osame M. Identity of HTLV-I-associated tropical spastic paraparesis and HTLV-I-associated myelopathy [letter]. Lancet 1988; i:651.
128. Osame M. Reveiw of WHO kagoshima meeting and diagnostic guidelines for HAM/TSP. In: Blattner W (ed). Human Retrovirology HTLV. New York: Raven Press, 1990, pp. 191–7.
129. Osame M, Matsumoto M, Usuku K, Izumo S, Ijichi N, Amitani H, et al. Chronic progressive myelopathy associated with elevated antibodies to human T-lymphotropic virus type I and adult T-cell leukemialike cells. Ann Neurol 1987; 21:117–22.
130. Osame M, Igata A, Matsumoto M, Kohka M, Usuku K, Izumo S. HTLV-I associated myelopathy (HAM), treatment trials, retrospective survey and clinical and laboratory findings. Hematol Rev 1990; 3:271–84.
131. Osame M, McArthur JC. Neurologic manifestations of infection with human T cell lymphotropic virus type I. In: Asburr AK, McKhann GM, McDonald WI (eds). Disease of the Nervous System: Clinical Neurobiology. Philadelphia: WB Saunders, 1990, pp. 1331–9.
132. McFarlin DE, Blattner WA. Non-AIDS retroviral infections in humans. Annu Rev Med 1991; 42:97–105.
133. Hollsberg P, Hafler D. Pathogenesis of diseases induced by human lymphotropic virus type I infection. N Engl J Med 1993; 328:1173–82.
134. Ceroni M, Piccardo P, Rodgers-Johnson P, Mora C, Asher DM, Gajdusek DC, Gibbs CJ, Jr. Intrathecal synthesis of IgG antibodies to HTLV-I supports an etiological role for HTLV-I in tropical spastic paraparesis. Ann Neurol 1988; 23:S188–91.
135. Link H, Cruz M, Gessain A, Gout O, de The G, Kam-Hansen S. Chronic progressive myelopathy associated with HTLV-I: oligoclonal IgG and anti-HTLV-I IgG antibodies in cerebrospinal fluid and serum. Neurology 1989; 39:1566–72.
136. Nomoto M, Utatsu Y, Soejima Y, Osame M. Neopterin in cerebrospinal fluid: a useful marker for diagnosis of HTLV-I-associated myelopathy/tropical spastic paraparesis. Neurology 1991; 41:457.
137. Mattson DH, McFarlin DE, Mora C, Zaninovic V. Central-nervous-system lesions detected by magnetic resonance imaging in an HTLV-I antibody positive symptomless individual [letter]. Lancet 1987; ii:49.

138. Cruickshank JK, Rudge P, Dalgleish AG, Newton M, McLean BN, Barnard RO, et al. Tropical spastic paraparesis and human T cell lymphotropic virus type 1 in the United Kingdom. Brain 1989; 112:1057–90.
139. Nakagawa M, Izumo S, Ijichi S, Kubota H, Arimura K, Kawabata M, Osame M. HTLV-I-associated myelopathy: analysis of 213 patients based on clinical features and laboratory findings. J Neurovirol 1995; 1:50–61.
140. Arimura K, Rosales R, Osame M, Igata A. Clinical electrophysiologic studies of HTLV-I-associated myelopathy. Arch Neurol 1987; 44:609–12.
141. Ludolph AC, Hugon J, Roman GC, Spencer PS, Schoenberg BS. A clinical neurophysiologic study of tropical spastic paraparesis. Muscle Nerve 1988; 11:392–7.
142. Arimura K, Arimura M, Yonenaga Y, Rosales R, Osame M. Clinical electrophoysiologic findings in patients with HTLV-I associated myelopathy. In: Roman GC, Vernant JC, Osame M (eds). HTLV-I and the Nervous System. New York: Alan R Liss, 1989, pp. 240–50.
143. Arimura K, Arimura Y, Moritoyo H, Tokimura Y, Takenaga S, Sonoda Y, et al. How helpful is thoracic paraspinal EMG in HAM/TSP? Muscle Nerve 1995; 18:248–50.
144. Kaplan JE, Osame M, Kubota H, Igata A, Nishitani H, Maeda Y, et al. The risk of development of HTLV-I-associated myelopathy/tropical spastic paraparesis among persons infected with HTLV-I. J Acquir Immune Defic Syndr 1990; 3:1096–101.
145. LaGrenade L, Hanchard B, Fletcher V, Carnston B, Blattner W. Infective dermatitis of Jamaican children: a marker for HTLV-I infection [see comments]. Lancet 1990; 336:1345–7.
146. Kanazawa H, Ijichi S, Eiraku N, Igakura T, Higuchi I, Nakagawa M, Kuriyama M, Tanaka S, Osame M. Behçet's disease and Sjogren syndrome in a patient with HTLV-I-associated myelopathy [letter]. J Neurol Sci 1993; 119:121–2.
147. Igakura T, Kawahigashi Y, Kanazawa H, Nakagawa M, Osame M. HTLV-I and Behcet's disease [letter]. J Rheumatol 1993; 20:2175–6.
148. Yoshida Y, Sakamoto Y, Yoshimine A, Maruyama Y, Ikegami N, Inose M, et al. Three cases of juvenile onset HTLV-I–associated myelopathy with pseudohypoparathyroidism. J Neurol Sci 1993; 118:145–9.
149. Takayanagui OM, Moura LS, Petean FC, Biscaro TA, Covas DT, Osame M. Human T-lymphotropic virus type I-associated myelopathy/tropical spastic paraparesis and systemic lupus erythematosus. Neurology 1997; 48:1469–70.
150. Watanabe T, Ono A, Mochizuki M. Analysis of the infiltrating cells of HTLV-I uveitis. AIDS Res Hum Retrovir 1994; 10:444.
151. Mochizuki M, Ono A, Ikeda E, Hikita N, Watanabe T, Yamaguchi K, et al. HTLV-I uveitis. J Acquir Immune Defic Syndr Hum Retrovirol 1996; 13:S50–6.
152. Hall WW, Liu CR, Schneewind O, Takahashi H, Kaplan MH, Roupe G, Vahlne A. Deleted HTLV-I provirus in blood and cutaneous lesions of patients with mycosis fungoides [see comments]. Science 1991; 253:317–20.
153. Nishimura M, Mingioli E, McFarlin DE, Jacobson S. Demonstration of human T-cell lymphotropic virus type I (HTLV-I) from an HTLV-I seronegative south Indian patient with chronic, progressive spastic paraparesis. Ann Neurol 1993; 34:867–70.
154. Rosenblatt JD, Giorgi JV, Golde DW, Ezra JB, Wu A, Winberg CD, et al. Integrated human T-cell leukemia virus II genome in $CD8^+$ T cells from a patient with "atypical" hairy cell leukemia: evidence for distinct T and B cell lymphoproliferative disorders. Blood 1988; 71:363–9.
155. Kaplan MH, Hall WW, Susin M, Pahwa S, Salahuddin SZ, Heilman C, et al. Syndrome of severe skin disease, eosinophilia, and dermatopathic lymphadenopathy in patients with HTLV-II complicating human immunodeficiency virus infection. Am J Med 1991; 91:300–9.
156. Bryz-Gornia V, Bushunow P, Amin R. Cutaneous T-cell lymphoma in a patient with HTLV-II and HIV. AIDS Res Hum Retrovir 1994; 10:474.

157. Modahl LE, Young KC, Varney KF, Khayam-Bashi H, Murphy EL. Are HTLV-II-seropositive injection drug users at increased risk of bacterial pneumonia, abscess, and lymphadenopathy? J Acquir Immune Defic Syndr Hum Retrovirol 1997; 16:169–75.
158. Berger JR, Svenningsson A, Raffanti S, Resnick L. Tropical spastic paraparesis-like illness occurring in a patient dually infected with HIV-1 and HTLV-II. Neurology 1991; 41:85–7.
159. Harrington WJ Jr, Sheremata W, Hjelle B, Dube DK, Bradshaw P, Foung SK, et al. Spastic ataxia associated with human T-cell lymphotropic virus type II infection. Ann Neurol 1993; 33:411–4.
160. Sheremata WA, Harrington WJ Jr, Bradshaw PA, Foung SK, Raffanti SP, Berger JR, et al. Association of '(tropical) ataxic neuropathy' with HTLV-II. Virus Res 1993; 29:71–7.
161. Jacobson S, Lehky T, Nishimura M, Robinson S, McFarlin DE, Dhib-Jalbut S. Isolation of HTLV-II from a patient with chronic, progressive neurological disease clinically indistinguishable from HTLV-I–associated myelopathy/tropical spastic paraparesis. Ann Neurol 1993; 33:392–6.
162. Hjelle B, Appenzeller O, Mills R, Alexander S, Torrez-Martinez N, Jahnke R, Ross G. Chronic neurodegenerative disease associated with HTLV-II infection. Lancet 1992; 339:645–6.
163. Zehender G, Meroni L, Varchetta S, De Maddalena C, Cavalli B, Gianotto M, et al. Human T-lymphotropic virus type 2 (HTLV-2) provirus in circulating cells of the monocyte/macrophage lineage in patients dually infected with human immunodeficiency virus type 1 and HTLV-2 and having predominantly sensory polyneuropathy. J Virol 1998; 72:7664–8.
164. Lefrere JJ, Courouce AM, Mariotti M, Wattel E, Prou O, Bouchardeau F, Lambin P. Rapid progression to AIDS in dual HIV-1/HTLV-I infection [letter]. Lancet 1990; 336:509.
165. Visconti A, Visconti L, Bellocco R, Binkin N, Colucci G, Vernocchi L, et al. HTLV-II/HIV-1 coinfection and risk for progression to AIDS among intravenous drug users. J Acquir Immune Defic Syndr 1993; 6:1228–37.
166. Usuku K, Sonoda S, Osame M, Yashiki S, Takahashi K, Matsumoto M, et al. HLA haplotype-linked high immune responsiveness against HTLV-I in HTLV-I-associated myelopathy: comparison with adult T-cell leukemia/lymphoma. Ann Neurol 1988; 23:S143–50.
167. Sonoda S, Fujiyoshi T, Yashiki S. Immunogenetics of HTLV-I/II and associated diseases. J Acquir Immune Defic Syndr Hum Retrovirol 1996; 13:S119–23.
168. Jeffery KJ, Usuku K, Hall SE, Matsumoto W, Taylor GP, Procter J, et al. HLA alleles determine human T-lymphotropic virus-I (HTLV-I) proviral load and the risk of HTLV-I-associated myelopathy. Proc Natl Acad Sci USA 1999; 96:3848–53.
169. Fogdell-Hahn A, Ligers A, Gronning M, Hillert J, Olerup O. Multiple sclerosis: a modifying influence of HLA class I genes in an HLA class II associated autoimmune disease. Tissue Antigens 2000; 55:140–8.
170. Nagai M, Usuku K, Matsumoto w, Kodama D, Takenouchi N, Moritoyo T, et al. Analysis of HTLV-I proviral load in 202 HAM/TSP patients and 243 asymptomatic HTLV-I carriers: high proviral load strongly predisposes to HAM/TSP. J Neurovirol 1998; 4:586–93.
171. Gessain A. Virological aspects of tropical spastic paraparesis/HTLV-I associated myelopathy and HTLV-I infection [see comments]. J Neurovirol 1996; 2:299–306.
172. Kubota R, Fujiyoshi T, Izumo S, Yashiki S, Maruyama I, Osame M, Sonoda S. Fluctuation of HTLV-I proviral DNA in peripheral blood mononuclear cells of HTLV-I-associated myelopathy. J Neuroimmunol 1993; 42:147–54.
173. Kira J, Koyanagi Y, Yamada T, Itoyama Y, Goto I, Yamamoto N, et al. Increased HTLV-I proviral DNA in HTLV-I-associated myelopathy: a quantitative polymerase chain reaction study [published erratum appears in Ann Neurol 1991 Apr;29(4):363]. Ann Neurol 1991; 29:194–201.
174. Hanon E, Hall S, Taylor GP, Saito M, Davis R, Tanaka Y, et al. Abundant tax protein expression in $CD4^+$ T cells infected with human T-cell lymphotropic virus type I (HTLV-I) is prevented by cytotoxic T lymphocytes. Blood 2000; 95:1386–92.

175. Furukawa Y, Osame M, Kubota R, Tara M, Yoshida M. Human T-cell leukemia virus type-1 (HTLV-1) Tax is expressed at the same level in infected cells of HTLV-1–associated myelopathy or tropical spastic paraparesis patients as in asymptomatic carriers but at a lower level in adult T-cell leukemia cells. Blood 1995; 85:1865–70.
176. Levin MC, Jacobson S. HTLV-I associated myelopathy/tropical spastic paraparesis (HAM/TSP): a chronic progressive neurologic disease associated with immunologically mediated damage to the central nervous system. J Neurovirol 1997; 3:126–40.
177. Piccardo P, Ceroni M, Rodgers-Johnson P, Mora C, Asher DM, Char G, et al. Pathological and immunological observations on tropical spastic paraparesis in patients from Jamaica. Ann Neurol 1988; 23:S156–60.
178. Izumo S, Usuku K, Osame M, Machigashira K, Johnson M, Hakagawa M. The neuropathology of HTLV-I associated myelopathy in Japan: report of an autopsy case and review of the literature. In: Roman GC, Vernant JC, Osame M (eds). HTLV-I and the Nervous System. New York: Alan R Liss, 1989, pp. 261–7.
179. Moore GR, Traugott U, Scheinberg LC, Raine CS. Tropical spastic paraparesis: a model of virus-induced, cytotoxic T-cell-mediated demyelination? Ann Neurol 1989; 26:523–30.
180. Yoshioka A, Hirose G, Ueda Y, Nishimura Y, Sakai K. Neuropathological studies of the spinal cord in early stage HTLV-I-associated myelopathy (HAM). J Neurol Neurosurg Psychiatry 1993; 56:1004–7.
181. Akizuki S, Yoshida S, Setoguchi M, et al. The neuropathology of human T cell lymphotropic virus type I-associated myelopathy. In: Roman GC, Vernant JC, Osame M, et al. (eds). HTLV-I and the Nervous System. New York: Alan R Liss, 1989, pp. 253–60.
182. Wu E, Dickson DW, Jacobson S, Raine CS. Neuroaxonal dystrophy in HTLV-1-associated myelopathy/tropical spastic paraparesis: neuropathologic and neuroimmunologic correlations. Acta Neuropathol 1993; 86:224–35.
183. Umehara F, Nakamura A, Izumo S, Kubota R, Ijichi S, Kashio N, et al. Apoptosis of T lymphocytes in the spinal cord lesions in HTLV-I-associated myelopathy: a possible mechanism to control viral infection in the central nervous system. J Neuropathol Exp Neurol 1994; 53:617–24.
184. Umehara F, Izumo S, Nakagawa M, Ronquillo AT, Takahashi K, Matsumuro K, et al. Immunocytochemical analysis of the cellular infiltrate in the spinal cord lesions in HTLV-I-associated myelopathy. J Neuropathol Exp Neurol 1993; 52:424–30.
185. Umehara F, Izumo S, Takeya M, Takahashi K, Sato E, Osame M. Expression of adhesion molecules and monocyte chemoattractant protein-1 (MCP-1) in the spinal cord lesions in HTLV-I-associated myelopathy. Acta Neuropathol 1996; 91:343–50.
186. Iwasaki Y. Pathology of chronic myelopathy associated with HTLV-I infection (HAM/TSP). J Neurol Sci 1990; 96:103–23.
187. Kira J, Itoyama Y, Koyanagi Y, Tateishi J, Kishikawa M, Akizuki S, et al. Presence of HTLV-I proviral DNA in central nervous system of patients with HTLV-I-associated myelopathy. Ann Neurol 1992; 31:39–45.
188. Ohara Y, Iwasaki Y, Izumo S, Kobayashi I, Yoshioka A. Search for human T-cell leukemia virus type I (HTLV-I) proviral sequences by polymerase chain reaction in the central nervous system tissue of HTLV-I-associated myelopathy. Arch Virol 1992; 124:31–43.
189. Jacobson S, Zaninovic V, Mora C, Rodgers-Johnson P, Sheremata WA, Gibbs CJ, Jr, et al. Immunological findings in neurological diseases associated with antibodies to HTLV-I: activated lymphocytes in tropical spastic paraparesis. Ann Neurol 1988; 23:S196–200.
190. Jacobson S, McFarlin DE, Robinson S, Voskuhl R, Martin R, Brewah A, et al. HTLV-I-specific cytotoxic T lymphocytes in the cerebrospinal fluid of patients with HTLV-I-associated neurological disease. Ann Neurol 1992; 32:651–7.
191. Jacobson S, Shida H, McFarlin DE, Fauci AS, Koenig S. Circulating $CD8^+$ cytotoxic T lymphocytes specific for HTLV-I pX in patients with HTLV-I associated neurological disease. Nature 1990; 348:245–8.

192. Elovaara I, Koenig S, Brewah AY, Woods RM, Lehky T, Jacobson S. High human T cell lymphotropic virus type 1 (HTLV-1)-specific precursor cytotoxic T lymphocyte frequencies in patients with HTLV-1-associated neurological disease. J Exp Med 1993; 177:1567–73.
193. Nagasato K, Nakamura T, Shirabe S, Shibayama K, Ohishi K, Ichinose K, et al. Presence of serum anti-human T-lymphotropic virus type I (HTLV-I) IgM antibodies means persistent active replication of HTLV-I in HTLV-I-associated myelopathy. J Neurol Sci 1991; 103:203–8.
194. Matsui M, Nagumo F, Tadano J, Kuroda Y. Characterization of humoral and cellular immunity in the central nervous system of HAM/TSP. J Neurol Sci 1995; 130:183–9.
195. Kuroda Y, Matsui M. Cerebrospinal fluid interferon-gamma is increased in HTLV-I-associated myelopathy. J Neuroimmunol 1993; 42:223–6.
196. Nakamura S, Nagano I, Yoshioka M, Shimazaki S, Onodera J, Kogure K. Detection of tumor necrosis factor-alpha-positive cells in cerebrospinal fluid of patients with HTLV-I-associated myelopathy. J Neuroimmunol 1993; 42:127–30.
197. Nishimoto N, Yoshizaki K, Eiraku N, Machigashira K, Tagoh H, Ogata A, et al. Elevated levels of interleukin-6 in serum and cerebrospinal fluid of HTLV-I-associated myelopathy/tropical spastic paraparesis. J Neurol Sci 1990; 97:183–93.
198. Tendler CL, Greenberg SJ, Blattner WA, Manns A, Murphy E, Fleisher T, et al. Transactivation of interleukin 2 and its receptor induces immune activation in human T-cell lymphotropic virus type I-associated myelopathy: pathogenic implications and a rationale for immunotherapy. Proc Natl Acad Sci USA 1990; 87:5218–22.
199. Tendler CL, Greenberg SJ, Burton JD, Danielpour D, Kim SJ, Blattner WA, et al. Cytokine induction in HTLV-I associated myelopathy and adult T-cell leukemia: alternate molecular mechanisms underlying retroviral pathogenesis. J Cell Biochem 1991; 46:302–11.
200. Matsuda M, Tsukada N, Miyagi K, Yanagisawa N. Increased levels of soluble vascular cell adhesion molecule-1 (VCAM-1) in the cerebrospinal fluid and sera of patients with multiple sclerosis and human T lymphotropic virus type-1-associated myelopathy. J Neuroimmunol 1995; 59:35–40.
201. Saarloos MN, Koenig RE, Spear GT. Elevated levels of iC3b and C4d, but not Bb, complement fragments from plasma of persons infected with human T cell leukemia virus (HTLV) with HTLV-I-associated myelopathy/tropical spastic paraparesis. J Infect Dis 1995; 172:1095–7.
202. Morimoto C, Matsuyama T, Oshige C, Tanaka H, Hercend T, Reinherz EL, Schlossman SF. Functional and phenotypic studies of Japanese adult T cell leukemia cells. J Clin Invest 1985; 75:836–43.
203. Kitajima I, Osame M, Izumo S, Igata A. Immunological studies of HTLV-I associated myelopathy. Autoimmunity 1988; 1:125–31.
204. Yasuda K, Sei Y, Yokoyama MM, Tanaka K, Hara A. Healthy HTLV-I carriers in Japan: the haematological and immunological characteristics. Br J Haematol 1986; 64:195–203.
205. Kramer A, Jacobson S, Reuben JF, Murphy EL, Wiktor SZ, Cranston B, et al. Spontaneous lymphocyte proliferation in symptom-free HTLV-I positive Jamaicans [letter]. Lancet 1989; 2:923–4.
206. Wiktor SZ, Jacobson S, Weiss SH, Shaw GM, Reuben JS, Shorty VJ, et al. Spontaneous lymphocyte proliferation in HTLV-II infection. Lancet 1991; 337:327–8.
207. Ijichi S, Machigashira K, Nagai M, Osame M, Osame M, Hall WW. Late phase spontaneous proliferation of cultured peripheral blood lymphocytes associated with HTLV-I infection: involvement of cellular responses against the infected cells. Jpn J Trop Med Hyg 1996; 24:143–9.
208. Eiraku N, Ijichi S, Yashiki S, Osame M, Sonoda S. Cell surface phenotype of in vitro proliferating lymphocytes in HTLV-I-associated myelopathy (HAM/TSP). J Neuroimmunol 1992; 37:223–8.
209. Machigashira K, Ijichi S, Nagai M, Yamano Y, Hall WW, Osame M. In vitro virus propagation and high cellular responsiveness to the infected cells in patients with HTLV-I-associated myelopathy (HAM/TSP). J Neurol Sci 1997; 149:141–5.

210. Itoyama Y, Minato S, Kira J, Goto I, Sato H, Okochi K, Yamamoto N. Spontaneous proliferation of peripheral blood lymphocytes increased in patients with HTLV-I-associated myelopathy. Neurology 1988; 38:1302–7.
211. Ijichi N, Eiraku N, Osame M, et al. Hypothetical pathogenesis of HAM/TSP: occurrence of proliferative response of lymphocytes in the central nervous system. In: Roman GC, Vernant JC, Osame M, (eds). HTLV-I and the Nervous System. New York: Alan R Liss, 1989, pp. 242–59.
212. Kannagi M, Matsushita S, Shida H, Harada S. Cytotoxic T cell response and expression of the target antigen in HTLV-I infection. Leukemia 1994; 8 Suppl 1:S54–9.
213. Jacobson S, McFarlin D, Robinson S. Demonstration of HTLV-I specific cytotoxic T lymphocytes in the cerebrospinal fluid of patients with HTLV-I associated neurologic disease. Ann Neurol 1992; 32:651–7.
214. Koenig S, Woods RM, Brewah YA, Newell AJ, Jones GM, Boone E, et al. Characterization of MHC class I restricted cytotoxic T cell responses to tax in HTLV-1 infected patients with neurologic disease. J Immunol 1993; 151:3874–83.
215. Parker CE, Daenke S, Nightingale S, Bangham CR. Activated, HTLV-1-specific cytotoxic T-lymphocytes are found in healthy seropositives as well as in patients with tropical spastic paraparesis. Virology 1992; 188:628–36.
216. Kannagi M, Harada S, Maruyama I, Inoko H, Igarashi H, Kuwashima G, et al. Predominant recognition of human T cell leukemia virus type I (HTLV-I) pX gene products by human $CD8^+$ cytotoxic T cells directed against HTLV-I-infected cells. Int Immunol 1991; 3:761–7.
217. Shida H, Tochikura T, Sato T, Konno T, Hirayoshi K, Seki M, et al. Effect of the recombinant vaccinia viruses that express HTLV-I envelope gene on HTLV-I infection. EMBO J 1987; 6:3379–84.
218. McFarland HF, Goodman A, Jacobson S. Virus-specific cytotoxic T cells in multiple sclerosis. Ann NY Acad Sci 1988; 532:273–9.
219. Plata F, Dadaglio G, Chenciner N, Hoffenbach A, Wain-Hobson S, Michel F, Langlade Demoyen P. Cytotoxic T lymphocytes in HIV-induced disease: implications for therapy and vaccination. Immunodefic Rev 1989; 1:227–46.
220. Zinkernagel RM, Doherty PC. Restriction of in vitro T cell-mediated cytotoxicity in lymphocytic choriomeningitis within a syngeneic or semiallogeneic system. Nature 1974; 248:701–2.
221. Townsend AR, Rothbard J, Gotch FM, Bahadur G, Wraith D, McMichael AJ. The epitopes of influenza nucleoprotein recognized by cytotoxic T lymphocytes can be defined with short synthetic peptides. Cell 1986; 44:959–68.
222. Townsend A, Bodmer H. Antigen recognition by class I-restricted T lymphocytes. Annu Rev Immunol 1989; 7:601–24.
223. Madden DR, Garboczi DN, Wiley DC. The antigenic identity of peptide-MHC complexes: a comparison of the conformations of five viral peptides presented by HLA-A2 [published erratum appears in Cell 1994 Jan 28; 76:following 410]. Cell 1993; 75:693–708.
224. Utz U, Koenig S, Coligan JE, Biddison WE. Presentation of three different viral peptides, HTLV-1 Tax, HCMV gB, and influenza virus M1, is determined by common structural features of the HLA-A2.1 molecule. J Immunol 1992; 149:214–21.
225. Parker KC, DiBrino M, Hull L, Coligan JE. The beta 2-microglobulin dissociation rate is an accurate measure of the stability of MHC class I heterotrimers and depends on which peptide is bound. J Immunol 1992; 149:1896–904.
226. Sakai K, Zamvil SS, Mitchell DJ, Hodgkinson S, Rothbard JB, Steinman L. Prevention of experimental encephalomyelitis with peptides that block interaction of T cells with major histocompatibility complex proteins. Proc Natl Acad Sci USA 1989; 86:9470–4.
227. Wraith DC, Smilek DE, Mitchell DJ, Steinman L, McDevitt HO. Antigen recognition in autoimmune encephalomyelitis and the potential for peptide-mediated immunotherapy. Cell 1989; 59:247–55.

228. Holoshitz J, Frenkel A, Ben-Nun A, Cohen IR. Autoimmune encephalomyelitis (EAE) mediated or prevented by T lymphocyte lines directed against diverse antigenic determinants of myelin basic protein. Vaccination is determinant specific. J Immunol 1983; 131:2810–3.
229. Klinman DM, Nutman TB. ELISPOT assay to detect cytokine-secreting murine and human cells. Klinman and Nutman, eds. Current Protocols in Immunology. London: John Wiley & Sons, 1994.
230. Kubota R, Kawanishi T, Matsubara H, Manns A, Jacobson S. Demonstration of human T lymphotropic virus type I (HTLV-I) tax-specific $CD8^+$ lymphocytes directly in peripheral blood of HTLV-I-associated myelopathy/tropical spastic paraparesis patients by intracellular cytokine detection. J Immunol 1998; 161:482–8.
231. Greten TF, Slansky JE, Kubota R, Soldan SS, Jaffee EM, Leist TP, et al. Direct visualization of antigen-specific T cells: HTLV-1 Tax11-19-specific CD8(+) T cells are activated in peripheral blood and accumulate in cerebrospinal fluid from HAM/TSP patients. Proc Natl Acad Sci USA 1998; 95:7568–73.
232. Bieganowska K, Hollsberg P, Buckle GJ, Lim DG, Greten TF, Schneck J, et al. Direct analysis of viral-specific $CD8^+$ T cells with soluble HLA- A2/Tax11–19 tetramer complexes in patients with human T cell lymphotropic virus-associated myelopathy. J Immunol 1999; 162:1765–71.
233. Horvat B, Loukides JA, Anandan L, Brewer E, Flood PM. Production of interleukin 2 and interleukin 4 by immune $CD4^-$ $CD8^+$ and their role in the generation of antigen-specific cytotoxic T cells. Eur J Immunol 1991; 21:1863–71.
234. Widmer MB, Acres RB, Sassenfeld HM, Grabstein KH. Regulation of cytolytic cell populations from human peripheral blood by B cell stimulatory factor 1 (interleukin 4). J Exp Med 1987; 166:1447–55.
235. Matsui M, Kuroda Y. Relevance of humoral and cellular immunity in the central nervous system in HAM/TSP. J Neuroimmunol 1994; 54:180.
236. Elovaara I, Utz U, Smith S, Jacobson S. Limited T cell receptor usage by HTLV-I tax-specific, HLA class I restricted cytotoxic T lymphocytes from patients with HTLV-I associated neurological disease. J Neuroimmunol 1995; 63:47–53.
237. Furukawa K, Mori M, Ohta N, Ikeda H, Shida H, Shiku H. Clonal expansion of $CD8^+$ cytotoxic T lymphocytes against human T cell lymphotropic virus type I (HTLV-I) genome products in HTLV-I-associated myelopathy/tropical spastic paraparesis patients. J Clin Invest 1994; 94:1830–9.
238. Kuroda Y, Matsui M, Kikuchi M, Kurohara K, Endo C, Yukitake M, et al. In situ demonstration of the HTLV-I genome in the spinal cord of a patient with HTLV-I-associated myelopathy. Neurology 1994; 44:2295–9.
239. Levin MC, Lehky TJ, Flerlage AN, Katz D, Kingma DW, Jaffe ES, et al. Immunologic analysis of a spinal cord-biopsy specimen from a patient with human T-cell lymphotropic virus type I-associated neurologic disease. N Engl J Med 1997; 336:839–45.
240. Offner H, Buenafe AC, Vainiene M, Celnik B, Weinberg AD, Gold DP, et al. Where, when, and how to detect biased expression of disease-relevant V beta genes in rats with experimental autoimmune encephalomyelitis. J Immunol 1993; 151:506–17.
241. Hara H, Morita M, Iwaki T, Hatae T, Itoyama Y, Kitamoto T, et al. Detection of human T lymphotrophic virus type I (HTLV-I) proviral DNA and analysis of T cell receptor V beta CDR3 sequences in spinal cord lesions of HTLV-I-associated myelopathy/tropical spastic paraparesis. J Exp Med 1994; 180:831–9.
242. Hoger TA, Jacobson S, Kawanishi T, Kato T, Nishioka K, Yamamoto K. Accumulation of human T lymphotropic virus (HTLV)-I-specific T cell clones in HTLV-I-associated myelopathy/tropical spastic paraparesis patients. J Immunol 1997; 159:2042–8.
243. Garboczi DN, Ghosh P, Utz U, Fan QR, Biddison WE, Wiley DC. Structure of the complex between human T-cell receptor, viral peptide and HLA-A2 [comment]. Nature 1996; 384:134–41.

244. Wucherpfenning KW, Hollsberg P, Richardson JH, Benjamin D, Hafler DA. T-cell activation by autologous human T-cell leukemia virus type I-infected T-cell clones. Proc Natl Acad Sci USA 1992; 89:2110–4.
245. Kubota R, Soldan SS, Martin R, Jacobson S. An altered peptide ligand antagonizes antigen-specific T cells of patients with human T lymphotropic virus type I-associated neurological disease. J Immunol 2000; 164:5192–8.
246. Ijichi S, Izumo S, Eiraku N, Machigashira K, Kubota R, Nagai M, et al. An autoaggressive process against bystander tissues in HTLV-I-infected individuals: a possible pathomechanism of HAM/TSP. Med Hypotheses 1993; 41:542–7.
247. Kubota R, Osame M, Jacobson S. Effects of microbes on the immune system. In: Cunningham MW, Fujinami RS (eds). Effects of Microbes on the Immune System. Philadelphia: Lippincott Williams & Wilkins, 2000, pp. 349–71.
248. Hollsberg P. Pathogenesis of chronic progressive myelopathy associated with human T-cell lymphotropic virus type I. Acta Neurol Scand Suppl 1997; 169:86–93.

8
HIV-Specific Neutralizing Antibodies

David C. Montefiori

INTRODUCTION

Infection with human immunodeficiency virus type 1 (HIV-1) generates cellular and humoral immune responses of various magnitudes to multiple virus-specific antigens. Perhaps the most beneficial B cell response is one that is directed against the surface gp120 and transmembrane gp41 envelope glycoproteins of the virus; both glycoproteins are major targets for the antibody-mediated neutralization of HIV-1 infectivity. To ensure its survival, the virus has evolved a number of immune-evasion strategies that limit the potential benefit of neutralizing antibodies. Chief among these is a high degree of genetic and antigenic variation exhibited by the gp120 and gp41, making the virus a constant moving target for immune surveillance. Critical neutralization epitopes may also be masked by *N*-linked glycans and other structural elements in the native oligomeric envelope glycoprotein complex of the virus. This chapter gives a general overview of how HIV-1 is neutralized by antibody, why the neutralizing antibody response fails to control infection and, finally, what is being done to develop an HIV-1 vaccine that has an effective antibody component.

NEUTRALIZATION MECHANISM AND EPITOPES

Antibody-mediated neutralization of HIV-1 is achieved when antibody binds with adequate avidity and appropriate specificity to the native viral envelope glycoprotein complex. This complex is synthesized as a gp160 precursor that is cleaved intracellularly by a cellular protease to generate the surface gp120 and transmembrane gp41 *(1–3)*. The gp120 molecule is bound noncovalently to gp41 in a trimolecular complex of gp120–gp41 heterodimers on the virus surface, where oligomerization of the heterodimers involves contacts in the gp41 ectodomain *(4–6)*. Both glycoproteins are heavily glycosylated to the extent that approx 50% of the molecular mass of gp120 is carbohydrate *(7,8)*. The gp120 molecule is further comprised of five regions containing relatively conserved amino acid sequences that are interspersed by five variable regions (Fig. 1). Although genetic variation occurs throughout the HIV-1 genome, it is most extensive in the envelope glycoproteins *(9,10)*. The high mutation rate of the HIV-1 genome is due to a lack of proofreading function in the virus-encoded reverse transcriptase, making the enzyme highly error prone *(11)*. HIV-1 has evolved a level of fitness that can tolerate an unusual degree of sequence variation in Env *(12)*.

From: *Retroviral Immunology: Immune Response and Restoration*
Edited by: Giuseppe Pantaleo and Bruce D. Walker © Humana Press Inc., Totowa, NJ

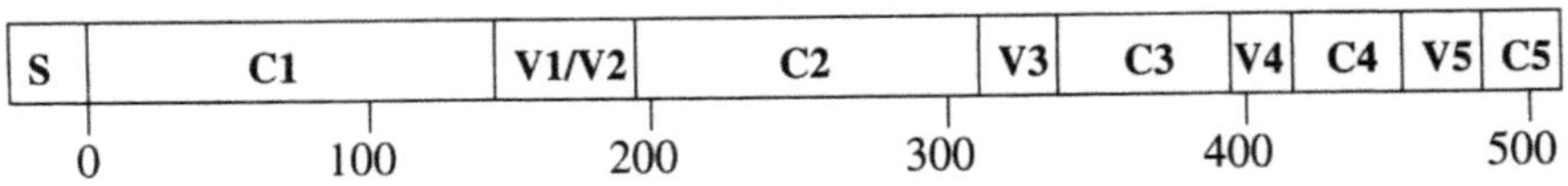

Fig. 1. Linear representation of the gp120 molecule showing regions of conserved and variable amino acid sequences. Conserved (C1-C5) and variable (V1-V5) regions of gp120 are shown in blocks. S represents the signal sequence. Numbering below the figure represents amino acid residues, begining with the initial methionine.

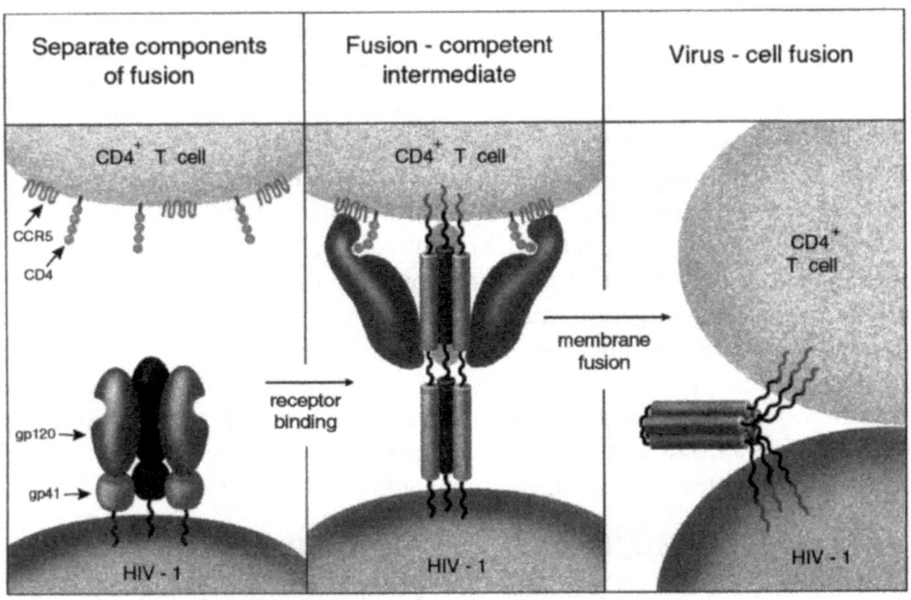

Fig. 2. Organization of the oligomeric envelope glycoprotein complex and its interactions with the cell surface during binding and fusion.

It is generally accepted that the physical presence of antibody on the native oligomeric envelope glycoprotein complex can block the virus's ability to bind and fuse with the cytoplasmic membrane, thereby preventing the virus from gaining entry into cells *(13–15)*. Binding and fusion is a multistep process (Fig. 2) that begins with a high-affinity interaction between gp120 and the HLA class II receptor molecule, CD4, on the cell surface *(16)*. After gp120 has engaged CD4, additional contacts are made between gp120 and a cellular coreceptor molecule that lead to exposure of the hydrophobic fusion domain of gp41. Insertion of the gp41 fusion peptide into the cellular membrane completes the fusion process *(17,18)*. Each of these steps may provide a means for antibody to neutralize the infectivity of the virus *(13,14,19–23)*.

Coreceptor usage is a major determinant of cellular tropism and, as will be explained later, can affect the outcome of neutralizing antibody assessments by influencing the choice of cells used to prepare virus stocks. Although a number of coreceptors have been shown to be utilized by HIV-1, CCR5 and CXCR4 are the two major coreceptors used in most cases *(24,25)*. CCR5 and CXCR4 belong to a class of seven-

Table 1
Two Categories of Culturable HIV-1

- *T cell line adapted (TCLA)*—Passaged multiple times in T-cell lines
- *Primary isolates*—Minimal passage in PBMC only

Table 2
Coreceptors Used by Strains of HIV-1 that Differ in Their Overall Sensitivity to Neutralization

HIV-1 category[a]	Phenotype[b]	Major coreceptor	Antibody-mediated neutralization
TCLA	SI	CXCR4	Sensitive
Primary	SI	CXCR4, CCR5/CXCR4	Difficult
Primary	NSI	CCR5	Difficult

[a] TCLA, T cell line adapted

[b] SI, syncytium-inducing; NSI, non-syncytium-inducing

transmembrane G-coupled proteins that serve as chemokine receptors during inflammation *(26,27).* The coexpression of CCR4 and CXCR4 on mitogen-stimulated, $CD4^+$ peripheral blood mononuclear cells (PBMCs) has made it possible to isolate viral variants that use either or both coreceptors. In contrast to PBMC, $CD4^+$ human T cell lines generally express only CXCR4.

Coreceptor usage is also used for classification purposes *(28)* and could be an important determinant of pathogenesis *(29–31).* Thus, most isolates obtained during early seroconversion through the period of clinical latency use CCR5 as their sole coreceptor (R5 strains). Isolates that use CXCR4 (X4 strains) or both coreceptors (R5/X4 strains) arise later in infection and may be adapted to replication efficiently in T-cell lines. X4 and R5/X4 strains are also said to have a syncytium-inducing (SI) phenotype by virtue of their ability to infect and induce syncytium formation in MT-2 cells. R5 strains are unable to infect T cell lines, including MT-2 cells, and are said to have a non-SI (NSI) phenotype.

Importantly, T cell line adapted (TCLA) variants and primary isolates of HIV-1 exhibit a striking dichotomy in their overall sensitivity to neutralization in vitro (Tables 1 and 2). By simple definition, TCLA refers to strains that have been passaged multiple times in $CD4^+$ T cell lines whereas primary isolates have been passaged a limited number of times in PBMCs exclusively. Repeated passage of HIV-1 in T-cell lines has the consequence of selecting virus variants that are highly sensitive to neutralization relative to primary isolates *(32,33).* A similar phenomenon has been described for other lentiviruses *(34,35),* including the simian immunodeficiency virus *(36).*

The early widespread use of TCLA strains for studies of HIV-1–specific neutralizing antibodies gave the misleading impression that neutralizing antibodies were of little clinical value. Questions were raised concerning the nature and relevance of the neutralization determinants on these two categories of virus once it was learned that the ability to neutralize TCLA strains did not predict the ability to neutralize primary iso-

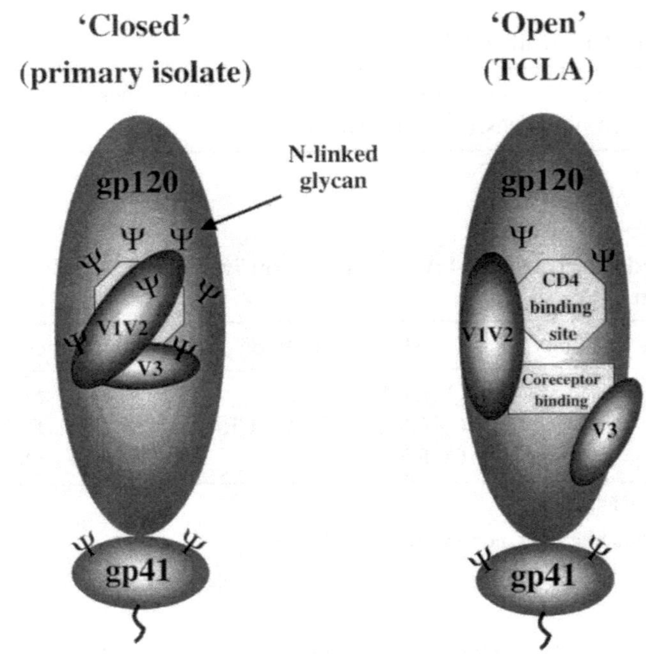

Fig. 3. Model of the structural elements in gp120 that infuence the sensitivity of HIV-1 to neutralization by antibody

lates *(37–39)*. It may be argued on the basis of passage history that primary isolates more closely resemble the targets of a biologically relevant antibody response.

One of the earliest questions to be asked was whether the dichotomy in neutralization between TCLA strains and primary isolates was related to coreceptor usage. For example, the majority of primary isolates were known to utilize CCR5 whereas all TCLA strains used CXCR4 and not CCR5. Studies with CXCR4-using primary isolates have since concluded that use of this coreceptor does not impart the neutralization-sensitive phenotype *(40–42)*. It now appears that the dichotomy in neutralization sensitivity is unrelated to coreceptor usage and is most likely determined by the structure of the native oligomeric gp120–gp41 envelope complex as it exists on the surface of these two categories of the virus *(17,18,43–45)*. As revealed by X-ray crystallography, the highly conserved binding domains for CD4 and coreceptor are conformation dependent and exist as recessed areas or "pockets" on the inner core of the gp120 molecule. The extent to which this region is recessed may limit the exposure of critical epitopes. The virus also casts a protective shield over the surface of the gp120 molecule in the form of *N*-linked glycans and variable loop structures (e.g., V1/V2) that may mask the receptor and coreceptor binding groves. Neutralization epitopes might be further occluded by subunit–subunit interactions in the quaternary structure of the oligomeric envelope glycoprotein complex. The relevance of this structural plasticity to antibody-mediated neutralization was first suggested by the observation that certain antibodies bind monomeric gp120 better than oligomeric Env *(46–49)*.

For a variety of reasons, the neutralization epitopes on TCLA strains are more accessible to antibody binding relative to their exposure on primary isolates (Fig. 3). Differential exposure of critical epitopes in the HIV-1 envelope glycoproteins was first suggested by the observation that TCLA strains are 200–2000 times more sensitive to inhibition by soluble CD4 *(37,50,51)*. It follows that if the CD4-binding domain of primary isolate gp120 is in a less favorable conformation to engage CD4 as compared to TCLA strains, this region might also be less accessible for antibody binding. In addition to the CD4 binding site, the third variable cystein-cystein loop (V3-loop) of gp120 exhibits dramatic differences in the exposure of epitopes *(52)*. The V3-loop plays an important role in binding and fusion *(13,53–55)*, making it an interesting a potentially beneficial target for neutralizing antibody induction. Unfortunately, whereas the V3 loop is highly exposed for efficient neutralization of TCLA strains, it is poorly exposed and rarely a target for the neutralization of primary isolates *(56,57)*. Finally, mutations that eliminate the addition of *N*-linked glycans at specific sites on the gp120 molecule have been shown to dramatically increase the neutralization sensitivity of HIV-1 *(58–61)* and SIV *(62–64)*.

The gp41 molecule is another potential target for neutralizing antibodies but only one gp41-specific neutralization epitope has been identified with certainty. That epitope is recognized by the human monoclonal antibody, 2F5, which binds a region of the gp41 ectodomain having the amino acid sequence ELDKWA *(65)*. The 2F5 epitope is highly conserved on multiple genetic variants of HIV-1 and, although it is a target for neutralization of diverse primary isolates *(66,67)*, it appears to be poorly immunogenic in HIV-1–infected individuals.

One may envision other gp120- and gp41-specific neutralization epitopes that are exposed during the intermediate stages of binding and fusion. An example would be the transient "prehairpin" conformation of gp41 that forms after gp120 engages CD4 and coreceptor *(18)*. Formation of this intermediate structure permits insertion of the amino (N)-terminal hydrophobic fusion domain of gp41 into the target cell membrane (Fig. 2). This gp41 intermediate must undergo further structural changes to draw the virus membrane into close proximity with the cytoplasmic membrane of the cell for fusion to take place *(18,68)*. Antibodies that bind the prehairpin intermediate could conceivably block the conformational changes that are needed for virus–cell fusion. Peptides with a similar mode of action have potent anti-HIV-1 activity in vitro *(69)* and have shown promising results in early clinical tests *(70)*. Part of the reason people fail to make antibodies to these putative gp41 fusion epitopes might be that the intermediate structures are short lived *(68)*. It also remains to be shown whether such intermembrane epitopes are physically accessible to the B-cell receptor and soluble antibody.

Primary isolates are not completely resistant to neutralization and, as a whole, exhibit a spectrum of neutralization sensitivity that is low as compared to TCLA strains. Epitopes for neutralizing antibody induction by primary isolates may be divided into three broad categories (Table 3). The first category consists of epitopes that generate a B-cell response in infected individuals (i.e., immunogenic) and are adequately exposed on the native envelope glycoprotein complex of primary isolates to permit efficient antibody binding (i.e., antigenic). These epitopes are highly variable and can be potent targets for strain-specific neutralization. For example, most primary isolates are neutralized potently by autologous serum samples obtained from the infected individual several months or more after the virus was isolated *(71–78)*. Those same serum samples neutralize only a fraction of isolates from other infected individuals (approx 25% on average), where the potency of neutralization is low *(75–78)*. The

Table 3
Three General Categories of Neutralization Epitopes Found on Primary HIV-1 Isolates

- Immunogenic and antigenic on the native envelope glycoprotein complex. *Antibodies to these epitopes are detected in cases where serum from an infected individual neutralizes a primary isolate. The antibodies may be generated either by monomers or oligomers and usually neutralize TCLA strains better than primary isolates.*
- Antigenically conserved but poorly immunogenic. (Examples are epitopes recognized by monoclonal antibodies IgG1b12, 2G12, and 2F5)
- Immunogenic but poorly antigenic on the native oligomeric envelope glycoprotein complex. (Most of these epitopes reside in the V3-loop of gp120 and are involved in the neutralization of TCLA strains but not primary isolates.)

location and structure of these strain-specific neutralization epitopes on primary isolates are currently unknown.

A second category of neutralization epitopes resides in relatively conserved regions of the gp120 and gp41 molecules. At least three examples of such epitopes are known to be present on TCLA strains as well as primary isolates. One example is the 2F5 epitope located in the gp41 ectodomain as described earlier. Another example is an epitope in the CD4-binding domain of gp120 recognized by monoclonal antibody IgG1b12 and that is sensitive to mutations in V2 and C3 *(79,80)*. A third example is an epitope recognized by monoclonal antibody 2G12. This latter monoclonal antibody recognizes an epitope comprised of amino acid residues in the C2–V4 regions of gp120 that involves sites of *N*-glycosylation *(79,81)*. The fact that serum samples from HIV-1–infected individuals rarely possess neutralizing activity equivalent to these monoclonal antibodies suggests that the cognate epitopes are poorly immunogenic.

A third category of neutralization epitopes on primary isolates is responsible for the production of antibodies that neutralize TCLA strains but not primary isolates. Most epitopes in this category are linear and reside in the V3 loop of gp120. B cells are thought to recognize these epitopes in the context of gp120 monomers that are released into circulation by cell-free virions and infected cells *(82)*. Such epitopes are thought to be occluded by subunit–subunit interactions, variable loop structures, or other tertiary folds in the gp120 molecule and to become exposed when gp120 dissociates from the oligomeric complex. The same epitopes would be similarly exposed on the surface of TCLA strains of the virus (Fig. 3).

NEUTRALIZING ANTIBODIES INDUCED BY HIV-1 INFECTION

The natural antibody response to HIV-1 fails to control virus replication and to prevent immunologic suppression and progression to AIDS even when combined with other immune-effector mechanisms induced by infection, such as HIV-1–specific $CD8^+$ cytotoxic T lymphocytes *(83,84)*. A major factor that limits the efficacy of neutralizing antibodies is the virus's ability to mutate to escape contemporaneous antibody specificities. Although the B cells eventually respond to make antibodies that neutralize an escape variant, the length of time needed for that response to mature provides the escape variant a wide window of opportunity to replicate unabated by antibodies;

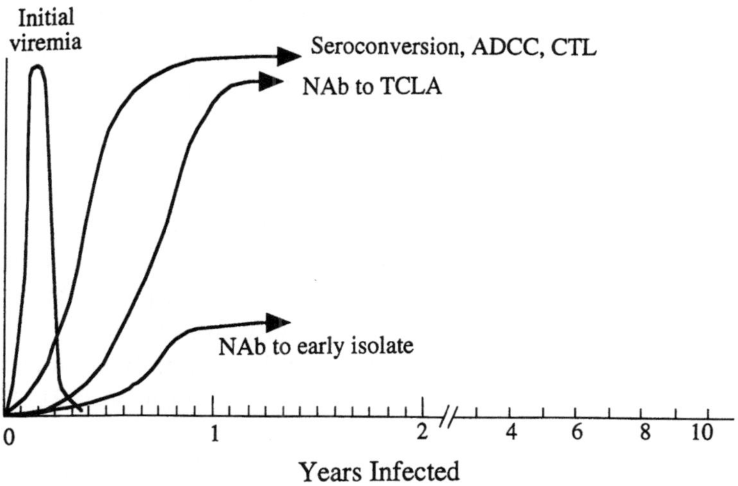

Fig. 4. Average time course for neutralizing antibody induction during the early stages of HIV-1 infection.

rough estimates indicate that this period of time varies considerably but averages approx 8 mo *(71–78)*. The fact that isolate-specific neutralizing antibodies can be detected for many years after they are generated *(71–74)* further suggests that the targeted variants are never completely suppressed but continue to persist at levels sufficient to maintain the strain-specific antibody response.

The earliest neutralizing antibodies to be detected in an HIV-1–infected individual are more strain-specific than those seen later in infection *(76,77)* and, in some cases, the early antibodies neutralize TCLA strains before they are capable of neutralizing the early autologous isolate *(75)*. These latter cases are additional evidence that primary patient isolates possess neutralization epitopes that are shared with TCLA strains but are not adequately exposed on the native envelope glycoprotein complex of the corresponding primary strain for that strain to be neutralized. The time when neutralizing antibodies first become detectable during primary infection does not correspond to the initial downregulation of plasma viremia (Fig. 4) *(75,76,78,85)*. This lack of correlation with the putative immunologic suppression of virus replication is consistent with the notion that other immune responses, primarily cytolytic T lymphocytes (CTLs), are responsible for the partial resolution of plasma viremia during the acute stage of HIV-1 infection *(83–85)*. It is conceivable that an accelerated neutralizing antibody response would alter the course of infection to favor the host, perhaps by slowing the initial spread of the virus until the CTL response has had sufficient time to mature. This is an important concept for vaccination. For example, vaccinated individuals who are not completely protected from infection might still benefit from a rapid anamnestic antibody response primed by the vaccine as long as the antibodies are able to neutralize the transmitted strain of virus.

No clear model has emerged to explain the poor immunogenicity of neutralization epitopes during HIV-1 infection. Some have suggested that long-term exposure to high doses of gp120 is required before antibody affinity can mature sufficiently to achieve neutralization *(86,87)*. Others have suggested that non-essential epitopes on gp120 act as "decoys," focusing the B-cell response on dispensable regions of the virus while avoiding B-cell recognition of more essential epitopes needed for neutralization *(88)*. A greater understanding of the immunologic basis for this phenomenon would greatly benefit vaccine development.

A small subset of HIV-1–infected individuals who tolerate infection for long periods of time without experiencing immunologic suppression or other clinical symptoms occasionally possess broadly cross-reactive neutralizing antibodies in their serum *(75,89–91)*. These infected individuals, who have come to be known as long-term non-progressors (LTNP), also have low virus loads in their peripheral blood and lymph nodes *(89,90)*. It has been suggested that their broadly cross-reactive neutralizing antibodies are the product of B cell responses to multiple neutralization-escape variants over long periods of time in the absence of immune suppression *(92)*. Although it is tempting to speculate that a vigorous neutralizing antibody response adds to the control of virus replication in these individuals, it is in fact difficult to know whether neutralizing antibodies are a cause of effect of long-term nonprogression. Indeed, LTNP are a heterogeneous group, where the role of neutralizing antibodies must be weighed with other factors, including potent cellular immune responses *(89,90,93–95)*, coreceptor polymorphisms *(96,97)*, and replication-defective virus variants *(98)* that also may contribute to long-term nonprogression. Nonetheless, the broadly cross-reactive neutralizing activity of their serum gives reason to believe that it will one day be possible to generate similar antibodies by vaccination.

VACCINES

Despite the limited value of neutralizing antibodies in established HIV-1 infection, it remains possible that preexisting immunity induced by vaccination will provide a significant clinical benefit. One way to predict the importance of neutralizing antibodies in the setting of vaccination is to perform passive immunization experiments in a relevant animal model. Infection with HIV-1 in chimpanzees *(99)*, and with simian immunodeficiency virus (SIV) in macaques *(100,101)*, are two classic models that have been exploited for this purpose in relationship to acquired immune deficiency syndrome (AIDS) vaccine development. A more recent model is the chimeric simian–human immunodeficiency virus (SHIV) infection of macaques. SHIV is a genetically engineered virus for which the envelope glycoproteins of HIV-1 were inserted into the backbone of an infectious molecular clone of SIV *(102–109)*. Envelope glycoproteins of TCLA variants and primary isolates of HIV-1 have been used for SHIV construction (see Table 4 for some examples). Being infectious and sometimes pathogenic in macaques, the SHIV model makes it possible to test the efficacy of candidate HIV-1 Env vaccines in a relevant animal model.

Passive infusion of appropriate virus-specific antibodies has provided solid protection against HIV-1 infection in chimpanzees *(110)*, and against highly virulent strains of SIV *(111,112)* and SHIV *(113–116)* in macaques. Those results confirm earlier reports *(117,118)* and support the notion that neutralizing antibody induction is a highly desirable goal for HIV-1 vaccines. Protection has correlated with the ability of passive antibody to neutralize the challenge virus in vitro at doses that are achieved in vivo, adding validity to the assays that are used to estimate the immunogenicity of candidate HIV-1 vaccines. Importantly, passive antibody experiments in macaques and

Table 4
SHIV Variants Used in Monkey Models

SHIV	Derivation	Pathogenic in monkeys
IIIB	T cell line adapted (TCLA) strain of HIV-1	No
KU-2	Monkey-passaged SHIV-IIIB	Yes
89.6	Primary isolate that is dual tropic for T cells and macrophages	No
89.6P	Monkey-passaged SHIV-89.6, isolated from cells	Yes
89.6PD	Monkey-passaged SHIV-89.6, isolated from plasma	Yes
KB9	Molecularly cloned SHIV-89.6P	Yes

hu-PBL-SCID mice have shown that antibodies capable of neutralizing one strain of virus but not another in vitro only protect against the former virus in vivo *(115,119–122)*. This outcome predicts that the neutralizing antibodies generated by an HIV-1 vaccine will need to be broadly cross-reactive to be effective against the numerous variants circulating within and between affected populations.

Various candidate HIV-1 vaccines have been tested since 1988 for safety and efficacy in phase I and II clinical trials *(83,123–126)*. A major goal has been to induce the production of HIV-1-specific CTL and neutralizing antibodies in healthy noninfected volunteers. Many candidate vaccines have included the viral envelope glycoproteins for neutralizing antibody induction. The envelope glycoproteins also have potential for CTL induction, where other viral subunits (e.g., Gag and Pol) have been included for CTL induction as well.

The majority of envelope glycoprotein subunit immunogens that have advanced to human clinical trials are based on monomeric, monovalent gp120 and gp160 from TCLA strains of virus. Only recently have a small number of primary isolate gp120 subunits entered human clinical trials *(127,128)*. The various envelope immunogens have been administered as either gp120 or gp160 protein, V3-loop peptides or live recombinant pox virus vectors (e.g., vaccinia and canarypox) expressing either gp120 or gp160. Titers of neutralizing antibodies generated by gp120 protein inoculation in adjuvant have been much higher than those generated by the recombinant vectors. Immunization with the recombinant vectors does, however, prime for an anamnestic (secondary) neutralizing antibody response that is seen after subunit boosting. The magnitude of the anamnestic response has in some cases surpasses the magnitude of neutralizing antibody induction achieved with protein alone (Fig. 5). B cell priming by recombinant vectors also has a dose-sparing benefit, where only one or two boosts with gp120 protein is needed to achieve the same level of neutralizing antibody induction that is seen with three or four inoculations with gp120 protein alone (Fig. 5). The gp120 made in mammalian cells performs better than products derived from yeast or insect cells, which might be due to a greater preservation of the structural integrity of the immunogen as dictated by the glycosylation pathways of the cells.

Titers of neutralizing antibodies in sera from vaccinated volunteers have in certain cases overlapped the titers seen in sera from infected individuals (Fig. 6). Unfortunately, the vaccine-induced neutralizing antibodies have been highly specific for the V3-loop of the vaccine strain of virus and, with rare exceptions, only neutralize that strain of virus (Fig. 6) *(19,129–131)*. This narrow specificity is a major concern for the

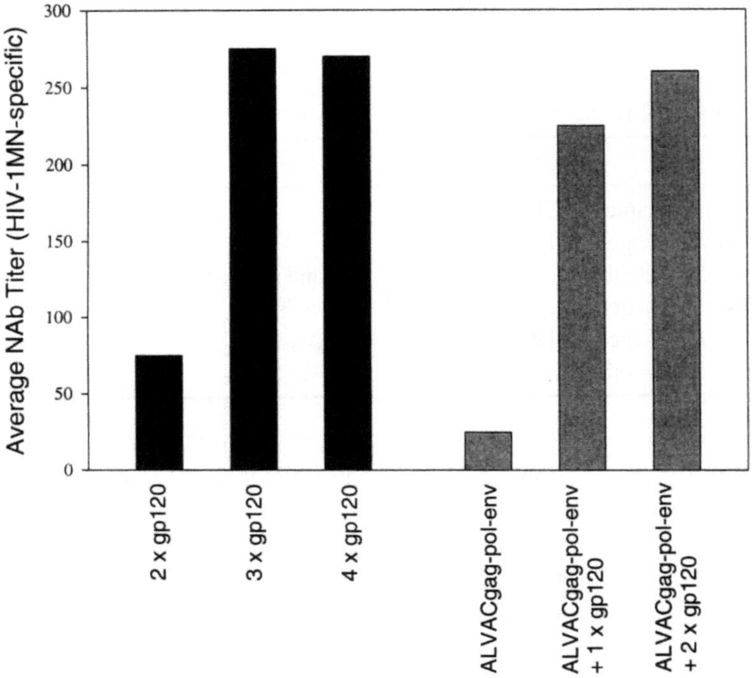

Fig. 5. Priming of an HIV-1MN-specific neutralizing antibody response by immunizing with recombinant canarypox vectors (ALVAC). Data are derived from multiple clinical trials in healthy noninfected volunteers.

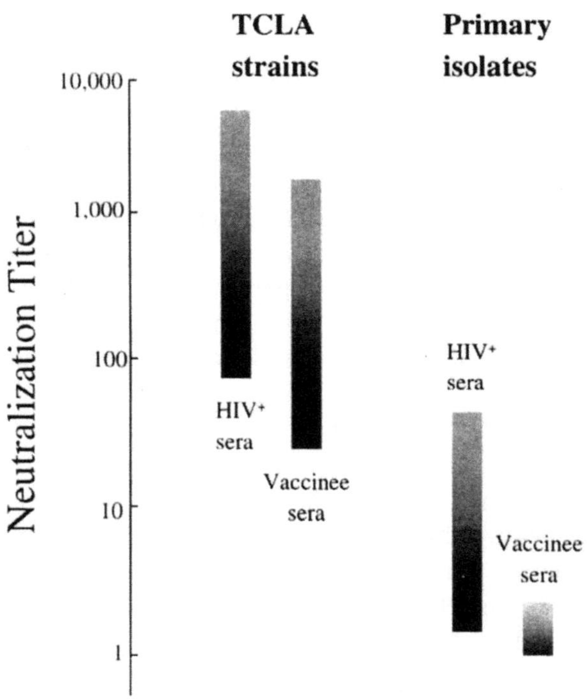

Fig. 6. Magnitude of neutralizing antibody induction in vaccinated volunteers as compared to HIV-1–infected individuals.

Table 5
New Experimental HIV-1 Vaccine Approaches for the Induction of Potent, Broadly Cross-reactive Neutralizing Antibodies

- Use of stable oligomers of uncleaved gp 140 and cleaved gp 120/gp41 heterodimers
- Use of a polyvalent mixture of primary isolate envelope glycoproteins (monomers or oligomers?).
- Introduce structural modifications in the envelope glycoproteins to expose cryptic epitopes:
  - Deletion of V1/V2 variable loops
  - Eliminate certain sites of *N*-linked glycan addition
  - Isolate or synthesize stable fusion intermediates of gp41

overall effectiveness of the antibody component of current HIV-1 vaccine candidates. Adding to this concern, at least 16 vaccinated volunteers participating in phase II studies of candidate gp120 vaccines became infected with HIV-1 through high risk behavior and showed no evidence that they were able to control their virus better than nonvaccinated individuals *(132–135)*.

Several alternate strategies to generate a more effective neutralizing antibody response are under investigation (Table 5). One approach is to immunize with oligomeric envelope glycoproteins with the goal of preserving the native structure of relevant epitopes. Initial efforts have focused on oligomers of uncleaved gp140 that lack the transmembrane region and cytoplasmic tail of gp41 so as to be secreted as a soluble product. To date, uncleaved oligomeric gp140s made from TCLA strains and primary isolates have shown no advantage over monomeric gp120 in terms of the magnitude and cross-reactivity of neutralizing antibody induction or the ability to protect against SHIV infection in macaques *(136)*. This disappointing outcome might be an early indication that preserving the native structure of the envelope glycoprotein complex from a single strain of virus will not solve the problem of cross-reactive neutralizing antibody induction. For example, antibodies generated by infection generally lack cross-reactive neutralizing activity despite the fact that native envelope glycoprotein complexes are present for B-cell recognition *(137)*. It remains possible that the structure of this first generation of uncleaved gp140s was not optimal for neutralizing antibody induction. A second generation of stable uncleaved gp140 oligomers, and cleaved gp120/gp41 heterodimers is under investigation *(138,139)*. It will be important to determine whether those products are capable of generating a cross-reactive neutralizing antibody response that is not predicted by the immune response to infection.

Another strategy focuses on the variable epitopes possessed by primary isolates that are known to be both immunogenic and antigenic. For example, cross-reactive neutralizing antibody induction might be achieved by immunizing with a polyvalent mixture of envelope glycoproteins from multiple strains of the virus (Table 3). The choice of strains to use in a polyvalent vaccine is an important consideration to assure an adequate level of cross-reactivity. An optimal cassette might contain the gp120 from each neutralization serotype of the virus. In this regard, efforts to identify the neutralization subtypes of HIV-1 might hasten the development of an effective HIV-1 vaccine. Our current knowledge of HIV-1 neutralization subtypes is extremely limited and, at the very least, the neutralization subtypes do not appear to correspond to the different genetic subtypes of the virus

(140–145). A polyvalent approach will also benefit from increased efforts to characterize the immunogenicity of primary isolate envelope glycoproteins.

Other novel approaches aim to alter the native structure of gp120 and gp41 in an effort to improve the immunogenicity of cryptic epitopes. An example is to remove *N*-linked glycans and variable loops (e.g., V1/V2) to expose the CD4-binding and coreceptor-binding sites for heightened B-cell recognition *(62)*. Another example would be to isolate or synthesize a stable configuration of the prehairpin intermediate of gp41 that forms prior to virus–cell fusion *(23,146)*. Approaches such as these are in early stages of development and afford fresh new avenues to pursue in the quest to design an appropriate immunogen for HIV-1–specific neutralizing antibody induction. Even with an optimal immunogen, however, it will be extremely difficult to sustain a high titer of neutralizing antibodies without regular boosting. The need to boost regularly would create major economic and logistic barriers to achieving long-term immunity in developing countries. An attractive alternative would be to aim for long-lasting B-cell priming by a recombinant vector to accelerate the production of neutralizing antibodies in response to infection *(147)*. The success of vector priming will ultimately depend on the availability of an appropriate immunogen for cross-reactive neutralizing antibody induction. It will also require that an anamnestic neutralizing antibody response be long lived and capable of preventing immune suppression and reducing the rate of virus transmission.

CONCLUDING REMARKS

The most feasible means to halt the global AIDS epidemic will be through vaccination. Although promising antiretroviral drugs are now available, their high cost prohibits their widespread use in developing countries that carry the heaviest burden of HIV-1 infections. Toxicities and emergence of resistant viruses are additional limiting factors for those who have access to drugs. A safe, broadly effective, stable and inexpensive vaccine is urgently needed. Conventional vaccine strategies, such as the use of whole killed and live attenuated virus preparations, are viewed by many as being too unsafe for a virus such as HIV-1 that integrates genetically, establishes a chronic infection, and is extremely difficult to evaluate for attenuation. The path to an HIV-1 vaccine has instead relied on recombinant viral subunits that are free of any potential infectivity. This shift from empiric testing of whole virus preparations to a more rational design approach to vaccine discovery has been accompanied by a heavy reliance on laboratory tests in place of efficacy trials to judge the potential worth of candidate HIV-1 vaccines during their early stages of development.

A major goal of the HIV-1 vaccine discovery process has been to identify in vitro correlates of protective immunity. As a result of concentrated efforts there is a growing concensus that a combination of CTL and neutralizing antibodies would provide the greatest benefit to an HIV-1 vaccine *(83,84,126,148,149)*. Helpful in this regard is the fact that assays to detect and quantify HIV-1–specific neutralizing antibodies have achieved a high level of standardization and validation. The complexities of these neutralization assays are also begining to be understood at a level that allow the results to be interpreted in a meaningful way. Results obtained to date strongly suggest that monovalent, monomeric envelope glycoproteins are poor immunogens to use for broadly cross-reactive neutralizing antibody induction. Efforts to improve the antibody component of candidate HIV-1 vaccines now focus on polyvalent Env and other immunogens that possess native or modified envelope glycoprotein structures. Only with large scale phase III efficacy trials will we learn the true value of in vitro assays and ultimately speed the development of future products.

REFERENCES

1. Allan JS, Coligan JE, Barin F, McLane MF, Sodroski JG, Rosen CA, et al. Major glycoprotein antigens that induce antibodies in AIDS patients are encoded by HTLV-III. Science 1985; 228:1091–4.
2. Veronese FM, DeVico AL, Copeland TD, Droszland S, Gallo RC, Sarngadharan MG. Characterization of gp41 as the transmembrane protein coded by the HTLV-III/LAV envelope gene. Science 1985; 229:1402–5.
3. McCune JM, Rabin LB, Feinberg MB, Lieberman M, Kosek JC, Reyes GR, Weissman IL. Endoproteolytic cleavage of gp160 is required for the activation of human immunodeficiency virus. Cell 1988; 53:55–67.
4. Earl PL, Doms RW, Moss B. Oligomeric structure of the human immunodeficiency virus type 1 envelope glycoprotein. Proc Natl Acad Sci USA 1990; 87:648–52.
5. Lu M, Blacklow SC, Kim PS. A trimeric structural domain of the HIV-1 transmembrane glycoprotein. Nat Struct Biol 1995; 2:1075–82.
6. Weissenhorn W, Wharton SA, Calder LJ, Earl PL, Moss B, Alirandis E, et al. The ectodomain of HIV-1 env subunit gp41 forms a soluble, alpha-helical, rod-like oligomer in the absence of gp120 and the N-terminal fusion peptide. EMBO J 1996; 15:1507–14.
7. Geyer H, Holschbach C, Hunsman C, Schneider J. Carbohydrates of human immunodeficiency virus: structures of oligosaccharides linked to the envelope glycoprotein gp120. J Biol Chem 1988; 263:11760–8.
8. Mizouchi T, Spellman MW, Larkin M, Solomon J, Basa LJ, Feizi T. Carbohydrate structures of the human immunodeficiency virus (HIV) recombinant envelope glycoprotein gp120 produced in Chinese hamster ovary cells. Biochem J 1988; 254:599–605.
9. Korber BTM, Allen EE, Farmer AD, Myers GL. Heterogeneity of HIV-1 and HIV-2. AIDS 1995; 9:Suppl A:S5–18.
10. Myers G, Pavlakis GN. Evolutionary potential of complex retroviruses. In: Levy JA. The Retroviruses. New York: Plenum, 1992; pp. 51–104.
11. Roberts JD, Bebenek K, Kunkel TA. The accuracy of reverse transcriptase from HIV-1. Science 1988; 242:1171–3.
12. Coffin JM. HIV viral dynamics. AIDS 1996; 10:Suppl 3:S75–84.
13. Ugolini S, Mondor I, Parren PWHI, Burton DR, Tilley SA, Klasse PJ, Sattentau QJ. Inhibition of virus attachment to $CD4^+$ target cells is a major mechanism of T cell line-adapted HIV-1 neutralization. J Exp Med 1997; 186:1287–98.
14. Valenzuela A, Blanco J, Krust B, Franco R, Hovanessian AG. Neutralizing antibodies against the V3 loop of human immunodeficiency virus type 1 gp120 block the CD4-dependent and -independent binding of virus to cells. J Virol 1997; 71:8289–98.
15. Parren PWHI, Naniche D, Mondor I, et al. Neutralization of HIV-1 by antibody to gp120 is determined primarily by occupancy of sites on the virion irrespective of epitope specificity. J Virol 1998; 72:3512–9.
16. Lasky LA, Nakamura G, Smith DH, Fennie C, Shimasaki C, Patzer E, et al. Delineation of a region of the human immunodeficiency virus gp120 glycoprotein critical for interaction with the CD4 receptor. Cell 1987; 50:975–85.
17. Wyatt R, Sodroski J. The HIV-1 envelope glycoproteins: fusogens, antigens, and immunogens. Science 1998; 280:1884–8.
18. Chan DC, Kim PS. HIV entry and its inhibition. Cell 1998; 93:681–4.

19. Montefiori DC, Graham BS, Zhou JT, Zhou JY, Bucco R, Cavacini LA, et al. V3-specific neutralizing antibodies in sera from HIV-1 gp160-immunized volunteers block virus fusion and act synergistically with human monoclonal antibody to the conformation-dependent CD4 binding region of gp120. J Clin Invest 1993; 92:840–7.
20. McDougal JS, Kennedy MS, Orloff SL, Nicholson, JKA, Spira TJ: Mechanism of human immunodeficiency virus type 1 (HIV-1) neutralization: irreversible inactivation of infectivity by anti-HIV-1 antibody. J Virol 1996; 70:5236–45.
21. Sullivan N, Sun Y, Sattentau Q, Thali M, Wu D, Denisova G, et al. CD4-induced conformational changes in the human immunodeficiency virus type 1 gp120 glycoprotein: consequences for virus entry and neutralization. J Virol 1998; 72:4694–703.
22. Salzwedel K, Smith ED, Dey B, Berger EA: Sequential CD4-coreceptor interactions in human immunodeficiency virus type 1 Env function: soluble CD4 activates Env for coreceptor-dependent fusion and reveals blocking activities of antibodies against cryptic conserved epitopes on gp120. J Virol 2000; 74:326–33.
23. LaCasse RA, Follis KE, Trahey M, Scarborough JD, Littman DR, Nunberg JH. Fusion-competent vaccines: broad neutralization of primary isolates of HIV. Science 1999; 283:357–62.
24. Wu L, Gerard N, Wyatt R, et al. CD4-induced interaction of primary HIV-1 gp120 glycoproteins with the chemokine receptor CCR-5. Nature 1996; 384:179–83.
25. Lapham CK, Ouyang J, Chandrasekhar B, Nguyen NY, Dimitrov DS, Golding H. Evidence for cell-surface association between fusion and the CD4-gp120 complex in human cell lines. Science 1996; 274:602–5.
26. Berger EA. HIV entry and tropism: the chemokine receptor connection. AIDS 1997; 11:Suppl A:S3–S16.
27. Moore JP, Trkola A, Dragic T. Co-receptors for HIV-1 entry. Curr Opin Immunol 1997; 9:551–62.
28. Berger EA, Doms RW, Fenyö E-M, Korber BTM, Littman DR, Moore JP, et al. HIV-1 phenotypes classified by co-receptor usage. Nature 1998; 391–240.
29. Koot M, Vos AHV, Keet RPM, De Goede REY, Dercksen FG, Terpstra MW, et al. HIV-1 biological phenotype in long-term infected individuals evaluated with an MT-2 cocultivation assay. AIDS 1992; 6:49–54.
30. Richman DD, Bozzette SA. The impact of the syncytium-inducing phenotype of human immunodeficiency virus on disease progression. J Infect Dis 1994; 169:968–74.
31. van't Wout AB, Kootstra NA, Mulder-Kampinga GA, Albrecht-van Lent N, Scherpbier HJ, Veenstra J, et al. Macrophage-tropic variants initiate human immunodeficiency virus type 1 infection after sexual, parenteral, and vertical transmission. J Clin Invest 1994; 94:2060–7.
32. Sawyer LSW, Wrin MT, Crawford-Miksza L, Potts B, Wu Y, Weber PA, et al. Neutralization sensitivity of human immunodeficiency virus type 1 is determined in part by the cell in which the virus is propagated. J Virol 1994; 68:1342–9.
33. Wrin T, Loh TP, Vennari JC, Schuitemaker H, Nunberg JH. Adaptation to persistent growth in the H9 cell line renders a primary isolate of human immunodeficiency virus type 1 sensitive to neutralization by vaccine sera. J Virol 1995; 69:39–48.
34. Baldinotti F, Matteucci D, Mazzetti P, et al. Serum neutralization of feline immunodeficiency virus is markedly dependent on passage history of the virus and host system. J Virol 1994; 68:4572–9.
35. Cook RF, Berger SL, Rushlow KE, et al. Enhnaced sensitivity to neutralizing antibodies in a variant of equine infectious anemia virus is linked to amino acid substitutions in the surface unit envelope glycoprotein. J Virol 1995; 69:1493–9.
36. Means RE, Greenough T, Desrosiers RC. Neutralization sensitivity of cell culture-passaged simian immunodeficiency virus. J Virol 1997; 71:7895–902.
37. Daar ES, Li XL, Moudgil T, Ho DD. High concentrations of recombinant soluble CD4 are required to neutralize primary human immunodeficiency virus type 1 isolates. Proc Natl Acad Sci USA 1990; 87:6574–8.

38. Montefiori DC, Zhou J, Barnes B, Lake D, Hersh EM, Masuho Y, Lefkowitz LB Jr. Homotypic antibody responses to fresh clinical isolates of human immunodeficiency virus. Virol 1991; 182:635–43.
39. Moore JP, Cao Y, Qing L, Sattentau QJ, Pyati J, Koduri R, et al. Primary isolates of human immunodeficiency virus type 1 are relatively resistant to neutralization by monoclonal antibodies to gp120, and their neutralization is not predicted by studies with monomeric gp120. J Virol 1995; 69:101–9.
40. Montefiori DC, Collman RG, Fouts TR, Zhou JY, Bilska M, Hoxie JA, et al. Evidence that antibody-mediated neutralization of human immunodeficiency virus type 1 by sera from infected individuals is independent of coreceptor usage. J Virol 1998; 72:1886–93.
41. Trkola A, Ketas T, KewalRamani VN, Endorf F, Binley JM, Katinger H, et al. Neutralization sensitivity of human immunodeficiency virus type 1 primary isolates to antibodies and CD4-based reagents is independent of their coreceptor usage. J Virol 1998; 72:1876–85.
42. LaCasse RA, Follis KE, Moudgil T, Trahey M, Binley JM, Planelles V, et al. Coreceptor utilization by human immunodeficiency virus type 1 is not a primary determinant of neutralization sensitivity. J Virol 1998; 72:2491–5.
43. Kwon PD, Wyatt R, Robinson J, Sweet RW, Sodroski J, Hendrickson WA. Structure of an HIV gp120 envelope glycoprotein in complex with the CD4 receptor and a neutralizing human antibody. Nature 1998; 393:648–59.
44. Weissenhorn W, Dessen A, Harrison SC, Skehel JJ, Wiley DC. Atomic structure of the ectodomain from HIV-1 gp41. Nature 1997; 387:426–30.
45. Chan DC, Fass D, Berger JM, Kim PS. Core structure of gp41 from the HIV envelope glycoprotein. Cell 1997; 89:263–73.
46. Fouts TR, Binley JM, Trkola A, Robinson JE, Moore JP. Neutralization of the human immunodeficiency virus type 1 primary isolate JR-FL by human monoclonal antibodies correlates with antibody binding to the oligomeric form of the envelope glycoprotein complex. J Virol 1997; 71:2779–85.
47. Roben P, Moore JP, Thali M, Sodroski J, Barbas CF, Burton DR. Recognition properties of a panel of human recombinant Fab fragments to the CD4 binding site of gp120 that show differing abilities to neutralize human immunodeficiency virus type 1. J Virol 1994; 68:4821–8.
48. Sattentau QJ, Moore JP. Human immunodeficiency virus type 1 neutralization is determined by epitope exposure on the gp120 oligomer. J Exp Med 1995; 182:185–96.
49. Stamatatos L, Zolla-Pazner S, Gorny MK, Cheng-Mayer C. Binding of antibodies to virion-associated gp120 molecules of primary-like human immunodeficiency virus type 1 (HIV-1) isolates: effect on HIV-1 infection of macrophages and peripheral blood mononuclear cells. Virology 1997; 229:360–9.
50. Moore JP, McKeating JA, Huang Y, Ashkenazi A, Ho DD. Virions of primary human immunodeficiency virus type 1 isolates resistant to soluble CD4 (sCD4) neutralization differ in sCD4 binding and glycoprotein gp120 retention from sCD4-sensitive isolates. J Virol 1992; 66:235–43.
51. Moore JP, Burkly LC, Connor RI, Cao Y, Tizard R, Ho DD, Fisher RA. Adaptation of two primary human immunodeficiency virus type 1 isolates to growth in transformed T-cell lines correlates with alterations in the responses of their envelope glycoproteins to soluble CD4. AIDS Res Hum Retrovir 1993; 9:529–39.
52. Bou-Habib DC, Roderiquez G, Oravecz T, Berman PW, Lusso P, Norcross MA. Cryptic nature of envelope V3 region epitopes protects primary monocytotropic human immunodeficiency virus type 1 from antibody neutralization. J Virol 1994; 68:6006–13.
53. Cocchi F, DeVico AL, Garzino-Demo A, Cara A, Gallo RC, Lusso P. The V3 domain of the HIV-1 gp120 envelope glycoprotein is critical for chemokine-mediated blockade of infection. Nat Med 1996; 2:1244–7.

54. Trkola A, Dragic T, Arthos J, Binley JM, Olson WC, Allaway GP, et al. CD4-dependent, antibody-sensitive interactions between HIV-1 and its co-receptor CCR-5. Nature 1996; 384:184–7.
55. Wu L, Gerard NP, Wyatt R, Choe H, Parolin C, Ruffing N, Borsetti A, et al. CD4-induced interaction of primary HIV-1 gp120 glycoproteins with the chemokine receptor CCR-5. Nature 1996; 384:179–83.
56. VanCott TC, Polonis VR, Loomis LD, Michael NL, Nara PL, Birx DL. Differential role of V3-specific antibodies in neutralization assays involving primary and laboratory-adapted isolates of HIV type 1. AIDS Res Hum Retrovir 1995; 11:1379–91.
57. Spenlehauer C, Saragosti S, Fleury HJA, Kirn A, Aubertin A-M, Moog C. Study of the V3 loop as a target epitope for antibodies involved in the neutralization of primary isolates versus T-cell-line-adapted strains of human immunodeficiency virus type 1. J Virol 1998; 72:9855–64.
58. Back NKT, Smit L, de Jong J-J, Keulen W, Schutten M, Goudsmit J, Tersmette M. An N-glycan within the human immunodeficiency virus type 1 gp120 V3 loop affects virus neutralization. Virology 1994; 199:431–8.
59. Schønning K, Jansson B, Olofsson S, Neilsen JO, Hansen J-ES. Resistance to V3-directed neutralization caused by an N-linked oligosaccharide depends on the quanternary structure of the HIV-1 envelope oligomer. Virology 1996; 218:134–40.
60. Schønning K, Jansson B, Olofsson S, Hansen J-ES. Rapid selection for an N-linked oligosacharide by monoclonal antibodies directed against the V3 loop of human immunodeficiency virus type 1. J Gen Virol 1996; 77:753–8.
61. Schønning K, Bolmstedt A, Novotny J, Søgaard Lund O, Olofsson S, Hansen J-ES. Induction of antiboides against epitopes inaccessible on the HIV type 1 envelope oligomer by immunization with recombinant monomeric glycoprotein 120. AIDS Res Hum Retrovir 1998; 16:1451–6.
62. Reitter JN, Means RE, Desrosiers RC. A role for carbohydrates in immune evasion in AIDS. Nat Med 1998; 4:679–84.
63. Chackerian B, Rudensey LM, Overbaugh J. Specific N-linked and O-linked glycosyaltion modifications in the envelope V1 domain of simian immunodeficiency virus variants that evolve in the host alter recognition by neutralizing antibodies. J Virol 1997; 71:7719–27.
64. Rudensey LM, Kimata JT, Long EM, Chackerian B, Overbaugh J. Changes in the extracellular envelope glycotprotein of variants that evolve during the course of simian immunodeficiency vurus SIV_{Mne} infection affect neutralizing antibdoy recognition, syncytium formation, and macrophage tropism but not replication, cytopathicity, or CCR-5 coreceptor recognition. J Virol 1998; 72:209–17.
65. Muster T, Guinea R, Trkola A, et al: Cross-neutralizing activity against divergent human immunodeficiency virus type 1 isolates induced by the gp41 sequence ELDKWAS. J Virol 1994; 68:4031–4.
66. D'Souza MP, Livnat D, Bradac JA, Bridges SH. Evaluation of monoclonal antibodies to human immunodeficiency virus type 1 primary isolates by neutralization assays: performance criteria for selecting candidate antibodies for clinical trials. J Infect Dis 1997; 175:1056–62.
67. Purtscher M, Trkola A, Grassauer A, Schultz PM, Klima A, Döpper S, et al. Restricted antigenic variability of the epitope recognized by the neutralizing gp41 antibody 2F5. AIDS 1996; 10:587–93.
68. Jones PL, Korte T, Blumenthal R. Conformational changes in cell surface HIV-1 envelope glycoproteins are triggered by cooperation between cell surface CD4 and co-receptors. J Biol Chem 1998; 273:404–9.
69. Wild CT, Shugars DC, Greenwell TK, McDanal CB, Matthews TJ. Peptides corresponding to a predicted α-helical domain of human immunodeficiency virus type 1 gp41 are potent inhibitors of virus infection. Proc Natl Acad Sci USA 1994; 91:9770–4.
70. Kilby JM, Hopkins S, Venetta TM, DiMassimo B, Cloud GA, Lee JY, et al. Potent suppression of HIV-1 replication in humans by T-20, a peptide inhibitor of gp41-mediated virus entry. Nat Med 1998; 4:1302–7.

71. Albert J, Abrahamsson B, Nagy K, Aurelius E, Gaines H, Nystrom G, Fenyo EM. Rapid development of isolate-specific neutralizing antibodies after primary HIV-1 infection and consequent emergence of virus variants which resist neutralization by autologous sera. AIDS 1990; 4:107–12.
72. Tremblay M, Wainberg MA. Neutralization of multiple HIV-1 isolates from a single subject by autologous sequential sera. J Infect Dis 1990; 162:735–7.
73. Arendrup M, Nielsen C, Stig Hanson J-E, Pedersen C, Mathiesen L, Nielsen JO. Autologous HIV-1 neutralizing antibodies: emergence of neutralization-resistant escape virus and subsequent development of escape virus neutralizing antibodies. J Acquir Immune Defic Syndr 1992; 5:303–7.
74. Wrin T, Crawford L, Sawyer L, Weber P, Sheppard HW, Hanson CV. Neutralizing antibody responses to autologous and heterologous isolates of human immunodeficiency virus. J Acquir Immune Defic Syndr 1994; 7:211–9.
75. Pilgrim AK, Pantaleo G, Cohen OJ, Fink LM, Zhou JY, Zhou JT, et al. Neutralizing antibody responses to human immunodeficiency virus type 1 in primary infection and long-term non-progressive infection. J Infect Dis 1997; 176:924–32.
76. Moog C, Fleury HJA, Pellegrin I, Kirn A, Aubertin AM. Autologous and heterologous neutralizing antibody responses following initial seroconversion in human immunodeficiency virus type 1-infected individuals. J Virol 1997; 71:3734–41.
77. Carotenuto P, Looij D, Keldermans L, de Wolf F, Goudsmit J. Neutralizing antibodies are positively associated with $CD4^+$ T-cell counts and T-cell function in long-term AIDS-free infection. AIDS 1998; 12:1591–600.
78. Pellegrin I, Legrand E, Neau D, Bonot P, Masquelier B, Pellegrin J-L, et al. Kinetics of appearance of neutralizing antibodies in 12 patients with primary or recent HIV-1 infection and relationship with plasma and cellular viral loads. J AIDS 1996; 11:438–47.
79. Burton DR, Montefiori DC. The antibody response in HIV-1 infection. AIDS 1997; 11:Suppl A:S87–S98.
80. Mo H, Stamatatos L, Ip JE, Barbas CF, Parren PWHI, Burton DR, et al. Human immunodeficiency virus type 1 mutants that escape neutralization by human monoclonal antibody IgG1b12. J Virol 1997; 71:6869–74.
81. Trkola A, Purtscher M, Muster T, Ballaun C, Buchacher A, Sullivan N, et al. Human monoclonal antibody 2G12 defines a distinctive neutralization epitope on the gp120 glycoprotein of human immunodeficiency virus type 1. J Virol 1996; 70:1100–8.
82. Burton DR. A vaccine for HIV type 1: the antibody perspective. Proc Natl Acad Sci USA 1997; 94:10018–23.
83. Letvin NL. Progress in the development of an HIV-1 vaccine. Science 1998; 280:1875–80.
84. Haynes BF, Pantaleo G, Fauci AS. Toward an understanding of the correlates of protective immunity to HIV infection. Science 1996; 271:324–8.
85. Koup RA, Safrit JT, Cao Y, Andrews CA, McLeod G, Borkowsky W, et al. Temporal association of cellular immune responses with the initial control of viremia in primary human immunodeficiency virus type 1 syndrome. J Virol 1994; 68:4650–5.
86. Montelaro RC, Cole KS, Hammond SA. Maturation of immune responses to lentivirus infection—implications for AIDS vaccine development. AIDS Res Hum Retrovir 1998; 14:Suppl 3:S255–9.
87. Cole KS, Murphey-Corb M, Narayan O, Joag SV, Shaw G, Montelaro RC. Common themes of antibody maturation to simian immunodeficiency virus, simian-human immunodeficiency virus, and human immunodeficiency virus type 1 infections. J Virol 1998; 72:7852–9.
88. Nara PL, Garrity R. Deceptive imprinting: a cosmopolitan strategy for complicating vaccination. Vaccine 1998; 16:1780–7.
89. Cao Y, Qin L, Zhang L, Safrit J, Ho DD. Virologic and immunologic characterization of long-term survivors of human immunodeficiency virus type 1 infection. N Engl J Med 1995; 332:201–8.

90. Pantaleo G, Menzo S, Vaccarezza M, Graziosi C, Cohen OJ, Demarest JF, et al. Studies in subjects with long-term nonprogressive human immunodeficiency virus infection. N Engl J Med 1995; 332:209–16.
91. Montefiori DC, Pantaleo G, Fink LM, Zhou JT, Zhou JY, Bilska M, et al. Neutralizing and infection-enhancing antibody responses to human immunodeficiency virus type 1 in long term non-progressors. J Infect Dis 1996; 173:60–7.
92. Bradney AP, Scheer S, Crawford JM, Buchbinder SP, Montefiori DC. Neutralization-escape in human immunodeficiency virus type 1-infected long-term nonprogressors. J Infect Dis 1999; 179:1264–7.
93. Klein MR, van Baalen CA. Kinetics of Gag-specific cytotoxic T lymphocyte responses during the clinical course of HIV-1 infection: a longitudinal analysis of rapid progressors and long-term asymptomatics. J Exp Med 1995; 181:1356–72.
94. Rinaldo C, Huang X-L, Fan Z, Ding M, Beltz L, Panicali D, et al. High levels of anti-human immunodeficiency virus type 1 (HIV-1) memory cytotoxic T-lymphocyte activity and low viral load are associated with lack of disease in HIV-1-infected long-term nonprogressors. J Virol 1995; 69:5838–42.
95. Harrer T, Harrer E, Kalams SA, Elbeik T, Staprans SI, Feinberg MB, et al. Strong cytotoxic T cell and weak neutralizing antibody responses in a subset of persons with stable nonprogressing HIV type 1 infection. AIDS Res Hum Retrovir 1996; 12:585–92.
96. Dean M, Carrington M, Winkler C, Huttley GA, Smith MW, Allikmets R, et al. Genetic restriction of HIV-1 infection and progression to AIDS by a deletion allele of the CKR5 structural gene. Science 1996; 273:1856–62.
97. Smith MW, Dean M, Carrington M, Winkler C, Huttley GA, Lomb DA, et al. Contrasting genetic influence of CCR2 and CCR5 variants on HIV-1 infection and disease progression. Science 1997; 277:959–65.
98. Kirchoff F, Greenough TC, Brettler DB, Sullivan JL, Desrosiers RC. Absence of intact *nef* sequences in a long-term survivor with nonprogressive HIV-1 infection. N Engl J Med 1995; 332:228–32.
99. Alter HJ, Eichberg JW, Masur H, Saxinger WC, Gallo RC, Macher AM, et al. Transmission of HTLV-III infection from human plasma to chimpanzees: an animal model for AIDS Science 1984; 226:549–52.
100. Desrosiers RC. The simian immunodeficiency viruses. Annu Rev Immunol 1990; 8:557–78.
101. Gardner MB. The history of simian AIDS. J Med Primatol 1996; 25:148–57.
102. Shiba R, Adachi A. SIV/HIV recombinants and their use in studying biological properties. AIDS Res Hum Retrovir 1992; 8:403–9.
103. Li J, Lord CI, Haseltine W, Letvin NL, Sodroski J. Infection of cynomolgus monkeys with a chimeric HIV-1/SIVmac virus that expresses the HIV-1 envelope glycoproteins. J Acq Immune Def Syndr 1993; 5:639–46.
104. Luciw PA, Pratt-Lowe E, Shaw KES, Levy JA, Cheng-Mayer C. Persistent infection of rhesus macaques with T-cell line-tropic and macrophage-tropic clones of simian/human immunodeficiency viruses (SHIV). Proc Natl Acad Sci USA 1995; 92:7490–4.
105. Li JT, Halloran M, Lord CI, Watson A, Ranchalis J, Fung M, et al. Persistent infection of macaques with simian-human immunodeficiency viruses. J Virol 1995; 69:7061–71.
106. Joag SV, Li Z, Foresman L, Stephens EB, Zhao LJ, Adany I, et al. Chimeric simian human immunodeficiency virus that causes progressive loss of $CD4^+$ T cells and AIDS in pig-tailed macaques. J Virol 1996; 70:3189–97.
107. Reimann KA, Li JT, Veazey R, Halloran M, Park I-W, Karlsson GB, et al. A chimeric simian/human immunodeficiency virus expressing a primary patient human immunodeficiency virus type 1 isolate *env* causes an AIDS-like disease after in vivo passage in rhesus monkeys. J Virol 1996; 70:6922–8.

108. Reimann KA, Li JT, Voss G, Lekutis C, Tenner-Racz K, Racz P, et al. An *env* gene derived from a primary HIV-1 isolate confers high in vivo replicative capacity to a chimeric simian/human immunodeficiency virus in rhesus monkeys. J Virol 1996; 70:3198–206.
109. Karlsson GB, Halloran M, Li J, Park I-W, Gomila R, Reimann KA, et al. Characterization of molecularly cloned simian-human immunodeficiency viruses causing rapid CD4+ lymphocyte depletion in rhesus monkeys. J Virol 1997; 71:4218–25.
110. Conley AJ, Kessler JA II, Boots LJ, McKenna PM, Schleif WA, Emini EA, et al. The consequence of passive administration of an anti-human immunodeficiency virus type 1 neutralizing monoclonal antibody before challenge of chimpanzees with a primary virus isolate. J Virol 1996; 70:6751–8.
111. Haigwood NL, Watson A, Sutton WF, McClure J, Lewis A, Ranchalis J, et al. Passive immune globulin therapy in the SIV/macaque model: early intervention can alter disease profile. Immunol Lett 1996; 51:107–14.
112. Clements JE, Montelaro RC, Zink MC, Amedee AM, Miller S, Trichel AM, et al. Cross-protective immune responses induced in rhesus macaques by immunization with attenuated macrophage-tropic simian immunodeficiency virus. J Virol 1995; 69:2737–44.
113. Mascola JR, Lewis MG, Stiegler G, Harris D, VanCott TC, Hayes D, et al. Protection of macaques against pathogenic simian/human immunodeficiency virus 89.6PD by passive transfer of neutralizing antibodies. J Virol 1999; 73:4009–18.
114. Mascola JR, Stiegler G, VanCott TC, Katinger H, Carpenter CB, Hanson CE, et al. Protection of macaques against vaginal transmission of a pathogenic HIV-1/SIV chimeric virus by passive infusion of neutralizing antibodies. Nat Med 2000; 6:207–10.
115. Shibata R, Igarashi T, Haigwood N, Buckler-White A, Ogert R, Ross W, et al. Neutralizing antibody directed against the HIV-1 envelope glycoprotein can completely block HIV-1/SIV chimeric virus infections of macaque monkeys. Nat Med 1999; 5:204–10.
116. Foresman L, Jia F, Li Z, Wang C, Stephens EB, Sahni M, et al. Neutralizing antibodies administered before, but not after, virulent SHIV prevent infection in macaques. AIDS Res Hum Retrovir 1998; 14:1035–43.
117. Prince AM, Reesink H, Pascual D, Horowitz B, Hewlett I, Murthy KM, et al. Prevention of HIV infection by passive immunization with HIV immunoglobulin. AIDS Res Hum Retrovir 1991; 7:971–3.
118. Emini EA, Schleiff WA, Nunberg JH, Conley AJ, Eda Y, Tokiyoshi S, et al. Prevention of HIV-1 infection in chimpanzees by gp120 V3 domain-specific monoclonal antibody. Nature 1992; 355:728–30.
119. Safrit JT, Fung MSC, Andrews CA, Braun DG, Sun WNC, Chang TW, Koup RA. hu-PBL-SCID mice can be protected from HIV-1 infection by passive transfer of monoclonal antibody to the principal neutralizing determinant of envelope gp120. AIDS 1993; 7:15–21.
120. Gauduin M-C, Safrit JT, Weir R, Fung MSC, Koup RA. Pre- and postexposure protection against human immunodeficiency virus type 1 infection mediated by a monoclonal antibody. J Infect Dis 1995; 171:1203–9.
121. Parren PWHI, Ditzel HJ, Gulizia RJ, Binley JM, Barbas CF III, Burton DR, Mosier DE. Protection against HIV-1 infection in hu-PBL-SCID mice by passive immunization with a neutralizing human monoclonal antibody against the gp120 CD4-binding site. AIDS 1995; 9:F1–6.
122. Gauduin M-C, Parren PWHI, Weir R, Barbas CF, Burton DR, Koup RA. Passive immunization with a human monoclonal antibody protects hu-PBL-SCID mice against challenge by primary isolates of HIV-1. Nat Med 1997; 3:1389–93.
123. Graham BS, Wright PF. Candidate AIDS vaccines. J Engl J Med 1995; 333:1331–9.
124. Walker M-C, Fast PE, Graham BS, Belshe R, Dolin R. Phase I/II preventive vaccine trial: conference summary. AIDS Res Hum Retrovir 1995; 11:1279–85.
125. Graham BS. Serologic responses to candidate AIDS vaccines. AIDS Res Hum Retrovir 1994; 10:Suppl. 2:S145–8.

126. Heilman CA, Baltimore D. HIV vaccines-where are we going? Nat Med 1998; 4:532–4.
127. Francis DP, Gregory T, McElrath MJ, Belshe RB, Gorse GJ, Migasena S, et al. Advancing AIDSVAX™ to phase 3. Safety, immunogenicity, and plans for phase 3. AIDS Res Hum Retrovir 1998; 14:S325–31.
128. Beddows S, Lister S, Cheingsong R, Bruck C, Weber J. Comparison of the antibody repertoire generated in healthy volunteers following immunization with a monomeric recombinant gp120 construct derived from a CCR5/CXCR4-using human immunodeficiency virus type 1 isolate with sera from naturally infected individuals. J Virol 1999; 73:1740–5.
129. Bures R, Gaitan, A, Zhu T, Graziosi C, McGrath K, Tartaglia J, et al. Immunization with recombinant canarypox vectors expressing membrane-anchored gp120 followed by soluble gp160 boosting fails to generate antibodies that neutralize R5 primary isolates of human immunodeficiency virus type 1. AIDS Res Hum Retrovir 2000; 16:2019–35.
130. Mascola JR, Snyder SW, Weislow OS, Belay SM, Belshe RB, Schwartz DH, et al. Immunization with envelope subunit vaccine products elicits neutralizing antibodies against laboratory-adapted but not primary isolates of human immunodeficiency virus type 1. J Infect Dis 1996; 173:340–8.
131. Belshe RB, Gorse GJ, Mulligan MJ, Evans TG, Keefer MC, Excler J-L, et al. Rapid induction of HIV-1 immune responses by canarypox (ALVAC) HIV-1 and gp120 SF2 recombinant vaccines in uninfected volunteers. AIDS 1998; 12:2407–15.
132. Connor RI, Korber BTM, Graham BS, Hahn BH, Ho DD, Walker BD, et al. Immunological and virological analyses of persons infected by human immunodeficiency virus type 1 while participating in trials of recombinant gp120 subunit vaccines. J Virol 1998; 72:1552–76.
133. Graham BS, McElrath MJ, Connor RI, Schwartz DH, Gorse GJ, Keefer MC, et al. Analysis of intercurrent human immunodeficiency virus type 1 infections in phase I and II trials of candidate AIDS vaccines. J Infect Dis 1998; 177:310–9.
134. McElrath JM, Corey L, Greenberg PD, Matthews TJ, Montefiori DC, Rowen L, et al. Human immunodeficiency virus type 1 infection despite prior immunization with a recombinant envelope vaccine regimen. Proc Natl Acad Sci USA 1996; 93:3972–7.
135. Kahn JO, Steimer KS, Baenziger J, Duliege A-M, Feinberg M, Elbeik T, et al. Clinical, immunologic, and virologic observations related to human immunodeficiency virus (HIV) type 1 infection in a volunteer in an HIV-1 vaccine clinical trial. J Infect Dis 1995; 171:1343–7.
136. Montefiori DC, Evans TG. Toward an HIV-1 vaccine that generates potent, broadly cross-reactive neutralizing antibodies. AIDS Res Hum Retrovir 1999; 15:689–98.
137. Montefiori DC, Reimann KA, Wyand MS, Manson K, Lewis MG, Collman RG, et al. Neutralizing antibodies in sera from macaques infected with chimeric simian-human immunodeficiency virus containing the envelope glycoproteins of either a laboratory-adapted variant or a primary isolate of human immunodeficiency virus type 1. J Virol 1998; 72:3427–31.
138. Binley JM, Sanders RW, Clas B, Schuelke N, Master A, Guo Y, et al. A recombinant human immunodeficiency virus type 1 envelope glycoprotein complex stabilized by an intramolecular disulfide bond between the gp120 and gp41 subunits is an antigenic mimic of the trimeric virion-associated structure. J Virol 2000; 74:627–43.
139. Yang X, Florin L, Farzan M, Kolchinsky P, Kwong PD, Sodroski J, Wyatt R. Modifications that stabilize human immunodeficiency virus envelope glycoprotein trimers in solution. J Virol 2000; 74:4746–54.
140. Louisirirotchanakul S, Beddows S, Cheingsong-Popov R, et al. Characterization of sera from subjects infected with HIV-1 subtypes B and E in Thailand by antibody binding and neutralization. J AIDS Hum Retrovirol 1998; 19:315–20.
141. Mascola JR, Louder MK, Surman SR, et al. Human immunodeficiency virus type 1 neutralizing antibody serotyping using serum pools and an infectivity reduction assay. AIDS Res Hum Retrovir 1996; 12:1319–28.

142. Nyambi PN, Nkengasong J, Lewi P, et al. Multivariate analysis of human immunodeficiency virus type 1 neutralization data. J Virol 1996; 70:6235–43.
143. Weber J, Fenyö E-M, Beddows S, Kaleebu P, Bjorndal A, the WHO Network for HIV Isolation and Characterization. Neutralization serotypes of human immunodeficiency virus type 1 field isolates are not predicted by genetic subtype. J Virol 1996; 70:7827–32.
144. Kostrikis LG, Cao Y, Ngai H, Moore JP, Ho DD. Quantitative analysis of serum neutralization of human immunodeficiency virus type 1 from subtypes A, B, C, D, E, F, and I: lack of direct correlation between neutralization serotypes and genetic subtypes and evidence for prevalent serum-dependent infectivity enhancement. J Virol 1996; 70:445–58.
145. Moore JP, Cao Y, Leu J, Qin L, Korber B, Ho DD. Inter-and intraclade neutralization of human immunodeficiency virus type 1: Genetic clades do not correspond to neutralization serotypes but partially correspond to gp120 antigenic serotypes. J Virol 1996; 70:427–44.
146. Montefiori DC, Moore JP. Magic of the occult? Science 1999; 283:336–7.
147. Ourmanov I, Bilska M, Hirsch VH, Montefiori DC. Recombinant modified vaccinia virus Ankara expressing the surface gp120 of simian immunodeficiency virus (SIV) primes for a rapid neutralizing antibody response to SIV infection in macaques. J Virol 2000; 74:2960–5.
148. Schmitz JE, Kuroda MJ, Santra S, Sasseville VG, Simon MA, Lifton MA, et al. $CD8^+$ lymphocytes control viremia in simian immunodeficiency virus infection. Science 1999; 283:857–60.
149. Jin X, Bauer DE, Tuttleton SE, Lewin S, Gettie A, Blanchard J, et al. Dramatic rise in plasma viremia after $CD8^+$ T cell depletion in simian immunodeficiency virus-infected macaques. J Exp Med 1999; 189:991–8.

9

Cytotoxic T-Cell Responses in Acute and Chronic HIV-1 Infection

Hugo Soudeyns and Giuseppe Pantaleo

INTRODUCTION

Cell-mediated immune responses can be broken down into three physically and temporally distinct phases: (1) uptake, processing, and presentation of soluble or cell-associated antigens at the surface of antigen-presenting cells, in association with proteins encoded by genes located within the major histocompatibility complex (MHC); (2) antigen recognition, which is mediated by the T-cell receptor (TCR); and (3) the effector phase, during which antigen-activated T cells express differentiated functions aimed at directly (cytolytic machinery) or indirectly (cytokine release) containing the pathogen.

Antigen Presentation and Recognition

Distinct processing pathways are mobilized depending on whether the antigens are produced extracellularly or intracellularly. Antigens sampled from the extracellular milieu associate with MHC class II heterodimers (*1–5,* reviewed in *6*). Conversely, endogenously produced antigens are degraded intracytoplasmically into peptides *(7,8),* shuttled into late endoplasmic reticulum, loaded onto class I heavy chain-β_2 microglobulin complexes, and transported to the cell surface *(9–14).* The polymorphism of MHC class I and class II genes is focussed in regions of the molecules that are directly involved in peptide binding, and defines the spectrum of peptides that can be produced, presented, and recognized by the host *(6),* thus influencing the susceptibility of individuals and populations to specific pathogens, including human immunodeficiency virus type 1 (HIV-1) *(15–17).*

As obligate intracellular parasites, all viruses require their gene products and constituents to be manufactured by the host cell. Peptides derived from nascent viral proteins, complexed with MHC class I molecules at the cell surface, flag virus-infected cells for attack by antigen-specific cytotoxic T lymphocytes (CTLs). T cell recognition of peptide-MHC class I complexes is mediated by the αβ TCR, a polymorphic, clonally distributed heterodimer expressed at the surface of T cells *(18).* Mature TCR genes are somatically rearranged from multiple, discontinuous gene segments (V, D, J) *(19,20).* TCR rearrangement involves processing of the germline DNA coding ends, resulting in a high level of diversification at the V(D)J junction (complementarity-determining region

From: *Retroviral Immunology: Immune Response and Restoration*
Edited by: Giuseppe Pantaleo and Bruce D. Walker © Humana Press Inc., Totowa, NJ

3, or CDR3) *(18)*. This is because amino acid residues encoded within CDR3 closely contact the antigenic peptide and directly mediate the recognition of peptide–MHC complexes *(21,22)*. Because of this, the TCRs of various T-cell clones responding to identical peptide–MHC complexes tend to exhibit structural similarities *(22–26)*.

The sum of TCR combinations and specificities within a host is termed the TCR repertoire. It can be analyzed by a number of methods, including flow cytometry, multiparallel polymerase chain reaction (PCR) and runoff-based assays such as the "immunoscope" *(27–33)*. The diversity and persistence of CTL responses can be monitored using TCR phenotyping, taking advantage of the fact that specific CTL clones express TCRs with unique CDR3 regions *(34)*. Thus, CDR3-specific PCR and TCR heteroduplex mobility shift assays have been successfully used to track antigen-specific CTLs in various clinical settings, including HIV infection *(35–39)*.

Effector Functions of Cytotoxic T Lymphocytes

Following recognition of MHC–peptide complexes by the TCR, transmembrane activation signals are transmitted to the T cell through the CD3 moiety of the Ti complex. These events result in the T cell acquiring an activated phenotype, characterized by (1) increased cell size and metabolic activity; (2) increased cell-surface expression of TCR, CD4, or CD8 accessory proteins, HLA-DR, as well as other markers associated with T-cell activation; (3) production of specific cytokines profiles; and (4) emergence of MHC-restricted antigen-specific effector function, that is, in the case of CTLs, cytocidal properties. The large majority of cells possessing CTL activity express the CD8 accessory molecule, and recognize antigen complexed with MHC class I molecules (i.e., derived from the endogenous antigen processing/presentation pathway). Interestingly, MHC class II-restricted $CD4^+$ CTLs have been detected in HIV-infected subjects *(40)*, in whom they have been hypothesized to act on cells having processed soluble HIV-1 antigens via the exogenous pathway *(41)*.

On target recognition, cell killing by $CD8^+$ CTLs can be mediated by two distinct pathways (Fig. 1). The first depends on the secretion of perforin and granzyme B by the CTLs. Perforin introduces pores into cytoplasmic membranes, therefore compromising the osmotic integrity of the target cell *(42,43)*. Studies on perforin-deficient mice have revealed that this mechanism of defense was essential to host resistance against intracellular parasites, including noncytopathic viruses such as lymphocytic choriomeningitis virus (LCMV) *(44,45)*. The presence of perforin also facilitates, but is not essential for, the penetration of the target cell by granzyme B, a protease capable of activating the caspase-mediated apoptotic cascade in target cells *(46,47)*. Granzyme A, also comprised within exocytosed cytotoxic granules, is also capable of inducing apoptosis of target cells, apparently through a caspase-independent mechanism *(48,49)*.

The second CTL killing pathway involves upregulation of the levels of expression of Fas-ligand (CD95L) at the surface of the CTL. On cognate cell–cell contact, CD95L interacts with Fas (CD95) on the surface of the target cell, to which potent transmembrane apoptotic signals are thereby delivered (Fig. 1) *(50–52)*. Apoptosis of target cells can also be triggered by soluble Fas-ligand (sCD95L) and tumor necrosis factor-α (TNF-α), both expressed by antigen-activated CTLs *(53)*. These two modes of CTL killing are not mutually exclusive, as multiple mechanisms may simultaneously contribute to the destruction and removal of target cells, thereby counteracting potential CTL escape strategies (see later).

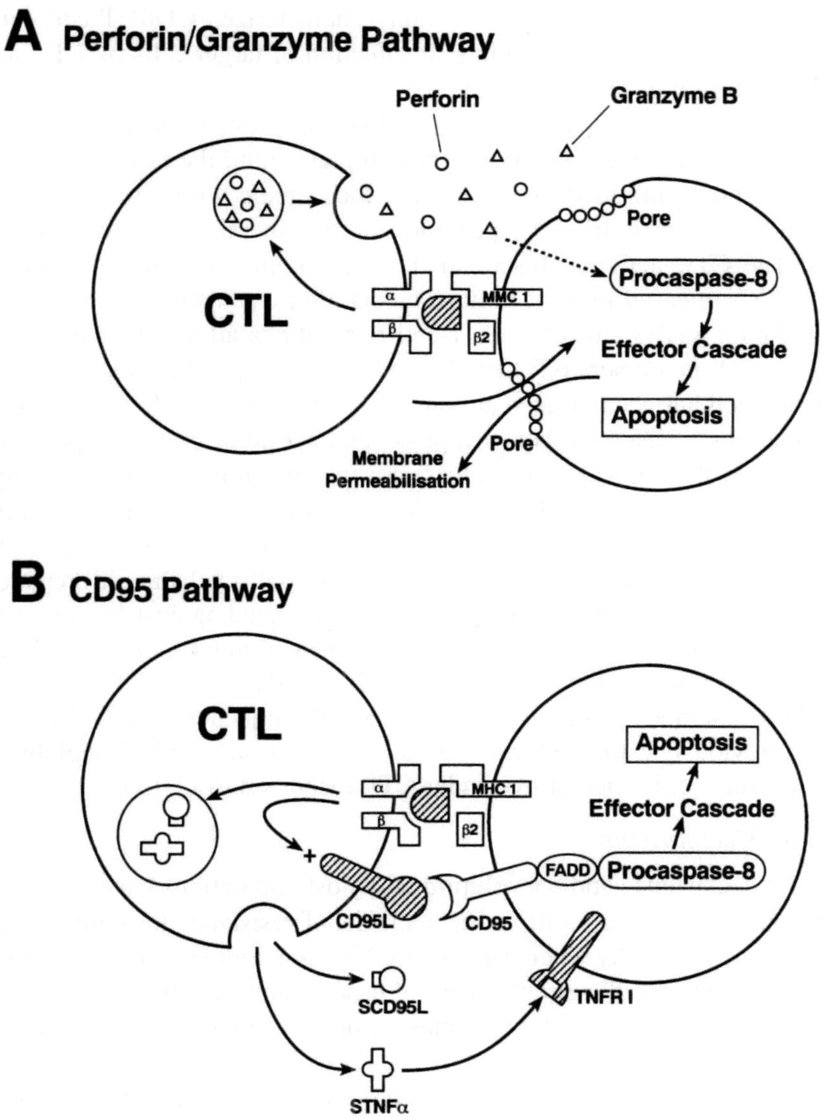

Fig. 1. Cell killing by CD8+ cytotoxic T lymphocytes (CTL) can be mediated by two distinct pathways. **A.** Following antigen-specific recognition, perforin introduces pores into cytoplasmic membranes, facilitating the penetration of the target cell by granzyme B, which in turn activates the caspase-mediated apoptotic cascade. **B.** Following antigen-specific recognition, levels of expression of Fas-ligand are up-regulated at the surface of the CTL. Interaction with Fas at the surface of the target cell triggers the apoptotic cascade.

In addition, antigen-specific CD8+ effectors can secrete pro-inflammatory cytokines such as interferon-γ (IFN-γ), TNF-α, and interleukin-16 (IL-16), which possess intrinsic antiviral and cytotoxic activities *(54–56)*. Furthermore, in the case of primary and chronic infection with HIV-1, CD8+ T cells have been shown to release a variety of β-chemokines (MIP-1α, MIP-1β, RANTES) that interact with HIV-1 fusion coreceptor CCR5 at the surface of CD4+ T cells and block fusion/internalization of R5 HIV-1 isolates *(57–59)*. As well, other incompletely characterized CD8+ T cell derived diffusible factors have been shown to inhibit infection of target cells by HIV, apparently via inhibition of viral gene transcription *(60–63)*.

Classical methods for measuring CTL activity rely on the labeling of target cells with radioactive ^{51}Cr, which remains in the cytoplasm until the osmotic integrity of the cell becomes compromised *(64)*. Targets are then mixed with effector T-cell populations expanded in vitro from suspensions of peripheral blood mononuclear cells (PBMCs). The CTL activity present in the cell sample is defined according to the amounts of ^{51}Cr released into the culture media after a standard incubation time *(64)*. Limiting dilution analysis of effector T-cell populations allows the calculation of the frequency of CTL precursors (CTLp) directed against a specific antigen *(65)*. Over the years, this method has accumulated an impressive track record. However, since effector T-cell populations necessarily require a prolonged period of in vitro expansion prior to the assay, it was thought that ^{51}Cr release assays and limiting dilution analysis seriously underestimated the actual frequencies of terminally differentiated antigen-specific effector CTL (CTLe), which possess only low proliferative potential. Recently, several new techniques have been developed that confirmed this discrepancy. These include: (1) intracellular staining with antibodies directed against IFN-γ, followed by flow cytometric analysis *(66,67)* or enzyme-linked immunospot (ELISPOT) assays *(68)*; and (2) staining with soluble tetramerized MHC class I–peptide complexes *(68,69)*. These methods have revealed that actual frequencies of CTLe were much higher than previously estimated, and have seriously questioned (although by no means excluded) the mere existence of bystander CTL responses *(68,70,71)*.

CTL Escape Mechanisms

Long-term coexistence and coevolution with host populations have resulted in retroviral pathogens developing multiple mechanisms of resistance to immune recognition and CTL killing. Especially when used in combination, these strategies have the potential to rapidly undermine the effectiveness of nascent and established CTL responses.

With regards to HIV-1, three broad classes of CTL escape mechanisms have been shown to be most significant:

1. Viral latency, in which the levels of expression of viral gene products is reduced, effectively prevents the presentation of viral peptides to the immune system. This strategy is common to retroviruses, which can integrate in the host cell chromosome and remain in a transcriptionally silent state for extended periods of time *(72)*. Latency also has the advantage of shielding the retroviral pathogen from the effects of antiretroviral therapy *(73,74)*.

2. Some viral gene products, including HIV-1 Nef, have the capacity to downregulate the levels of expression of MHC class I molecules at the surface of primary CD4+ T lymphocytes, directly interfering with antigen presentation and rendering HIV-infected cells markedly harder to recognize by HIV-specific CTL, at least in vitro *(75)*. Interestingly, this property of Nef appears to be selectively restricted to HLA-A and -B alleles and not HLA-C and -E, to allow HIV-infected cells to avoid cytotoxic attacks mediated by natural killer (NK) cells *(76)*. Nef has also been shown to be able to increase the expression levels of Fas ligand by HIV-infected CD4+ T cells, indirectly triggering Fas-mediated apoptosis in responding HIV-specific CTL *(77)*.

3. A critical factor affecting the efficacy and persistence of CTL responses is the emergence of viral variants expressing mutated CTL epitopes, leading to loss of recognition by T cells *(78)*. This mechanism has been observed in multiple viral infections of animals (LCMV and MHV-JHM in the mouse *(79,80)*) and humans (EBV, HBV, HCV *(81–83)*), including HIV-1 *(78,84–87)*. MHC peptide binding residues in the epitope can be mutated as well, leading to failure of antigen presentation to the T cell *(88)*. In some cases, epitope variation has been shown to result in the creation of proteasome cleavage sites, resulting in the destruction of the epitope and absence of specific peptide presentation *(89)*. Epitope mutation can also lead to the presentation of antagonist peptides, which, through altered TCR signaling, might modulate or even abrogate CTL responses to the wild-type peptide *(82,90–94)*. However, the potential impact of this escape strategy on in vivo CTL responses and on the outcome of pathological processes associated with infectious diseases has yet to be convincingly demonstrated. Mutations mapping outside of the epitope itself can equally influence CTL responses, for example, by reducing the efficacy of a given proteolytic cleavages required for proper antigen processing, transport and/or presentation *(95–97)* (Fig. 2). The study of synonymous vs nonsynonymous (ds/dn) mutations rates clearly demonstrates that it is the selective pressure applied by epitope-specific CTL clones which drives diversification of the primary sequence of the virus *(84,98)*. Immune selection of preexisting variants present in the circulating virus pool gives rise to complex equilibrium dynamics that can result in a high rate of viral escape from CTL responses *(99–101)*. The striking differences in HIV-1 quasispecies diversity profiles seen between long-term nonprogressors (LTNP) and patients with progressive disease well illustrates this point *(102)*. Because of their relative importance in the induction of immune responses, understanding the kinetics of epitope variation within immunodominant regions will have a definite impact on the development of an HIV vaccine.

CTL RESPONSES IN PRIMARY HIV INFECTION

Shortly following initial infection of the host with HIV-1, a large proportion of patients experience a mononucleosis-like illness of varying severity, which has been termed acute retroviral syndrome or primary HIV infection (PI) *(103–106)*. These acute symptoms coincide with transient, high-level HIV-1 viremia, and with a sudden transitory drop in the levels of circulating $CD4^+$ T cells, which results in an inversion of the normal $CD4^+$:$CD8^+$ T cell ratio *(105,107–109)*. It is during this phase of the disease that viral dissemination of and seeding of peripheral lymphoid organs is thought to occur *(110,111)*. Symptoms of PI alleviate with the curtailment of initial HIV-1 viremia, which has been postulated to simply reflect viral population dynamics, that is, the depletion of the pool of highly susceptible target cells capable of producing large amounts of progeny virus *(112)*. However, several lines of evidence convincingly implicate the host's emerging cell-mediated immune responses in this process:

1. PI is commonly characterized by a significant rise in absolute $CD8^+$ T cell count, which contributes to the rapid inversion of the CD4:CD8 ratio. A large proportion of these expanded $CD8^+$ T cells display cell-surface activation markers such as HLA-DR, CD25, and CD28, indicative of their ongoing involvement in antigen-specific or bystander cell-mediated immune responses *(110,111)*. As well, major expansions of T cells expressing specific TCRBV determinants have been observed in a large propor-

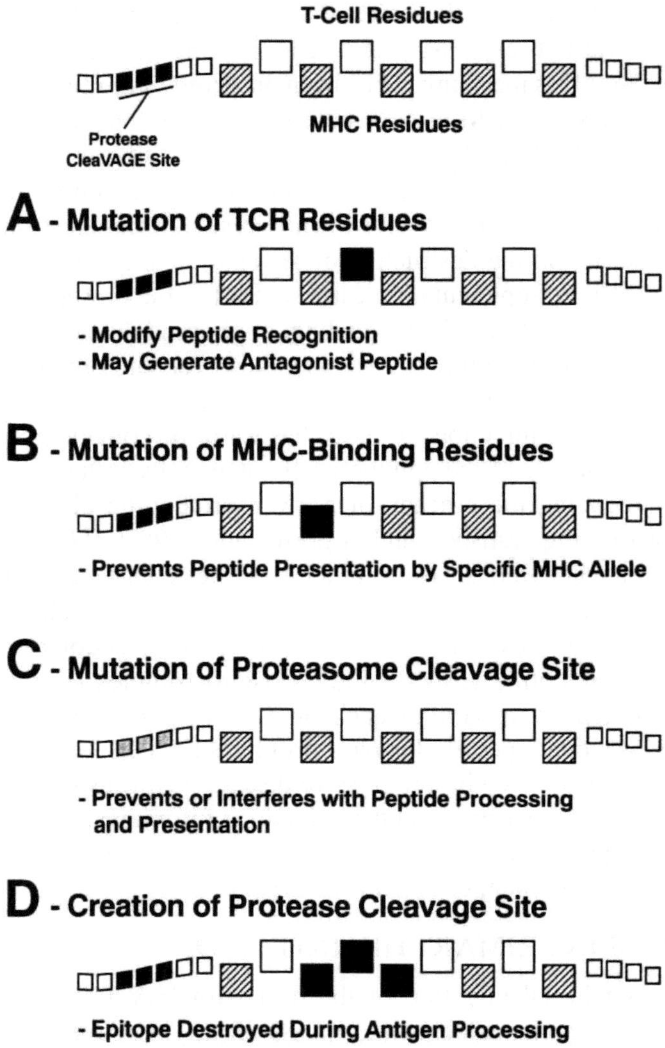

Fig. 2. Proposed mechanisms by which epitope mutation can lead to the loss of antigen recognition by cytotoxic T lymphocytes.

tion of patients with PI *(113)*. Expanded cell subsets were invariably comprised of activated CD8$^+$ T cells exhibiting MHC-restricted HIV-specific CTL activity *(35,113)*, a seminal finding that has since then been confirmed using tetrameric MHC-peptide complexes *(114)*. Clonal diversity analysis using TCR β-chain phenotyping revealed that these CD8$^+$ T-cell populations were comprised of multiple expanded T-cell clones, and that the CDR3 region of their TCRs often exhibited a degree of structural homology consistent with antigen-driven selection processes *(23,35,113,115)*. TCRBV-specific expansions of T cells have also been observed during acute infection with Epstein–Barr virus (EBV) *(116,117)* and measles virus *(118)*, and might therefore represent a commonplace mechanism of CD8$^+$ T-cell recruitment during primary immune responses to viral pathogens (Fig. 3).

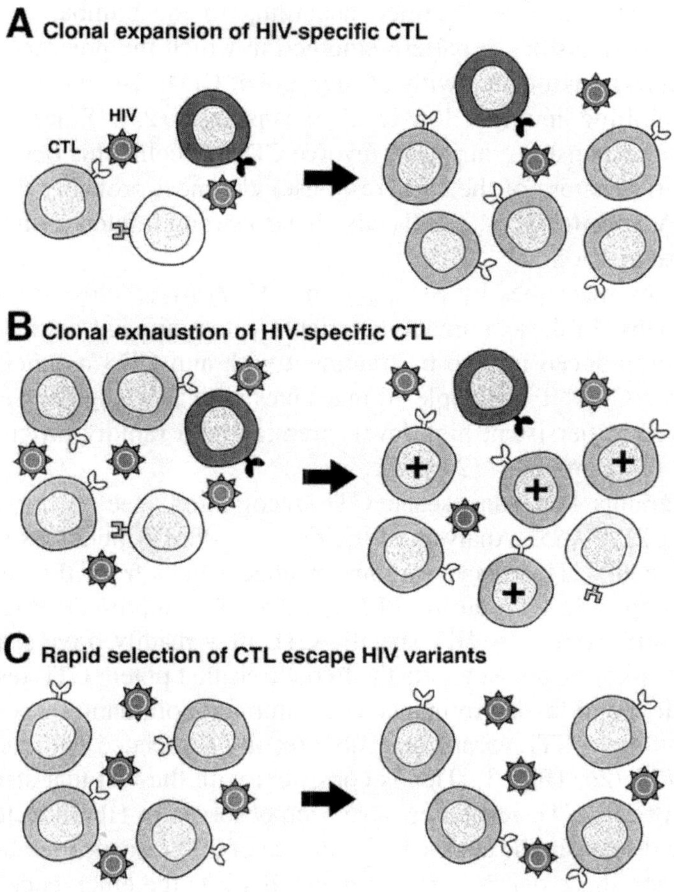

Fig. 3. Dynamics of the HIV-specific CTL responses during primary HIV infection **(A)** High levels of antigen causes the mono-oligoclonal expansion of HIV-specific CTL, leading to a down-regulation of initial viremia. **(B)** Elevated and persistent levels of HIV antigens drive a portion of HIV-specific CTL clones into clonal exhaustion (exhaustive induction). **(C)** Selective pressure exerted by HIV-specific CTL drives the rapid emergence of CTL escape HIV-1 variants, which in turn leads to a partial loss of viral recognition by the host and may contribute to HIV persistence.

2. Several groups have reported that the timing of this massive mobilization of HIV-specific $CD8^+$ CTL, but not that of the HIV-specific humoral response, closely coincided with the rapid downregulation of circulating HIV-1 levels observed during PI *(119–122)*.

3. The magnitude of the initial HIV-1–specific CTL response is predictive of the rate of HIV disease progression: subjects in whom higher frequencies of HIV Env-specific (but not Gag- or Pol-specific) CTL precursors were observed during PI exhibited significantly lower levels of plasma HIV-1 RNA and infectious HIV-1 titers in PBMCs over the first 18 mo following infection *(122)*. These patients also showed mildly reduced rates of $CD4^+$ T-cell decline over this period *(122)*.

4. When PI patients were stratified according to the number and magnitude of TCRBV-specific expansions, a pattern emerged in which the presence of single, high-level expansions was associated with a faster rate of $CD4^+$ T-cell decline than that seen in patients exhibiting multiple low-level expansions *(123)*. Since most, if not all, TCRBV-specific expansions during PI involve $CD8^+$ T cells, this observation suggests that the qualitative nature of the CTL response, and most probably the level of clonal diversity of HIV-specific $CD8^+$ T cells, also have a strong influence on the initial rate of HIV disease progression.

5. PI of rhesus macaques by SIV_{mac251} or $SHIV_{MD14YE}$ closely resembles that of HIV PI in humans. In these animals, a variable yet significant degree of $CD8^+$ T-cell depletion can be induced in vivo by treatment with anti-CD8 monoclonal antibodies. Infection of such $CD8^+$ T cell depleted macaques with SIV_{mac251} or $SHIV_{MD14YE}$ consistently resulted in persistent high-level viremia and a rapidly progressive course of SIV disease in these animals *(124,125)*.

6. HIV-1 variants that can escape CTL recognition (see earlier) can be readily detected during PI *(84,85)*. Analysis of the rates of dS/dN mutations revealed that the rapid emergence of CTL escape variants resulted solely from the selective pressure applied by HIV-specific CTL during PI *(84,85,98)*. This represents direct evidence that the initial pressure exerted by HIV-specific CTL may readily drive sequence variation within targeted epitopes, and supports the hypothesis that potent CTL responses directed against specific peptide determinants (i.e., immunodominant responses) are more directly susceptible to CTL escape and more readily associated with the progression of HIV disease *(123,126)* (Fig. 3). This is consistent with the fact that stable but broadly-directed HIV-specific CTL responses have been observed in HIV-infected subjects with nonprogressive disease in the absence of evidence of CTL escape mutation *(127,128)*.

Taken together, these data strongly suggest that it is the emergence of HIV-specific CTLs which is principally responsible for the downregulation of HIV viremia during PI, and that achieving early control of viral replication is critical in order to delay the progression of HIV disease.

Control of primary HIV-1 viremia by the emerging CTL response may be effected through the reduction in the numbers of HIV-infected activated $CD4^+$ T lymphocytes, which represent the main cellular reservoir for production of rapidly replicating virus *(129,130)*. On MHC-restricted antigen-specific activation, $CD8^+$ T cells have also been shown to produce an array of soluble factors with antiviral or HIV-blocking activity, including β-chemokines MIP-1α, MIP-1β, and RANTES which can antagonize infection of $CD4^+$ T cells by R5 HIV-1 isolates via coreceptor blockade and/or induction of coreceptor internalization *(57–61)*.

In several PI patients, highly amplified HIV-specific CTL clones were shown to disappear with rapid kinetics directly following their expansion phase (*35,* Pantaleo et al., *unpublished results*). Furthermore, longitudinal DNA sequence analysis of HIV isolated from plasma revealed that the deletion occurred prior to the appearance of significant amino acid variation within the cognate CTL epitopes *(35,98)*. This phenomenon is highly reminiscent of antigen-driven clonal exhaustion observed in murine models of acute/persistent viral infections *(131,132)*. According to this model, persistingly high levels of antigen circulating throughout the lymphoid system drive the expansion and subsequent deletion of antigen-specific CTL clones *(131,132)*. Since this depletion takes place early on in the course of HIV disease, it is thought to reduce the size and the clonal diversity of the T cell repertoire available to recognize given peptide–MHC combinations, and may interfere with the ability of the host to maintain long-term immunological control of viral replication (Fig. 3). Finally, while potent virus-specific CTL responses are present in most cases during the initial phase of HIV infection, it is clear that these responses almost invariably fail in preventing establishment of persistent infection and the transition between PI and chronic HIV disease (reviewed in *133*).

CTL RESPONSES DURING CHRONIC AND PROGRESSIVE HIV INFECTION

Using limiting-dilution analysis and cytotoxicity testing, HIV-specific, MHC-restricted CTLs can be easily detected in HIV-infected subjects throughout the course of chronic HIV disease *(134–136),* including clinical AIDS *(137).* As it is the case with PI, HIV-specific CTL responses are closely associated with the control of viral replication during chronic HIV infection. First, viral load and loss of $CD4^+$ T cells are inversely correlated to CTL activity and the frequency of CTLe in HIV-infected subjects *(138,139);* second, when compared with progressors, long-term asymptomatics exhibit higher levels of HIV-specific CTL activity *(140,142);* third, gradual decrease in HIV-specific CTL activity is a robust predictor of progression to AIDS *(140,143);* fourth, passive transfer of ex vivo-expanded HIV-specific CTL induces a transient reduction in the levels of HIV-infected $CD4^+$ T cells in HIV-infected subjects *(129),* while transfer of such cells in HIV-infected severe combined immunodeficiency (SCID) mice results in a 1-log reduction in circulating plasma viremia *(144);* lastly, monoclonal antibody-mediated depletion of $CD8^+$ T cells in SIV-infected rhesus macaques causes a major reactivation of circulating SIV levels *(145).*

CTL responses can be detected in multiple tissues, including the peripheral blood, lymph nodes *(146),* spleen *(147),* pulmonary alveolar fluid *(146,148),* and cerebrospinal fluid *(149,150).* CTL activity can be directed against a wide range of HIV-1 antigens, including peptide determinants located within Gag p17, Gag p24, Gag p15, Env gp120, and Env gp41, but also within Pol, Rev, and Nef, as the response is by no means limited to structural virion proteins. The distribution of CTL epitopes is not regular amongst HIV-1 proteins, as multiple overlapping epitopes cluster within so-called "immunodominant" regions *(151,152).* HIV-specific CTL responses have been shown to be restricted by a variety of HLA-A, -B, and -C alleles (reviewed in *153–155*). Accordingly, individual HIV-1–infected subjects generally exhibit a heterogeneous pattern of simultaneous CTL responses to a variety of HIV antigens, a pattern that may be further complicated by multiple rounds of HIV CTL escape mutation *(99,156).*

In the absence of effective antiretroviral treatment, the complexity and the size of the CTL response appear to decrease as HIV disease progresses towards its terminal stages, underscoring yet again the importance of CTL responses in host resistance to HIV *(146).* Multiple nonmutually exclusive mechanisms have been proposed to account for this progressive decline of HIV-specific CTL responses: (1) HIV-specific helper responses mediated by activated $CD4^+$ T cells might become heavily depleted during early HIV disease, resulting in the progressive loss of cognate helper function required to maintain a high-level of HIV-specific CTL response *(157);* (2) destruction of lymph node architecture has been associated with chronic progressive HIV infection *(158,159),* and may compromise antigen presentation to HIV-specific CD8+ CTL and CD4+ T helper (Th) cells; (3) in late HIV disease, CD8+ T cells have themselves been shown to become susceptible to HIV infection and to carry a significant viral load, consistent with impaired function of this cell subset *(160,161);* and (4) antigen-driven clonal exhaustion of HIV-specific CTLs, which has been shown to occur during primary HIV infection *(35),* could also take place during chronic HIV disease to further restrict the HIV-specific CTL repertoire. These various mechanisms are consistent with the incremental decline in the numbers and activity of CD8+ HLA-DR+ anti-HIV CTLs observed among HIV-infected patients, and with the reduced clonogenic potential of these cells *(162,163).* This progressive deterioration of CTL responses appears to be unique to HIV infection, as CTL responses to EBV and hepatitis B virus (HBV), for example, remain stable for long periods, even in subjects coinfected with HIV *(137,164).* Ultimately, these mechanisms of CTL depletion, in combination with multiple viral strategies of CTL escape, provide an explanation for the almost systematic failure of the cell-mediated immune response in preventing the development of HIV disease and the progression to AIDS.

EFFECTS OF ANTIRETROVIRAL THERAPY ON CTL RESPONSES

The development of combination antiretroviral regimens containing inhibitors of the HIV-1 protease, that is, highly active antiretroviral therapy (HAART), has had a considerable impact on the clinical outcome of chronic HIV disease. These regimens have been credited with the recently recorded declines in the incidence of HIV-related morbidity and mortality *(165).* As a general rule, introduction of HAART during chronic HIV infection induces a rapid reduction in circulating levels of HIV-1 RNA, typically to below the detection limit of most virological assays. Concomitant increases in CD4+ T cell counts are observed in most subjects, which are mainly the product of cellular redistribution *(166,167).* HAART also results in a variable but generally significant degree of improvement in immune function, that is, proliferative responses of CD4+ T cells to stimulation with mitogens or recall antigens *(66,168,169).* Treatment of chronic infection with HAART leads to an early increase (i.e., up to 8 wk post-induction) in CD8+ T-cell counts, which then progressively decline with continuing effective suppression of viral activity *(168,170).* This decline mainly involves CD8+ T cells expressing memory markers (CD45RO+), and is correlated with an overall reduction in the levels of CD8+ T cells exhibiting an activated cell-surface phenotype (HLA-DR+, CD38+) *(168).* Presumably, these reflect decreasing numbers of virus-specific CTL, but also a reduction in the extent of bystander CD8+ T cell activation *(170).* In the long term (i.e., >24 wk), an increase in CD8+ T cells coexpressing CD28 and exhibiting a naive phenotype (CD45RA+) can also be noted in most subjects, consistent with resumption of *de novo* T-cell production and with progressive reemergence of functional cell-mediated immunocompetence *(66,170–172).*

Using MHC–peptide tetramer staining, Ogg et al. have confirmed that the frequency of HIV-peptide specific CTL effectors in peripheral blood declines following initiation of HAART, a finding that has since then been corroborated by others *(138,173,174).* The early decline of CTLs is markedly irregular, consistent with rapid redistribution of these cells between various lymphoid subcompartments *(173,174).* However, in one small cohort, late decay (i.e., >2 wk following initiation of HAART) was shown to proceed with a half-life of 45 d *(173).* It is unclear whether the value of this half-life will be confirmed when clinical and immunological parameters can be more closely controlled in larger study groups. Furthermore, whether the frequencies of CTLe measured using MHC–peptide tetramers significantly correlate with reductions in HIV-1 viral load and with bulk HIV peptide specific CTL activity still remains a hotly debated issue *(138,174)*. Finally, preliminary data indicate that this decline in CTLe frequencies is not observed within lymph nodes, and may in fact be restricted to the peripheral blood, underlining yet again the importance of studying different lymphoid subcompartments to obtain a global picture of the dynamics of immune responses [Pantaleo et al., *manuscript in preparation*].

With respect to the levels of clonality of T-cell populations, initiation of antiretroviral therapy induces a remakable yet incomplete normalization of both the CD4$^+$ and the CD8$^+$ T cell repertoires *(175–177)*. High-level mono-oligoclonal TCRBV-specific expansions of HIV-specific CD8$^+$ T cells, routinely observed in chronically infected patients, were not readily swayed by initiation of therapy. In fact, the overall restriction in T cell diversity was only shown to slowly and progressively improve with time, with no major changes taking place before at least 6 mo *(176,177)*. This likely reflects a reduction of virus-specific and bystander immune activation, the progressive decay of HIV-specific memory CTL populations, and a resumption of thymopoiesis leading to a gradual regeneration of a diversified naive CD8$^+$ T-cell repertoire. The characterization of the effects of antiretroviral therapy on the antigenic specificity, dynamics, clonal diversity, and persistence of this reemerging naive CTL repertoire is currently unclear, and will warrant further investigation.

In the case of PI, standard clinical management now mandates immediate initiation of antiretroviral therapy *(178,179)*, with the combined objectives of (1) rapidly suppressing HIV replication; (2) attempting to prevent and/or limit spreading of virus throughout the peripheral lymphoid system; (3) shortening the symptomatic phase of PI; (4) rapidly restoring CD4$^+$ T cell counts and the CD4$^+$/CD8$^+$ ratio; and (5) preserving host virus-specific CD4$^+$ helper T-cell responses, which, according to some authors, may at least in part become irreversibly compromised during PI *(157,180,181)*. As mentioned above, PI is characterized by high-level expansion of HIV-specific CTL, which are instrumental in reducing peripheral viral load. Following PI, acute CD8$^+$ T cell lymphocytosis subsides, but CD8 counts nevertheless remain abnormally elevated throughout a large part of chronic HIV infection *(103,110)*. There is evidence that this reduction in CD8 counts is accompanied by a commensurate decline of HIV-specific CTL, due in part to the decline in circulating viral load, to clonal exhaustion, and to redistribution/recirculation of CTL within the lymphoid system *(35,36)*. Whether HAART treatment during PI can influence transition-associated HIV-specific CTL decline will require further investigation. However, preliminary data suggest that TCR repertoire stabilization, which is associated with reduced CD8$^+$ T-cell oligoclonality and with differential mobilization of the CTL pool, occurs more rapidly in PI patients treated with HAART than in those left untreated (Soudeyns and Pantaleo, *unpublished observations*). Since T-cell repertoire diversity has been shown to markedly influence the progression of HIV disease *(123)*, rapid normalization of the CD8$^+$ repertoire might represent an additional argument in support of aggressive treatment of PI with potent combinations of antiretrovirals *(182)*.

In summary, there is now growing evidence that introduction of suppressive antiretroviral regimen in primary and chronic HIV infection can result in a progressive decline in the frequency of HIV-specific CTL. In view of the need for prolonged treatment with HAART to maintain virological response and reinforce immunocompetence, there is concern that a decline in virus-specific cell-mediated immune responses might lead to a loss of control of residual viral replication, and, indirectly, to the emergence of drug-resistant HIV variants. This potential "catch-22" situation has led to the suggestion of introducing therapeutic breaks in HAART regimen, to allow in vivo repriming of CTL responses with autologous viral isolates (structured therapy interruptions). Another manner to avoid this predicament would be to combine HAART with immunomodulator treatments or therapeutic vaccination, to artificially boost cell-mediated immune responses while at the same time maintaining HIV replication under tight pharmacological control *(183)*.

CONCLUDING REMARKS

Because cell-mediated immune responses, and, in particular, antigen-specific CTLs, play a central role in host defense against HIV, this virus has integrated a number of CTL escape mechanisms into its lifestyle. These strategies are aimed at facilitating the establishment and maintenance of persistent infection in the host, and are effective both during primary and chronic HIV infection. CTL-induced mutation of viral epitopes represents a serious obstacle to the development of a successful vaccine to prevent HIV infection. Expansion of the pharmacological armementarium has recently led to the introduction of several therapeutic combinations capable of achieving long-term suppression of HIV replication. However, there is evidence that effective control of viremia leads to a progressive decline in HIV-specific CTLs, at least in peripheral blood. Since this decline may become incompatible with the maintenance of effective levels of HIV-specific cell-mediated immunity, HAART may need to be supplemented with effective immunomodulatory regimen.

REFERENCES

1. Fremont DH, Hendrickson WA, Marrack P, Kappler J. Structures of an MHC class II molecule with covalently bound single peptides. Science 1996; 272:1001–4.
2. Roche PA, Cresswell P. Invariant chain association with HLA-DR molecules inhibits immunogenic peptide binding. Nature 1990; 345:615–8.
3. Guagliardi LE, Koppelman B, Blum JS, Marks MS, Cresswell P, Brodsky FM. Co-localization of molecules involved in antigen processing and presentation in an early endocytic compartment. Nature 1990; 343:133–9.
4. Peterson M, Miller J. Antigen presentation enhanced by the alternatively spliced invariant chain gene product p41. Nature 1992; 357:596–8.
5. Sherman MA, Weber DA, Jensen PE. DM enhances peptide binding to class II MHC by release of invariant chain-derived peptide. Immunity 1995; 3:197–205.
6. Germain RN. MHC-dependent antigen processing and peptide presentation: providing ligands for T lymphocyte activation. Cell 1994; 76:287–99.
7. Townsend A, Bastin J, Gould K, Brownlee G, Andrew M, Coupar B, Boyle D, Chan S, Smith G. Defective presentation to class I-restricted cytotoxic T lymphocytes in vaccinia-infected cells is overcome by enhanced degradation of antigen. J Exp Med 1988; 168:1211–24.
8. Goldberg AL, Rock KL. Proteolysis, proteasomes and antigen presentation. Nature 1992; 357:375–9.
9. Bjorkman PJ, Saper MA, Samraoui B, Bennett WS, Strominger JL, Wiley DC. Structure of the human class I histocompatibility antigen, HLA-A2. Nature 1987; 329:506–12.

10. Bjorkman PJ, Saper MA, Samraoui B, Bennett WS, Strominger JL, Wiley DC. The foreign antigen binding site and T cell recognition regions of class I histocompatibility antigens. Nature 1987; 329:512–8.
11. Garrett TPJ, Saper MA, Bjorkman PJ, Strominger JL, Wiley DC. Specificity pockets for the side chains of peptide antigens in HLA-Aw68. Nature 1989; 342:692–6.
12. Kleijmeer MJ, Kelly A, Geuze HJ, Slot JW, Townsend A, Trowsdale J. Location of MHC-encoded transporters in the endoplasmic reticulum and *cis*-golgi. Nature 1992; 357:342–4.
13. Van Kaer L, Ashton-Rickardt PG, Ploegh HL, Tonegawa S. TAP1 Mutant mice are deficient in antigen presentation, surface class I molecules, and CD4-8+ T Cells Cell 1992; 71:1205–14.
14. Grandea AG, Androlewicz MJ, Athwal RS, Geraghty DE, Spies T. Dependence of peptide binding by MHC class I molecules on their interaction wit TAP. Science 1995; 270:105–8.
15. Hill AVS, Allsopp CEM, Kwiatkowski D, Anstey NM, Twumasi P, Rowe PA, Bennett S, Brewster D, McMichael AJ, Greenwood BM. Common West African HLA antigens are associated with protection from severe malaria. Nature 1991; 352:595–600.
16. Gilbert SC, Plebanski M, Gupta S, Morris J, Cox M, Aidoo M, Kwiatkowski D, Greenwood BM, Whittle HC, Hill AVS. Association of malaria parasite population structure HLA, and immunological antagonism. Science 1998; 279:1173–7.
17. Carrington M, Nelson GW, Martin MP, Kissner T, Vlahov D, Goedert JJ, Kaslow R, Buchbinder S, Hoots K, O'Brien SJ. HLA and HIV-1: Heterozygote advantage and B*35-Cw*04 disadvantage. Science 1999; 283:1748–52.
18. Davis MM, Bjorkman PJ. T-cell antigen receptor genes and T-cell recognition. Nature 1998; 334:395–401.
19. Tonegawa S. Somatic generation of antibody diversity. Nature 1983; 302:575–81.
20. Siu G, Clark SP, Yoshikai Y, Malissen M, Yanagi Y, Strauss E, Mak TW, Hood L. The human T cell antigen receptor is encoded by variable, diversity, and joining gene segments that rearrange to generate a complete V gene. Cell 1984; 37:393–401.
21. Jorgensen JL, Esser U, Fazekas de St. Groth B, Reay PA, Davis MM. Mapping T-cell receptor-peptide contacts by variant peptide immunization of single-chain transgenics. Nature 1992; 355:224–30.
22. Garcia KC, Degano M, Pease LR, Huang M, Peterson PA, Teyton L, Wilson IA. Structural basis of plasticity in T cell receptor recognition of a self peptide-MHC antigen. Science 1998; 279:1166–72.
23. McHeyzer-Williams MG, Davis MM. Antigen-specific development of primary and memory T cells in vivo. Science 1995; 268:106–11.
24. Moss PAH, Moots RJ, Rosenberg WMC, Rowland-Jones SJ, Bodmer HC, McMichael AJ, Bell JI. Extensive conservation of α and β chains of the human T-cell antigen receptor recognizing HLA-A2 and influenza A matrix peptide. Proc Natl Acad Sci USA 1991; 88:8987–90.
25. Bowness P, Moss PAH, Rowland-Jones S, Bell JI, McMichael AJ. Conservation of T cell receptor usage by HLA B27-restricted influenza-specific cytotoxic T lymphocytes suggests a general pattern for antigen-specific major histocompatibility complex class I-restricted responses. Eur J Immunol 1993; 23:1417–21.
26. Lehner PJ, Wang ECY, Moss PAH, Williams S, Platt K, Friedman SM, Bell JI, Borysiewicz LK. Human HLA-A0201-restricted cytotoxic T lymphocyte recognition of influenza A is dominated by T cells bearing the Vβ17 gene segment. J Exp Med 1995; 181:79–91.
27. Posnett DN, Romagne F, Necker A, Kotzin BL, Sékaly R-P. First human TCR monoclonal antibody workshop. The Immunologist 1996; 4(1):5–8.
28. Choi Y, Kotzin B, Herron L, Callahan J, Marrack P, Kappler J. Interaction of staphylococcus aureus toxin "superantigens" with human T cells. Proc Natl Acad Sci USA 1989; 86:8941–5.
29. Labrecque N, McGrath H, Subramanyam M, Huber BT, Sékaly R-P. Human T cells respond to mouse mammary tumor virus-encoded superantigens: Vβ restriction and conserved evolutionary features. J Exp Med 1993; 177:1735–43.

30. Rebai N, Pantaleo G, Demarest JF, Ciurli C, Soudeyns H, Adelsberger JW, Vaccarezza M, Walker RE, Sékaly RP, Fauci AS. Analysis of the T-cell receptor β-chain variable-region (Vβ) repertoire in monozygotic twins discordant for human immunodeficiency virus: evidence for perturbations of specific Vβ segments in $CD4^+$ T cells of the virus-positive twin. Proc Natl Acad Sci USA 1994; 91:1529–33.
31. Pannetier C, Cochet M, Darche S, Casrouge A, Zoller M, Kourilsky P. The sizes of the CDR3 hypervariable regions of the murine T-cell receptor beta chains vary as a function of the recombined germ-line segments. Proc Natl Acad Sci USA 1993; 90:4319–23.
32. Pannetier C, Even J, Kourilsky P. T-cell repertoire diversity and clonal expansions in normal and clinical samples. Immunol Today 1995; 16:176–81.
33. Soudeyns H, Rebai N, Pantaleo GP, Ciurli C, Boghossian T, Sékaly R-P, Fauci AS. The T cell receptor Vβ repertoire in HIV-1 infection and disease. Sem Immunol 1993; 5:175–85.
34. MacDonald HR, Casanova J-L, Maryanski JL, Cerottini J-C. Oligoclonal expansion of major histocompatibility complex class i-restricted cytolytic T lymphocytes during a primary immune response in vivo: direct monitoring by flow cytometry and polymerase chain reaction. J Exp Med 1993; 177:1487–92.
35. Pantaleo G, Soudeyns H, Demarest JF, Vaccarezza M, Graziosi C, Paolucci S, Daucher M, Cohen OJ, Denis F, Biddison W, Sekaly R-P, Fauci AS. Evidence for rapid disappearance of initially expanded HIV-specific $CD8^+$ T cell clones during primary infection. Proc Natl Acad Sci USA 1997; 94:9848–53.
36. Pantaleo G, Soudeyns H, Demarest JF, Vaccarezza M, Graziosi C, Paolucci S, Daucher M, Cohen OJ, Denis F, Biddison W, Sekaly R-P, Fauci AS. Accumulation of Human Immunodeficiency Virus-specific cytotoxic T lymphocytes away from the predominant site of virus replication during primary infection. Eur J Immunol 1997; 27:3166–73.
37. Wack A, Montagna D, Dellabona P, Casorati G. An improved PCR-heteroduplex method permits high-sensitivity detection of clonal expansions in complex T cell populations. J Immunol Methods 1996; 196:181–92.
38. Vavassori M, Maccario R, Moretta A, Comoli P, Wack A, Locatelli F, Lanzavecchia A, Maserati E, Dellabona P, Casorati G, Montagna D. Restricted TCR repertoire and long-term persistence of donor-derived antigen-experienced $CD4^+$ T cells in allogeneic bone marrow transplantation recipients. J Immunol 1996; 157:5739–47.
39. Shen DF, Doukhan L, Kalams S, Delwart E. High-resolution analysis of the T-cell receptor β-chain repertoires using heteroduplex tracking: generally stable, clonal $CD8^+$ expansions in all healthy young adults. J Immunol Methods 1998; 215:113–21.
40. Siliciano RF, Lawton T, Knall C, Karr RW, Berman P, Gregory T, Reinherz EL. Analysis of host-virus interactions in AIDS with anti-gp120 T cell clones: Effect of HIV sequence variation and a mechanism for $CD4^+$ cell depletion. Cell 1998; 54:561–75.
41. Hammond SA, Bollinger RC, Stanhope PE, Quinn TC, Schwartz D, Clements ML, Siliciano RF. Comparative clonal analysis of Human Immunodeficiency Virus type 1 (HIV-1)-specific $CD4^+$ and $CD8^+$ cytolytic T lymphocytes isolated from seronegative humans immunized with candidate HIV-1 vaccines. J Exp Med 1992; 176:1531–42.
42. Young JD, Hengartner H, Podack ER, Cohn ZA. Purification and characterization of a cytolytic pore-forming protein from granules of cloned lymphocytes with natural killer activity. Cell 1986; 44:849–59.
43. Lichtenheld MG, Olsen KJ, Lu P, Lowrey DM, Hameed A, Hengartner H, Podack ER. Structure and function of human perforin. Nature 1988; 335:448–51.
44. Kagi D, Ledermann B, Burki K, Seiler P, Odermatt B, Olsen KJ, Podack E, Zinkernagel RM, Hengartner H. Cytotoxicity mediated by T cells and natural killer cells is greatly impaired in perforin-deficient mice. Nature 1994; 369:31–7.

45. Kagi D, Ledermann B, Burki K, Hengartner H, Zinkernagel RM. CD8+ T cell mediated protection against an intracellular bacterium by perforin-dependent cytotoxicity. Eur J Immunol 1994; 24:3068–72.
46. Heusel JW, Wesselschmidt RL, Shresta S, Russell JH, Ley TJ. Cytotoxic lymphocytes require granzyme B for the rapid induction of DNA fragmentation and apoptosis in allogeneic target cells. Cell 1994; 76:977–87.
47. Darmon AJ, Nicholson DW, Bleackley RC. Activation of the apoptotic protease CPP32 by cytotoxic T-cell-derived granzyme B. Nature 1995; 377:446–8.
48. Shresta S, Graubert TA, Thomas DA, Raptis SZ, Ley TJ. Granzyme A initiates an alternative pathway for granule-mediated apoptosis. Immunity 1999; 10:595–605.
49. Beresford PJ, Xia Z, Greenberg AH, Lieberman J. Granzyme A loading induces rapid cytolysis and a novel form of DNA damage independently of caspase activation. Immunity 1999; 10:585–94.
50. Itoh N, Yonehara S, Ishii A, Yonehara M, Mizushima S-I, Sameshima M, Hase A, Seto Y, Nagata S. The polypeptide encoded by the cDNA for human cell surface antigen Fas can mediate apoptosis. Cell 1991; 66:233–43.
51. Suda T, Takahashi T, Goldstein P, Nagata S. Molecular cloning and expression of the Fas ligand, a novel member of the tumor necrosis factor family. Cell 1993; 75:1169–78.
52. Lowin B, Hahne M, Mattmann C, Tschopp J. Cytolytic T-cell cytotoxicity is mediated through perforin and Fas lytic pathways. Nature 1994; 370:650–2.
53. Arai KI, Lee F, Miyajima A, Miyatake S, Arai N, Yokota T. Cytokines: coordinators of immune and inflammatory responses. Ann Rev Biochem 1990; 59:783–836.
54. Berke G. The CTL's kiss of death. Cell 1995; 81:9–12.
55. Zou P, Goldstein S, Devadas K, Tewari D, Notkins AL. Human CD4+ T cells transfected with IL-16 cDNA are resistant to HIV-1 infection: inhibition of mRNA expression. Nature Medicine 1997; 3:659–64.
56. Guidotti LG, Ishikawa T, Hobbs MV, Matzke B, Schreiber R, Chisari FV. Intracellular inactivation of the hepatitis B virus by cytotoxic T lymphocytes. Immunity 1996; 4:25–36.
57. Cocchi F, DeVico A, Garzino-Demo A, Arya S, Gallo R, Lusso P. Identification of RANTES, MIP-1α, and MIP-1β as the major HIV-suppressive factors produced by CD8+ T cells. Science 1995; 270:1811–5.
58. Yang OO, Kalams SA, Trocha A, Cao H, Luster A, Johnson RP, Walker BD. Suppression of Human Immunodeficiency Virus type 1 replication by CD8+ cells: evidence for HLA class I-restricted triggering of cytolytic and non-cytolytic mechanisms. J Virol 1997; 71:3120–8.
59. Van Baalen CA, Schutten M, Huisman RC, Boers PHM, Grutters RA, Osterhaus ADME. Kinetics of antiviral activity by Human Immunodeficiency Virus type 1-specific cytotoxic T lymphocytes (CTL) and rapid selection of CTL escape virus in vitro. J Virol 1998; 72:6851–7.
60. Walker CM, Moody DJ, Stites DP, Levy JA. CD8+ Lymphocytes can control HIV infection in vitro by suppressing virus replication. Science 1986; 234:1563–6.
61. Walker CM, Erickson AL, Hsueh FC, Levy JA. Inhibition of Human Immunodeficiency Virus replication in acutely infected CD4+ cells by CD8+ cells involves a noncytotoxic mechanism. J Virol 1991; 65:5921–7.
62. Moriuchi H, Moriuchi M, Combadiere C, Murphy PM, Fauci AS. CD8+ T-cell-derived soluble factor(s), but not β-chemokines RANTES, MIP-1α, and MIP-1β, suppress HIV-1 replication in monocyte/macrophages. Proc Natl Acad Sci USA 1996; 93:15341–5.
63. Mackewicz CE, Blackbourn DJ, Levy JA. CD8+ T cells suppress Human Immunodeficiency Virus replication by inhibiting viral transcription. Proc Natl Acad Sci USA 1995; 92:2308–12.
64. Brunner KT, Mauel J, Cerottini JC, Chapuis B. Quantitative assay of the lytic action of immune lymphoid cells on 51-Cr-labelled allogeneic target cells in vitro; inhibition by isoantibody and by drugs. Immunology 1968; 14:181–96.

65. Taswell C. Limiting dilution assays for the determination of immunocompetent cell frequencies. I. Data analysis. J Immunol 1981; 126:1614–9.
66. Komanduri KV, Viswanathan MN, Wieder ED, Schmidt DK, Bredt BM, Jacobson MA, McCune JM. Restoration of cytomegalovirus-specific CD4+ T-lymphocyte responses after ganciclovir and highly active antiretroviral therapy in individuals infected with HIV-1. Nature Medicine 1998; 4:953–6.
67. Kern F, Surel IP, Brock C, Freistedt B, Radtke H, Scheffold A, Blsczyk R, Reinke P, Schneider-Mergener J, Radbruch A, Walden P, Volk H-D. T-cell epitope mapping by flow cytometry. Nature Medicine 1998; 4:975–8.
68. Murali-Krishna K, Altman JD, Suresh M, Sourdive DJD, Zajac AJ, Miller JD, Slansky J, Ahmed R. Counting antigen-specific CD8 T cells: A reevaluation of bystander activation during viral infection. Immunity 1998; 8:177–87.
69. Altman JD, Moss P, Goulder P, Barouch DH, McHeyzer-Williams M, Bell JI, McMichael AJ, Davis MM. Phenotypic analysis of antigen-specific T lymphocytes. Science 1996; 274:94–6.
70. Tough DF, Borrow P, Sprent J. Induction of bystander T cell proliferation by viruses and type I interferon in vivo. Science 1996; 272:1947–50.
71. Doherty PC. The numbers game for virus-specific CD8+ T cells. Science 1998; 280:227.
72. Butera ST, Roberts BD, Lam L, Hodge T, Folks TM. Human Immunodeficiency Virus type 1 RNA expression by four chronically infected cell lines indicates multiple mechanisms of latency. J Virol 1994; 68:2726–30.
73. Finzi D, Hermankova M, Pierson T, Carruth LM, Buck C, Chaisson RE, Quinn TC, Chadwick K, Margolick J, Brookmeyer R, Gallant J, Markowitz M, Ho DD, Richman DD, Siliciano RF. Identification of a reservoir for HIV-1 in patients on highly active antiretroviral therapy. Science 1997; 278:1295–300.
74. Wong JK, Hezareh M, Günthard HF, Havlir DV, Ignacio CC, Spina CA, Richman DD. Recovery of replication-competent HIV despite prolonged suppression of plasma viremia. Science 1997; 278,1291–5.
75. Collins KL, Chen BK, Kalams SA, Walker BD, Baltimore D. HIV-1 nef protein protects infected primary cells against killing by cytotoxic T lymphocytes. Nature 1998; 391:397–401.
76. Cohen GB, Gandhi RT, Davis DM, Mandelboim O, Chen BK, Strominger JL, Baltimore D. The selective downregulation of class I major histocompatibility complex proteins by HIV-1 protects HIV-infected cells from NK cells. Immunity 1999; 10:661–71.
77. Xu, X-N, Laffert B, Screaton GR, Kraft M, Wolf D, Kolanus W, Mongkolsapay J, McMichael AJ, Baur AS. Induction of Fas ligand expression by HIV involves the interaction of Nef with the T cell receptor ζ chain. J Exp Med 1999; 189:1489–96.
78. Phillips RE, Rowland-Jones S, Nixon DF, Gotch FM, Edwards JP, Ogunlesi AO, Elvin JG, Rothbard JA, Bangham CRM, Rizza CR, McMichael AJ. Human Immunodeficiency Virus genetic variation that can escape cytotoxic T cell recognition. Nature 1991; 354:453–9.
79. Pewe L, Xue S, Perlman S. Infection with cytotoxic T-lymphocyte escape mutants results in increased mortality and growth retardation in mice infected with a neurotropic coronavirus. J Virol 1998; 72:5912–8.
80. Aebischer T, Moskophidis D, Rohrer UH, Zinkernagel RM, Hengartner H. In vitro selection of lymphocytic choriomeningitis virus escape mutants by cytotoxic T lymphocytes. Proc Natl Acad Sci USA 1991; 88:11047–51.
81. Bertoletti A, Costanzo A, Chisari FV, Levrero M, Artini M, Sette A, Penna A, Giuberti T, Fiaccadori F, Ferrari C. Cytotoxic T lymphocyte response to a wild type hepatitis B virus epitope in patients chronically infected by variant viruses carrying substitutions within the epitope. J Exp Med 1994; 180:933–43.
82. Tsai S-L, Chen Y-M, Chen M-H, Huang C-Y, Sheen I-S, Yeh C-T, Huang J-H, Kuo GC, Liaw Y-F. Hepatitis C virus variants circumventing cytotoxic T lymphocyte activity as a mechanism of chronicity. Gastroenterology 1998; 115:954–66.

83. de Campos-Lima PO, Levitsky V, Brooks J, Lee SP, Hu LF, Rickinson AB, Masucci MG. T cell responses and virus evolution: loss of HLA A11-restricted CTL epitopes in Epstein-Barr virus isolates from highly A11-positive populations by selective mutation of anchor residues. J Exp Med 1994; 179:1297–305.
84. Price DA, Goulder PJR, Klenerman P, Sewell AK, Easterbrook PJ, Troop M, Bangham CRM, Phillips RE. Positive selection of HIV-1 cytotoxic T lymphocyte escape variants during primary infection. Proc Natl Acad Sci USA 1997; 94:1890–5.
85. Borrow P, Lewicki H, Wei X, Horwitz MS, Peffer N, Meyers H, Nelson JA, Gairin JE, Hahn BH, Oldstone MBA, Shaw GM. Antiviral pressure exerted by HIV-1-specific cytotoxic T lymphocytes (CTLs) during primary infection demonstrated by rapid selection of CTL escape virus. Nature Medicine 1997; 3:205–11.
86. Mortara L, Letourneur F, Gras-Masse H, Venet A, Guillet JG, Bourault-Villada I. Selection of virus variants and emergence of virus escape mutants after immunization with an epitope vaccine. J Virol 1998; 72:1403–10.
87. Koenig S, Conley AJ, Brewah YA, Jones GM, Leath S, Boots LJ, Davey V, Pantaleo G, Demarest JF, Carter C, Wannebo C, Yannelli JR, Rosenberg SA, Lane HC. Transfer of HIV-1-specific cytotoxic T lymphocytes to an AIDS patient leads to selection for mutant HIV variants and subsequent disease progression. Nature Medicine 1995; 1:330–6.
88. Couillin I, Culmann-Penciolelli B, Gomard E, Choppin J, Levy J-P, Guillet J-G, Saragosti S. Impaired cytotoxic T lymphocyte recognition due to genetic variations in the main immunogenic region of the Human Immunodeficiency Virus 1 NEF protein. J Exp Med 1994; 180:1129–34.
89. Ossendorp F, Eggers M, Neisig A, Ruppert T, Groettrup M, Sijts A, Mengedé E, Kloetzel P-M, Neefjes J, Koszinowski U, Melief C. A single residue exchange within a viral CTL epitope alters proteasome-mediated degradation resulting in lack of antigen presentation. Immunity 1996; 5:115–24.
90. Klenerman P, Rowland-Jones S, McAdam S, Edwards J, Daenke S, Lalloo D, Kóppe B, Rosenberg W, Boyd D, Edwards A, Giangrande P, Phillips RE, McMichael AJ. Cytotoxic T-cell activity antagonized by naturally occurring HIV-1 gag variants. Nature 1994; 369:403–7.
91. Meier U-C, Klenerman P, Griffin P, James W, Koppe B, Larder B, McMichael A, Phillips R. Cytotoxic T lymphocyte lysis inhibited by viable HIV mutants. Science 1995; 270:1360–2.
92. Bertoletti A, Sette A, Chisari FV, Penna A, Levrero M, De Carli M, Fiaccadori F, Ferrari C. Natural variants of cytotoxic epitopes are T-cell receptor antagonists for antiviral cytotoxic T cells. Nature 1994; 369:407–10.
93. Madrenas J, Wange RL, Wang JL, Isakov N, Samelson LE, Germain RN. ζ phosphorylation without ZAP-70 activation induced by TCR antagonists or partial agonists. Science 1995; 267:515–8.
94. Reis e Sousa C, Levine EH, Germain RN. Partial signaling by $CD8^+$ T cells in response to antagonist ligands. J Exp Med 1996; 184:149–57.
95. Eisenlohr LC, Yewdell JW, Bennink JR. Flanking sequences influence the presentation of an endogenously synthetized peptide to cytotoxic T lymphocytes. J Exp Med 1992; 175:481–487.
96. Bodmer HC, Gotch FM, McMichael AJ. Class I cross-restricted T cells reveal low responder allele due to processing of viral antigen. Nature 1989; 337:653–5.
97. Del Val M, Schlicht HJ, Ruppert T, Reddehase MJ, Koszinowski UH. Efficient processing of an antigenic sequence for presentation by MHC class I molecules depends on its neighboring residues in the protein. Cell 1991; 66:1145–53.
98. Soudeyns H, Paolucci S, Chappey C, Daucher M, Graziosi C, Vaccarezza M, Cohen OJ, Fauci AS, Pantaleo G. Selective pressure exerted by immunodominant human immunodeficiency virus type 1-specific cytotoxic T lymphocyte responses during primary infection drives genetic variation restricted to the cognate epitope. Eur J Immunol 1999; 29:3629–35.
99. Nowak MA, May RM, Phillips RE, Rowland-Jones S, Lalloo DG, McAdam S, Klenerman P, Köppe B, Sigmund K, Bangham CRM, McMichael AJ. Antigenic oscillations and shifting immunodominance in HIV-1 infections. Nature 1995; 375:606–11.

100. Wolinsky SM, Korber BTM, Neumann AU, Daniels M, Kunstman KJ, Whetsell AJ, Furtado MR, Cao Y, Ho DD, Safrit JT, Koup RA. Adaptive evolution of Human Immunodeficiency Virus-type 1 during the natural course of infection. Science 1996; 272:537–42.
101. Coffin JM. HIV population dynamics in vivo: implications for genetic variation, pathogenesis, and therapy. Science 1995; 267:483–9.
102. Delwart EL, Sheppard HW, Walker BD, Goudsmit J, Mullins JI. Human Immunodeficiency Virus type 1 evolution in vivo tracked by DNA heteroduplex mobility assays. J Virol 1994; 68:6672–83.
103. Fauci AS. The human immunodeficiency virus: infectivity and mechanisms of pathogenesis. Science 1988; 239:617–22.
104. Tindall B, Hing M, Edwards P, Barnes T, Mackie A, Cooper DA. Several clinical manifestations of primary hiv infection. AIDS 1989; 3:747–9.
105. Clark SJ, Saag MS, Decker WD, Campbell-Hill S, Roberson JL, Veldkamp PJ, Cappes JC, Hahn BH, Shaw GM. High titers of cytopathic virus in plasma of patients with symptomatic primary HIV-1 infection. New Engl J Med 1991; 324:954–60.
106. Kinloch-de-Loës S, de Saussure P, Saurat JH, Stalder H, Hirschel B, Perrin L. Symptomatic primary infection due to Human Immunodeficiency Virus type 1: review of 31 cases. Clin Infect Dis 1993; 17:59–65.
107. Daar ES, Moudgil T, Meyer RD, Ho DD. Transient high levels of viremia in patients with primary Human Immunodeficiency Virus type 1 infection. New Engl J Med 1991; 324:961–4.
108. Piatak M, Saag MS, Yang LC, Clark SJ, Kappes JC, Luk K-C, Hahn BH, Shaw GM, Lifson JD. High levels of HIV-1 in plasma during all stages of infection determined by competitive PCR. Science 1993; 259:1749–54.
109. Graziosi C, Pantaleo G, Butini L, Demarest JF, Saag MS, Shaw GM, Fauci AS. Kinetics of Human Immunodeficiency Virus type 1 (HIV-1) DNA and RNA synthesis during primary HIV-1 infection. Proc Natl Acad Sci USA 1993; 90:6405–9.
110. Pantaleo G, Graziosi C, Fauci AS. The immunopathogenesis of Human Immunodeficiency Virus infection. New Engl J Med 1993; 328:327–35.
111. Pantaleo G and Fauci AS. New concepts in the immunopathogenesis of HIV infection. Ann Rev Immunol 1995; 13:487–512.
112. Phillips AN. Reduction of HIV concentration during acute infection: independence from a specific immune response. Science 1996; 271:497–9.
113. Pantaleo GP, Demarest JF, Soudeyns H, Graziosi C, Denis F, Adelsberger JW, Borrow P, Saag MS, Shaw GM, Sékaly R-P, Fauci AS. Major expansion of $CD8^+$ T lymphocytes with a predominant Vβ usage during the primary immune response to HIV. Nature 1994; 370:463–7.
114. Wilson JDK, Ogg GS, Allen RL, Goulder PJR, Kelleher A, Sewell AK, O'Callaghan CA, Rowland-Jones SL, Calla MFC, McMichael AJ. Oligoclonal expansions of $CD8^+$ T cells in chronic HIV infection are antigen-specific. J Exp Med 1998; 188:785–90.
115. Rock EP, Sibbald PR, Davis MM, Chien Y-H. CDR3 length in antigen-specific immune receptors. J Exp Med 1994; 179:323–8.
116. Smith TJ, Terada N, Robinson CC, Gelfand EW. Acute infectious mononucleosis stimulates the selective expression/expansion of Vβ6.1-3 and Vβ7 T cells. Blood 1993; 81:1521–6.
117. Callan MFC, Steven N, Krausa P, Wilson JDK, Moss PAH, Gillespie GM, Bell JI, Rickinson AB, McMichael AJ. Large clonal expansions of $CD8^+$ T cells in acute infectious mononucleosis. Nature Medicine 1996; 2:906–11.
118. Mongkolsapaya J, Jaye A, Callan MFC, Magnusen AF, McMichael AJ, Whittle HC. Antigen-specific expansion of cytotoxic T lymphocytes in acute measles virus infection. J Virol 1999; 73:67–71.
119. Borrow P, Lewicki H, Hahn BH, Shaw GM, Oldstone MB. CTL activity associated with control of viremia in primary HIV-1 infection. J Virol 1994; 68:6103–10.

120. Koup RA, Safrit JT, Cao Y, Andres CA, McLeod G, Borkowsky W, Farthing C, Ho DD. Temporal association of cellular immune responses with the initial control of viremia in primary human immunodeficiency virus type 1 syndrome. J Virol 1994; 68:4650–5.
121. Safrit JT, Andrews CA, Zhu T, Ho DD, Koup RA. Characterization of Human Immunodeficiency Virus type 1-specific cytotoxic T lymphocyte clones isolated during acute seroconversion: recognition of autologous virus sequences within a conserved immunodominant epitope. J Exp Med 1994; 179:463–72.
122. Musey L, Hughes J, Schacker T, Shea T, Corey L, McElrath MJ. Cytotoxic T cell responses, viral load, and disease progression in early Human Immunodeficiency Virus type 1 infection. New Engl J Med 1997; 337:1267–74.
123. Pantaleo G, Demarest JF, Schacker T, Vaccarezza M, Cohen OJ, Daucher M, Graziosi C, Schnittman SS, Quinn TJ, Shaw GM, Perrin L, Tambussi G, Lazzarin A, Sekaly R-P, Soudeyns H, Corey L, Fauci AS. The qualitative nature of the primary immune response to HIV infection is a prognosticator of disease progression independent of the initial level of plasma viremia. Proc Natl Acad Sci USA 1997; 94:254–8.
124. Schmitz JE, Kuroda MJ, Santra S, Sasseville VG, Simon MA, Lifton M. A, Racz P, Tenner-Racz K, Dalesandro M, Scallon BJ, Ghrayeb J, Forman MA, Montefiori DC, Rieber EP, Letvin NL, Reitmann KA. Control of viremia in simian immunodeficiency virus infection by $CD8^+$ lymphocytes. Science 1999; 283:857–60.
125. Matano T, Shibata R, Siemon C, Connors M, Lane HC, Martin MA. Administration of an anti-CD8 monoclonal antibody interferes with the clearance of chimeric Simian/Human Immunodeficiency Virus during primary infection of rhesus macaques. J Virol 1998; 72:164–9.
127. Goulder PJ, Phillips RE, Colbert RA, McAdam S, Ogg G, Nowak MA, Giangrande P, Luzzi G, Morgan B, Edwards A, McMichael AJ, Rowland-Jones, S. Late escape from an immunodominant cytotoxic T-lymphocyte response associated with progression to AIDS. Nat Med 1997; 3:212–7.
128. Brander C, Hartman KE, Trocha AK, Jones NG, Johnson RP, Korber B, Wentworth P, Buchbinder SP, Wolinsky S, Walker BD, Kalams SA. Lack of strong immune selection pressure by the immunodominant, HLA-A*0201-restricted cytotoxic T lymphocyte response in chronic human immunodeficiency virus-1 infection. J Clin Invest 1998; 101:2559–66.
129. Harrer T, Harrer E, Kalams SA, Barbosa P, Trocha A, Johnson RP, Elbeik T, Feinberg MB, Buchbinder SP, Walker BD. Cytotoxic T lymphocytes in asymptomatic long-term nonprogressing HIV-1 infection. Breadth and specificity of the response and relation to in vivo viral quasispecies in a person with prolonged infection and low viral load. J Immunol 1996; 156:2616–23.
130. Finzi D, Siliciano RF. Viral dynamics in HIV-Infection. Cell 1998; 93:665–71.
131. Moskophidis D, Lechner F, Pircher H, Zinkernagel RM. Virus pesistence in acutely infected immunocompetent mice by exhaustion of antiviral cytotoxic effector T cells. Nature 1993; 362:758–61.
132. Oxenius A, Zinkernagel RM, Hengartner H. Comparison of activation versus induction of unresponsiveness of virus-specific $CD4^+$ and $CD8^+$ T cells upon acute versus persistent viral infection. Immunity 1998; 9:449–57.
133. Soudeyns H, Pantaleo G. The moving target: mechanism of HIV persistence during primary infection. Immunol. Today 1999; 20:446–50.
134. Walker BD, Chakrabarti S, Moss B, Paradis TJ, Flynn T, Durno AG, Blumberg RS, Kaplan JC, Hirsch MS, Schooley RT. HIV-specific cytotoxic T lymphocytes in seropositive individuals. Nature 1987; 328:345–8.
135. Walker BD, Flexner C, Birch-Limberger K, Fisher L, Paradis TJ, Aldovini A, Young R, Moss B, Schooley RT. Long-term culture and fine specificity of human cytotoxic T-lymphocyte clones reactive with Human Immunodeficiency Virus type 1. Proc Natl Acad Sci USA 1989; 86:9514–8.

136. Takahashi K, Dai L-C, Fuerst TR, Biddison WE, Earl PL, Moss B, Ennis FA. Specific lysis of Human Immunodeficiency Virus type 1-infected cells by a HLA-A3.1-restricted CD8+ cytotoxic T-lymphocyte clone that recognizes a conserved peptide sequence within the gp41 subunit of the envelope protein. Proc Natl Acad Sci USA 1991; 88:10277–81.
137. Carmichael A, Jin X, Sissons P, Borysiewicz L. Quantitative analysis of the Human Immunodeficiency Virus type 1 (HIV-1)-specific cytotoxic T lymphocyte (CTL) response at different stages of HIV-1 infection: differential CTL responses to HIV-1 and Epstein-Barr Virus in late disease. J Exp Med 1993; 177:249–56.
138. Ogg GS, Jin X, Bonhoeffer S, Dunbar PR, Nowak MA, Monard S, Segal JP, Cao Y, Rowland-Jones SL, Cerundolo V, Hurley A, Markowitz M, Ho DD, Nixon DF, McMichael AJ. Quantitation of HIV-1-specific cytotoxic T lymphocytes and plasma load of viral RNA. Science 1998; 279:2103–6.
139. Greenough TC, Brettler DB, Somasundaran M, Panicali DL, Sullivan, JL. Human Immunodeficiency Virus type 1-specific cytotoxic T lymphocytes (CTL), virus load, and CD4+ T cell loss: evidence supporting a protective role for CTL in vivo. J Infect Dis 1997; 176:118–25.
140. Klein MR, van Baalen CA, Holwerda AM, Kerkhof Garde SR, Bende RJ, Keet IPM, Eeftinck-Schattenkerk J-KM, Osterhaus ADME, Schuitemaker H, Miedema F. Kinetics of gag-specific cytotoxic T lymphocyte responses during the clinical course of HIV-1 infection: a longitudinal analysis of rapid progressors and long-term asymptomatics. J Exp Med 1995; 181:1365–72.
141. Pantaleo G, Menzo S, Vaccarezza M, Graziosi C, Cohen OJ, Demarest JF, Montefiori D, Orenstein JM, Fox C, Schrager LK, Margolick JB, Buchbinder S, Giorgi JV, Fauci AS. Studies in subjects with long-term nonprogressive Human Immunodeficiency Virus infection. New Engl J Med 1995; 332:209–16.
142. Dyer WB, Ogg GS, Demoitie M-A, Jin X, Geczy AF, Rowland-Jones SL, McMichael AJ, Nixon DF, Sullivan JS. Strong Human Immunodeficiency Virus (HIV)-specific cytotoxic T-lymphocyte activity in Sidney blood bank cohort patients infected with nef-defective HIV type 1. J Virol 1999; 73:436–43.
143. Kvale D, Aukrust P, Osnes K, Muller F, Froland SS. CD4+ and CD8+ lymphocytes and HIV RNA in HIV infection: high baseline counts and in particular rapid decrease of CD8+ lymphocytes predict AIDS. AIDS 1999; 13:195–201.
144. McKinney DM, Lewinsohn DA, Riddell SR, Grenberg PD, Mosier DE. The antiviral activity of HIV-specific CD8+ CTL clones is limited by elimination due to encounter with HIV-infected targets. J Immunol 1999; 163:861–7.
145. Jin X, Bauer DE, Tuttleton SE, Lewin S, Gettie A, Blanchard J, Irwin CE, Safrit JT, Mittler J, Weinberger L, Kostrikis LG, Zhang L, Perelson AS, HO DD. Dramatic rise in plasma viremia after CD8+ T cell depletion in Simian Immunodeficiency Virus-infected macaques. J Exp Med 1999; 189:991–8.
146. Hoffenbach A, Langlade-Demoyen P, Dadaglio G, Vilmer E, Michel F, Mayaud C, Autran B, Plata F. Unusually high frequencies of HIV-specific cytotoxic T lymphocytes in humans. J Immunol 1989; 142:452–62.
147. Cheynier R, Henrichwark S, Hadida F, Pelletier E, Oksenhendler E, Autran B, Wain-Hobson S. HIV and T cell expansion in splenic white pulps is accompanied by infiltration of HIV-specific cytotoxic T lymphocytes. Cell 1994; 78:373–87.
148. Plata F, Autran B, Martins LP, Wain-Hobson S, Raphael M, Mayaud C, Denis M, Guillon J-M, Debré P. AIDS virus-specific cytotoxic T lymphocytes in lung disorders. Nature 1987; 328:348–51.
149. Sethi KK, Naher H, Stroehmann I. Phenotypic heterogeneity of cerebrospinal fluid-derived HIV-specific and HLA-restricted cytotoxic T-cell clones. Nature 1988; 335:178–81.

150. Jassoy C, Johnson RP, Navia BA, Worth J, Walker BD. Detection of a vigorous HIV-1-specific cytotoxic T lymphocyte response in cerebrospinal fluid from infected persons with AIDS dementia complex. J Immunol 1992; 149:3113–9.
151. Venet A, Walker BD. Cytotoxic T-cell epitopes in HIV/SIV infection. AIDS 1993; 7(S1):S117–26.
152. Johnson RP, Trocha A, Buchanan TM, Walker BD, Identification of overlapping HLA class I-restricted cytotoxic T cell epitopes in a conserved region of the Human Immunodeficiency Virus type 1 envelope glycoprotein: definition of minimum epitopes and analysis of the effects of sequence variation. J Exp Med 1992; 175:961–71.
153. McMichael AJ, Walker BD. Cytotoxic T lymphocyte epitopes: implications for HIV vaccines. AIDS 1994; 8(S1):S155–73.
154. Gotch FM, Koup RA, Safrit JT. New observations on cellular immune responses to HIV and T-cell epitopes. AIDS 1997; 11(SA):S99–107.
155. Korber BTM, Walker BD, Brander C, Koup RA, Moore JP, Haynes BF, Editors. HIV molecular immunology database. Los Alamos National Laboratory: Theoretical Biology and Biophysics, Los Alamos, New Mexico. 1997.
156. Johnson RP, Trocha A, Yang L, Mazzara GP, Panicali DL, Buchanan TM, Walker BD. HIV-1 gag-specific cytotoxic T lymphocytes recognize multiple highly conserved epitopes. fine specificity of the gag-specific response defined by using unstimulated peripheral blood mononuclear cells and cloned effector cells. J Immunol 1991; 147:1512–21.
157. Rosenberg ES, Billingsley JM, Caliendo AM, Boswell SL, Sax PE, Kalams SA, Walker BD. Vigorous HIV-1-specific $CD4^+$ T cell responses associated with control of viremia. Science 1997; 278:1447–50.
158. Pantaleo G, Graziosi C, Demarest JF, Butini L, Montroni M, Fox CH, Orenstein JM, Kotler DP, Fauci AS. HIV infection is active and progressive in lymphoid tissue during the clinically latent stage of disease. Nature 1993; 362:355–8.
159. Embretson J, Zupancic M, Ribas JL, Burke A, Racz P, Tenner-Racz K, Haase AT. Massive covert infection of helper T lymphocytes and macrophages by HIV during the incubation period of AIDS. Nature 1993; 362:359–62.
160. De Maria A, Pantaleo G, Schnittman SM, Greenhouse JJ, Baseler M, Orenstein JM, Fauci AS. Infection of $CD8^+$ T lymphocytes with HIV. Requirement for interaction with infected $CD4^+$ cells and induction of infectious virus from chronically infected $CD8^+$ cells. J Immunol 1991; 146:2220–6.
161. Livingstone WJ, Moore M, Innes D, Bell JE, Simmonds P. Frequent infection of peripheral blood CD8-positive T-lymphocytes with HIV-1. Edinburgh heterosexual transmission study group. Lancet 1996; 348:649–4.
162. Pantaleo G, Koenig S, Baseler M, Lane HC, Fauci AS. Defective clonogenic potential of $CD8^+$ T lymphocytes in patients with AIDS. Expansion in vivo of a nonclonogenic $CD3^+CD8^+DR^+CD25^-$ T cell population. J Immunol 1990; 144:1696–704.
163. Pantaleo G, DeMaria A, Koenig S, Butini L, Moss B, Baseler M, Lane HC, Fauci AS. $CD8^+$ T lymphocytes of patients with AIDS maintain a normal broad cytolytic function despite the loss of Human Immunodeficiency Virus-specific cytotoxicity. Proc Natl Acad Sci USA 1990; 87:4818–22.
164. Rehermann B, Fowler P, Sidney J, Person J, Redeker A, Brown M, Moss B, Sette A, Chisari FV. The cytotoxic T lymphocyte response to multiple Hepatitis B Virus polymerase epitopes during and after viral hepatitis. J Exp Med 1995; 181:1047–58.
165. Palella FJ, Delaney KM, Moorman AC, Loveless MO, Fuhrer J, Satten GA, Aschman DJ, Holmberg SD. Declining morbidity and mortality among patients with advanced human immunodeficiency virus infection. HIV outpatient study investigators. N Engl J Med 1998; 338:853–60.

166. Bucy RP, Hockett RD, Derdeyn CA, Saag MS, Squires K, Sillers M, Mitsuyasu RT, Kilby JM. Initial increase in blood CD4+ lymphocytes after HIV antiretroviral therapy reflects redistribution from lymphoid tissues. J Clin Invest 1999; 103:1391–8.
167. Fleury S, de Boer RJ, Rizzardi GP, Wolthers KC, Otto SA, Welbon CC, Graziosi C, Knabenhans C, Soudeyns H, Bart P-A, Gallant S, Corpataux J-M, Gillet M, Meylan P, Schnyder P, Meuwly J-Y, Spreen W, Glauser MP, Miedema F, Pantaleo G. Limited CD4+ T-cell renewal in early HIV-1 infection: effect of highly active antiretroviral therapy. Nat Med 1998; 4:794–801.
168. Autran B, Carcelain G, Li TS, Blanc C, Mathez D, Tubiana R, Katlama C, Debre P, Leibowitch J. Positive effects of combined antiretroviral therapy on CD4+ T cell homeostasis and function in advanced HIV disease. Science 1997; 277:112–6.
169. Pakker NG, Kroon EDMB, Roos MTL, Otto SA, Hall D, Wit FW NM, Hamann D, van der Ende ME, Claessen FAP, Kauffmann RH, Koopmans PP, Kroon FP, ten Napel CHH, Sprenger HG, Weigel HM, Montaner JSG, Lange JMA, Reiss P, Schellekens PTA, Miedema F. Immune restoration does not invariably occur following long-term HIV-1 suppression during antiretroviral therapy. AIDS 1998; 13:203–12.
170. Pakker NG, Notermans DW, de Boer RJ, Roos MTL, de Wolf F, Hill A, Leonard JM, Danner SA, Miedema F, Schellekens PTA. Biphasic kinetics of peripheral blood T cells after triple combination therapy in HIV-1 infection: a composite of redistribution and proliferation. Nat Med 1998; 4:208–14.
171. Angel JB, Kumar A, Parato K, Filion LG, Diaz-Mitoma F, Daftarian P, Pham B, Sun E, Leonard JM, Cameron DW. Improvement in cell-mediated immune function during potent anti-human immunodeficiency virus therapy with ritonavir plus saquinavir. J Infect Dis 1998; 177:898–904.
172. O'Sullivan CE, Drew WL, McMullen DJ, Miner R, Lee JY, Kaslow RA, Lazar JG, Saag MS. Decrease of cytomegalovirus replication in human immunodeficiency virus infected-patients after treatment with highly active antiretroviral therapy. J Infect Dis 1999; 180:847–9.
173. Ogg GS, Jin X, Bonhoeffer S, Moss P, Nowak MA, Monard S, Segal JP, Cao Y, Rowland-Jones SL, Hurley A, Markowitz M, Ho DD, McMichael AJ, Nixon DF. Decay kinetics of Human Immunodeficiency Virus-specific effector cytotoxic T lymphocytes after combination antiretroviral therapy. J Virol 1999; 73:797–800.
174. Gray CM, Lawrence J, Schapiro JM, Altman JD, Winters MA, Crompton M, Loi M, Kundu SK, Davis MM, Merigan TC. Frequency of class I HLA-restricted anti-HIV CD8+ T cells in individuals receiving highly active antiretroviral therapy (HAART). J Immunol 1999; 162:1780–8.
175. Connors M, Kovacs JA, Krevat S, Gea-Banacloche JC, Sneller MC, Flanigan M, Metcalf JA, Walker RE, Falloon J, Baseler M, Stevens R, Feuerstein I, Masur H, Lane HC. HIV infection induces changes in CD4+ T-cell phenotype and depletions within the CD4+ T-cell repertoire that are not immediately restored by antiviral or immune-based therapies. Nat Med 1997; 3:533–40.
176. Gorochov G, Neumann AU, Kereveur A, Parizot C, Li T, Katlama C, Karmochkine M, Raguin G, Autran B, Debré P. Perturbations of CD4+ and CD8+ T-cell repertoires during progression to AIDS and regulation of the CD4+ repertoire during antiviral therapy. Nat Med 1998; 4:215–21.
177. Martinon F, Michelet C, Peguillet I, Taoufik Y, Lefebvre P, Goujard C, Guillet J-G, Delfraissy J-F, Lantz O. Persistent alterations in T-cell repertoire cytokine and chemokine receptor gene expression after 1 year of highly active antiretroviral therapy. AIDS 1999; 13:185–94.
178. Tindall B, Cooper DA. Primary HIV infection: host responses and intervention strategies. AIDS 1991; 5:1–14.
179. Kinloch-de Loës S, Hirschel BJ, Hoen B, Cooper DA, Tindall B, Carr A, Saurat J-H, Clumeck N, Lazzarin A, Mathiesen L, Raffi F, Antunes F, von Overbeck J, Luthy R, Glauser M, Hawkins D, Baumberger C, Yerly S, Perneger TV, Perrin L. A controlled trial of zidovudine in primary human immunodeficiency virus infection. New Engl J Med 1995; 333:408–13.

180. Pitcher CJ, Quittner C, Peterson DM, Connors M, Koup RA, Maino VC, Picker LJ. HIV-1-specific CD4+ T cells are detectable in most individuals with active HIV-1 infection, but decline with prolonged viral suppression. Nat Med 1999; 5:518–25.
181. Plana M, Garcia F, Gallart T, Miro JM, Gatell JM. Lack of T-cell proliferative response to HIV-1 antigens after 1 year of highly active antiretroviral treatment in early HIV-1 disease. The Lancet 1998; 352:1194–5.
182. Ho DD. Time to hit HIV, early and hard. New Engl J Med 1995; 333:450–1.
183. Pantaleo G. How immune-based intervention can change HIV therapy. Nat Med 1997; 3:483–6.

10
Characterization of the HIV-1–Specific T-Helper Cell Response

Bruce D. Walker

INTRODUCTION

Human immunodeficiency virus type 1 (HIV-1) is associated with persistent and progressive infection in the majority of untreated persons, with an average time of 10 yr until the development of acquired immune deficiency syndrome (AIDS). However, longitudinal cohort studies have now identified persons who have been infected for >20 yr without the development of disease. In fact, a small number of untreated infected persons have maintained viral loads at or below the limits of detection by the most sensitive assays now available, normal CD4 cell counts, and have had no evidence of disease manifestations related to HIV. Other human viral infections such as Epstein–Barr virus (EBV) and Cytomegalovirus (CMV) persist for the life of an infected person, but are held in check by a persistent and effective immune response. The existence of persons with chronic controlled HIV-1 infection suggests that a state of immunologic control may be achievable in this infection as well.

In the past 2 yr the critical role of the immune system in determining the viral set point and in influencing disease progression has become apparent from both in vivo and in vitro studies. Emerging data suggest that this immune control may be critically dependent on the presence of virus-specific T-helper cell responses, which are the focus of this chapter.

IMMUNE CONTROL IN VIRAL INFECTIONS

Numerous recent studies indicate that virus-specific cytolytic T lymphocytes (CTLs) are capable of massive expansion when generated in response to infection, and that the magnitude of these cells can be associated with control of viremia (reviewed in *1*). CTLs can mediate potent antiviral effects, killing virus-infected cells before progeny virions are produced *(2,3)*. However, not all chronic viral infections are equally capable of inducing and maintaining strong CTL responses. In both HIV and HCV infection, meager CTL responses are often generated, and at least in HIV infection, these responses do not persist. Loss of CTLs is temporally associated with HIV-1 disease progression *(4–6)*. These observations raise the important question as to what controls the magnitude, activation state, and persistence of CTLs.

From: *Retroviral Immunology: Immune Response and Restoration*
Edited by: Giuseppe Pantaleo and Bruce D. Walker © Humana Press Inc., Totowa, NJ

The best studied model to address maintenance of CTL function during the chronic phase of an infection is the lymphocytic chroriomeningitis virus (LCMV) model of chronic viral infection, and these studies reveal that virus-specific T-helper cells are likely to be the key to long-term immune control. LCMV is actually a family of related viruses that have quite different pathogenic potential (reviewed in *7*). With less virulent strains of LCMV such as the Armstrong strain, experimental virus infection is cleared in 8–10 d in the presence or absence of CTL *(8–10)*. In fact, studies have shown that T-helper cell responses are not required for the induction phase of CTL *(8,9)*. However, when mice are experimentally infected with more pathogenic strains of virus, CD4 T-helper cells are required to prevent the exhaustion of CTLs. One of these more pathogenic viruses, clone 13, shares 99.8% homology with the Armstrong strain, yet exhibits 10–50-fold enhanced replicative capacity *(10)*. If CD4 T cells are even transiently depleted at the time of infection, this leads to complete loss of functional CTLs and to a chronic infection in which the virus is not immunologically contained *(10)*. Similar results have been obtained in CD4 knockout mice and in mice transiently depleted of CD4 cells by administration of monoclonal anti-CD4 antibodies *(11)*, and mice deficient in CD4 cells are less protected by immunization against pathogens that are typically controlled by CTL *(12)*.

The need for T-helper cell responses to maintain CTL-mediated control is not limited to the LCMV model, but has been observed in γ-herpesvirus infections *(13)* and Friend virus infections *(14)*, among others. A similar need for help in maintaining immunologic control in human viral infections comes from recent studies in persons with hepatitis C virus (HCV) infection, in whom loss of T-helper cell responses is associated with loss of control of viremia *(15)*. The precise factors contributed by T-helper cells that allow CTLs to function more efficiently have been elusive, but are likely to include a number of soluble products produced by these cells on activation. Interactions between CD4 cells and antigen-presenting cells mediated through CD40–CD40 ligand interactions lead to enhanced APC function, and this likely facilitates maintenance of CTL function *(16,17)*. In addition, CD4 cells in some viral infections have been reported to be directly cytolytic for virus-infected cells.

Evidence of Immune Containment of HIV Infection

Increasing evidence points to a central role of the immune response in determining the viral set point at steady state in HIV infection. The most direct evidence comes from a macaque model of AIDS virus infection, in which CD8 cell depletion was associated with a dramatic increase in viral load in chronically infected animals *(18,19)*. When similar CD8 depletion was performed in naïve animals that were subsequently challenged with pathogenic virus, peak viremia was sustained, providing direct evidence that the initial drop in viremia is dependent on immunologic pressure exerted by CD8 cells *(18)*. The fact that increases in viral load correlated with decreases in antigen-specific CD8 cells as determined by direct visualization using major histocompatibility complex (MHC)–tetrameric complexes supports the conclusion that CTLs are an essential component of control. Other evidence pointing to a role for CTL come from cross-sectional studies showing that the magnitude of CD8 cells directed against a dominant A2 Gag epitope is negatively correlated with viral load *(20)*, and the observation that the decline in HIV-1 viremia is associated with the appearance of HIV-1–

specific CTLs *(21,22)*. Other studies show that CTL responses decline with disease progression *(4,5)*, providing additional support for the notion that CTLs are a key regulatory factor. The major question that has not been readily answered is why these CTLs, which appear to be so potent in vitro and correlate with control in vivo, are neither able to eradicate the virus nor to maintain persistent effective control.

T-HELPER CELLS IN HIV INFECTION

One of the most dramatic holes in the immune repertoire in HIV infection has been the relative lack of virus-specific T-helper cells (reviewed in *23*). HIV infects CD4 cells, and acute infection is associated with transient decrease in CD4 cell number, but these numbers usually recover. However, despite apparently near normal levels of CD4 cells during the asymptomatic phase of infection, the vast majority of infected persons do not have detectable virus-specific T-helper cell responses. Early in the epidemic it was noted that persons with AIDS-defining illness had a defect in their peripheral blood mononuclear cells in terms of ability to respond to soluble antigen, although the abililty to respond to mitogen remained intact *(24)*. Although the ability to proliferate in response to HIV antigens was impaired, CD4 cells could nevertheless produce measureable levels of interleukin-2 (IL-2) in response to stimulation with HIV envelope protein in vitro *(25)*. It was initially suspected that HIV, perhaps via direct interaction with the CD4 cell surface molecule, might be able to circumvent the induction of T-helper cell responses.

Detailed studies in a unique subset of persons who spontaneously control HIV without the need for antiviral therapy have now led to the conclusive demonstration that HIV can indeed induce T-helper cell responses *(26,27)*. As would be predicted from the LCMV model of chronic viral infection, the ability of these persons to contain viremia is dependent on both virus-specific T-helper cell responses and CTL responses *(28)*. In infected persons who control infection without the need for treatment, strong T-helper cell responses have been observed, with initial anecdotal cases now shown to be the norm in persons who control viremia. In those with high viral loads, these responses are typically completely undetectable. However, short-term stimulation with viral protein and intracellular staining for interferon-γ (IFN-γ) suggest that persons with progressive infection maintain a subset of CD4 cells that can react to HIV-1 proteins, but may not be able to proliferate and expand *(29)*. This observation supports earlier studies suggesting that there may be functional deficits in the subset of cells that can responds to HIV.

T-helper cell responses have been divided into different subsets depending on the cytokine profiles of the stimulated cells. Th1 type responses are associated with the production of IFN-γ and supportive of cellular immune responses, and as one might predict the robust T-helper cell responses found in persons who spontaneously control HIV secrete IFN-γ *(27)*. These cells also produce other cytokines upon stimulation with viral antigen, including the antiviral β-chemokines MIP-1α, MIP-1β, and RANTES *(27)*. Production of these particular cytokines in HIV-infected persons may in fact contribute to the beneficial effects of these cells by providing a direct antiviral effect in the local microenvironment where progeny virions may have been produced. Further studies are needed to determine the full range of cytokines produced by these cells.

Recent studies have confirmed the negative relationship between HIV-1–specific T-helper cell responses and control of viremia *(28)*. In our studies of a large cohort of persons with untreated HIV-1 infection, we have consistently found that strong Gag-specific proliferative responses are seen in persons who spontaneously control viremia without the need for drug therapy. Studies in macaques infected with attenuated simian immunodeficiency virus (SIV) constructs have also shown the presence of strong virus-specific T-helper cell responses in these animals that not only control viremia but are also protected from challenge with pathogenic virus *(30)*.

Targets of the T-Helper Cell Response in Infected Persons

T-helper cells recognize viral proteins that have been taken up by endocytosis, processed within vacuoles, and then complexed with MHC class II molecules. In theory one would expect that any viral protein would be able to be targeted by this response, and yet the available data suggest that the viral Gag protein may be the major target. The Gag protein is highly conserved among different HIV-1 isolates, and thus there may be a highly likelihood of homology between the infecting strain of virus and the cloned strains from which the testable immunogens have been derived. Our own studies have focused primarily on measuring T-helper cell responses to the Gag and Env proteins. We have detected Env-specific responses in only a subset of infected persons, and have yet to identify a person who has a stronger Env-specific proliferative response than their Gag-specific responses. That the target antigens for CTLs and T-helper cells are different is clear from the studies performed thus far. We have identified persons in whom Gag-specific T-helper cell responses are present, yet in whom no Gag-specific CTL can be detected.

Before accepting Gag as the major target for virus-specific T helper cells in HIV infection, more work will need to be done. Importantly, comprehensive studies using soluble proteins to all expressed HIV-1 proteins will need to be conducted, and these will need to include persons in all stages of disease.

Relationship Between T-Help and CTL in HIV Infection

As noted previously in the LCMV model, persistence of CTL in chronic viral infections is dependent on the presence of virus-specific T-helper cell responses *(7)*. If HIV follows rules similar to other viruses, then one would anticipate that persistent CTL responses would be observed in those who maintain virus-specific T help. To investigate a potential link between these responses, we examined functional HIV-1–specific memory CTL precursor frequencies and p24-specific proliferative responses in a cohort of infected untreated persons with a wide range of viral loads and CD4 cell counts *(28)*. Levels of p24-specific proliferative responses positively correlated with levels of Gag-specific CTL precursors and negatively correlated with levels of plasma HIV-1 RNA. Trends were observed in terms of the relationship between CTLs directed against other viral proteins and T helper cell responses. All persons with help had evidence of strong CTLs, but the converse was not always true—in other words, some persons had CTLs detectable in assays of precursor cells without detectable T-helper cell responses. One possible explanation for this apparent discrepancy is that the necessary addition of IL-2 to limiting dilution assays corrected the in vivo defect conferred by the lack of T-helper cell responses. These data link the levels of HIV-specific CTLs with

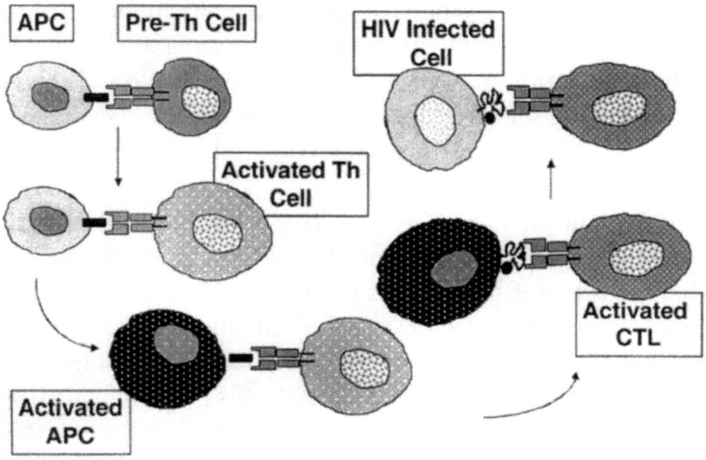

Fig. 1. Proposed model of CD4 T helper cell induction. Pre-T-helper cells are induced by interaction with antigen presenting cells, leading to their activation. This activation would normally lead to reciprocal activation of the APC, which in turn would activate CTL that would go on to lyse infected cells. A problem in HIV infection is that activation of CD4 cells renders them susceptible to lysis or activation-induced cell death in the presence of high levels of virus that are typical of acute infection. Impaired T-helper cell function may then lead to impaired CTL function.

virus-specific helper cell function during chronic viral infection, and provide a rationale for attempts to boost these responses with therapeutic immunization.

Potential Reasons for Lack of T-Helper Cell Responses in Most Infected Persons

The fact that the majority of persons who become HIV infected do not have persistent virus-specific T-helper cell responses remains an important unanswered question. There is now no question that HIV can indeed induce strong virus-specific T-helper cell responses, but these are not readily detected in the vast majority of infected persons, particularly when proliferation assays are used to assess for the presence of these cells. A number of possibilities have to be considered. One attractive hypothesis is based on the distinct property of HIV-1 to infect activated CD4 cells. One can hypothesize that as virus-specific T-helper cells are being generated in response to infection, these cells may become selectively targeted at a time when viral load is at its highest. Infection and loss of these cells would then result in lack of strong T helper cell responses to HIV (Fig. 1). However, other virus-specific T-helper cell responses, for example, against CMV, would be expected to remain intact, as this subset of cells would not be activated during acute HIV infection. Support for this hypothesis would be provided by data indicating that HIV-1–specific T-helper cells are preferentially targeted in acute infection, but thus far such data do not exist.

There are a number of additional potential explanations, all of which likewise lack experimental confirmation. Activation-induced cell death is one possibility, and may be supported by the extremely high viral loads seen in acute infection. In our studies of persons with acute HIV infection identified prior to or at the time of seroconversion, the average viral load was >10 million copies. The persistent stimulation of developing

T-helper cells with high levels of viral protein may lead to apoptosis of these cells, and prevent the effective establishment of a memory population *(31)*. Other proposed explanations include induction of anergy *(32)*, T-cell exhaustion *(33)*, and altered peptide ligands existing among the developing viral quasispecies *(34)*. Each of these possibilities needs to be investigated, as this issue is extremely important in the design of strategies to correct this deficit.

Any attempt to explain the lack of virus-specific T-helper cell responses in chronic HIV infection must also take into account observations in other chronic human viral infections in which a lack of T-helper cells has been postulated to contribute to chronic infection. The most apparent example is HCV infection, which like HIV results in chronic uncontrolled infection in the majority of infected persons *(35)*. In addition, HCV infection is associated with extremely high levels of viremia *(36)*. Recent studies in a chimpanzee model of acute HCV infection have shown that successful clearance of viremia can be achieved and is associated with a strong and broadly directed CTL response *(37)*. Although T-helper cell responses were not assessed in those studies, recent studies in successfully cleared acute HCV infection in humans have shown that persistent resolution of viremia is associated with strong and persistent CTL and T-helper cell responses *(15)*. The induction and maintenance of HCV-specific T-helper cell responses has been shown to be associated with clearance of HCV viremia in humans Lechner, 2000 #3456. The lack of strong T-helper cell responses in HCV infection is thus also associated with progressive infection. Here again the mechanism of loss of virus-specific T-helper cell responses is not known, but raises the question as to whether there may be a common mechanism. Because HCV has not been shown to infect CD4 cells, it is unlikely that this would be the common mechanism. However, as both HIV and HCV infection are associated with extremely high viral loads, activation-induced cell death in the presence of persistent high level viremia could serve as a common mechanism.

Effects of Antiviral Therapy on Virus-Specific T-Helper Cell Responses

The hypothesis that HIV-1–specific T-helper cells might be generated and lost in acute infection has now been tested experimentally, and provides encouraging evidence that all persons have the ability to induce this response. Persons with acute HIV infection presenting prior to seroconversion have been treated with potent combination antiviral regimens. This has led to the rapid decline in viremia in most infected persons, and has been consistently associated with the development of strong Gag-specific T-helper cell responses *(27)*. These responses have persisted in all persons in whom viremia could be contained. Thus these studies show that all persons have the capacity to generate these responses, but that they are likely lost in the earliest stages of infection in most persons. Other anecdotal studies have shown that persons with treated acute infection who have subsequently discontinued medications have on occasion controlled viremia without further therapy *(38,39)*, but the extent to which this is a predictable response to early therapy remains to be determined.

Prospects for Augmenting HIV-1–Specific T-Helper Cell Responses

A major question regarding therapeutic interventions in HIV infection is whether HIV-1–specifc immune responses can be restored on treatment, and whether this would have a beneficial effect on disease progression. An early indication that highly aggressive antiretroviral therapy (HAART) might result in some measure of immune reconstitution came from studies of CD4 cell number in persons in whom viral load was persistently suppressed by antiviral drug therapy. Often dramatic increases in CD4 cell counts have been observed. The fact that these increases in CD4 cell number were accompanied by a decreased risk of opportunistic infections and death suggested that they might be functionally relevant. More detailed quantitation of naive cells by Autran et al. in persons initiating HAART has revealed a progressive increase in these cells over the course of treatment, even in persons with advanced stage disease *(40)*. In the first few weeks of treatment there is typically a rapid rise in CD4 cell number, which subsequently continues as a slow but persistent rise. This increase is predominantly due to memory cells during the first 4 mo on treatment, but is then followed by significant rise in naive CD4 cells in most persons. These rises in naive CD4 cells are associated with overall decreases in CD4 cell activation markers, consistent with interruption of ongoing viral replication. Although increases in T-cell proliferative responses to recall antigens and mitogens are observed, treatment with HAART has generally not been associated with increases in HIV-1–specific T-cell responses. Although increases in HIV-1–specific immune responses have been observed in some studies, these have been quite modest *(41,42)*.

The HAART-induced increases in naive cells are encouraging, particularly if these cells can be educated to target HIV. Other recent studies suggest that there may also be restoration of a broader T-cell repertoire with HAART, although this has not always been observed *(43)*. Other recent studies also suggest that HAART may lead to recovery of functional immune responses to certain pathogens such as CMV.

Approaches to Augmenting HIV-Specific T-Helper Cell Responses

The fact that T-helper cell responses are associated with control of viremia, and the clear association between functional CTL responses and control of chronic viral infections provide compelling rationale for attempts to augment these responses in infected persons. One can hypothesize that restoration of these responses would lead to an increase in CTL responses, which in turn might lead to enhanced control of viremia. Although this remains a hypothesis without direct supporting evidence, a number of approaches are presently being pursued. Of approaches that can be implemented immediately, therapeutic vaccination may be the most promising *(44)*. A number of studies have already shown that whole inactivated viral vaccines as well as subunit vaccines can induce T-helper cell responses *(44)*. The fact that viremia can be controlled during the induction phase of immunization provides optimism that the responses induced may be inducible by a number of approaches presently being pursued. These include the use of subunit vaccines, whole inactivated, envelope-depleted vaccine, canarypox vectors, polynucleotide vaccines, and various combinations of these.

Other approachs that should be testable within the next year is the use of autologous dendritic cells that have been pulsed with either apoptotic cells or with soluble proteins *(45)*. Structured treatment interruption, designed to exposed the infected person to a regulated dose of replicating autologous virus, is another approach currently being tested, but for which there are concerns regarding the development of drug resistance.

An optimistic view is that restoring T-helper cell responses alone might lead to augmentation of effective CTL responses, particularly given that CTL may lack effector function in situations in which T help is limiting. However, the extent to which therapeutic vaccine approaches, or combinations of these approaches, will be effective will likely depend to the extent to which both CTL and T-helper cells can be induced.

Although there is enormous optimism regarding effective immune reconstitution, there are a number of potential obstacles. Not the least of these is the finding that even persons with long-term nonprogressing infection who have strong T-helper cell responses and CTL responses can progress after years of controlled infection. One observation of particular concern was the observed drop in CD4 cells in a long-term nonprogressor years after infection, which occurred in the absence of detectable rise in viremia *(46)*. This suggests that continued cellular destruction may be occurring even at undetectable viral loads, and indicates that long-term immune control will be a difficult challenge. Another potential obstacle for therapeutic vaccination related to what has been termed original antigenic sin. First described for antibody responses, recent studies suggest that a similar phenomenon may occur with T-cell responses. Basically, despite viral sequence variation and lack of ability of T cells to effectively recognize a new variant with mutation in the CTL epitope, there may be enough cross recognition to continue to sustain the now obsolete CTL response *(47)* Kalams, 1996 #1613. Such possibilities underscore the need to induce new immune responses.

CONCLUSIONS

The emerging view of HIV infection is that it is controlled by a partially effective immune response that wanes over time. The major measurable effectors contributing to control of viremia are CTLs, but for effective functioning these cells require virus-specific T-helper cells. All persons who become HIV infected have the capacity to generate T-helper cell responses, which can be reliably generated with successful therapy of acute infection. Although Gag is a major inducer of T-helper cell responses, other antigens likely also play a role. There is a clear rationale for attempts to boost HIV-specific T helper cell responses in persons with chronic infection, but the extent to which effective immunity can be restored remains to be determined. Nevertheless, the data accumulated thus far indicate that HIV follows the same biological rules that govern other viral infections, and identification of the defects in immunity are an important first step in the road to immune reconstitution.

REFERENCES

1. Goulder PJR, Rowland SL, McMichael AJ, Walker BD. Anti-HIV cellular immunity: recent advances towards vaccine design. AIDS 1999; 13:s121–s36.
2. Yang OO, Kalams SA, Rosenzweig M, Trocha A, Jones N, Koziel M, et al. Efficient lysis of human immunodeficiency virus type 1-infected cells by cytotoxic T lymphocytes. J Virol 1996; 70:5799–806.
3. Yang OO, Tran AC, Kalams SA, Johnson RP, Roberts MR, Walker BD. Lysis of HIV-1-infected cells and inhibition of viral replication by universal receptor T cells. Proc Natl Acad Sci USA 1997; 94:11478–83.
4. Klein MR, van Baalen CA, Holwerda AM, Kerkhof Garde SR, Bende RJ, Keet IP, et al. Kinetics of Gag-specific cytotoxic T lymphocyte responses during the clinical course of HIV-1 infection: a longitudinal analysis of rapid progressors and long-term asymptomatics. J Exp Med 1995; 181:1365–72.

5. Rinaldo C, Huang X-L, Fan Z, Ding M, Beltz L, Logar A, et al. High levels of anti-human immunodeficiency virus type 1 (HIV-1) memory cytotoxic T-lymphocyte activity and low viral load are associated with lack of disease in HIV-1-infected long-term nonprogressors. J Virol 1995; 69:5838–42.
6. Harrer T, Harrer E, Kalams SA, Barbosa P, Trocha A, Johnson RP, et al. Cytotoxic T lymphocytes in asymptomatic long-term nonprogressing HIV-1 infection. Breadth and specificity of the response and relation to in vivo viral quasispecies in a person with prolonged infection and low viral load. J Immunol 1996; 156:2616–23.
7. Kalams SA, Walker BD. The critical need for CD4 help in maintaining effective cytotoxic T lymphocyte responses [comment]. J Exp Med 1998; 188:2199–204.
8. Ahmed R, Butler LD, Bhatti L. $T4^+$ T helper cell function in vivo: differential requirement for induction of antiviral cytotoxic T-cell and antibody responses. J Virol 1988; 62:2102–6.
9. Rahemtulla A, Fung-Leung WP, Schilham MW, Kundig TM, Sambhara SR, Narendran A, et al. Normal development and function of $CD8^+$ cells but markedly decreased helper cell activity in mice lacking CD4. Nature 1991; 353:180–4.
10. Matloubian M, Concepcion RJ, Ahmed R. $CD4^+$ T cells are required to sustain $CD8^+$ cytotoxic T-cell responses during chronic viral infection. J Virol 1994; 68:8056–63.
11. Battegay M, Moskophidis D, Rahemtulla A, Hengartner H, Mak TW, Zinkernagel RM. Enhanced establishment of a virus carrier state in adult $CD4^+$ T-cell-deficient mice. J Virol 1994; 68:4700–4.
12. von Herrath MG, Yokoyama M, Dockter J, Oldstone MB, Whitton JL. CD4-deficient mice have reduced levels of memory cytotoxic T lymphocytes after immunization and show diminished resistance to subsequent virus challenge. J Virol 1996; 70:1072–9.
13. Cardin RD, Brooks JW, Sarawar SR, Doherty PC. Progressive loss of $CD8^+$ T cell-mediated control of a gamma-herpesvirus in the absence of $CD4^+$ T cells. J Exp Med 1996; 184:863–71.
14. Hasenkrug KJ, Brooks DM, Dittmer U. Critical role for CD4(+) T cells in controlling retrovirus replication and spread in persistently infected mice. J Virol 1998; 72:6559–64.
15. Gerlach JT, Diepolder HM, Jung MC, Gruener NH, Schraut WW, Zachoval R, et al. Recurrence of hepatitis C virus after loss of virus-specific CD4(+) T-cell response in acute hepatitis C [see comments]. Gastroenterology 1999; 117:933–41.
16. Bennett SR, Carbone FR, Karamalis F, Flavell RA, Miller JF, Heath WR. Help for cytotoxic-T-cell responses is mediated by CD40 signalling [see comments]. Nature 1998; 393:478–80.
17. Schoenberger SP, Toes RE, van der Voort EI, Offringa R, Melief CJ. T-cell help for cytotoxic T lymphocytes is mediated by CD40-CD40L interactions [see comments]. Nature 1998; 393:480–3.
18. Schmitz JE, Kuroda MJ, Santra S, Sasseville VG, Simon MA, Lifton MA, et al. Control of viremia in simian immunodeficiency virus infection by $CD8^+$ lymphocytes. Science 1999; 283:857–60.
19. Jin X, Bauer DE, Tuttleton SE, Lewin S, Gettie A, Blanchard J, et al. Dramatic Rise in plasma viremia after CD8(+) T cell depletion in simian immunodeficiency virus-infected macaques. J Exp Med 1999; 189:991–8.
20. Ogg GS, Jin X, Bonhoeffer S, Dunbar PR, Nowak MA, Monard S, et al. Quantitation of HIV-1-specific cytotoxic T lymphocytes and plasma load of viral RNA. Science 1998; 279:2103–6.
21. Koup RA, Hesselton RM, Safrit JT, Somasundaran M, Sullivan JL. Quantitative assessment of human immunodeficiency virus type 1 replication in human xenografts of acutely infected Hu-PBL-SCID mice. AIDS Res Hum Retrovir 1994; 10:279–84.
22. Borrow P, Lewicki H, Hahn BH, Shaw GM, Oldstone MBA. Virus-specific $CD8^+$ cytotoxic T-lymphocyte activity associated with control of viremia in primary human immunodeficiency virus type 1 infection. J. Virol 1994; 68:6103–10.

23. Rosenberg ES, Walker BD. HIV type 1-specific helper T cells: a critical host defense. AIDS Res Hum Retrovir 1998; 14:Suppl 2:S143–7.
24. Lane HC, Depper JM, Greene WC, Whalen G, Waldmann TA, Fauci AS. Qualitative analysis of immune function in patients with the acquired immunodeficiency syndrome. Evidence for a selective defect in soluble antigen recognition. N Engl J Med 1985; 313:79–84.
25. Clerici M, Stocks NI, Zajac RA, Boswell RN, Bernstein DC, Mann DL, et al. Interleukin-2 production used to detect antigenic peptide recognition by T-helper lymphocytes from asymptomatic HIV-seropositive individuals. Nature 1989; 339:383–5.
26. Schwartz D, Sharma U, Busch M, Weinhold K, Matthews T, Lieberman J, et al. Absence of recoverable infectious virus and unique immune responses in an asymptomatic HIV^+ long-term survivor. AIDS Res Hum Retrovir 1994; 10:1703–11.
27. Rosenberg ES, Billingsley JM, Caliendo AM, Boswell SL, Sax PE, Kalams SA, et al. Vigorous HIV-1-specific $CD4^+$ T cell responses associated with control of viremia. Science 1997; 278:1447–50.
28. Kalams SA, Buchbinder SP, Rosenberg ES, Billingsley JM, Colbert DS, Jones NG, et al. Association between virus-specific cytotoxic T-lymphocyte and helper responses in human immunodeficiency virus type 1 infection. J Virol 1999; 73:6715–20.
29. Pitcher CJ, Quittner C, Peterson DM, Connors M, Koup RA, Maino VC, et al. HIV-1-specific $CD4^+$ T cells are detectable in most individuals with active HIV-1 infection, but decline with prolonged viral suppression [see comments]. Nat Med 1999; 5:518–25.
30. Gauduin MC, Glickman RL, Ahmad S, Yilma T, Johnson RP. Characterization of SIV-specific $CD4^+$ T-helper proliferative responses in macaques immunized with live-attenuated SIV. J Med Primatol 1999; 28:233–41.
31. Abbas AK. Die and let live: eliminating dangerous lymphocytes. [Review] [15 refs]. Cell 1996; 84:655–7.
32. Milich DR, Linsley PS, Hughes JL, Jones JE. Soluble CTLA-4 can suppress autoantibody production and elicit long term unresponsiveness in a novel transgenic model. J Immunol 1994; 153:429–35.
33. Moskophidis D, Lechner F, Pircher H, Zinkernagel RM. Virus persistence in acutely infected immunocompetent mice by exhaustion of antiviral cytotoxic effector T cells [see comments]. Nature 1993; 362:758–61.
34. Klenerman P, Meier UC, Phillips RE, McMichael AJ. The effects of natural altered peptide ligands on the whole blood cytotoxic T lymphocyte response to human immunodeficiency virus. Eur J Immunol 1995; 25:1927–31.
35. Liang TJ, Rehermann B, Seeff LB, Hoofnagle JH. Pathogenesis, natural history, treatment, and prevention of hepatitis C. Ann Intern Med 2000; 132:296–305.
36. Neumann AU, Lam NP, Dahari H, Gretch DR, Wiley TE, Layden TJ, et al. Hepatitis C viral dynamics in vivo and the antiviral efficacy of interferon-alpha therapy. Science 1998; 282:103–7.
37. Cooper S, Erickson AL, Adams EJ, Kansopon J, Weiner AJ, Chien DY, et al. Analysis of a successful immune response against hepatitis C virus. Immunity 1999; 10:439–49.
38. Lisziewicz J, Rosenberg E, Lieberman J, Jessen H, Lopalco L, Siliciano R, et al. Control of HIV despite the discontinuation of antiretroviral therapy [letter]. N Engl J Med 1999; 340:1683–4.
39. Ortiz. Containment of breakthrough HIV plasma viremia in the absence of antiretroviral therapy is associated with a broad and vigorous HIV-specific CTL response. In: 6th Conference on Retroviruses and Opportunistic Infections, 1999; Chicago, 1999.
40. Autran B, Carcelain G, Li TS, Blanc C, Mathez D, Tubiana R, et al. Positive effects of combined antiretroviral therapy on $CD4^+$ T cell homeostasis and function in advanced HIV disease. Science 1997; 277:112–6.
41. Kelleher AD, Carr A, Zaunders J, Cooper DA. Alterations in the immune response of human immunodeficiency virus (HIV)-infected subjects treated with an HIV-specific protease inhibitor, ritonavir. J Infect Dis 1996; 173:321–9.

42. Angel JB, Kumar A, Parato K, Filion LG, Diaz-Mitoma F, Daftarian P, et al. Improvement in cell-mediated immune function during potent anti-human immunodeficiency virus therapy with ritonavir plus saquinavir. J Infect Dis 1998; 177:898–904.
43. Connors M, Kovacs JA, Krevat S, Gea-Banacloche JC, Sneller MC, Flanigan M, et al. HIV infection induces changes in CD4+ T-cell phenotype and depletions within the CD4+ T-cell repertoire that are not immediately restored by antiviral or immune-based therapies [see comments]. Nat Med 1997; 3:533–40.
44. Gotch F, Hardy G, Imami N. Therapeutic vaccines in HIV.1 infection. Immunol Rev 1999; 170:173–82.
45. Dhodapkar MV, Steinman RM, Sapp M, Desai H, Fossella CF, Krasovsky J, et al. Rapid generation of broad T-cell immunity in humans after a single injection of maturation dendritic cells. J Clin Invest 1999; 104:173–80.
46. Greenough TC, Sullivan JL, Desrosiers RC. Declining CD4 T-cell counts in a person infected with nef-deleted HIV-1 [letter]. N Engl J Med 1999; 340:236–7.
47. Klenerman P, Zinkernagel RM. Original antigenic sin impairs cytotoxic T lymphocyte responses to viruses bearing variant epitopes [see comments]. Nature 1998; 394:482–5.

11
Immune Responses to Nonhuman Primate Lentiviruses

Amitinder Kaur, Marie-Claire Gauduin, and R. Paul Johnson

INTRODUCTION

The primate subgroup of lentiviruses is made up of an expanding number of related viruses that display a remarkably diverse range of effects on their hosts. At present, 18 different primate lentiviruses have been described in naturally infected African primates, and more are likely to be identified *(1)*. Five main groupings of primate lentiviruses have been described: human immunodeficiency virus type 1 (HIV-1)/simian immunodeficiency virus (SIV)cpz, HIV-2/SIVsm, SIVagm, SIVsykes, and SIVmandrill. Each of these groups can be further subdivided into different subgroups, which are named according to the species in which they were identified (Table 1). Primate lentiviruses share similar genetic organization and have similar biological characteristics, such as the use of CD4 as a primary receptor for virus entry, tropism for $CD4^+$ T lymphocytes, and the ability to induce chronic, persistent infection *(2)*.

However, the outcome of infection with primate lentiviruses varies widely. In their natural hosts, primate lentiviruses are generally nonpathogenic. For instance, sooty mangabeys, a species found in West Africa that is naturally infected with SIVsm, maintain relatively high levels of viremia (10^5–10^7 RNA copies per milliliter of plasma) *(3)* yet remain healthy without $CD4^+$ T-cell depletion or immunodeficiency. Similarly, SIV can be readily cultured from African green monkeys, another naturally infected species that exhibits no signs of SIV-induced immunodeficiency *(4)*. Indirect evidence suggests the natural hosts of primate lentiviruses have been infected for extended periods of time. For instance, the genetic phylogeny of the SIVagm subgroups closely parallels that of the geographically distinct subfamilies of African green monkeys, an observation that supports the conclusion that African green monkeys have been infected with SIVagm for thousands of years and that each subspecies of virus has coevolved with the subspeciation of the host *(1)*.

In multiple instances, induction of acquired immune deficiency syndrome (AIDS) by primate lentiviruses has occurred as a result of transmission of a primate lentivirus from its natural host to a susceptible species. AIDS has occurred following transmission of SIVsm from sooty mangabeys to captive Asian macaques (resulting in SIVmac) *(5)* and most likely to humans (resulting in HIV-2) *(6)*. Similarly, based on phyloge-

From: *Retroviral Immunology: Immune Response and Restoration*
Edited by: Giuseppe Pantaleo and Bruce D. Walker © Humana Press Inc., Totowa, NJ

Table 1
Classification of Primate Lentiviruses

Virus	Species infected
SIVcpz	
HIV-1	Human
SIVcpz	Chimpanzee *(Pan troglodytes troglodytes, P. troglodytes schweinfurthii)*
SIVsm	
HIV-2	Human
SIVmac	Macaques *(Macaca mulatta, M. fascicularis, M. nemestrina)*
SIVsm	Sooty mangabey *(Cercocebus atys)*
SIVagm	
SIVagmGri	Grivet monkey *(Chlorocebus aethiops)*
SIVagmSab	Green monkey *(C. sabaeus)*
SIVagmTan	Tantalus monkey *(C. tantalus)*
SIVagm Ver	Vervet monkey *(C. pygerythrus)*
SIVmnd	
SIVmnd	Mandrill *(Mandrillus sphinx)*
SIVlhoest	L'Hoest monkey *(Cercopithecus lhoesti)*
SIVsun	Sun-tailed monkey *(C. solatus)*
SIVsyk	Sykes' Monkey *(Cercopithecus albogularis)*

Viruses are grouped based on phylogenetic lineages (see ref. *1* for detailed listing) and do not include a number of nonhuman lentiviruses for which detailed sequence and phylogenetic information is not yet available. HIV-1, HIV-2, and SIVmac arose as the result of relatively recent cross-species transmission. The other viruses listed are likely to have coevolved with their hosts for extended periods of time and do not appear to induce disease in their natural hosts.

netic similarities and geographic distribution, HIV-1 is believed to have originated as a result of cross-species transmission of SIVcpz from chimpanzees to humans *(1,7)*.

Experimental analysis of infection of nonhuman primates with SIV has become an increasingly valuable tool for AIDS research *(8)*. Dissection of immune responses to SIV infection in natural hosts and comparison of these responses to those in hosts that develop AIDS may shed light on mechanisms of immunodeficiency. Nonhuman primate models have also been extensively utilized for the evaluation of AIDS vaccines *(9)* and for analysis of AIDS pathogenesis. Nonhuman primate studies have also proved useful in the analysis of therapeutic strategies for AIDS, including efforts to reconstitute immune function *(10)*.

All of these factors have heightened the importance of expanding our knowledge of immune responses to primate lentiviruses in nonhuman primates. This chapter addresses studies on immune responses in the setting of experimental lentivirus infection of nonhuman primates, as well as the more limited studies on the natural hosts of SIV. AIDS vaccine studies in macaques and chimpanzees are not discussed in detail; several recent reviews have addressed this topic *(11,12)*.

MACAQUES

Rhesus macaques *(Macaca mulatta)* are Old World primates of Asian origin. Although infection with primate lentiviruses is common among African nonhuman primates, Asian nonhuman primates,including macaques, are not naturally infected with SIV *(1)*. Two years after the discovery of HIV in humans *(13)*, reports of outbreaks of opportunistic infections in captive macaques at the New England and California Regional Primate Centers in the early 1980s led to the description of simian AIDS and subsequent identification of SIVmac *(14)*. The relatively close phylogenetic relationship of SIVmac with SIVsm suggested the possibility that sooty mangabeys may have transmitted SIVsm to rhesus macaques while in captivity. Although it has not been possible to document a specific event that resulted in the cross-species transmission leading to SIVmac, inoculation of rhesus macaques with tissue homogenates from sooty mangabeys at the Tulane Regional Primate Research Center independently produced a pathogenic virus (SIVsmDelta B670) that is similar to SIVmac *(15)*.

A variety of different Asian macaque species have been used for AIDS research, including rhesus macaques *(Macaca mulatta)*, cynomolgus macaques *(M. fascicularis)*, and pig-tailed macaques *(M. nemestrina)*. Multiple different viruses have also been used for infection of macaques, including SIVmac, SIVsm, and HIV-2 strains. HIV-1 does not infect Asian macaques, except for pig-tailed macaques, who develop low viral loads without immunodeficiency *(16)*. The specific virus and species chosen for study can have dramatic effects on disease progression. For instance, SIVmac-induced disease is usually slower in cynomolgus macaques than rhesus macaques. Newer chimeric lentiviruses (designated SHIVs) have been created by inserting the HIV-1 envelope into a pathogenic molecular clone of SIVmac, thereby allowing analysis of HIV-1 envelope vaccines in rhesus macaques. The pathogenicity of SHIVs varies widely from nonpathogenic viruses with relatively low virus loads *(17)* to highly pathogenic viruses leading to $CD4^+$ T-cell depletion in <4 wk *(18)*. Of these various models, the most commonly used and best characterized model with respect to disease course and immune responses is that of rhesus macaques infected with SIVmac, and the subsequent discussion focuses on this model.

Clinical Manifestations of SIVmac Infection

SIVmac exhibits a number of similarities to HIV, including a comparable genetic organization, tropism for $CD4^+$ T lymphocytes and macrophages, and the requirement of specific coreceptors for virus entry *(2)*. The clinical course of SIV infection in macaques is generally similar to that of HIV-1 infection in humans, although with a more rapid rate of progression. For commonly used pathogenic strains of SIVmac in rhesus macaques, average survival is 12–24 mo, compared with 10 yr in untreated HIV-infected people *(2)*. After either intravenous or mucosal infection, an initial burst of plasma viremia is generally seen 9–16 d after infection, followed by a widespread dissemination of the virus and the development of virus-specific immune responses *(19)*. One to three weeks after SIV infection, macaques develop a transient rash on the face, trunk, and groin that is similar to that described in HIV-1–infected humans in early infection *(20)*. Macaques may also develop transient axillary and inguinal lymphadenopathy, followed by immune abnormalities similar to those seen in HIV-infected individuals *(21)*. The absolute $CD4^+$ T-cell number in peripheral blood gradually declines over time and an AIDS-like disease state develops *(14,21,22)*. Macaques typically die with weight loss, diarrhea, and opportunistic infections such as disseminated cytomegalovirus, *Mycobacterium avium*, and *Pneumocystis carinii* pneumonia. Other common disease manifestations include encephalitis and lymphoid malignancies *(23)*.

Immune Responses in SIV-infected Macaques

Phenotypic Analysis of Lymphocyte Subsets

Many of the observed changes in lymphocyte subsets in SIV-infected macaques mirror those in HIV-infected people. Acute SIV infection results in a transient decrease in circulating $CD4^+$ T lymphocytes followed by a rebound and a subsequent increase in the percentage of $CD8^+$ T cells in peripheral blood *(19)*. Depletion of $CD4^+$ T lymphocytes following infection with pathogenic strains of SIVmac generally occurs over a period of 2–12 mo and is ultimately accompanied by a disruption of T-cell homeostasis resulting in decreases in all circulating $CD3^+$ lymphocytes *(19,24)*, as has been reported in HIV-infected human subjects progressing to AIDS *(25)*. However, there are several notable differences in lymphocyte subset changes in lentivirus-infected humans and monkeys. Increases in expression of CD38 on lymphocytes, which occurs during HIV infection and has equal or better prognostic value than $CD4^+$ T-cell counts or viral load *(26)*, have not been observed in SIV-infected macaques *(24,27)*. Similarly, although HIV infection in humans is associated with a loss of naive phenotype $CD4^+$ and $CD8^+$ lymphocytes expressing both CD45RA and CD62L *(28)*, SIV-infected macaques develop a selective loss of $CD45RA^-$ memory phenotype lymphocytes, resulting in an enrichment or preservation of $CD45RA^+$ $CD62L^+$ cells *(24,29)*.

Humoral Responses

As in HIV-infected humans *(30)*, virus-binding antibodies arise early in the course of SIV infection, shortly after the peak in viral replication *(19)*. The kinetics of neutralizing antibody responses in SIV-infected macaques are dependent on the specific assay employed. Using a SIVmac strain that is relatively susceptible to neutralization, neutralizing antibody responses can be detected within 3–5 wk after infection with pathogenic SIVmac strains, whereas antibodies able to neutralize more resistant strains of virus (e.g., SIVmac239) either never develop or are present only at low titer after 6 mo or more *(19,31)*. Several changes in the characteristics of virus-specific antibodies occur during the course of SIV infection, including increases in the titer of virus-binding antibodies, increases in the avidity of antibodies, and a decrease in the ratio of antibodies able to recognize conformational vs linear epitopes *(32)*. These changes, which have also been observed in HIV-infected humans, have been termed a maturation of the SIV-specific antibody response and, in animals infected with attenuated SIV strains, appear to correlate temporally with the onset of protective immunity *(33)*.

SIV-Specific CTL Responses

Using standard ^{51}Cr-release assays, SIV-specific cytolytic T lymphocyte (CTL) activity can be detected as early as 7 d after SIV infection *(19)* and generally peaks coincident with the decline in plasma viremia, similar to the pattern observed in acute HIV infection *(34)*. SIV-specific CTL activity is mediated by classical $CD8^+$ lymphocytes, which lyse target cells in a major histocompatibility complex (MHC)-restricted manner, although lysis of target cells expressing envelope may take place by both MHC-restricted and unrestricted pathways *(35)*. As is characteristic of HIV-specific

CTL responses, the SIV-specific CTL response is generally polyclonal and is directed against multiple SIV proteins, including Gag, Pol, Env, Nef, and Rev *(36)*. A number of different SIV-specific CTL epitopes have been identified, including a relatively immunodominant peptide (p11 C-M) *(37)* in Gag that is restricted by the Mamu-A*01 class I molecule, which is present in about 30% of rhesus macaques. Analysis of SIV-specific $CD8^+$ responses using tetramers of the Mamu-A*01 molecule complexed with peptide p11 C-M have proved to be a rapid and quantitative means to assess cell-mediated immune responses in macaques *(38)*.

A number of observations strongly suggest that $CD8^+$ T lymphocytes play a key role in inhibiting SIV replication in vivo. These include: (1) The close temporal association between the onset of CTL activity and the decline in plasma viremia in acute SIV infection *(19)*, (2) positive correlations between the strength of SIV-specific CTL responses and prolonged survival *(39)*, (3) the strong selective pressure for the emergence of escape mutations in SIV CTL epitopes *(40)*, and (4) the observed increases in plasma viremia following transient in vivo depletion of $CD8^+$ lymphocytes using monoclonal antibodies *(41,42)*.

$CD8^+$ T-Lymphocyte–Mediated Antiviral Activity

Two years after the initial report that $CD8^+$ T lymphocytes from HIV-infected humans could inhibit viral replication *(43)*, a report appeared documenting similar activity in SIV-infected macaques *(44)*. As in HIV infection, this $CD8^+$-lymphocyte–mediated activity consists of at least two components: an MHC-restricted activity that occurs when $CD8^+$ cells are in direct contact with infected cells and an MHC-unrestricted activity that is mediated by soluble factors *(45,46)*. Although it is clear that SIV-specific CTL are able to inhibit SIV replication *(45,46)*, it is not known whether a population of $CD8^+$ cells exists that is able to inhibit viral replication but is not able to mediate CTL activity. $CD8^+$ T-lymphocyte–mediated antiviral activity has been described in animals infected with wild-type pathogenic SIV strains, as well as attenuated SIV strains and vaccinated animals *(45–47)*. Inhibition of SIV replication by soluble factors is in part mediated by the β-chemokines RANTES, MIP-1α, and MIP-1β, and there appear to be factors other than these β-chemokines that mediate inhibition of SIV replication *(46,48)*. In several studies, production of β-chemokines by stimulated $CD8^+$ lymphocytes from vaccinated macaques has correlated with protection against challenge *(48,49)*. However, the precise nature of the $CD8^+$ lymphocyte population mediating this activity and the immunologic mechanisms involved in the induction of this response by vaccines that do not typically induce CTL responses remain to be defined.

$CD4^+$ T-Helper Responses

As in most HIV-infected people *(50)*, macaques infected with pathogenic strains of SIV generally have low to absent SIV-specific proliferative responses *(51,52)* (Fig. 1). The absence of these responses appears directly related to high levels of SIV replication. Macaques infected with either attenuated SIV strains *(52,53)* or a nonpathogenic strain of HIV-2 *(51)* develop SIV-specific proliferative responses, which in the case of animals infected with the attenuated virus SIVmac239Δnef, can be quite vigorous with stimulation indices exceeding 60 (Fig. 1). SIV-specific proliferative responses have also been detected following antiretroviral therapy early in the course of SIV infection

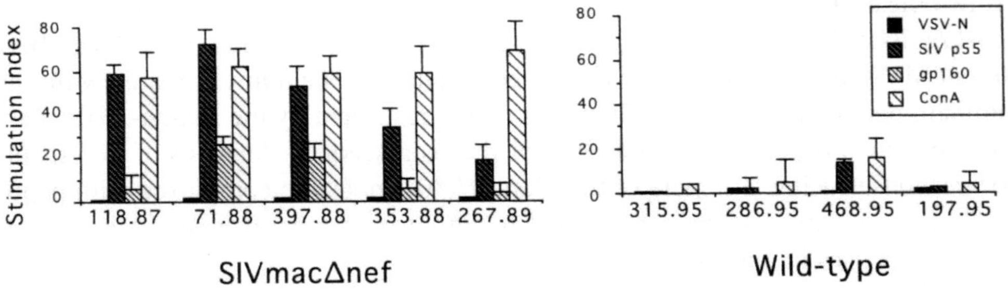

Fig. 1. Absence of SIV-specific proliferative responses in animals infected with pathogenic SIV strains. Proliferative responses to SIV antigens were assessed using a standard [^{3}H] thymidine incorporation assay. Data are modified from *(52)*.

(54). Loss of SIV-specific T helper responses may occur as a result of cytopathic infection of CD4$^+$ T cells by SIV-infected antigen-presenting cells, a phenomenon that has been described in vitro for HIV-infected antigen presenting cells *(54a)*. This scenario is supported by the observation that vaccinated macaques that had SIV-specific proliferative responses prior to challenge with pathogenic SIVmac and were not protected, lost these responses *(51,55)*. Only limited data are available on cytokine responses in macaques infected with pathogenic SIV strains. Assessment of responses by either reverse transcriptase-polymerase chain reaction (RT-PCR) or intracellular cytokine staining suggest that transient, low level interleukin-2 (IL-2) and interferon-γ (IFN-γ) responses are generated during acute SIV infection, in some cases in association with IL-4 and IL-10 as well *(24,56)*. In contrast, animals chronically infected with live attenuated SIV have a strong and sustained T helper-1 (Th1) response, characterized by production of IL-2, IFN-γ, and the β-chemokines MIP-1α, MIP-1β, and RANTES following antigen-specific stimulation *(52)*.

Protective Immunity

Considerable effort has been expended to determine which specific immune responses are able to protect against lentivirus infection in the macaque model. However, this effort has been complicated by several factors. AIDS vaccine trials in monkeys have been carried out using a diverse array of different species and viruses. Protection can readily be achieved using relatively nonpathogenic and easy-to-neutralize SIV strains, but has been quite challenging to induce using difficult-to-neutralize strains that are more characteristic of primary HIV-1 isolates. Examination of the role of cellular immune responses in protective immunity has been significantly constrained by the inability to perform adoptive transfer experiments and the limited ability to deplete specific lymphocyte subsets in vivo using murine monoclonal antibodies. In addition, the correlates of protection are likely to vary depending on the specific virus and species selected for study, the route of challenge (intravenous vs mucosal), the specific vaccine approach, and a variety of other factors.

Neutralizing Antibodies

Multiple properties of primate lentiviruses confound the ability of antibodies to neutralize viral replication. These include oligomerization of the viral envelope, extensive glycosylation which serves to inhibit antibody recognition of gp120, the fact that most virus-specific antibodies recognize monomeric forms of gp120 (viral debris), the relative inaccessibility of critical functional domains of gp120 to antibodies, and the considerable antigenic variation that occurs in the most antigenic domains of envelope *(57,58)*. Not surprisingly, antibody-mediated protection has been relatively difficult to obtain, although it has been observed in selective circumstances such as chimpanzees challenged with HIV-1 *(59)* and macaques challenged with nonpathogenic or easy-to-neutralize strains of SIV or SHIV *(60,61)*. Protection against pathogenic SHIV strains or against a SHIV strain expressing the envelope of a primary HIV-1 isolate has been demonstrated, but has required either high-titer neutralizing antibodies *(62)* or a cocktail of HIV-1–specific neutralizing antibodies *(63)*, which are atypical of responses generated either with natural infection or following vaccination. In the setting of challenge with pathogenic strains of SIV that are relatively resistant to neutralization, passive transfer experiments using polyclonal antiserum have generally been unsuccessful *(64,65)*, although there are exceptions *(66)*. However, infusion of immunoglobulin from an SIV-infected long term nonprogressor macaque immediately after SIV infection has resulted in lower levels of viral replication and improved survival *(67)*. In addition, reports of a correlation between protection induced by attenuated SIV and either neutralizing antibodies *(68)* or the development of high titer, high avidity antibodies *(33,66)* have supported a role for antibody responses in protective immunity. Taken together, these data suggest that induction of antibody responses able to neutralize pathogenic SIV strains is difficult to achieve, but that antibody responses may play a role in preventing or containing SIV infection in selected circumstances.

However, there are multiple instances where protection against challenge has been demonstrated in the absence of neutralizing antibodies against the challenge strain. Many of these involve the use of chimeric viruses expressing highly divergent envelope proteins. For instance, animals vaccinated with attenuated SIVmac strains are relatively resistant to infection with SHIV strains expressing the HIV-1 envelope *(69,70)* or to a SIV-murine leukemia virus hybrid *(71)*. Conversely, immunization with a nonpathogenic SHIV strain resulted in protection from vaginal challenge with SIVmac *(72)*. In each of these cases, absolute or relative protection was observed in the absence of detectable neutralizing antibodies. Finally, immunization with the highly attenuated strain SIVmac239Δ4, which does not induce any detectable neutralizing antibody responses, has resulted in partial protection against vaginal challenge with SIVmac251 *(73)*.

CTL Responses

The ability of attenuated SIV strains to induce protection against heterologous viruses in the absence of neutralizing antibodies has suggested the possibility that CTL directed against the SIVmac backbone shared by the attenuated virus and the chimeric SHIV may play a significant role in mediating protection. Further observations that support a role for CTL responses include the fact that induction of an early, strong SIV-specific CTL responses in SIVmac239Δ4-vaccinated animals was associated with protection *(73)* and that less protection against challenge was observed using a virus (SIVsmE660) with a heterologous backbone that is less likely to be recognized by CTL specific for structural proteins such as Gag and Pol. A correlation between CTL activity and protection has also been observed in nonpathogenic SHIV-immunized animals vaginally challenged with SIVmac239 and in animals mucosally exposed to subinfectious doses of HIV-2 *(74)* or SIV *(75)*. An inverse correlation between the level of CTL activity induced by a recombinant vaccinia virus expressing SIV Nef and the levels of viremia after challenge has also been observed *(76)*. Taken together, these observations support a role for CTL in protective immunity. However, CTL responses alone are not sufficient to mediate protection *(77)*, and more definitive studies on the role of $CD8^+$ T cells in vaccine-mediated protection need to be carried out, such as the depletion of $CD8^+$ cells in vaccinated animals with monoclonal antibodies *(41,42)*.

SOOTY MANGABEYS

Natural History of SIV Infection in Sooty Mangabeys

Sooty mangabeys *(Cercocebus atys)* are Old World primates indigenous to Central and West Africa that naturally harbor SIV without developing AIDS *(78)*. SIV infection is widely prevalent in free-ranging feral sooty mangabeys *(79)* and captive sooty mangabeys housed at zoos and regional primate research centers in the United States *(78,80)*. Seroprevalence rates of SIV infection in captive sooty mangabeys range between 30% and 62% *(15,78,80)*. The colony of captive sooty mangabeys at the Yerkes Regional Primate Research Center was established with wild-born animals in 1968; SIV seropositivity was documented in sera collected as early as 1981 and so far, immunodeficiency has not been documented in SIV-infected sooty mangabeys (*81* and H. McClure, personal communication). The rate of seroprevalence increases with age and is higher among female mangabeys *(78)*. In this serosurvey, >80% of mangabeys >5 yr of age were SIV seropositive, while <20% of mangabeys <1 yr of age were seropositive *(78)*. The pattern of SIV infection in sooty mangabeys, that of commonly being prevalent in adults and uncommon or absent in juveniles and infants, suggests that horizontal transmission, probably via the sexual route, is the common mode of natural intraspecies transmission *(78,79)*.

Why Do SIV-Infected Sooty Mangabeys Not Develop AIDS?

Despite investigation of viral and host factors, the basis for nonpathogenic SIV infection in sooty mangabeys has not been established. In HIV-infected humans and SIV-infected rhesus macaques, disease progression is positively correlated with the level of viral replication *(82,83)*. In contrast, sooty mangabeys maintain a high level of set-point viremia and yet remain asymptomatic. Thus, their disease-resistant state is not due to decreased susceptibility to infection or effective control of viral replication.

VIRAL FACTORS

Analysis of the virologic characteristics of SIVsm infection in sooty mangabeys have not revealed any obvious factors that account for the lack of disease in its natural host. SIV isolates from asymptomatic sooty mangabeys are pathogenic and induce AIDS when inoculated into rhesus *(M. mulatta)* and pig-tailed *(M. nemestrina)* macaques *(84)*. Levels of plasma viral RNA in naturally infected sooty mangabeys range between 10^5 and 10^7 copies/mL and approximate those detected in SIV-infected macaques with end-stage AIDS *(3,24)*. SIV can be easily isolated from peripheral blood mononuclear cells (PBMCs) and plasma of naturally infected sooty mangabeys *(85)*. Moreover, CD4+ T lymphocytes and macrophages of sooty mangabeys support SIV replication in vitro to the same or greater extent than cells from rhesus macaques *(86)*. There is also evidence for a rapid turnover of virus-producing cells in naturally SIV-infected mangabeys, as demonstrated by a rapid decline in plasma viremia after administration of the potent antiviral drug (R)–9–(2–phosphonylmethoxypropyl) adenine (PMPA) (R. Grant et al; unpublished data). In this study, the mean half-life of virus-producing cells in the initial rapid decay phase was 0.8 d, which is comparable to that reported in SIV-infected macaques and HIV-infected humans *(87,88)*. Thus, the absence of immunodeficiency in the presence of a high viral load in SIV-infected sooty mangabeys is not due to noncytopathic infection or a slow, low level of viral replication.

HOST FACTORS

Chemokine Receptor Usage

Differences in coreceptor usage of alterations in the CD4 molecule do not account for the lack of disease progression in sooty mangabeys *(89–91)*. Since disease does not occur despite high levels of viral replication, it seems unlikely that host "resistance" genes that confer decreased susceptibility to SIV infection would play a major role in preventing immunodeficiency in sooty mangabeys. Similar to SIVmac isolates, primary SIVsm isolates use CCR5, BOB and Bonzo coreceptors for infection *(89)*. However, unlike SIVmac, they replicate poorly in CEMx174 cells *(89)*. The sequence of the CCR5 molecule from sooty mangabeys is highly homologous to those in rhesus macaques and humans *(89,91)*. Sooty mangabeys have a second allele of CCR5 that has a 24-bp deletion (CCR5Δ24). Heterozygotes for this allele have reduced surface expression of CCR5, yet their viral loads are comparable to mangabeys homozygous for wild-type CCR5 *(91)*. The allelic frequency of heterozygous CCR5Δ24 ranges between 0.04% and 4.1% *(91,92)*, making it an unlikely contributor to resistance against infection. Homozygous CCR5Δ24 with a high allelic frequency of 86.6% is found in red-capped sooty mangabeys *(92)*. However, such mangabeys are also SIV-infected and their SIV isolates efficiently use CCR2b instead of CCR5 as a coreceptor *(92)*.

Immune Responses in SIV-Infected Sooty Mangabeys

An expanding body of evidence over the past decade has provided a detailed characterization of both humoral and cellular immune responses in SIV-infected sooty mangabeys. A number of differences between SIV-infected mangabeys and macaques have been described, including differences in lymphocyte phenotype, neutralizing antibody, and CTL responses.

Phenotypic Analysis of Lymphocyte Subsets

Although sooty mangabeys naturally infected with SIV do not develop AIDS, infection with SIV does manifest in some perturbation of T lymphocyte subsets in mangabeys. In a cross-sectional analysis, lower percentages of circulating CD4+ T lymphocytes and naive CD4+ and CD8+ T lymphocytes were observed in naturally SIV-infected sooty mangabeys as compared to uninfected animals (Table 2). However, in contrast to SIV-infected rhesus macaques, SIV-infected sooty mangabeys main-

Table 2
Phenotype of Peripheral Blood Lymphocytes in Normal and SIV-Infected Sooty Managabeys and Rhesus Macaques

	Sooty mangabey		Rhesus macaque	
	SIV^-	$^aSIV^+$	SIV^-	$^bSIV^+$
	(n = 7)	(n = 11)	(n = 8)	(n = 3)
Percent lymphocytes that are				
$CD3^+$	67.6 ± 3.4	72.9 ± 10.8	72.8 ± 4.9	51.3 ± 18.5
$CD4^+$	45.9 ± 6.6	25.6 ± 8.4	43.4 ± 5.0	12.3 ± 6.4
$CD3^+8^+$	34.1 ± 5.8	38.6 ± 6.7	27.5 ± 4.5	35.7 ± 13.8
$CD3^+4^-8^-$	13.7 ± 2.4	14.7 ± 4.9	4.6 ± 6.0	10.0 ± 5.6
NK ($CD3^-8^+$)	2.4 ± 1.0	4.4 ± 2.4	10.5 ± 6.4	16.3 ± 15.5
Percent $CD3^+8^+$ that are				
$CD45RA^+CD62L^+$	54.1 ± 10.6	24.5 ± 10.6	36.3 ± 16.1	24.0 ± 8.0
$CD45RA^-CD62L^-$	14.4 ± 5.3	23.2 ± 8.6	19.3 ± 8.6	11.0 ± 10.0
$CD45RA^+CD62L^-$	28.9 ± 7.1	46.8 ± 13.8	37.0 ± 7.4	61.3 ± 2.1
$CD45RA^-CD62L^+$	2.6 ± 0.5	5.9 ± 5.4	7.8 ± 5.2	2.5 ± 2.5
Percent $CD4^+$ that are				
$CD45RA^+CD62L^+$	73.7 ± 3.9	34.7 ± 13.3	30.3 ± 10.9	35.0 ± 10.8
$CD45RA^-CD62L^-$	9.1 ± 1.2	23.1 ± 7.5	26.6 ± 6.4	13.3 ± 9.8
$CD45RA^+CD62L^-$	8.4 ± 2.6	33.2 ± 13.4	10.7 ± 3.4	49.7 ± 4.2
$CD45RA^-CD62L^+$	8.7 ± 2.0	9.4 ± 4.9	32.4 ± 8.2	2.7 ± 2.5

[a] Naturally SIV-infected sooty mangabeys.

[b] SIVmac239-infected rhesus macaques infected for more than 8 mo.

tained T-cell homeostasis, as evidenced by a normal fraction of $CD3^+$ T lymphocytes (Table 2 and *93*).

Several phenotypic differences between lymphocytes of uninfected rhesus macaques and sooty mangabeys have been described. These include an elevated $CD8^+$ T-lymphocyte count, lower CD4/CD8 ratio, and a higher frequency of CD25 and HLA-DR expressing $CD8^+$ T lymphocytes in sooty mangabeys as compared with rhesus macaques *(94)*. More recent studies *(24)* using three- and four-color flow cytometry have revealed several additional differences between uninfected sooty mangabeys and rhesus macaques, including: (1) an expanded population of $CD3^+CD4^-CD8^-$ lymphocytes in uninfected sooty mangabeys, (2) a lower percentage of $CD3^-CD8^+$ natural killer (NK) cells in sooty mangabeys, and (3) a greater fraction of naive phenotype ($CD45RA^+CD62L^+$) $CD4^+$ and $CD8^+$ T lymphocytes in uninfected adult sooty mangabeys compared to adult rhesus macaques (Table 2). It is not clear how these phenotypic differences may contribute to apathogenic infection. The observation of a significant population of double negative T lymphocytes in sooty mangabeys is intriguing. Such double-negative T lymphocytes are rarely seen in normal macaques *(24)*. In humans, a subset of this population is characterized by an oligoclonal T-cell receptor (TCR) repertoire, usage of an invariant TCR Vα chain, secretion of both Th2 (IL-4) and Th1 (INF-γ) cytokines, and recognition of the nonpolymorphic MHC class I-like CD1d molecules *(95)*.

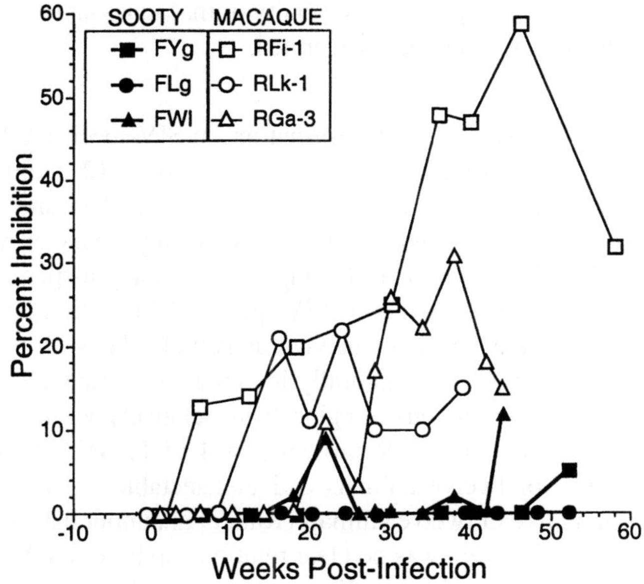

Fig. 2. Longitudinal analysis of neutralizing antibodies to SIV in three sooty mangabeys and three rhesus macaques infected with SIVmac239. Percent inhibition of SIVmac239 with sera at 1:20 dilution is shown. Reproduced with permission from *(24)*.

Humoral Immunity

In naturally infected mangabeys, virus-specific antibodies have been readily identified by ELISA using whole HIV-2 *(85)*. Antibody titers were relatively low compared to SIV-infected rhesus macaques with high viral loads *(85)*. By Western blot or radioimmunoprecipitation assays, sera from naturally SIV-infected sooty mangabeys cross-reacted with most SIV proteins, and the pattern was similar to that obtained with sera from SIV-infected rhesus and pig-tailed macaques *(78)*.

Early studies on sooty mangabeys reported weak or undetectable neutralizing antibodies to SIV in naturally SIV-infected sooty mangabeys using standard neutralization assays *(81,85)*. In a more recent study, we evaluated SIV-specific neutralizing antibodies using a sensitive assay that detects SIV replication using cells containing a reporter gene (secreted alkaline phosphatase) under the control of a Tat-responsive promoter *(96)*. SIV-specific neutralizing antibodies were evaluated longitudinally in sooty mangabeys and rhesus macaques infected with SIVmac239. Neutralizing antibodies to SIVmac239 were not detected in the sera of any of three SIVmac239-infected sooty mangabeys up to 1 yr after SIV infection *(24)*. In contrast, two of three macaques concurrently infected with SIVmac239 showed rising neutralizing antibody titers starting at 20 wk after SIV infection (Fig. 2). SIV-specific virus binding antibodies measured by enzyme-linked immunosorbent assay (ELISA) were detectable at equal levels in the sooty mangabeys and rhesus macaques after 12 wk of infection, and in the sooty mangabeys, high levels of anti-SIV antibodies were detected at time points when neutralizing antibodies were not detected *(24)*. In a cross-sectional analysis, sera from five naturally infected mangabeys did not neutralize SIVmac239, SIVmac251, or SIVsmE660 (R. Means, personal communication). Detailed studies of specific epitopes recognized by antibodies from sooty mangabeys and analysis of differences in the ability of macaques and mangabeys to recognize neutralizing epitopes have not been performed.

CD8+ T-Cell Responses

Several recent reports have provided information on SIV-specific CTL activity using standard ^{51}Cr-release assays. In a cross-sectional analysis of 12 naturally SIV-infected sooty mangabeys with plasma viremia ranging between 10^5 and 10^7 viral RNA copies/mL, SIV-specific CTL activity was not detected in primary ex vivo CTL assays using unstimulated PBMC. However, following in vitro antigen-specific stimulation to expand CTL precursors, variable levels of SIV-specific CTL activity could be detected *(97),* indicating absent or low levels of in vivo activated CTL with preservation of an expandable pool of memory CTL in naturally infected sooty mangabeys. The SIV-specific CTL response was heterogenous, ranging from relatively vigorous activity (>20% specific lysis against one or more SIV proteins) in 4 of 12 animals, to weak activity (10–20% lysis) in three of twelve animals and undetectable (<10% specific lysis) or inconsistently present in five of twelve animals (Kaur et al., unpublished observations). In this cross-sectional analysis, there was no clear relationship between the strength of CTL activity and the level of plasma viremia (Kaur et al., unpublished observation), suggesting an ineffective in vivo immune response. Interestingly, reduction of the viral load in naturally infected mangabeys with the antiretroviral drug PMPA resulted in a three- to -sixfold rise in SIV-specific CTL precursor frequency (as measured by limiting dilution assays) in three of three mangabeys at the time of peak decline in viral loads (A. Kaur, R. Grant, unpublished observations). One explanation of this observation is that the high levels of SIV replication in naturally infected sooty mangabeys may inhibit SIV-specific CTL activity, either via a direct effect on $CD8^+$T cells or by suppressing $CD4^+$T-helper responses, which may play a role in maintaining virus-specific CTL responses *(98).* Similar results documenting transient increases in HIV-specific CTL precursors have been observed in HIV-infected subjects after institution of highly active antiretroviral therapy, although prolonged therapy results in a decrease in CTL activity *(99).*

Inoculation of SIV-naive sooty mangabeys with the pathogenic molecular clone SIVmac239 resulted in a vigorous and polyclonal memory CTL response that was associated with low viral loads at set point *(24).* Thus, the weaker or ineffective CTL response in naturally infected sooty mangabeys is not due to an innate inability of sooty mangabeys to process or respond to SIV antigen. In both models of SIV infection in sooty mangabeys, high set-point viremia with weak CTL activity in naturally infected mangabeys, and low set-point viremia with vigorous CTL activity in SIVmac239-infected sooty mangabeys, the animals remain asymptomatic and do not develop immunodeficiency *(24).*

Immunodominant SIV-specific CTL epitopes mapping to conserved regions of the SIV Gag, Nef, and Env protein have been identified in both naturally infected and SIVmac239-infected sooty mangabeys *(97).* Similar CTL epitopes were recognized by both naturally infected and SIVmac239-infected mangabeys that shared class I MHC alleles *(97).*

$CD8^+$ T cells from naturally infected sooty mangabeys secrete a soluble factor that can inhibit in vitro SIV replication of exogenously infected PBMC *(100),* similar to the activity described in HIV-infected people and SIV-infected macaques *(43,45).*

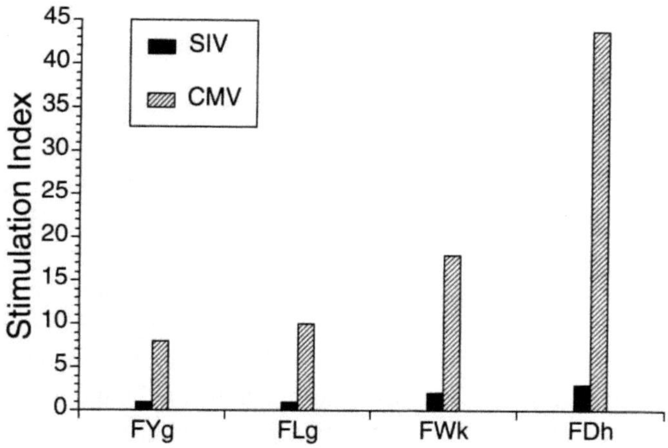

Fig. 3. Intact CMV-specific and absent SIV-specific T proliferative activity in four SIV-infected sooty mangabeys. FYg and FLg were infected with SIVmac239, while FWk and FDh were naturally infected sooty mangabeys.

The limited quantitative information obtained from bulk CTL assays or from assays of soluble antiviral factors precludes any clear conclusions regarding comparative differences in SIV-specific $CD8^+$ T-cell responses between mangabeys and macaques. The advent of improved techniques for the quantitation of cell-mediated immune responses, such as enzyme-linked immunospot (ELISPOT) and the use of MHC-tetramers, should facilitate such cross-species comparisons.

$CD4^+$ T-Cell Responses

Proliferative responses in SIV-infected sooty mangabeys have been detected when autologous macrophages pulsed with ultraviolet-irradiated inactivated SIV were used as antigen-presenting cells *(101,102)*. However, these responses were weaker compared to those elicited in SIV-infected rhesus macaques.

Using standard proliferation assays, we have been unable to detect SIV-specific proliferative responses to p55 antigen in either naturally infected or experimentally infected mangabeys (Fig. 3). However, relatively vigorous CMV-specific proliferative responses were observed in these animals demonstrating that cell-mediated immune response against other viruses are intact.

Cytokine Secretion by $CD4^+$ T Lymphocytes

The combination of relatively high virus loads coupled with weak or ineffective cell-mediated immune responses has led to speculation that naturally infected sooty mangabeys may manifest a Th2 response, analogous to the Th2 response observed in patients with lepromatous leprosy *(103)*. Cytokine secretion profiles of cloned T-cell lines from normal and SIV-infected animals have demonstrated a predominantly Th1 type pattern in rhesus macaques and a Th2 pattern in sooty mangabeys *(104)*. Longitudinal ex vivo analysis of unstimulated PBMC in a SIVmac239-infected sooty mangabey revealed secretion of IL-10 and IL-4, but not IL-2 or IFN-γ *(24)*. This limited information supports the concept of a Th2 bias in mangabeys, but more data need to be obtained to confirm this view, including information of cytokine responses in fresh PBMC following stimulation with SIV antigens.

T-Cell Turnover in SIV-Infected Sooty Mangabeys

Several pieces of indirect evidence suggest that sooty mangabeys naturally infected with SIV might have increased levels of $CD4^+$ and $CD8^+$ T-cell turnover, as has previously been reported in SIV-infected macaques *(105,106)* and HIV-infected people *(107)*. Sooty mangabeys naturally infected with SIV have lower peripheral $CD4^+$ T-lymphocyte counts as compared to uninfected mangabeys (*93* and Table 2). Moreover, the rapid decay of plasma viremia following PMPA therapy (R. Grant, unpublished data) strongly suggests that SIV-infected $CD4^+$T lymphocytes in mangabeys have a short half-life in vivo, similar to SIV-infected macaques *(87)* and HIV-infected people *(108)*. Surprisingly, recent studies on T-lymphocyte turnover in sooty mangabeys using the proliferation marker Ki-67 *(93)*, or the nucleoside analog bromodeoxyuridine (Kaur et al., manuscript in preparation) show that unlike pathogenic SIV infection in rhesus macaques, $CD4^+$ and $CD8^+$ T-lymphocyte turnover is not increased in SIV-infected sooty mangabeys. Chakrabarti et al. showed that the percentage of proliferating $CD4^+$ and $CD8^+$ T lymphocytes did not differ between SIV-naive and SIV-infected sooty mangabeys and was three to fivefold higher in SIV-infected rhesus macaques compared to sooty mangabeys *(93)*. Moreover, thymic function as assessed by measurement of T-cell receptor excisional circles (TREC) was affected to a comparable extent in SIV-infected sooty mangabeys and rhesus macaques *(93)*. Thus, the difference between the AIDS-susceptible rhesus macaques and the AIDS-resistant sooty mangabeys appears to be related to the extent of T-lymphocyte turnover induced by SIV infection, rather than an enhanced regenerative capacity. In the setting of high viral loads, the association of increased T-lymphocyte proliferation in pathogenic infection suggests that death of uninfected cells (indirect cell death) may be an important mechanism of immunodeficiency and that sooty mangabeys may fail to develop immunodeficiency because of lower levels of indirect cell death *(93)*.

In summary, SIV infection in sooty mangabeys is characterized by high levels of viral replication, cytopathic infection and weak or ineffective host immune responses, features that are shared by pathogenic lentiviral infections. However, unlike pathogenic lentiviral infections, SIV-infection in sooty mangabeys does not result in progressive $CD4^+$ T lymphocytopenia, loss of T-lymphocyte homeostasis, or immunodeficiency and is not associated with increased T-lymphocyte turnover. Because there is rapid turnover of infected cells, the absence of increased turnover of $CD4^+$ and $CD8^+$ lymphocytes in SIV-infected sooty mangabeys implies an absence of bystander (uninfected) cell proliferation in mangabeys, and increased bystander cell turnover in pathogenic lentivirus infections. If so, the failure of immunodeficiency to develop in mangabeys may be a reflection of decreased bystander cell destruction in SIV-infected sooty mangabeys.

CHIMPANZEES

Chimpanzees were the first animals that could be experimentally infected with HIV-1 and remain the nonhuman primate species that can be most readily infected with HIV-1 *(8)*. Reports from multiple groups documented infection of chimpanzees with laboratory-adapted strains of HIV-1 (HIV-1 Lai or IIIB), which resulted in seroconversion and persistent infection, but without depletion of CD4+ T lymphocytes or evidence of immunodeficiency *(109,110)*. Lack of disease could not be attributed to the use of laboratory-adapted HIV-1 strains, since accidental infection of laboratory workers with HIV-1 Lai has resulted in CD4+ T-lymphocyte depletion and AIDS *(111)*. The exception to the well-documented apathogenic course of experimental HIV-1 infection in chimpanzees is an animal that had been sequentially inoculated with three different HIV-1 strains (SF-2, LAV, NDK). An initial report documented transient thrombocytopenia and mild lymphopenia 3 yr after the first infection *(112)*, which subsequently resolved. However, 5–7 yr later, this animal developed persistent thrombocytopenia and depletion of CD4+ T lymphocytes (< 100/mm^3) accompanied by an increase in plasma viremia to 10^5 RNA equivalents/ml and chronic diarrhea, ultimately requiring euthanasia of the animal *(113)*. The development of the disease appeared to in large part reflect evolution of the virus, since inoculation of a second chimpanzee with blood from the initial affected chimpanzee resulted in high viral loads and CD4+ T-lymphocyte depletion within 4 wk.

Increasing knowledge regarding the prevalence and phylogenetic relationships of primate lentiviruses led to speculation in the 1980s that chimpanzees might represent the natural host for the primate lentivirus that served as the origin of HIV-1. Initial efforts to assess the extent of natural infection of chimpanzees with lentiviruses were hindered by the limited ability to obtain blood samples from chimpanzees in the wild. However, over the past decade surveys of captive chimpanzees ultimately identified several cases of chimpanzees naturally infected with a primate lentivirus that is phylogenetically related to HIV-1 and that has been designated SIVcpz, *(7,114,115)*. The distant phylogenetic relationship of the initial isolate, SIVcpz (ANT), with HIV-1 strains *(114)* and the low prevalence of antibodies to HIV-1 in feral chimpanzees in the wild *(116,117)* initially cast doubt on whether SIVcpz was the source for HIV-1 infection in humans. However, the identification of additional instances of SIVcpz infection in chimpanzees, and a reanalysis of the phylogenetic relationship of the SIVcpz strains based on the new sequences have strengthened the hypothesis that HIV-1 infection is likely to have originated from a subspecies of chimpanzees, *Pan troglodytes troglodytes,* that is naturally infected with SIVcpz *(1,7,115)*. Unfortunately, little information is available on viral loads and immunological effects of natural SIVcpz infection in chimpanzees. Most of the available data on naturally infected chimpanzees are derived from a single chimpanzee that was imported from Zaire and has been studied for > 9 yr at the Biomedical Primate Research Center in the Netherlands *(116,118)*. This animal has developed thrombocytopenia but not CD4+ T-lymphocyte depletion or opportunistic infections and is otherwise well.

Virologic Factors Associated with Lack of Immunodeficiency in HIV/SIV-Infected Chimpanzees

Several findings suggest chimpanzees are not intrinsically resistant to AIDS. Chimpanzees express the chemokine receptors CCR5 and CXCR4 on T lymphocytes *(119,120)* and are susceptible to cytopathic infection in vitro *(121)*. More compelling is the observation that the ability of experimental HIV-1 infection to cause disease in chimpanzees can be serially passaged from one animal to another *(113)*. The lack of disease in chimpanzees experimentally infected with HIV is likely to be due to the relatively low levels of viral replication in vivo, as demonstrated by a variety of different assays. Quantitative limiting dilution cultures of PBMC have revealed relatively low levels of virus-infected cells compared with HIV-infected subjects of SIVmac-infected macaques, and efforts to culture virus from plasma have generally been unsuccessful *(110,122)*. More precise quantitative data have been recently obtained using nucleic acid based measurements of plasma RNA. In experimentally infected animals for which data are available, levels of steady state (set point) viral RNA have generally been low (10^2–10^3 genome equivalents per milliliter) *(113,123)* whereas levels of 10^5 copies/mL were observed in the two chimpanzees with pathogenic experimental infection *(113)*. Levels of HIV-1 proviral DNA in experimentally infected chimpanzees have also been reported to be low (1:1000–1:25,000 cells) *(124)*, although higher levels have been reported in lymph nodes *(125)*. Plasma viral RNA levels in naturally infected chimpanzees are in the range of 10^4 copies per milliliter (*126*, J. Heeney, personal communication), and virus has been cultured from plasma *(118,122)*.

Another factor proposed to be associated with nonprogression in chimpanzees is the lack of monocyte tropism *(124)*. Efforts to isolate macrophage-tropic HIV-1 strains from experimentally infected animals have been unsuccessful, and chimpanzee monocyte-derived macrophages are resistant to infection with macrophage-tropic HIV-1 strains *(124)*. These authors postulate that the lack of infection of antigen-presenting cells may preserve immune function in chimpanzees.

Immunological Factors Associated with Lack of Immunodeficiency in HIV-Infected Chimpanzees

A variety of different immunologic factors have been proposed to account for the lack of disease in most HIV-1–infected chimpanzees (Table 3). Interpretation of the importance of any of these factors is considerably complicated by the fact that viral loads in the majority of experimentally infected chimpanzees are low and would be expected to be associated with minimal HIV-induced immune pathology. It is therefore likely that many of the immunologic characteristics described below primarily reflect the consequences of low levels of HIV-1 replication, and do not play a causal role in the lack of immunodeficiency in chimpanzees. More detailed examination of immune responses in naturally infected chimpanzees should be revealing in offering insights to immunologic factors associated with nonprogression but has been quite limited owing to the small number of naturally infected animals in captivity available for study.

$CD8^+$ T-Cell Responses

Many early efforts to identify HIV-1 specific CTL activity in experimentally infected chimpanzees were unsuccessful, leading to speculation that the lack of a cytotoxic T-cell response played a role in the lack of immunodeficiency *(127)*. However, two recent studies have provided convincing evidence for HIV-specific CTL activity in experimentally infected chimpanzees *(123,128)*. The use of more quantitative assays of cell-mediated immunity (intracellular cytokine staining or ELISPOTs) will be required to compare how these CTL responses compare with those observed in pathogenic and nonpathogenic primate lentivirus infection in other species.

$CD8^+$ T lymphocytes from experimentally infected chimpanzees are able to suppress HIV-1 replication in vitro *(129,130)*. One report has suggested uninfected chimpanzees also have $CD8^+$ lymphocyte mediated antiviral activity *(129)* but this was not confirmed in a subsequent study *(130)*. Again, the significance of this finding is uncertain and is compli-

Table 3
Immunologic Factors Associated with Lack of Immunodeficiency in HIV-Infected Chimpanzees

Immunologic Factor	Reference
$CD4^+$ T-lymphocyte responses	
Preservation of	
• Antigen-specific responses	*118*
• HIV-specific proliferative responses	*132*
$CD8^+$ T-lymphocyte responses	
Production of	
• Soluble antiviral factors	*129*
	118
• HIV-specific CTL	*123*
	128
Apoptosis	
Decreased susceptibility to	
• Tat-induced apoptosis	*133*
• gp120-induced apoptosis	*134*
• T cell receptor-induced apoptosis	*135*
• Fas-induced apoptosis	*136*
	137
Decreased expression of Fas on $CD4^+$ T lymphocytes	*133*
General	
Decreased expression of activation markers (HLA-DR, CD38)	*133*
Preservation of antigen-presenting cell function	*124*
Anergy	
Less susceptibility to gp120-induced anergy	*134*
Natural killer responses	
Preserved NK activity	*118*

cated by difficulties in the precise quantitation of antiviral activity, especially across different species. The role of β-chemokines, IL-16, or other specific molecules in mediating inhibition of viral replication by chimpanzee $CD8^+$ cells is unknown.

$CD4^+$ T-Cell Responses

Although studies are limited, available data suggest that $CD4^+$ T-cell responses are relatively preserved in HIV-infected chimpanzees. In contrast to HIV-1–infected humans *(131),* antigen-specific proliferative responses to recall antigens such as candida are similar in HIV-1–infected and uninfected chimpanzees *(118).* Proliferative responses to HIV-1 antigens can also be readily detected in infected chimpanzees *(132).*

Immune Activation and Apoptosis

One of the characteristic features of pathogenic lentivirus infection in humans and Asian macaques has been increases in levels of T-cell activation and apoptosis *(104).*

Not surprisingly, analysis of HIV-1–infected chimpanzees documents no significant increase in levels of T cells expressing activation markers or undergoing apoptosis. Analysis of activation markers on T lymphocytes from HIV-infected chimpanzees has shown no evidence for increases in expression of DR, CD38, or Fas as compared with uninfected chimpanzees *(133)*. As compared with HIV-1–infected humans, chimpanzees experimentally infected with HIV-1 show a low level of T-cell apoptosis induced by a variety of stimuli including Fas/Fas ligand interactions *(133)*, gp120 binding *(134)*, CD3-mediated stimulation *(135,136)*, and HIV-1 Tat *(137)*.

In the HIV-infected chimpanzee that developed AIDS, increased levels of T cell activation associated with increases in viral load were observed *(113)*, suggesting that the absence of immune activation and apoptosis in asymptomatic chimpanzees is more likely a consequence of low viral loads than the primary factor responsible for the lack of immune deficiency in chimpanzees.

Humoral Responses in HIV-Infected Chimpanzees

Conflicting reports have appeared on antibodies able to mediate antibody-dependent cell-mediated cytotoxicity (ADCC) in chimpanzees. One group has reported low to absent ADCC activity in experimentally infected chimpanzees *(138)*, while another group has reported levels that are comparable to those in HIV-infected people *(139)*. The reasons for these discrepant findings are not clear, but may be related to differences in the target cells used for these assays. Analysis of neutralizing antibody responses in chimpanzees experimentally infected with HIV-1 has demonstrated early development of type-specific responses followed later by group-specific responses *(140,141)*. Interestingly, serial analysis of neutralization of autologous virus isolates in a naturally infected chimpanzee have suggested the cyclic emergence of escape variants, a pattern not observed in experimentally infected chimpanzees *(122)*.

AFRICAN GREEN MONKEYS

African green monkeys (AGMs; genus *Chlorocebus*) are distributed throughout subsaharan Africa and are another natural host for simian immunodeficiency viruses. They comprise the largest reservoir of SIV in the wild, with seroprevalence rates ranging between 27% and 60% in different surveys *(142,143)*. Four subspecies of SIV-infected AGMs with natural habitats in distinct geographical regions of Africa have been identified. These are the vervet monkeys (*C. pygerythrus*) resident from Southern Ethiopia to South Africa and Angola, grivet monkeys (*C. aethiops*) limited to Ethiopia and Sudan, tantalus monkeys (*C. tantalus*) in Central Africa, and sabaeus or green monkeys (*C. sabaeus*) which reside exclusively in West Africa *(142)*. These four subspecies of AGMs are phenotypically and geographically distinct and are believed to have diverged from a common ancestor a long time ago.

SIVagm

SIV isolates from the different subspecies of AGMs (SIVagm) are characterized by marked genetic variability, suggesting that SIV has been in the AGM population for a long time and that the virus has coevolved with its host, with each subspecies harboring its own distinct virus *(144–147)*. Sequence data from portions of the *pol* and *env* gene have revealed interspecies amino acid sequence differences ranging roughly between

19% and 40% *(145,147)*. Phylogenetic tree analysis also reveals a distinct separation of West African and East African SIVagm sequences within the SIVagm superfamily and indicates that the grivet and vervet viruses are coevolutionarily more closely related to each other than the sabaeus monkey viruses *(145)*. Genetic diversity is further documented by size differences of the Gag, Pol, and Env proteins among SIVagm isolates from different species *(146)*.

Irrespective of the sequence diversity, SIVagm from all the subspecies share certain common properties. SIVagm uses CD4 as a receptor for cell entry and can infect macrophages *(148,149)*. It is cytopathic for permissive cells but replicates poorly in many $CD4^+$ cell lines *(4)*. SIVagm isolates from vervets and sabaeus monkeys differ from SIVmac251, in that poor or no virus replication occurs in the HUT78 and CEMx174 CD4-positive cell lines *(144,145)*. SIVagm isolates replicate efficiently in SupT1, Molt4 (clone8), MT-4, Jurkat, U937, and AA2 CD4-positive cell lines *(144,145)*. This is in contrast to SIVmac strains that do not replicate well in SupT1, Jurkat-T, and U937 cells *(144)*. These data indicate that coreceptor usage of SIVagm is likely to differ from other SIV strains.

Natural SIVagm Infection

AGMs residing in Africa have a high prevalence of SIV infection in the wild. Twenty-six percent to 60% of AGMs in the wild are SIV seropositive *(142,143,150)*. Interestingly, AGMs resident in the Caribbeans (Barbados AGM) are not SIV infected *(151)*. These were shipped from Africa to the Caribbean around the seventeenth century. The absence of SIV infection could indicate that SIV was introduced into African-resident AGMs after the seventeenth century or that the Caribbean AGMs are progeny of SIV-uninfected AGMs *(151)*.

Transmission of SIV within the AGM population in the wild has been studied in grivets residing near the Awash National Park in Ethiopia. Seropositivity is age related. Thus, it is almost universal in females of breeding age and in older males, and it is virtually absent in young, sexually inactive animals *(152)*. The predominant mode of transmission appears to be via the sexual route, since both sexes remain almost entirely SIVagm negative until sexual maturity *(152)*. More than 80% of females of breeding age are seropositive, and SIV is almost completely absent in nonbreeding age groups *(152)*.

Although AGMs constitute a large reservoir of natural SIV infection, there is only limited cross-species transmission to other primates in the wild and no evidence that natural cross-species transmission results in AIDS. Natural cross-species transmission of SIVagm has been reported in patas monkeys and baboons *(150,153)*.

Pathogenicity of SIVagm

In early studies experimental inoculation of uncloned SIVagm was shown to produce immunosuppression in pig-tailed macaques, but not in rhesus macaques *(154)*. Species-specific differences in pathogenicity of SIVagm appears to be related to the extent of in vivo SIV replication *(155)*. Thus, in contrast to SIVagm infection in rhesus macaques, infection of pig-tailed macaques with SIVagm is associated with high viral load in plasma and tissues *(155)*.

The basis of apathogenic SIVagm infection in AGMs does not appear to be due to a low level of virus replication, since SIV DNA is detected in PBMCs by PCR (5–50 copies per 10^5 cells), infectious SIV can be readily isolated from PBMCs, and SIV RNA can be detected in peripheral blood by *in situ* hybridization *(156,157)*. However, unlike pathogenic SIV infection, the viral load in lymph nodes and PBMCs is comparable, the architecture of lymph nodes is normal and SIV-reactive cells are not detected by immunohistochemistry or *in situ* hybridization *(156)*. There is currently little information on levels of plasma SIV RNA in naturally infected AGMs. In one study, adult AGMs experimentally inoculated with the molecular clone SIVagm3 had plasma SIV RNA levels ranging between 4×10^4 and 1.6×10^5 copies/mL at 59–95 wk after infection *(158)*. In a recent study, set-point plasma viremia in five SIV-AGMs experimentally inoculated with plasma or PBMC from a naturally SIV-infected AGM ranged between 2×10^3 and 2×10^5 RNA copies/mL *(159)*. These levels are lower than or in the low range of values observed in naturally-infected sooty mangabeys.

Since SIV-seronegative adult AGMs have low $CD4^+$ T-lymphocyte counts, it is possible that a limited target cell population may limit the extent of viral replication and contribute to apathogenicity. This was tested by experimental infection of AGMs at birth, since >60% of peripheral lymphocytes in neonates are $CD4^+$ *(158)*. Neonatal AGMs did not develop AIDS after SIVagm infection, and, surprisingly, had significantly delayed onset of viral replication compared to infected adults *(158)*.

Immune Responses to SIV in AGMs

Phenotype of Peripheral Blood Lymphocytes

Adult AGMs differ from macaques and sooty mangabeys in having lower $CD4^+$ and higher $CD8^+$ lymphocyte counts and a low CD4/CD8 ratio *(158,160)*. At birth, AGMs have >60% circulating $CD4^+$ T lymphocytes. These steadily decline to 10–20% by adulthood *(158)*. $CD4^+$ and $CD8^+$ lymphocyte counts are similar in adult SIV-infected and SIV uninfected AGMs *(158,160)*. A peculiar feature in AGMs, irrespective of their SIV infection status, is the high frequency of $CD4^+$ cells in peripheral blood that also express low levels of the CD8 molecule *(158)*.

Humoral Immunity

In SIV-infected AGMs, SIV-specific antibodies are readily detected by an HIV-2 ELISA. The antibody profile of naturally infected AGMs is generally characterized by detectable antibodies to gp140 and gp45 but not to Gag or Pol proteins *(146,147)*. Weak p24 reactivity to autologous virus isolates can be detected in some animals *(146)*.

In immunoblots, using lysates derived from the SIVagm3 isolate, serum from naturally infected East African AGMs reacted predominantly with gp140 and gp45. In contrast, serum from a pig-tailed macaque infected with uncloned SIVagm3 virus reacted with all major viral proteins *(161)*. In the same study, when uninfected AGMs were inoculated intravenously with cell-free SIVagm, they seroconverted within 4 wk and mounted a strong antibody response against all major SIV proteins (Gag and Env). This was in contrast to reactivity of sera from naturally infected AGMs and indicates that the absence of Gag-specific antibodies in naturally infected AGMs is not due to a defect in host response *(161)*. Sera of naturally infected West African sabaeus monkeys reacts with the gp120, gp41, p24, and p17 of SIVagm(sab) isolates. They do not recognize p17 of SIVagm(gri-1), SIVagm(tyo-1), or SIVmac251 and react weakly with transmembrane and p24 proteins of these isolates *(145)*. Thus, there is interspecies variability in the SIV-specific humoral response among AGMs.

In earlier studies, neutralization antibodies were absent or detected at low levels in naturally infected AGMs *(148)*. In a recent study, a comprehensive analysis showed that the detection of neutralizating antibodies in sera of naturally infected AGMs is dependent on the strain of SIVagm and the type of cells used for detection *(162)*. Using SupT1 cells and a laboratory-passaged SIV isolate derived from one naturally infected AGM, 50% neutralization antibody titers ranging from 1:54 to 1:7983 were detected in all 20 naturally infected AGMs. However, when the same sera were tested against the same virus using Molt-4/Clone 8 cells neutralizing antibodies could not be detected. Neutralizing antibodies were also not detected against two other SIVagm isolates, irrespective of the type of cell used in the assay. However, they were detected to variable and sometimes very high levels against SIVmac251 and SIVsmB670, but not against SIVsmE660. Although neutralizing antibodies can be detected in vitro, whether they neutralize virus in vivo remains to be determined.

Using peptide ELISA, immunodominant regions in the transmembrane region of the envelope that are group-specific antigenic determinants of SIV have been identified *(163,164)*. These regions induce strong humoral responses in almost all naturally infected captive or wild-caught AGMs that were tested *(164)*.

Antibody-dependent cellular cytotoxicity has been reported in naturally infected AGMs *(148)* and in AGMs vaccinated with whole inactivated SIVagm *(165)*. However, it was not sufficient to protect vaccinated AGMs from experimental infection.

Cellular Immunity

There is only limited published information on cellular immunity in SIV-infected AGMs. In vitro SIVagm replication is enhanced by 1–3 logs following depletion of $CD8^+$ T lymphocytes *(160)*. The suppressive activity of $CD8^+$ T lymphocytes from naturally infected AGMs was shown to be mediated by a soluble factor, subsequently identified as IL-16, which was also able to inhibit HIV-1 replication in vitro *(160,161)*. Whether the $CD8^+$ lymphocyte mediated SIV-suppressive effect is essential for apathogenic infection in AGMs is not known.

Protection Against Experimental Infection in AGMs

Even though SIV infection does not result in AIDS in AGMs, study of experimental infection in this species may help elucidate what arm of the immune response is effective for controlling viral replication. AGMs infected with SIVagm at birth do not develop AIDS. In contrast to infection in adults, neonatal infection results in delayed detection of viremia (more than two months after inoculation) and lower viral loads *(158)*. The reason for this is not clear.

There are two studies reporting results of experimental infection in AGMs after different vaccination strategies. Vaccination of AGMs with an inactivated whole SIVagm virus resulted in induction of SIV-specific antibodies, neutralizing antibodies, and ADCC, but did not protect against challenge with the homologous SIVagm virus *(165)*. AGMs vaccinated with a live attenuated nef-deleted variant of SIVagm had lower viral loads after challenge with wild-type *(166)*. Challenged AGMs had undetectable antibody levels prior to challenge, but were able to mount an anamnestic antibody response after challenge. Neutralizing antibodies were not detected and cellular immune responses were not reported *(166)*. The immune correlates of protection remain to be determined.

CONCLUSION

The diverse spectrum of primate lentivirus infection in different species offers the opportunity to try to identify specific immunologic mechanisms that may play a role in the etiology of AIDS. Interpretation of disease resistance in HIV-1–infected chimpanzees is complicated by the low levels of viremia in experimentally infected animals and the paucity of information on naturally infected animals. The fact that experimental HIV-1 infection in chimpanzees can in some cases lead to high viral loads and AIDS demonstrates they are not intrinsically resistant to disease, a finding that contrasts with sooty mangabeys and AGMs. The mechanisms as to how natural hosts such as sooty mangabeys and AGMs escape the consequences of immunodeficiency in spite of persistent high antigenic load remain unknown. The cellular reservoirs for SIV replication in sooty mangabeys and AGMs have not been precisely defined, but if the dominant cell type infected in vivo is the $CD4^+$ T lymphocyte, one would expect that sustained high levels of cytopathic viral replication in $CD4^+$ T lymphocytes would in time lead to loss of T-helper function. However, naturally infected sooty mangabeys maintain $CD4^+$ T lymphocyte counts and have preserved T-helper cell function to other viruses, like CMV. The ability of sooty mangabeys to maintain normal immune function in the face of continued high level viremia may potentially reflect differences in rates of indirect and direct cell death induced by SIV, a hypothesis that is supported by emerging evidence of normal T cell turnover in SIV-infected sooty mangabeys *(93)*. Further elucidation of mechanisms underlying the ability of natural hosts of primate lentiviruses to resist SIV-induced immunodeficiency may ultimately yield clues to the immunopathogenesis of AIDS in HIV-infected people.

ACKNOWLEDGMENTS

The authors would like to thank Ron Desrosiers for critical review of the manuscript and Carolyn A. O'Toole for manuscript preparation. This work was supported by AI43890, AI45314, and RR00168 (National Institutes of Health).

REFERENCES

1. Hahn BH, Shaw GM, De Cock KM, Sharp PM. AIDS as a zoonosis: scientific and public health implications. Science 2000; 287:607–14.
2. Desrosiers RC. Nonhuman Lentiviruses. In: Knipe DM, Howley DM (eds). Fields Virology, 4th edit. New York: Lippincott-Raven, 2000.
3. Rey-Cuille MA, Berthier JL, Bomsel-Demontoy MC, et al. Simian immunodeficiency virus replicates to high levels in sooty mangabeys without inducing disease. J Virol 1998; 72:3872–86.
4. Kraus G, Werner A, Baier M, et al. Isolation of human immunodeficiency virus-related simian immunodeficiency viruses from African green monkeys. Proc Natl Acad Sci USA 1989; 86:2892–6.
5. Mansfield KG, Lerche NW, Gardner MB, Lackner AA. Origins of simian immunodeficiency virus infection in macaques at the New England Regional Primate Research Center. J Med Primatol 1995; 24:116–22.
6. Chen Z, Telfer P, Gettie A, et al. Genetic characterization of new West African simian immunodeficiency virus SIVsm: geographic clustering of household-derived SIV strains with human immunodeficiency virus type 2 subtypes and genetically diverse viruses from a single feral sooty mangabey troop. J Virol 1996; 70:3617–27.

7. Gao F, Bailes E, Robertson DL, et al. Origin of HIV-1 in the chimpanzee *Pan troglodytes troglodytes*. Nature 1999; 397:436–41.
8. Kindt TJ, Hirsch VM, Johnson PR, Sawasdikosol S. Animal models for acquired immunodeficiency syndrome. Adv Immunol 1992; 52:425–75.
9. Schultz AM, Stott EJ. Primate models for AIDS vaccines. AIDS 1994; 8:S203–12.
10. Wyand MS. The use of SIV-infected rhesus monkeys for the preclinical evaluation of AIDS drugs and vaccines. AIDS Res Hum Retrovir 1992; 8:349–56.
11. Warren JT, Levinson MA. AIDS preclinical vaccine development: biennial survey of HIV, SIV, and SHIV challenge studies in vaccinated nonhuman primates. J Med Primatol 1999; 28:249–73.
12. Hulskotte EG, Geretti AM, Osterhaus AD. Towards an HIV-1 vaccine: lessons from studies in macaque models. Vaccine 1998; 16:904–15.
13. Barre-Sinoussi F, Chermann JC, Rey R, et al. Isolation of a T-lymphotrophic retrovirus from a patient at risk for acquired immunodeficiency syndrome (AIDS). Science 1983; 220:868–71.
14. Daniel MD, Letvin NL, King NW, et al. Isolation of T-cell tropic HTLV-III-like retrovirus from macaques. Science 1985; 228:1201–4.
15. Murphey-Corb M, Martin LN, Rangan SRS, et al. Isolation of an HTLV-III-related retrovirus from macaques with simian AIDS and its possible origin in asymptomatic mangabeys. Nature 1986; 321:435–7.
16. Agy MB, Frumkin LR, Corey L, et al. Infection of *Macaca nemestrina* by human immunodeficiency virus type-1. Science 1992; 257:103–6.
17. Igarashi T, Shibata R, Hasebe F, et al. Persistent infection with SIVmac chimeric virus having *tat, rev, vpu, env* and *nef* of HIV type 1 in macaque monkeys. AIDS Res Hum Retrovir 1994; 10:1021–9.
18. Reimann KA, Li JT, Veazey R, et al. A chimeric simian/human immunodeficiency virus expressing a primary patient HIV-1 isolate env causes an AIDS-like disease after in vivo passage in rhesus monkeys. J Virol 1996; 70:6922–8.
19. Reimann KA, Tenner-Racz K, Racz P, et al. Immunopathogenic events in acute infection of rhesus monkeys with simian immunodeficiency virus of macaques. J Virol 1994; 68:2362–70.
20. Ringler DJ, Murphy GF, King NW, Jr. An erythematous maculopapular eruption in macaques infected with an HTLV-III-like virus (STLV-III). J Invest Dermatol 1986; 87:674–7.
21. Letvin NL, Daniel MD, Sehgal PK, et al. Induction of AIDS-like diseases in macaque monkeys with T-cell tropic retrovirus STLV-III. Science 1985; 230:71–3.
22. Desrosiers RC. The simian immunodeficiency viruses. Ann Rev Immunol 1990; 8:557–8.
23. Lackner A. Pathology of simiam immunodeficiency virus induced disease. Curr Top Microbiol Immunol 1994; 188:35–59.
24. Kaur A, Grant RM, Means RE, McClure H, Feinberg M, Johnson RP. Diverse host response and outcome following SIVmac239 infection in sooty mangabeys and rhesus macaques. J Virol 1998; 72:9597–611.
25. Margolick JB, Munoz A, Ponnenberg AD, Park LP, Galai N, Giorgi JV, et al. Failure of T-cell homeostasis preceding AIDS in HIV-I infection. Nat Med 1995; 1:674–80.
26. Giorgi JV, Hultin LE, McKeating JA, et al. Shorter survival in advanced human immunodeficiency virus type 1 infection is more closely associated with T lymphocyte activation than with plasma virus burden or virus chemokine coreceptor usage. J Infect Dis 1999; 179:859–70.
27. Giorgi JV, Hultin LE, Desrosiers RC. The immunopathogenesis of retroviral diseases: no immunophenotypic alterations in T, B, and NK cell subsets in SIVmac239-challenged rhesus macaques protected by SIV delta nef vaccination. J Med Primatol 1996; 25:186–91.
28. Roederer M, Dubs JG, Anderson MT, Raju PA, Herzenberg LA, Herzenberg LA. CD8 naive T cell counts decrease progressively in HIV-infected adults. J Clin Invest 1995; 95:2061–6.

29. Veazey RS, Tham IC, Mansfield KG, et al. Identifying the target cell in primary simian immunodeficiency virus (SIV) infection: highly activated memory CD4+ T cells are rapidly eliminated in early SIV infection in vivo. J Virol 2000; 74:57–64.
30. Moore JP, Cao Y, Ho DD, Koup RA. Development of the anti-gp120 antibody response during seroconversion to human immunodeficiency virus type. J Virol 1994;68:5142–55.
31. Montefiori DC, Baba TW, Li A, Bilska M, Ruprecht RM. Neutralizing and infection-enhancing antibody responses do not correlate with the differential pathogenicity of SIVmac239 in adult and infant rhesus monkeys. J Immunol 1996; 157:5528–35.
32. Cole KS, Murphey-Corb M, Narayan O, Joag SV, Shaw GM, Montelaro RC. Common themes of antibody maturation to simian immunodeficiency virus, simian-human immunodeficiency virus, and human immunodeficiency virus type 1 infections. J Virol 1998; 72:7852–9.
33. Cole KS, Rowles JL, Jagerski BA, et al. Evolution of envelope-specific antibody responses in monkeys experimentally infected or immunized with simian immunodeficiency virus and its association with the development of protective immunity. J Virol 1997; 71:5069–79.
34. Koup RA, Safrit JT, Cao Y, et al. Temporal association of cellular immune responses with the initial control of viremia in primary human immunodeficiency virus type 1 syndrome. J Virol 1994; 68:4650–55.
35. Yamamoto H, Miller MD, Watkins DI, et al. Two distinct lymphocyte populations mediate simian immunodeficiency virus envelope-specific target cell lysis. J Immunol 1990; 145:3740–6.
36. Venet A, Bourgault I, Aubertin A-M, Kieny M-P, Levy J-P. Cytotoxic T lymphocyte response against multiple simian immunodeficiency virus (SIV) proteins in SIV-infected macaques. J Immunol 1992; 148:2899–908.
37. Allen TM, Sidney J, delGuercio M-F, et al. Characterization of the peptide binding motif of a rhesus MHC class I molecule (Mamu-A*01) that binds an immunodominant CTL epitope from SIV. J Immunol 1998; 160:6062–71.
38. Kuroda M, Schmitz JE, Barouch DH, et al. Analysis of gag-specific cytotoxic T lymphocytes in simian immunodeficiency virus-infected rhesus monkeys by cell staining with a tetrameric major histocompatibility complex class I-peptide complex. J Exp Med 1998; 187:1373–81.
39. Bourgault I, Villefroy P, Beyer C, Aubertin AM, Levy JP, Venet A. Cytotoxic T-cell response and AIDS-free survival in simian immunodeficiency virus-infected macaques. AIDS 1993; 7:S73–9.
40. Evans DT, O'Connor DH, Jing P, et al. Virus-specific cytotoxic T-lymphocyte responses select for amino-acid variation in simian immunodeficiency virus Env and Nef. Nat Med 1999; 5:1270–6.
41. Schmitz JE, Kuroda MJ, Santra S, et al. Control of viremia in simian immunodeficiency virus infection by CD8+ lymphocytes. Science 1999; 283:857–60.
42. Jin X, Bauer DE, Tuttleton SE, et al. Dramatic rise in plasma viremia after CD8(+) T cell depletion in simian immunodeficiency virus-infected macaques. J Exp Med 1999; 189:991–8.
43. Walker CM, Moody DJ, Stites DP, Levy JA. CD8+ lymphocytes can control HIV replication in vitro by suppressing virus replication. Science 1986; 234:1563–6.
44. Kannagi M, Chalifoux LV, Lord CI, Letvin NL. Suppression of SIV replication in vitro by CD8+ lymphocytes. J Immunol 1988; 140:2237–42.
45. Tsubota H, Lord CI, Watkins DI, Morimoto C, Letvin NL. A cytotoxic T lymphocyte inhibits AIDS virus replication in peripheral blood lymphocytes. J Exp Med 1989; 169:1421–34.
46. Gauduin M-C, Glickman RL, Means R, Johnson RP. Inhibition of simian immunodeficiency virus (SIV) replication by CD8+ T lymphocytes from macaques immunized with live attenuated SIV. J Virol 1998; 72:6315–24.
47. Lehner T, Wang Y, Cranage M, et al. Protective mucosal immunity elicited by targeted iliac lymph node immunization with a subunit SIV envelope and core vaccine in macaques. Nat Med 1996; 2:767–75.

48. Wang Y, Tao L, Mitchell E, et al. Generation of CD8 suppressor factor and beta chemokines, induced by xenogeneic immunization, in the prevention of simian immunodeficiency virus infection in macaques. Proc Natl Acad Sci USA 1998; 95:5223–8.
49. Heeney JL, Teeuwsen VJ, van Gils M, et al. Beta-chemokines and neutralizing antibody titers correlate with sterilizing immunity generated in HIV-1 vaccinated macaques. Proc Natl Acad Sci USA 1998; 95:10803–8.
50. Wahren B, Morfeld L, Biberfeld G, et al. Characteristics of the specific cell-mediated immune response in human immunodeficiency virus infection. J Virol 1987; 61:2017–23.
51. Dittmer U, Luke W, Stahl-Hennig C, et al. Early helper T-cell dysfunction in simian immunodeficiency virus but not in human immunodeficiency virus type-2-infected macaques. J Med Primatol 1994; 23:298–303.
52. Gauduin M-C, Glickman RL, Ahmad S, Yilma T, Johnson RP. Immunization with live attenuated simian immunodeficiency virus induces strong type 1 T helper responses and β-chemokine production. Proc Natl Acad Sci USA 1999; 96:14,31–6.
53. Dittmer U, Nisslein T, Bodemer W, et al. Cellular immune response of rhesus monkeys infected with a partially attenuated nef deletion mutant of the simian immunodeficiency virus. Virology 1995; 212:392–7.
54. Lifson JD, Rossio JL, Arnaout R, et al. Containment of simian immunodeficiency virus infection: cellular immune responses and protection from rechallenge following transient postinoculation antiretroviral treatment. J Virol 2000; 74:2584–93.
54a. Margolick JB, Volkman DJ, Folks TM, Fauci AS. Amplification of HTLV-III/LAV infection by antigen-induced activation of T cells and direct suppression by virus of lymphocyte blastogenic responses. J Immunol 1987; 138:1719–23.
55. Voss G, Nick S, Stahl-Hennig C, et al. Potential significance of the cellular immune response against the macaque strain of simian immunodeficiency virus (SIVmac) in immunized and infected rhesus macaques. J Gen Virol 1992; 73:2273–81.
56. Benveniste O, Vaslin B, Le Grand R, et al. Comparative interleukin (IL-2)/interferon IFN-gamma and IL-4/IL-10 responses during acute infection of macaques inoculated with attenuated nef-truncated or pathogenic SIcmac251 virus. Proc Natl Acad Sci USA 1996; 93:3658–63.
57. Burton DR. A vaccine for HIV type 1: the antibody perspective. Proc Natl Acad Sci USA 1997; 94:10018–23.
58. Wyatt R, Sodroski J. The HIV-1 envelope glycoproteins: fusogens, antigens, and immunogens. Science 1998; 280:1884–8.
59. Emini EA, Schleif WA, Nunberg JH, et al. Prevention of HIV-1 infection in chimpanzees by gp120 V3 domain-specific monoclonal antibody. Nature 1992; 355:728–30.
60. Lewis MG, Elkins WR, McCutchan FE, et al. Passively transferred antibodies directed against conserved regions of SIV envelope protect macaques from SIV infection. Vaccine 1993; 11:1347–55.
61. Baba TW, Liska V, Hofmann-Lehmann R, et al. Human neutralizing monoclonal antibodies of the IgG1 subtype protect against mucosal simian-human immunodeficiency virus infection. Nat Med 2000; 6:200–6.
62. Shibata R, Igarashi T, Haigwood N, et al. Neutralizing antibody directed against the HIV-1 envelope glycoprotein can completely block HIV-1/SIV chimeric virus infections of macaque monkeys. Nat Med 1999; 5:204–10.
63. Mascola JR, Lewis MG, Stiegler G, et al. Protection of macaques against pathogenic simian/human immunodeficiency virus 89.6PD by passive transfer of neutralizing antibodies. J Virol 1999; 73:4009–18.
64. Gardner M, Rosenthal A, Jennings M, Yee J, Antipa L, Robinson EJ. Passive immunization of rhesus macaques against SIV infection and disease. AIDS Res Hum Retrovir 1995; 11:843–54.

65. Kent KA, Kitchin P, Mills KHG, et al. Passive immunization of cynomolgus macaques with immune sera or a pool of neutralizing monoclonal antibodies failed to protect against challenge with SIVmac251. AIDS Res Hum Retrovir 1994; 10:189–94.
66. Clements JE, Montelaro RC, Zink MC, et al. Protective immune responses induced in rhesus macaques by immunization with attenuated macrophage-tropic simian immunodeficiency virus. J Virol 1995; 69:2737–44.
67. Haigwood NL, Watson A, Sutton W, et al. Passive immune globulin therapy in the SIV/macaque model: early intervention can alter disease profile. Immunol Lett 1996; 51:107–14.
68. Wyand MS, Manson KH, Garcia-Moll M, Montefiori D, Desrosiers RC. Vaccine protection by a triple deletion mutant of simian immunodeficiency virus. J Virol 1996; 70:3724–33.
69. Shibata R, Siemon C, Czajak SC, Desrosiers RC, Martin MA. Live, attenuated simian immunodeficiency virus vaccines elicit potent resistance against a challenge with a human immunodeficiency virus type 1 chimeric virus. J Virol 1997; 71:8141–8.
70. Wyand MS, Manson K, Montefiori DC, Lifson JD, Johnson RP, Desrosiers RC. Protection by live, attenuated simian immunodeficiency virus against heterologous challenge. J Virol 1999; 73:8356–63.
71. Gundlach BR, Reiprich S, Sopper S, et al. Env-independent protection induced by live, attenuated simian immunodeficiency virus vaccines. J Virol 1998; 72:7846–51.
72. Miller CJ, McChesney MB, Lu X, et al. Rhesus macaques previously infected with simian/human immunodeficiency virus are protected from vaginal challenge with pathogenic SIVmac239. J Virol 1997; 71:1911–21.
73. Johnson RP, Lifson JD, Czajak SC, et al. Highly attenuated vaccine strains of simian immunodeficiency virus protect against vaginal challenge: inverse relationship of degree of protection with level of attenuation. J Virol 1999; 73:4952–61.
74. Putkonen P, Makitalo B, Bottiger D, Biberfeld G, Thorstensson R. Protection of human immunodeficiency virus type 2-exposed seronegative macaques from mucosal simian immunodeficiency virus transmission. J Virol 1997; 71:4981–4.
75. Murphey-Corb M, Wilson LA, Trichel AM, et al. Selective induction of protective MHC class I-restricted CTL in the intestinal lamina propria of rhesus monkeys by transient SIV infection of the colonic mucosa. J Immunol 1999; 162:540–9.
76. Gallimore A, Cranage M, Cook N, et al. Early suppression of SIV replication by $CD8^+$ *nef*-specific cytotoxic T cells in vaccinated macaques. Nat Med 1995; 1:1167–73.
77. Yasutomi Y, Koenig S, Woods RM, et al. A vaccine-elicited, single viral epitope-specific cytotoxic T lymphocyte response does not protect against intravenous, cell-free simian immunodeficiency virus challenge. J Virol 1995; 69:2279–84.
78. Fultz PN, Gordon TP, Anderson DC, McClure HM. Prevalence of natural infection with simian immunodeficiency virus and simian T-cell leukemia virus type I in a breeding colony of sooty mangabey monkeys. AIDS 1990; 4:619–25.
79. Chen Z, Telfer P, Reed P, et al. Isolation and characterization of the first simian immunodeficiency virus from a feral sooty mangabey *(Cercocebus atys)* in West Africa. J Med Primatol 1995; 24:108–15.
80. Lowenstine LJ, Pedersen NC, Higgins J, et al. Seroepidemiologic survey of captive old-world primates for antibodies to human and simian retroviruses, and isolation of a lentivirus from sooty mangabeys *(Cercocebus atys)*. Int J Cancer 1986; 38:563–74.
81. Fultz PN, McClure HM, Anderson DC, Swenson RB, Anand R, Srinivasan A. Isolation of a T-lymphotropic retrovirus from naturally infected sooty mangabey monkeys *(Cercocebus atys)*. Proc Natl Acad Sci USA 1986; 83:5286–90.
82. Lifson JD, Nowak MA, Goldstein S, et al. The extent of early viral replication is a critical determinant of the natural history of simian immunodeficiency virus infection. J Virol 1997; 71:9508–14.

83. Mellors JW, Rinalso CR, Jr., Gupta P, White RM, Todd JA, Kingsley LA. Prognosis in HIV-1 infection predicted by the quantity of virus in plasma. Science 1996; 272:1167–70.
84. McClure HM, Anderson DC, Fultz PN, Ansari AA, Lockwood E, Brodie A. Spectrum of disease in macaque monkeys chronically infected with SIV/SMM. Vet Immunol Immunopathol 1989; 21:13–24.
85. Fultz PN, Stricker RB, McClure HM, Anderson DC, Switzer WM, Horaist C. Humoral Response to SIV/SMM infection macaque and mangabey monkeys. J Acquir Immune Defic Syndr 1990; 3:319–29.
86. Yehuda-Cohen T, Powell JD, Villinger F, McClure HM, Sell KW, Ahmed-Ansari A. Comparison of SIV/SMM replication in $CD4^+$ T cell and monocyte/macrophage cultures from rhesus macaques and sooty mangabeys. J Med Primatol 1990; 19:251–67.
87. Nowak MA, Lloyd AL, Vasquez GM, et al. Viral dynamics of primary viremia and antiretroviral therapy in simian immunodeficiency virus infection. J Virol 1997; 71:7518–25.
88. Perelson AS, Neumann AU, Markowitz M, Leonard JM, Ho DD. HIV-1 dynamics in vivo: virion clearance rate, infected cell life-span, and viral generation time. Science 1996; 271:1582–6.
89. Chen Z, Gettie A, Ho DD, Marx PA. Primary SIVsm isolates use the CCR5 coreceptor from sooty mangabeys naturally infected in West Africa: a comparison of coreceptor usage of primary SIVsm, HIV-2, and SIVmac. Virology 1998; 246:113–24.
90. Fomsgaard A, Hirsch VM, Johnson PR. Cloning and sequences of primate CD4 molecules: diversity of the cellular receptor for simian immunodeficiency virus/human immunodeficiency virus. Eur J Immunol 1992; 22:2973–81.
91. Palacios E, Digilio L, McClure HM, et al. Parallel evolution of CCR5-null phenotypes in humans and in a natural host of simian immunodeficiency virus. Curr Biol 1998; 8:943–6.
92. Chen Z, Kwon D, Jin Z, et al. Natural infection of a homozygous delta24 CCR5 red-capped mangabey with an R2b-tropic simian immunodeficiency virus. J Exp Med 1998; 188:2057–65.
93. Chakrabarti LA, Lewin SR, Zhang L, et al. Normal T-cell turnover in sooty mangabeys harboring active simian immunodeficiency virus infection. J Virol 2000; 74:1209–23.
94. Ahmed-Ansari A, Brodie AR, Fultz PN, Anderson DC, Sell KW, McClure HM. Flow microfluorometric analysis of peripheral blood mononuclear cells from nonhuman primates: correlation of phenotype with immune function. Am J Primatol 1989; 17:107–31.
95. Exley M, Garcia J, Balk SP, Porcelli S. Requirements for CD1d recognition by human invariant Valpha24$^+$ $CD4^-$ $CD8^-$ T cells. J Exp Med 1997; 186:109–20.
96. Means RE, Greenough T, Desrosiers RC. Neutralization sensitivity of cell culture-passaged simian immunodeficiency virus. J Virol 1997; 71:7895–902.
97. Kaur A, Yang J, Hempel D, et al. Identification of multiple simian immunodeficiency virus (SIV)-specific CTL epitopes in sooty mangabeys with natural and experimentally acquired SIV infection. J Immunol 2000; 164:934–43.
98. Kalams SA, Walker BD. The critical need for CD4 help in maintaining effective cytotoxic T lymphocyte responses. J Exp Med 1998; 188:2199–204.
99. Kalams SA, Goulder PJ, Shea AK, et al. Levels of human immunodeficiency virus type 1-specific cytotoxic T-lymphocyte effector and memory responses decline after suppression of viremia with highly active antiretroviral therapy. J Virol 1999; 73:6721–8.
100. Powell JD, Yehuda-Cohen T, Villinger F, McClure HM, Sell KW, Ahmed-Ansari A. Inhibition of SIV/SMM replication in vitro by $CD8^+$ cells from SIV/SMM infected seropositive clinically asymptomatic sooty mangabeys. J Med Primatol 1990; 19:239–49.
101. Powell JD, Villinger F, Yehuda-Cohen T, et al. Identification of SIV/SMM viral proteins that induce T cell response in experimentally infected rhesus macaques and naturally infected sooty mangabeys by the cellular Western blot assay. J Med Primatol 1990; 19:227–38.
102. Ahmed-Ansari A, Powell JD, Jensen PE, et al. Requirements for simian immunodeficiency virus antigen-specific in vitro proliferation of T cells from infected rhesus macaques and sooty mangabeys. AIDS 1990; 4:399–407.

103. Yamamura M, Uyemura K, Deans RJ, et al. Defining protective responses to pathogens: cytokine profiles in leprosy lesions. Science 1991; 254:277–9.
104. Villinger F, Folks TM, Lauro S, et al. Immunological and virological studies of natural SIV infection of disease-resistant nonhuman primates. Immunol Lett 1996; 51:59–68.
105. Rosenzweig M, DeMaria M, Harper DM, Friedrich S, Jain RK, Johnson RP. Increased rates of $CD4^+$ and $CD8^+$ T lymphocyte turnover in simian immunodeficiency virus-infected macaques. Proc Natl Acad Sci USA 1998; 95:6388–93.
106. Mohri H, Bonhoeffer S, Monard S, Perelson AS, Ho DD. Rapid turnover of T lymphocytes in SIV-infected rhesus macaques. Science 1998; 279:1223–7.
107. Hellerstein M, Hanley MB, Cesar D, et al. Directly measured kinetics of circulating T lymphorytes in normal and HIV-I infected humans. Nat Med 1999; 5:83–9.
108. Ho DD, Neumann AU, Perelson AS, Chen W, Leonard JM, Markowitz M. Rapid turnover of plasma virions and CD4 lymphocytes in HIV-1 infection. Nature 1995; 373:123–6.
109. Alter HJ, Eichberg JW, Masur H, et al. Transmission of HTLV-III infection from human plasma to chimpanzees: an animal model for AIDS. Science 1984; 226:549–52.
110. Fultz PN, McClure HM, Swenson RB, et al. Persistent infection of chimpanzees with human T-lymphotropic virus type III/lymphadenopathy-associated virus: a potential model for acquired immunodeficiency syndrome. J Virol 1986; 58:116–24.
111. Weiss SH, Goedert JJ, Gartner S, et al. Risk of human immunodeficiency virus (HIV-1) infection among laboratory workers. Science 1988; 239:68–71.
112. Fultz PN, Siegel RL, Brodie A, et al. Prolonged $CD4^+$ lymphocytopenia and thrombocytopenia in a chimpanzee persistently infected with human immunodeficiency virus type 1. J Infect Dis 1991; 163:441–7.
113. Novembre FJ, Saucier M, Anderson DC, et al. Development of AIDS in a chimpanzee infected with human immunodeficiency virus type 1. J Virol 1997; 71:4086–91.
114. Huet T, Cheynier R, Meyerhans A, Roelants G, Wain-Hobson S. Genetic organization of a chimpanzee lentivirus related to HIV-1. Nature 1990; 345:356–9.
115. Corbet S, Muller-Trutwin MC, Versmisse P, et al. Env sequences of simian immunodeficiency viruses from chimpanzees in Cameroon are strongly related to those of human immunodeficiency virus group N from the same geographic area. J Virol 2000; 74:529–34.
116. Peeters M, Fransen K, Delaporte E, et al. Isolation and characterization of a new chimpanzee lentivirus (simian immunodeficiency virus isolate cpz-ant) from a wild-captured chimpanzee. AIDS 1992; 6:447–51.
117. Janssens W, Fransen K, Peeters M, et al. Phylogenetic analysis of a new chimpanzee lentivirus SIVcpz-gab2 from a wild-captured chimpanzee from Gabon. AIDS Res Hum Retrov 1994; 10:1191–2.
118. Kestens L, Vingerhoets J, Peeters M, et al. Phenotypic and functional parameters of cellular immunity in a chimpanzee with a naturally acquired simian immunodeficiency virus infection. J Infect Dis 1995; 172:957–63.
119. ten Haaft PJ, Murthy KK, Verstrepen BE, Eichberg JW, Heeney JL. Intact CCR-5 coreceptors in HIV-1-infected chimpanzees [letter]. AIDS 1997; 11:1291–3.
120. Benton PA, Timanus DK, Shearer MH, White GL, Lee DR, Kennedy RC. Analysis of nonhuman primate peripheral blood mononuclear cells for susceptibility to HIV-1 infection and HIV coreceptor expression. Dev Comp Immunol 1999; 23:97–105.
121. Watanabe M, Ringler DJ, Fultz JJ, et al. A chimpanzee-passaged human immunodeficiency virus isolate is cytopathic for chimpanzee cells but does not induce disease. J Virol 1991;6 5:3344–3348.
122. Peeters M, Janssens W, Vanden Haesevelde M, et al. Virologic and serologic characteristics of a natural chimpanzee lentivirus infection. Virology 1995; 211:312–5.
123. Santra S, Fultz PN, Letvin NL. Virus-specific cytotoxic T lymphocytes in human immunodeficiency virus type 1-infected chimpanzees. J Virol 1999; 73:7065–9.

124. Schuitemaker H, Meyaard L, Kootstra NA, et al. Lack of T cell dysfunction and programmed cell death in human immunodeficiency virus type 1-infected chimpanzees correlates with absence of monocytotropic variants. J Infect Dis 1993; 168:1140–7.
125. Saksela K, Muchmore E, Girard M, Fultz P, Baltimore D. High viral load in lymph nodes and latent human immunodeficiency virus (HIV) in peripheral blood cells of HIV-1-infected chimpanzees. J Virol 1993; 67:7423–7.
126. Heeney JL. AIDS: a disease of impaired Th-cell renewal? Immunol Today 1995; 16:515–20.
127. Zarling JM, Ledbetter JA, Sias J, et al. HIV-infected humans, but not chimpanzees, have circulating cytotoxic T lymphocytes that lyse uninfected CD4+ cells. J Immunol 1990; 144:2992–8.
128. Balla-Jhagjhoorsingh SS, Koopman G, Mooij P, et al. Conserved CTL epitopes shared between HIV-infected human long-term survivors and chimpanzees. J Immunol 1999; 162:2308–14.
129. Castro BA, Walker CM, Eichberg JW, Levy JA. Suppression of human immunodeficiency virus replication by CD8+ cells from infected and uninfected chimpanzees. Cell Immunol 1991; 132:246–55.
130. Husch B, Eibl MM, Mannhalter JW. CD3, CD8 double-positive cells from HIV-1-infected chimpanzees show group-specific inhibition of HIV-1 replication. AIDS Res Hum Retrovir 1993; 9:405–13.
131. Clerici M, Stocks NI, Zajac RA, et al. Detection of three distinct patterns of T helper cell dysfunction in asymptomatic, human immunodeficiency virus-seropositive patients: Independence of CD4+ cell numbers and clinical staging. J Clin Invest 1989; 84:1892–9.
132. Eichberg JW, Zarling JM, Alter HJ, et al. T-cell responses to human immunodeficiency virus (HIV) and its recombinant antigens in HIV-infected chimpanzees. J Virol 1987; 61:3804–8.
133. Gougeon ML, Lecoeur H, Boudet F, et al. Lack of chronic immune activation in HIV-infected chimpanzees correlates with the resistance of T cells to Fas/Apo-1 (CD95)-induced apoptosis and preservation of a T helper 1 phenotype. J Immunol 1997; 158:2964–76.
134. Di Rienzo AM, Furlini G, Olivier R, Ferris S, Heeney J, Montagnier L. Different proliferative response of human and chimpanzee lymphocytes after contact with human immunodeficiency virus type 1 gp 120. Eur J Immunol 1994; 24:34–40.
135. Gougeon ML, Garcia S, Heeney J, et al. Programmed cell death in AIDS-related HIV and SIV infections. AIDS Res Hum Retrovir 1993; 9:553–63.
136. Estaquier J, Idzioek T, DeBels F, et al. Programmed cell death and AIDS: Significance of T-cell apoptosis in pathogenic and nonpathogenic primate lentiviral infections. Proc Natl Acad Sci USA 1994; 91:9431–5.
137. Ehret A, Westendorp MO, Herr I, et al. Resistance of chimpanzee T cells to human immunodeficiency virus type 1 Tat-enhanced oxidative stress and apoptosis. J Virol 1996; 70:6502–7.
138. Ferrari G, Humphrey W, McEurath MJ, et al. Clade B-based HIV-1 vaccines elicit cross-clade cytotoxic T lymphocyte reactivities in uninfected volunteers. Proc Natl Acad Sci USA 1997; 94:1396–401.
139. Broliden K, Hinkula J, Tolfvenstam T, Niphuis H, Heeney J. Antibody-dependent cellular cytotoxicity to clinical isolates of HIV-1 and SIVcpz: comparison of human and chimpanzees. AIDS 1996; 10:1199–204.
140. Nara PL, Robey WG, Arthur LO, et al. Persistent infection of chimpanzees with human immunodeficiency virus: serological responses and properties of reisolated viruses. J Virol 1987; 61:3173–80.
141. Goudsmit J, Debouck C, Meloen RH, et al. Human immunodeficiency virus type 1 neutralization epitope with conserved architecture elicits early type-specific antibodies in experimentally infected chimpanzees. Proc Natl Acad Sci USA 1988; 85:4478–82.
142. Hayami M, Ido E, Miura T. Survey of simian immunodeficiency virus among nonhuman primate populations. Curr Top Microbiol Immunol 1994; 188:1–20.

143. Jolly C, Phillips-Conroy JE, Turner TR, Broussard S, Allan JS. SIVagm incidence over two decades in a natural population of Ethiopian grivet monkeys *(Cercopithecus aethiops aethiops).* J Med Primatol 1996; 25:78–83.
144. Daniel MD, Li Y, Naidu YM, et al. Simian immunodeficiency viruses from African green monkeys. J Virol 1988; 62:4123–8.
145. Allan JS, Short M, Taylor ME, et al. Species-specific diversity among simian immunodeficiency viruses from African green monkeys. J Virol 1991; 65:2816–28.
146. Allan JS, Kanda P, Kennedy RC, Cobb EK, Anthony M, Eichberg JW. Isolation and characterization of simian immunodeficiency viruses from two subspecies of African green monkeys. AIDS Res Hum Retrovir 1990; 6:275–85.
147. Muller MC, Saksena NK, Nerrienet E, et al. Simian immunodeficiency viruses from central and western Africa: evidence for a new species-specific lentivirus in tantalus monkeys. J Virol 1993; 67:1227–35.
148. Norley SG, Kraus G, Ennen J, Bonilla J, Konig H, Kurth R. Immunological studies of the basis for the apathogenicity of simian immunodeficiency virus from African green monkeys. Proc Natl Acad Sci USA 1990; 87:9067–71.
149. Werner A, Winskowsky G, Cichutek K, Norley SG, Kurth R. Productive infection of both $CD4^+$ and $CD4^-$ human cell lines with HIV-1, HIV-2 and SIVagm. AIDS 1990; 4:537–44.
150. Bibollet-Ruche F, Brengues C, Galat-Luong A, et al. Genetic diversity of simian immunodeficiency viruses from West African green monkeys: evidence of multiple genotypes within populations from the same geographical locale. J Virol 1997; 71:307–13.
151. Daniel MD, Letvin NL, Sehgal PK, et al. Prevalence of antibodies to 3 retroviruses in a captive colony of macaque monkeys. Int J Cancer 1988; 41:601–8.
152. Phillips-Conroy JE, Jolly CJ, Petros B, Allan JS, Desrosiers RC. Sexual transmission of SIVagm in wild grivet monkeys. J Med Primatol 1994; 23:1–7.
153. Kodama T, Silva DP, Daniel MD, et al. Prevalence of antibodies to SIV in baboons in their native habitat. AIDS Res Hum Retrovir 1989; 5:337–43.
154. Johnson PR, Goldstein S, London WT, Fomsgaard A, Hirsch VM. Molecular clones of SIVsm and SIVagm: experimental infection of macaques and african green monkeys. J Med Primatol 1990; 19:279–86.
155. Hirsch VM, Dapolito G, Johnson PR, et al. Induction of AIDS by simian immunodeficiency virus from an African green monkey: species-specific variation in pathogenicity correlates with the extent of in vivo replication. J Virol 1995; 69:955–67.
156. Beer B, Scherer J, zur Megede J, Norley S, Baier M, Kurth R. Lack of dichotomy between virus load of peripheral blood and lymph nodes during long-term simian immunodeficiency virus infection of African green monkeys. Virology 1996; 219:367–75.
157. Hartung S, Boller K, Cichutek K, Norley SG, Kurth R. Quantitation of a lentivirus in its natural host: simian immunodeficiency virus in African green monkeys. J Virol 1992; 66:2143–9.
158. Beer B, Denner J, Brown CR, et al. Simian immunodeficiency virus of African green monkeys is apathogenic in the newborn natural host. J AIDS Hum Retrovir 1998; 18:210–20.
159. Diop O, Gueye A, Dias-Tavares M, et al. High levels of viral replication during primary simian immunodeficiency virus SIVagm infection are rapidly and strongly controlled in African green monkeys. J Virol 2000; 74:7538–47.
160. Ennen J, Findeklee H, Dittmar MT, Norley S, Ernst M, Kurth R. $CD8^+$ T lymphocytes of African green monkeys secrete an immunodeficiency virus-suppressing lymphokine. Proc Natl Acad Sci USA 1994; 91:7207–11.
161. Baier M, Werner A, Cichutek K, et al. Molecularly cloned simian immunodeficiency virus SIVagm3 is highly divergent from other SIVagm isolates and is biologically active in vitro and in vivo. J Virol 1989; 63:5119–23.

162. Gicheru MM, Otsyula M, Spearman P, et al. Neutralizing antibody responses in Africa green monkeys naturally infected with simian immunodeficiency virus (SIVagm). J Med Primatol 1999; 28:97–104.
163. Miller MA, Murphey-Corb M, Montelaro RC. Identification of broadly reactive continuous antigenic determinants of simian immunodeficiency virus glycoproteins. AIDS Res Hum Retrovir 1992; 8:1153–64.
164. Siegel F, Norley S, Hartung S, Kurth R. B-cell epitope mapping of the entire SIVagm envelope glycoprotein including fine mapping of immunogenic regions. J Acquir Immun Defic Syndr 1992; 5:583–90.
165. Siegel F, Kurth R, Norley S. Neither whole inactivated virus immunogen nor passive immunoglobulin transfer protects against SIVagm infection in the African green monkey natural host. J Acquir Immune Defic Syndr Hum Retrovir 1995; 8:217–26.
166. Beer B, Baier M, zur Megede J, Norley S, Kurth R. Vaccine effect using a live attenuated nef-deficient simian immunodeficiency virus of African green monkeys in the absence of detectable vaccine virus replication in vivo. Proc Natl Acad Sci USA 1997; 94:4062–7.

12
Intrahost Selective Pressure and HIV-1 Heterogeneity During Progression to AIDS

Vladimir V. Lukashov, and Jaap Goudsmit

INTRODUCTION

One of the most striking characteristics of human immunodeficiency virus type 1 (HIV-1) is the immense genetic variation of this virus. Within a single individual, HIV-1 population exists at any given time point as a swarm of mutant viruses, in which all viruses are genetically related yet virtually every virus is unique (intrahost heterogeneity) and is changing over time on almost a daily basis (intrahost evolution). Moreover, infected individuals within a human population harbour distinct viruses (interhost or population-wide heterogeneity). The majority of HIV-1 strains could be grouped into genetic subtypes A–J of HIV-1 group M, based on phylogenetic analysis of their sequences *(1–9)*. Many viruses have been shown to have mosaic genomes, in which different genes or gene regions are related to distinct HIV-1 subtypes *(10,11)*. A few dozens of HIV-1 strains described so far belong to more distant HIV-1 groups O and N *(12)*.

HIV-1 variation is determined by multiple simultaneously acting virus and host factors. HIV-1 replication is a highly error-prone process, mainly due to lack of proofreading activity of the reverse transcription *(13–17)*. The rate of nucleotide substitutions introduced by reverse transcriptase is approx 10^{-4} per nucleotide per cycle of replication, which means that every newly produced virus genome has on average one nucleotide substitution compared to the parental genome (the size of HIV-1 genome is approx 9.7 kb) *(13–18)*. In addition, insertions, deletions, duplications, and recombinations contribute to genetic heterogeneity of HIV-1 *(10,19–22)*. The extreme mutation rate of HIV, together with short replication times and high virus loads, are resulting in continual creation of random complex mixtures of antigenically and phenotypically different virus strains, which compete among themself for survival. Although most of these mutants are replication defective or less adapted to the given intrahost environment (less fit), some of them will have by chance a higher fitness and preferentially overgrow. Subsequent overgrowth of a certain virus strain is largely determined by its replicative properties, cellular tropism, ability to escape from host immune response and antiretroviral therapy as well as by stochastic processes like bottleneck events. In addition to selective forces that arise within host and include receptor availability, cell permissiveness, immune and drug pressures, the virus quasispecies is also shaped by

From: *Retroviral Immunology: Immune Response and Restoration*
Edited by: Giuseppe Pantaleo and Bruce D. Walker © Humana Press Inc., Totowa, NJ

events occurring during host-to-host transmission, which may depend on the transmission route and the dose of the inoculum.

Natural infection of HIV-1 is characterized by a highly variable incubation period between the moment of infection and the development of acquired immune deficiency syndrome (AIDS), which can last (without antiretroviral therapy) from several months or a few years in fast progressors to 10–15 yr and more in slow or nonprogressors. The rates of HIV-1 production and clearance in the host, as measured by HIV-1 load in plasma or serum, is one of decisive factors in AIDS progression *(23–38)*. The higher HIV-1 load is, the faster the virus causes immunodeficiency and AIDS. The difference in plasma virus loads between fast and slow progressors can be seen early in infection, when other AIDS prognostic markers, like CD4 cell counts, are still similar in both groups *(29,39)*. The duration of the AIDS-free period is determined by multiple factors of virus–host interaction, including antiviral immune response. The level of virus production in a host may be understood as a measure of the efficiency of a continuous virus adaptation to the versatile intrahost environment. Independently of virus load, the evolution of biological phenotype of HIV-1 from non-syncytium-inducing (NSI) to syncytium-inducing (SI) is also an important element in predicting disease progression. Specific mutations within HIV-1 genome determine the ability of virus to escape from host immune surveillance, to spread within human body by occupying new types of target cells and tissues, and to confront antiretroviral therapy.

The ability of a certain virus strain to maintain its high load in the host is one of the key elements determining advantage of this strain in its competition with other virus strains in the host, or virus fitness. At the same time, virus load can be used as a measure of HIV-1 virulence, that supposes that there is a relation between virus fitness and virulence. Yet, it seems to be incorrect to directly measure fitness of an HIV-1 strain based on its load in the host, as this parameter depends on a number of other factors, including peculiarities of the immune response, target cell availability, virus tropism, etc.

Among the HIV-1 genes, the genomic region coding for the HIV-1 envelope glycoprotein gp120, particularly, the third variable domain (the V3 region) of gp120, is of special interest for studying intrahost heterogeneity of HIV. The V3 region contains recognition sites for both humoral and cellular immune responses *(40–45)* and is implicated in a number of biological properties of the virus, including cell tropism, infectivity, and cytopathicity *(46–50)*.

INTRAHOST EVOLUTION OF HIV

HIV-1 Transmission

From the documented cases of HIV-1 transmission, it has become apparent that HIV-1 populations in newly infected recipients are relatively homogeneous and may represent a major or a minor virus subpopulation present in the donors *(8,51–57)*. Although these observations are evident for a limitation of virus heterogeneity occurring during transmission, the mechanisms of this process is not yet fully understood. The main question which remains to be answered is whether the nature of this process is random, and the probability of any virus strain present in the donor to be transmitted to the recipient by chance is similar, or a specific selection is operational during transmission, and only viruses with certain phenotype could establish infections in new hosts. The understanding of the mechanism of selection during transmission is especially difficult, as these mechanisms could differ for different transmission routes *(52,58)*.

Certainly, massive random population bottlenecks are occurring during transmission, since the inoculum never contains the whole repertoire of virus strains present in the donor. On the other hand, selection of virus phenotype during transmission is supported by observations that the NSI viruses are present in the majority of infected individuals during the early stages of the HIV-1 infection following vertical, sexual, and parenteral transmission, even after transmission of a phenotypically mixed SI/NSI virus population *(55,59,60)*. However, these observations could be influenced by a fact that SI viruses are present only in HIV-infected individuals who are at the latest stages of the disease and do not cause the majority of new infections. Moreover, owing to the peculiarities of experimental methods *(61)*, even in individuals who are characterized as carrying the SI phenotype, the majority of clonal viruses in the bulk isolate (up to 95%) could have indeed the NSI phenotype.

Evolution of HIV-1 Phenotype

HIV-1 phenotype is routinely characterized by cocultivation of patient lymphocytes with established cell lines or peripheral blood mononuclear cells (PBMCs) taken from uninfected donors. Several classification systems are used to characterize the virus phenotype. Historically, the first system was based on peculiarities of growth kinetics in cell cultures, defining viruses as slow/low or rapid/high *(62)*. Another system defines virus tropism as infectivity for macrophages (M tropic) or T cells (T tropic). The third system classifies viruses according to their ability to grow in MT-2 cells, causing multinucleated giant cells, or syncytia (SI, vs NSI viruses). Although the three systems are not strictly equivalent, there is a definite overlap between them, that is, the rapid/high viruses are usually SI and T tropic, while the slow/low viruses are usually NSI and M tropic. It is important to point out that, because of the peculiarities of experimental methods, a mixed SI/NSI virus population will be characterized in bulk culture as an SI, even when the majority of the viruses has the NSI phenotype *(61)*. To characterize the phenotypic heterogeneity of virus populations, biological cloning is often used. The SI phenotype is strongly associated with the presence of positively charged amino acids at positions 306 and/or 320 of the gp120 V3 region *(46–50)*. In addition, certain sequence changes within the V2 domain may contribute to a switch of virus phenotype from NSI to SI *(63,64)*. A most recent classification of the HIV-1 phenotype is based on the virus ability to use certain secondary receptors for entry into cells *(65)*. The NSI viruses tend to use primarily CCR5 for viral entry, while the SI viruses are generally capable to use CXCR4 or both CXCR4 and CCR5.

The M-tropic NSI viruses are present in the vast majority of infected individuals during the early stages of the HIV-1 infection, irrespective to the route of infection *(55,59,60)*. Some of infected individuals maintain exclusively NSI viruses in the course of infection, while in others SI viruses emerge *(66)*. The rates of appearance of SI viruses vary markedly among infected populations in relation to risk group and virus genetic subtype. In the Amsterdam cohorts, SI viruses have been found in 54% of homosexual men versus 21% of injecting drug users at the moment of AIDS diagnosis *(67)*. In another study, SI viruses have been shown to be extremely rare among AIDS patients in Ethiopia, infected with HIV-1 subtype C *(67a)*.

A switch of virus phenotype from NSI to SI (again, in most of the cases to the mixed NSI/SI population) is associated with more rapid $CD4^+$ cell depletion and faster disease progression as well as with a reduced survival time after AIDS diagnosis *(24,27,66,68–70)*. The mechanism by which SI viruses in combination with NSI viruses cause faster disease progression, compared to NSI viruses along, is not fully understood *(71)*, and thought to be related to a higher cytopathicity and broader cell tropism of SI viruses. SI viruses infect both naive and memory CD4 cells, while NSI viruses infect only memory CD4 cells *(72)*.

Compartmentalization of HIV-1 in the Host

In addition to HIV-1 diversity in serum and blood cells, HIV-1 strains in other tissues contribute to the intrahost heterogeneity of the virus. HIV-1 is present in a variety of human organs and tissues, and multiple studies have shown that HIV-1 populations in blood generally differ from those derived simultaneously from other tissues, including spleen, the central nervous system, semen, vaginal secretion, lung lavage, intestinal tissues, etc. *(52,73–77)*. Yet, because of their cross-sectional design, most of the studies could not address the main question of whether the differences between tissue-specific virus populations are the results of independent evolution during virus adaptation to particular tissues or the consequences of random founder effects and time-related uneven distribution of virus strains within the host. Although independent HIV-1 evolution in different tissues and existence of tissue-specific genotypic patterns of HIV-1 have been hypothesized in some studies, the data on these issues are inconsistent. A longitudinal study of serum- and intestinum-derived viruses obtained over a period of several years from three individuals has revealed that virus strains which are present in the intestinum and are absent in serum at a certain time point, could be found in serum at another time point (L. van der Hoek, V. V. Lukashov, and J. Goudsmit, *unpublished observations*). This indicates that differences in HIV-1 populations between different tissue compartments (at least between serum and intestinum) may be largely determined by random founder effects and sampling biases.

ANTIVIRAL IMMUNE RESPONSE AND INTRAHOST EVOLUTION OF HIV-1

In a few weeks to months after the moment of infection, human hosts are developing humoral and cellular immune response against the virus *(25,26)*. Among various virus proteins, the gp120 V3 domain is one of the most antigenic, being a target for neutralizing antibodies, although often cryptic in primary isolates *(78)*, and containing recognition sites for T-cell response *(40–45,79)*. Antibodies produced early in infection have been shown to bind efficiently in vitro to synthetic peptides mimicking the amino acid sequence of the V3 region of the virus present at seroconversion *(80,81)* and to block infection by HIV-1 strains with similar V3 regions in cell cultures *(82)*. A longitudinal study of the V3 sequences and the anti-V3 antibody response has revealed that the in vitro specificity of the early antibodies is reflecting accurately the virus population present in individual hosts around seroconversion *(81)*. After 5 yr of infection, the early antibody specificity has been preserved in the majority of individuals, but not the early virus populations. As a result, a poor correlation between the V3 sequences and the anti-V3 antibody reactivity has been observed after five years of infection *(81)*.

Naturally occurring amino acid changes within the V3 region have been shown to lead to antigenic variation *(80)*. In vitro and in vivo experiments have demonstrated, that, under the selective pressure of antibodies on different virus proteins, neutralization escape mutants are arising *(80,83–89)*. Taken together, these data suggest that humoral immune response may serve as a driving force for intrahost evolution of HIV-1. A virus may escape V3 antibodies by mutations within the V3 region as well as outside the V3 region, but within the gp120, and even by mutations within a separate, but structurally linked protein, gp41 *(79,80,89–91)*.

The role of neutralizing antibodies in postponing the development of AIDS has been supported by the observations of a distinct neutralizing antibody response in slow progressors compared to fast progressors *(29,92–94)*. Ability of anti-HIV antibodies to eliminate infectious virus from blood has experimentally been shown *(95)*. However, in several studies no difference has been observed between fast and slow progressors in the anti-V3 or anti-gp120 antibody titers *(29,96)* or the ability to neutralize primary HIV-1 isolates *(97,98)*. Antibody-mediated enhancement of the HIV-1 infection has also been demonstrated *(99,100)*. The question of whether quantitative and qualitative characteristics of the humoral immune response are important in controlling virus infection, is still under debate *(94)*.

Recently, the role of the T-cell (cytolytic T lymphocyte [CTL]) response in controlling virus infection has been strongly suggested *(98,101–105)*. It has been shown that partial virus clearance following primary HIV-1 infection coincides with the development of a CTL response, and precedes the appearance of antiviral antibodies *(106,107)*. Several studies have provided evidences for virus evolution related to escaping from the CTL response *(108–112)*, which indicates the ability of CTLs to exert selection pressure. An analysis of an individual with CTL response against an HIV-1 epitope within gp160 has revealed that in 4 mo the initial homogeneous virus population has been replaced by a population that had a single amino acid change within this epitope, while no accumulation of the amino acid changes outside this epitope has been observed *(108)*. In another study *(109)*, an immunodominant epitope has been identified in virus populations of six individuals. In the two donors, who progressed to AIDS, an amino acid change within this epitope was observed during disease progression. A persistent gag-specific CTL response in nonprogressors, declining during AIDS progression, has been demonstrated *(101)*. These data suggest that CTL responses may provide an additional selection pressure on the virus and that virus evolution associated with escape from CTL response may play a role in the development of AIDS.

THE ROLE OF HIV-1 EVOLUTION IN VIRUS PATHOGENESIS: THE MODEL OF CONTINUOUS VIRUS ADAPTATION

The error-prone mechanism of HIV-1 replication constantly produces multiple virus mutants, which results in virus populations representing complex mixtures of different virus strains at any given time point. In evolutionary studies, such a complex virus population can be described by characterizing the most abundant, or the consensus, sequence (by direct sequencing of the whole virus population) and the complexity of the population (the mean or the range of the nucleotide distances between the individual sequences in the population). Both the consensus sequence and the complexity of virus populations are changing in the course of the individual HIV-1 infection. The patterns and the rate of intrahost evolution of HIV-1 is governed by selective forces operational within the host as well as random processes. A powerful tool to study the relative input of selection-driven versus random processes in HIV-1 intrahost evolution is separate analysis of nonsynonymous (those that result in amino acid changes) and synonymous (those that do not change the amino acids) substitutions. Both the nonsynonymous and synonymous substitutions are appearing in newly produced virus genomes with the same rate during each replication cycle. Yet, subsequent fate of virus mutants with nonsynonymous and synonymous substitutions is determined by different processes. Since synonymous substitutions do not change the amino acids, they do not alter antigenic or phenotypic properties of the mutant virus. The number of synonymous substitution fixed in population is determined by the rate of their appearance, or HIV-1 variability. These mutation are considered to be selectively neutral and the probability of their fixation in the population is independent of selective forces operational within the host. In contrast, amino acid changes caused by nonsynonymous substitutions may alter antigenic or phenotypic characteristics of the virus and therefore are subjected to positive (if this alteration is advantageous) or negative (if it is deleterious) selection. It has been shown that the patterns of the HIV-1 synonymous and nonsynonymous intrahost evolution vary for different proteins or protein regions in relation to their function and immunogenicity. Within the immunodominant regions, like the gp120 V3 domain, the rate of fixation of nonsynonymous substitutions in the virus populations is generally higher than that of synonymous substitutions. In contrast, nucleotide substitutions accumulating within the *pol* gene of HIV-1 are predominantly synonymous.

To explain the possible role of virus intrahost variation in the destruction of the immune system and disease progression, several *a priori* hypotheses have been put forward, which consider a number of antigenically different virus strains simultaneously present in the host at a given time point as a direct cause of disease progression *(113–115)*. Subsequently obtained experimental data, however, have been found to be inconsistent with earlier thoughts and led to a principle reevaluation of this issue *(116)*. In our own study *(117)*, the intrahost evolution of the gp120 V3 region was analyzed during a 5-yr period following seroconversion in 44 individuals, of whom 13 had developed AIDS during this period. As a measure of antigenic diversity, the numbers of nonsynonymous substitutions accumulated over 5 yr have been studied in comparison to the numbers of synonymous substitutions. The rates of intrahost nonsynonymous evolution (the number of nonsynonymous substitutions that become fixed in the population per year) were significantly higher in nonprogressors, compared to progressors, while the rates of synonymous evolution were similar in both groups. Because the rate of synonymous evolution is a measure of virus ability to produce mutants, one should conclude, that in progressors and nonprogressors, virus variability (ability to produce mutants) is the same, yet the variation (evolution), which reflects the probability of new mutants to be fixed in the population, is different. Importantly, the numbers of nonsynonymous substitutions fixed in virus populations over 5 yr were proportional to the duration of the immunocompetent period of infection, which was measured as time between seroconversion and the moment of $CD4^+$ cells drop below 200 (Fig. 1). This observation indicates, that during the immunocompetent period, the rates of nonsynonymous evolution are similar in subsequent progressors and nonprogressors. The higher nonsynonymous

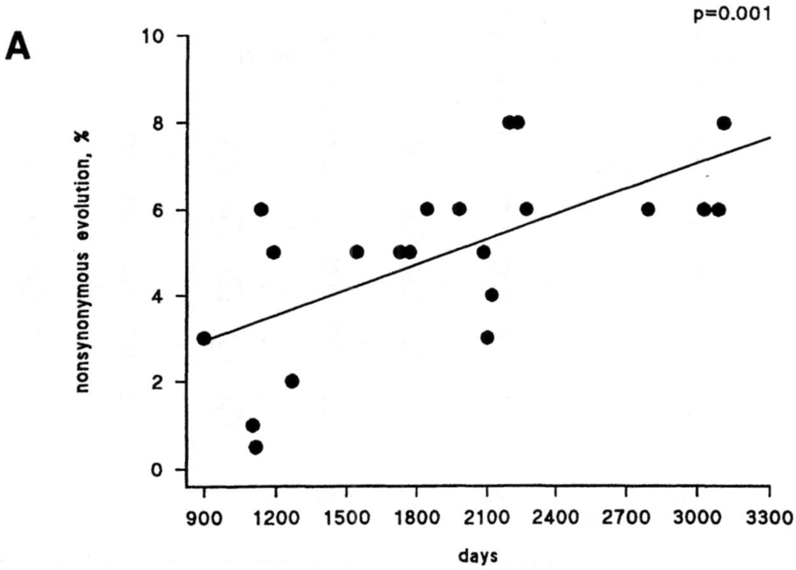

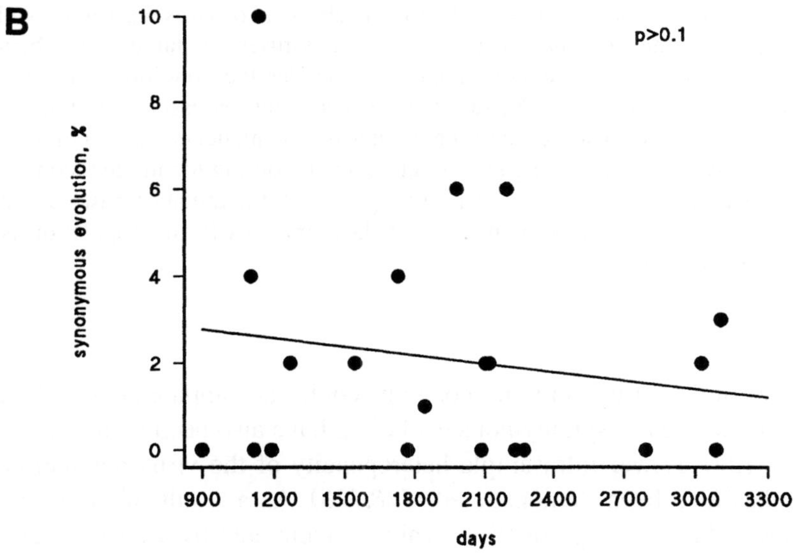

Fig. 1. Nonsynonymous **(A)**, but not synonymous **(B)** evolution of the HIV-1 gp120 V3 region over a 5-yr period is related to the length of the immunocompetent period in HIV-1 infection *(117)*. The V3 sequences were obtained from 21 individuals at seroconversion and 5 yr thereafter. The nonsynonymous and synonymous distances between the seroconversion and the 5-yr sequences from the same individual are shown in relation to the duration of the period (in days) during which the individual had remained immunocompetent (with CD4+ cell counts >200). Statistics: **A,** $p = 0.001$, $r = 0.64$, $r^2 = 0.41$; **B,** $p > 0.1$.

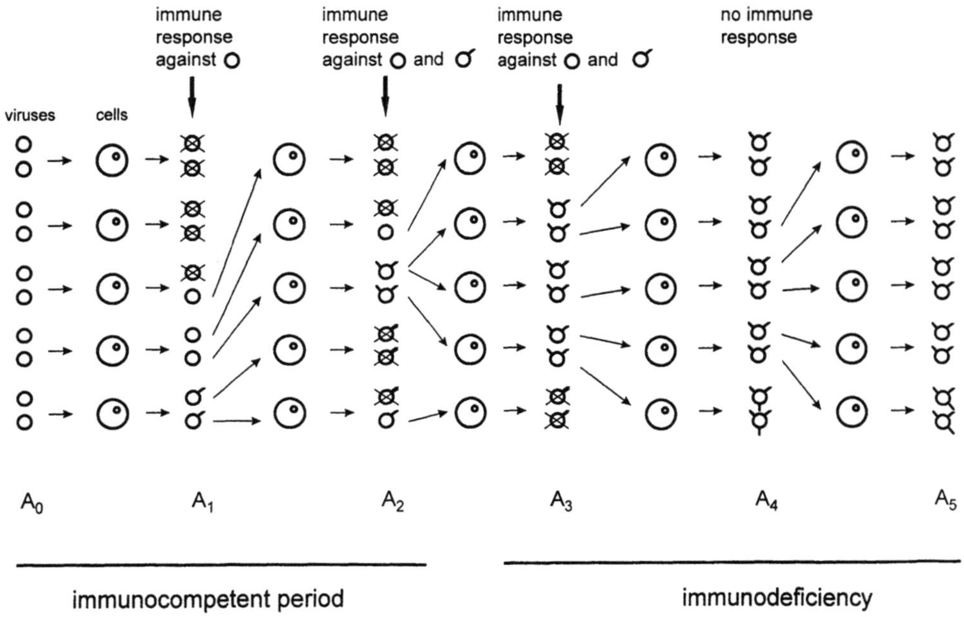

Fig. 2. The model of continuous virus adaptation demonstrates intrahost evolution of a virus population under the immune pressure and after immune collapse *(116)*. In a homogeneous virus population A_0, mutant viruses are produced during each round of virus replication with the same rate per infected cell, and compete with the original viruses for target cells, being initially present as a very minority in the virus population. Under the conditions of a host immune response against virus population A_0 (as it is seen in nonprogressors), escape mutants will preferentially grow out as a result of their higher fitness. The model explains a rapid virus evolution ($A_0 \Rightarrow A_1 \Rightarrow A_2 \Rightarrow A_3$) and a high virus heterogeneity during the immunocompetent period *(117,118)*. After immune collapse (as seen in progressors), the mutant viruses are arising with the same rate, but the probability of fixation of these mutants in the population is low. This results in evolutionary stasis.

evolution rates of the viruses in immunocompetent hosts compared to rapid progressors, as well as similar rates of synonymous evolution, have also been demonstrated in other studies *(118–127)*. Lower intrasample heterogeneity of the virus populations in rapid progressors has also been demonstrated *(118,128)*. As a result of these experimental findings, longitudinal virus production, which is facilitated by a continuous adaptation of the virus to the versatile intrahost environment, is thought to be more important in the development of AIDS, than a number of antigenically different virus strains simultaneously present in the host. These experimental data and ideas has recently been recapitulated in the model of continuous virus adaptation *(116)*.

To elaborate this model *(116)*, let us trace the evolution of a homogeneous virus population A_0 present in a host (Fig. 2). The first cycle of replication of this virus population will produce a variety of mutants, denote as A_1', A_1'' A_1''', etc., some of which will contain nonsynonymous substitutions altering their antigenic properties. Originally, each of these mutants is present as a very minority in the virus population, and is likely to be lost in an immunocompromized host, without having a selective advantage, that explain a slow virus evolution and relative homogeneity of the virus population in the immunocompromized host *(117,118)*. However, in an immunocompetent host immune pressure is directed against virus population A_0. Under these conditions, some escape mutants, say, A_1' and A_1'', will have selective advantages and preferentially grow out. As a result, after a certain period, the homogeneous virus population A_0 will be replaced by the heterogeneous virus population A_1, which contains both the A_1' and A_1'' strains. It is important to point out, that heterogeneity of A_1 is not a necessary factor in the model, it could contain a single virus strain. Thus, intrasample variation is unrelated to virulence. The process of the replacement of the virus population A_0 by A_1 coincides with a continuous virus production and a further destruction of host immune system. If, in spite of a continuous immune deterioration, the host is still able to produce a virus-specific immune response against A_1, continuing virus replication will result in production of new mutants and replacements of the virus population A_1 by populations A_2, A_3, etc. The preferential overgrowth of a mutant virus variant is additionally facilitated by a generally smaller virus population size in an immunocompetent host. The process of continuous replacements of virus populations will last until the final collapse of the immune system, thus explaining the numbers of nonsynonymous changes fixed during individual infections being proportional to the duration of the period during which the immune system of the host is relatively intact *(117)*. The observation of a generally higher virus heterogeneity in immunocompetent hosts is considered to be a reflection of continuous replacements of different virus populations. This level of intrasample virus heterogeneity is not necessarily increasing over time, and by itself is not decisive in the disease progression.

For simplicity, all antigenically different mutants in Fig. 2 are assumed to have the same replication rate and phenotype, including cell tropism, which means that all viruses have the same fitness and therefore the genetic differences between them are selectively neutral in the absence of immune response. In this case, the probability of fixation of a newly arising selectively neutral mutant is low, taking into account its initial low frequency in virus population, and the conditional fixation time is long. In the immunocompetent host, such a mutant could have selective advantage and better chances to be fixed in virus population in a shorter time, as a result of its competition with the original virus population for the same target cells. When the mutant virus has different cell tropism, longitudinal coexistence of the mutant and original viruses is possible, since the mutant and the original virus do not compete for target cells. A good example is virus evolution after the appearance of the SI viruses, when both the NSI and SI virus populations are present in an infected individual for years, each occupying a specific ecological niche (cell type). It is remarkable, that in contrast to slower evolution of virus antigenic properties, the incidence of appearance of SI viruses is the same or higher in immunocompromized hosts, compared to immunocompetent hosts (M. Koot et al., *unpublished observations*). This observation additionally supports the conclusion that virus ability to produce mutants is the same in progressors and nonprogressors, while the fixation probability is different and determined by their relative fitness in the presence or absence of the immune response and necessity to compete for target cells.

The main feature of the model of continuous virus adaptation *(116)* is its reevaluation of the weight of the respective contribution of host-specific vs virus-specific factors in the development of AIDS. This model considers a diverse virus population as a (passive) consequence of the host immune competence, rather than a factor leading to the development of AIDS, and explains the development of AIDS as a longitudinal process of the deterioration of the immune system by the virus, during which persistent virus production and continuous virus adaptation to the changing environment is taking place.

REFERENCES

1. Hahn BH, Gonda MA, Shaw GM, et al. Genomic diversity of the acquired immune deficiency syndrome virus HTLV-III: different viruses exhibit greatest divergence in their envelope genes. Proc Natl Acad Sci USA 1985; 82:4813–7.
2. Wong-Staal F, Shaw GM, Hahn BH, et al. Genomic diversity of human T-lymphotropic virus type III (HTLV-III). Science 1985; 229:759–62.
3. Kuiken CL, Zwart G, Baan E, Coutinho RA, Van den Hoek JAR, Goudsmit J. Increasing antigenic and genetic diversity of the V3 variable domain of the human immunodeficiency virus envelope protein in the course of the AIDS epidemic. Proc Natl Acad Sci USA 1993; 90:9061–5.
4. Kuiken CL, Lukashov VV, Baan E, Dekker J, Leunissen JAM, Goudsmit J. Evidence for limited within-person evolution of the V3 domain of the HIV-1 envelope in the Amsterdam population. AIDS 1996; 10:31–7.
5. Kalish ML, Luo C-C, Weniger BG, et al. Early HIV type 1 strains in Thailand were not responsible for the current epidemic. AIDS Res Hum Retrovir 1994; 10:1573–5.
6. Ou C-Y, Takebe Y, Weniger BG, et al. Independent introduction of two major HIV-1 genotypes into distinct high-risk populations in Thailand. Lancet 1993; 341:1171–4.
7. Lukashov VV, Cornelissen MTE, Goudsmit J, et al. Simultaneous introduction of distinct HIV-1 subtypes into different risk groups in Russia, Byelorussia and Lithuania. AIDS 1995; 9:435–9.
8. Zhu T, Mo H, Wang N, et al. Genotypic and phenotypic characterization of HIV-1 in patients with primary infection. Science 1993; 261:1179–81.
9. Lukashov VV, Kuiken CL, Boer K, Goudsmit J. HIV type 1 subtypes in The Netherlands circulating among women originating from AIDS endemic regions. AIDS Res Hum Retrovir 1996; 12:951–3.
10. Robertson DL, Sharp PM, McCutchan FE, Hahn BH. Recombination in HIV-1. Nature 1995; 374:124–6.
11. Cornelissen M, Kampinga G, Zorgdrager F, Goudsmit J, The UNAIDS Network for HIV Isolation and Characterization. Human immunodeficiency virus type 1 subtypes defined by env show high frequency of recombinant gag genes. J Virol 1996; 70:8209–12.
12. Peeters M, Gueye A, Mboup S, et al. Geographical distribution of HIV-1 group O viruses in Africa. AIDS 1997; 11:493–8.
13. Roberts JD, Bebenek K, Kunkel TA. The accuracy of reverse transcriptase from HIV-1. Science 1988; 242:1171–3.
14. Bebenek K, Abbotts J, Roberts JD, Wilson SN, Kunkel TA. Specificity and mechanism of error-prone replication by human immunodeficiency virus-1 reverse transcriptase. J Biol Chem 1989; 264,28:16948–56.
15. Roberts JD, Preston BD, Johnston LA, Soni A, Loeb LA, Kunkel TA. Fidelity of two retroviral reverse transcriptases during DNA-dependent DNA synthesis in vitro. Mol Cell Biol 1989; 9:469–76.
16. Preston BD, Poiesz BJ, Loeb LA. Fidelity of HIV-1 reverse transcriptase. Science 1988; 242:1168–71.
17. Ricchetti M, Buc H. Reverse transcriptases and genomic variability: the accuracy of DNA replication is enzyme specific and sequence dependent. EMBO J 1990; 9,5:1583–93.
18. Nowak M. HIV mutation rate. Nature 1990; 347:522.
19. Hu W, Temin HM. Retroviral recombination and reverse transcription. Science 1990; 250:1227–33.

20. Pathak VK, Temin HM. Broad spectrum of in vivo forward mutations, hypermutations and mutational hotspots in a retroviral shuttle vector after a single replication cycle: substitutions, frameshifts, and hypermutations. Proc Natl Acad Sci USA 1990; 87:6019–23.
21. Pulsinelli GA, Temin HM. Characterization of large deletions occurring during a single round of retrovirus vector replication: novel deletion mechanism involving errors in strand transfer. J Virol 1991; 65:4786–97.
22. Hu W-S, Temin HM. Retroviral recombination and reverse transcription. Science 1990; 250:1227–33.
23. Piatak M, Saag MS, Yang LC, et al. High levels of HIV-1 in plasma during all stages of infection determined by competitive PCR. Science 1993; 259:1749–54.
24. Connor RI, Mohri H, Cao Y, Ho DD. Increased viral burden and cytopathicity correlate temporally with CD4+ T-lymphocyte decline and clinical progression in human immunodeficiency virus type-1 infected individuals. J Virol 1993; 67:1772–7.
25. Daar ES, Moudgil T, Meyer RD, Ho DD. Transient high levels of viremia in patients with primary human immunodeficiency virus type 1 infection. N Engl J Med 1991; 324:961–4.
26. Graziosi C, Pantaleo G, Butini L, et al. Kinetics of human immunodeficiency virus type 1 (HIV-1) DNA and RNA synthesis during primary HIV-1 infection. Proc Natl Acad Sci USA 1993; 90:6405–9.
27. Jurriaans S, Van Gemen B, Weverling GJ, et al. The natural history of HIV-1 infection: virus load and virus phenotype independent determinants of clinical course? Virology 1994; 204:223–33.
28. Jurriaans S, Weverling GJ, Goudsmit J, et al. Distinct changes in HIV type 1 RNA versus p24 antigen levels in serum during short-term zidovudine therapy in asymptomatic individuals with and without progression to AIDS. AIDS Res Hum Retrovir 1995; 11:473–9.
29. Hogervorst E, Jurriaans S, De Wolf F, et al. Predictors for non- and slow progression in human immunodeficiency virus type 1 infection: low viral RNA copy numbers in serum and maintenance of high HIV-1 p24-specific, but not V3-specific antibody levels. J Infect Dis 1995; 171:811–21.
30. Mellors JW, Kingsley LA, Rinaldo CR Jr, Todd JA, Hoo BS, Kokka RP, Gupta P. Quantitation of HIV-1 RNA in plasma predicts outcome after seroconversion. Ann Intern Med 1995; 122:573–9.
31. Mellors JW, Rinaldo CR, Gupta P, White RM, Todd JA, Kingsley LA. Prognosis in HIV-1 infection predicted by the quantity of virus in plasma. Science 1996; 272:1167–70.
32. Gupta P, Kingsley L, Armstrong J, Ding M, Cottrill M, Rinaldo C. Enhanced expression of human immunodeficiency virus type 1 correlates with development of AIDS. Virology 1993; 196:586–95.
33. Schechter MT, Neumann PW, Weaver MS, et al. Low HIV-1 proviral DNA burden detected by negative polymerase chain reaction in seropositive individuals correlates with slower disease progression. AIDS 1991; 5:373–9.
34. Spijkerman IJ, Prins M, Goudsmit J, et al. Early and late HIV-1 RNA level and its association with other markers and disease progression in long-term AIDS-free homosexual men. AIDS 1997; 11:1383–8.
35. Keet IP, Janssen M, Veugelers PJ, et al. Longitudinal analysis of CD4 T cell counts, T cell reactivity, and human immunodeficiency type 1 RNA levels in persons remaining AIDS-free despite CD4 cell counts <200 for >5 years. J Infect Dis 1997; 176:665–71.
36. Goudsmit J, De Ronde A, Ho DD, Perelson AS. Human immunodeficiency virus fitness in vivo: calculation based on a single zidovudine resistance mutation at codon 215 of reverse transcriptase. J Virol 1996; 70:5662–4.
37. Blaak H, Brouwer M, Ran LJ, De Wolf F, Schuitemaker H. In vitro replication kinetics of human immunodeficiency virus type 1 (HIV-1) variants in relation to virus load in long-term survivors of HIV-1 infection. J Infect Dis 1998; 177:600–10.
38. Blaak H, De Wolf F, Van't Wout AB, et al. Temporal relationship between human immunodeficiency virus type 1 RNA levels in serum and cellular infectious load in peripheral blood. J Infect Dis 1997; 176:1383–7.

39. De Wolf F, Spijkerman I, Schellekens PT, et al. AIDS prognosis based on HIV-1 RNA, CD4+ T-cell count and function: markers with reciprocal predictive value over time after seroconversion. AIDS 1997; 11:1799–806.
40. Goudsmit J, Debouck C, Meloen RH, et al. Human immunodeficiency virus type 1 neutralization epitope with conserved architecture elicits early type-specific antibodies in experimentally infected chimpanzees. Proc Natl Acad Sci USA 1988; 85:4478–82.
41. Palker TJ, Clark ME, Langlois AJ, et al. Type-specific neutralization of the human immunodeficiency virus with antibodies to env-encoded synthetic peptides. Proc Natl Acad Sci USA 1988; 85:1932–6.
42. Safrit JT, Lee AY, Andrews CA, Koup RA. A region of the third variable loop of HIV-1 gp120 is recognized by HLA-B7-restricted CTLs from two acute seroconversion patients. J Immunol 1994; 153:3822–30.
43. Rusche JR, Javaherian K, McDanal C, et al. Antibodies that inhibit fusion of human immunodeficiency virus-infected cells bind a 24-amino acid sequence of the viral envelope, gp120. Proc Natl Acad Sci USA 1988; 85:3198–202.
44. Takahashi H, Cohen J, Hosmalin A, et al. An immunodominant epitope of the human immunodeficiency virus envelope glycoprotein gp160 recognized by class I major histocompatibility complex molecule-restricted murine cytotoxic T lymphocytes. Proc Natl Acad Sci USA 1988; 85:3105–9.
45. Takahashi H, Germain RN, Moss B, Berzofsky JA. An immunodominant class I-restricted cytotoxic T lymphocyte determinant of human immunodeficiency virus type 1 induces CD4 Class II-restricted help for itself. J Exp Med 1990; 171:571–6.
46. De Jong JJ, Goudsmit J, Keulen W, et al. Human immunodeficiency virus type 1 clones chimeric for the envelope V3 domain differ in syncytium formation and replication capacity. J Virol 1992; 66:757–65.
47. Kuiken CL, De Jong JJ, Baan E, Keulen W, Tersmette M, Goudsmit J. Evolution of the V3 envelope domain in proviral sequences and isolates of human immunodeficiency virus type 1 during transition of the viral biological phenotype. J Virol 1992; 66:4622–7.
48. De Jong JJ, De Ronde A, Keulen W, Tersmette M, Goudsmit J. Minimal requirements for the human immunodeficiency virus type 1 V3 domain to support the syncytium-inducing (SI) phenotype: analysis by single amino acid substitution. J Virol 1992; 66:6777–80.
49. Fouchier RAM, Groenink M, Kootstra NA, et al. Phenotype associated sequence variation in the third variable domain of the human immunodeficiency virus type 1 gp120 molecule. J Virol 1992; 66:3183–7.
50. De Wolf F, Hogervorst E, Goudsmit J, et al. Syncytium-inducing and non-syncytium-inducing capacity of human immunodeficiency virus type 1 subtypes other than B: phenotypic and genotypic characteristics. AIDS Res Hum Retrovir 1994; 10:1387–400.
51. Wolfs TFW, Zwart G, Bakker M, Goudsmit J. HIV-1 genomic RNA diversification following sexual and parental virus transmission. Virology 1992; 189:103–10.
52. Zhu T, Wang N, Carr A, et al. Genetic characterization of human immunodeficiency virus type 1 in blood and genital secretions: evidence for viral compartmentalization and selection during sexual transmission. J Virol 1996; 70:3098–107.
53. Zhang LQ, Mackenzie P, Cleland A, Holmes EC, Leigh Brown AJ, Simmonds P. Selection for specific sequences in the external envelope protein of human immunodeficiency virus type 1 upon primary infection. J Virol 1993; 67:3345–56.
54. Wolinsky SM, Wike CM, Korber BTM, et al. Selective transmission of human immunodeficiency virus type-1 variants from mothers to infant. Science 1992; 255:1134–7.
55. Cornelissen M, Mulder-Kampinga G, Veenstra J, et al. Syncitium-inducing (SI) phenotype suppression at seroconversion after intramuscular inoculation of a non-syncytium-inducing/SI phenotypically mixed human immunodeficiency virus population. J Virol 1995; 69:1810–8.

56. Mulder-Kampinga GA, Kuiken C, Dekker J, Scherpbier HJ, Boer K, Goudsmit J. Genomic human immunodeficiency virus type 1 RNA variation in mother and child following intra-uterine virus transmission. J Gen Virol 1993; 74:1747–56.
57. McNearney T, Hornickova Z, Markham R, et al. Relationship of human immunodeficiency virus type 1 sequence heterogeneity to stage of disease. Proc Natl Acad Sci USA 1992; 89:10247–51.
58. Goudsmit J, Lukashov VV, Van Ameijden EJ, Zorgdrager F, Van den Burg R, Cornelissen M. Impact of sexual versus parenteral transmission events on the evolution of the gag and env genes of HIV type 1. AIDS Res Hum Retrovir 1998; 14:1483–6.
59. Schuitemaker H, Kootstra NA, De Goede REY, De Wolf F, Miedema F, Tersmette M. Monocytotropic human immunodeficiency virus type 1 (HIV-1) variants detectable in all stages of HIV-1 infection lack T-cell line tropism and syncytium-inducing ability in primary T-cell culture. J Virol 1991; 65,1:356–63.
60. Van't Wout AB, Kootstra NA, Mulder-Kampinga GA, et al. Macrophage-tropic variants initiate human immunodeficiency virus type 1 infection after sexual, parenteral and vertical transmission. J Clin Invest 1994; 94:2060–7.
61. Lukashov VV, Goudsmit J. Increasing genotypic and phenotypic selection from the original genomic RNA populations of HIV-1 strains LAI and MN (NM) by peripheral blood mononuclear cell culture, B-cell-line propagation and T-cell-line adaptation. AIDS 1995; 9:1307–11.
62. Åsjö B, Morfeldt-Månson L, Albert J, et al. Replicative capacity of human immunodeficiency virus from patients with varying severity of HIV infection. Lancet 1986; ii:660–2.
63. Groenink M, Fouchier RAM, Broersen S, et al. Relation of phenotype evolution of HIV-1 to envelope V2 configuration. Science 1993; 260:1513–6.
64. Groenink M, Andeweg AC, Fouchier RAM, et al. Phenotype-associated env gene variation among eight related human immunodeficiency virus type 1 clones: evidence for in vivo recombination and determinants of cytotropism outside the V3 domain. J Virol 1992; 66:6175–80.
65. Berger EA, Doms RW, Fenyo EM, et al. A new classification for HIV-1 [letter]. Nature 1998; 391:240.
66. Koot M, Keet IPM, Vos AHV, et al. Prognostic value of HIV-1 syncytium-inducing phenotype for rate of CD4+ cell depletion and progression of AIDS. Ann Intern Med 1993; 118:681–8.
67. Spijkerman IJB, Koot M, Prins M, et al. Lower prevalence and incidence of HIV-1 syncytium-inducing phenotype among injecting drug users compared with homosexual men. AIDS 1995; 9:1085–92.
67a. Abebe A, Demissie D, Goudsmit J, Brouwer M, Kuiken CL, Pollakis G, et al. HIV-1 subtype C syncytium- and non-syncytium-inducing phenotypes and coreceptor usage among Ethiopian patients with AIDS. AIDS 1999; 13:1305–11.
68. Tersmette M, Lange JMA, De Goede REY, et al. Association between biological properties of human immunodeficiency virus variants and risk for AIDS and AIDS mortality. Lancet 1989; i:983–5.
69. Tersmette M, Gruters RA, De Wolf F, et al. Evidence for a role of virulent human immunodeficiency virus (HIV) variants in the pathogenesis of acquired immunodeficiency syndrome: studies on sequential HIV isolates. J Virol 1989; 63:2118–25.
70. Schuitemaker H, Koot M, Kootstra NA, et al. Biological phenotype of human immunodeficiency virus type 1 clones at different stages of infection: progression of disease is associated with a shift from monocytotropic to T-cell-tropic virus populations. J Virol 1992; 66:1354–60.
71. Fouchier RAM, Schuitemaker H. Molecular determinants of human immunodeficiency virus type 1 phenotype variability. Eur J Clin Invest 1996; 26:175–85.
72. Fouchier RA, Meyaard L, Brouwer M, Hovenkamp E, Schuitemaker H. Broader tropism and higher cytopathicity for CD4+ T cells of a syncytium-inducing compared to a non-syncytium-inducing HIV-1 isolate as a mechanism for accelerated CD4+ T cell decline in vivo. Virology 1996; 219:87–95.

73. Cheng-Mayer C, Weiss C, Seto D, Levy JA. Isolates of human immunodeficiency virus type 1 from the brain may constitute a special group of the AIDS virus. Proc Natl Acad Sci USA 1989; 86:8575–9.
74. Epstein LG, Kuiken C, Blumberg BM, et al. HIV-1 V3 domain variation in brain and spleen of children with AIDS: tissue-specific evolution within host-determined quasispecies. Virology 1991; 180:583–90.
75. Kuiken CL, Goudsmit J, Weiller GF, et al. Differences in human immunodeficiency virus type 1 V3 sequences from patients with and without AIDS dementia complex. J Gen Virol 1995; 76:175–80.
76. Van der Hoek L, Sol CJA, Maas J, Lukashov VV, Kuiken CL, Goudsmit J. Genetic differences between human immunodeficiency virus type 1 subpopulations in faeces and serum. J Gen Virol 1998; 79:259–67.
77. Van der Hoek L, Sol CJA, Snijders F, Bartelsman JFW, Boom R, Goudsmit J. Human immunodeficiency virus type 1 RNA populations in faeces with higher homology to intestinal populations than to blood populations. J Gen Virol 1996; 77:2415–25.
78. Bou-Habib DC, Roderiquez G, Oravecz T, Berman PW, Lusso P, Norcross MA. Cryptic nature of envelope V3 region epitopes protects primary monocytotropic human immunodeficiency virus type 1 from antibody neutralization. J Virol 1994; 68:6006–13.
79. Hogervorst E, De Jong JJ, Van Wijk A, et al. Insertion of primary syncytium-inducing (SI) and non-SI envelope V3 loops in human immunodeficiency virus type 1 LAI (HIV-1LAI) reduces neutralization sensitivity to autologous, but not heterologous HIV-1 antibodies. J Virol 1995; 69:6342–51.
80. Wolfs TFW, Zwart G, Bakker M, Valk M, Kuiken CL, Goudsmit J. Naturally occurring mutations within HIV-1 V3 genomic RNA lead to antigenic variation dependent on a single amino acid substitution. Virology 1991; 185:195–205.
81. Zwart G, Wolfs TFW, Valk M, Van der Hoek L, Kuiken CL, Goudsmit J. Characterization of the specificity of the human antibody response to the V3 neutralization domain of HIV-1. AIDS Res Hum Retrovir 1992; 8:1897–908.
82. Zwart G, Langedijk H, Van der Hoek L, et al. Immunodominance and antigenic variation of the principal neutralization domain of HIV-1. Virology 1991; 181:481–9.
83. Arendrup M, Nielsen C, Hansen J-ES, Pedersen C, Mathiesen L, Nielsen JO. Autologous HIV-1 neutralizing antibodies: emergence of neutralization-resistant escape virus and subsequent development of escape virus neutralizing antibodies. J AIDS 1992; 5:303–7.
84. Arendrup M, Sönnerborg A, Svennerholm B, et al. Neutralizing antibody response during human immunodeficiency virus type 1 infection: type and group specificity and viral escape. J Gen Virol 1993; 74:855–63.
85. Watkins BA, Buge S, Aldrich K, et al. Resistance of human immunodeficiency virus type 1 to neutralization by natural antisera occurs through single amino acid substitutions that cause changes in antibody binding at multiple sites. J Virol 1996; 70:8431–7.
86. Sirko DA, Ehrlich GD. Genotypic and phenotypic characterization of a neutralization-resistant breakthrough population of HIV-1. Virology 1997; 218:238–42.
87. Bongertz V, Costa CI, Santos VG, Filho EC, Galvao-Castro B, Morgado MG. Correlation between susceptibility of primary HIV-1 isolates to autologous and heterologous neutralizing antibodies. AIDS 1997; 11:969–75.
88. Tsang ML, Evans LA, McQueen P, et al. Neutralizing antibodies against sequential autologous human immunodeficiency virus type 1 isolates after seroconversion. J Infect Dis 1994; 170:1141–7.
89. Yoshida K, Nakamura M, Ohno T. Mutations of the HIV type 1 V3 loop under selection pressure with neutralizing monoclonal antibody NM-01. AIDS Res Hum Retrovir 1997; 13:1283–90.
90. Back NKT, Smit L, De Jong JJ, et al. An N-glycan within the human immunodeficiency virus type 1 gp120 V3 loop affects virus neutralization. Virology 1994; 199:431–8.

91. Back NKT, Smit L, Schutten M, Nara PL, Tersmette M, Goudsmit J. Mutations in HIV-1 gp41 affect sensitivity to neutralization by gp120 antibodies and soluble CD4. J Virol 1993; 67:6897–902.
92. Cao Y, Qing L, Zhang L, Safrit J, Ho DD. Virologic and immunologic characterization of long-term survivors of human immunodeficiency virus type 1 infection. N Engl J Med 1995; 332:201–8.
93. Pantaleo G, Menzo S, Vaccarezza M, et al. Studies in subjects with long-term nonprogressive human immunodeficiency virus infection. N Engl J Med 1995; 332:209–16.
94. Carotenuto P, Looij D, Keldermans L, De Wolf F, Goudsmit J. Neutralizing antibodies are positively associated with $CD4^+$ T-cell counts and T-cell function in long-term AIDS-free infection. AIDS 1998; 12:1591–600.
95. Igarashi T, Brown C, Azadegan A, et al. Human immunodeficiency virus type 1 neutralizing antibodies accelerate clearance of cell-free virions from blood plasma. Nat Med 1999; 5:211–6.
96. Zwart G, Van der Hoek L, Valk M, et al. Antibody responses to HIV-1 envelope and gag epitopes in HIV-1 seroconverters with rapid versus slow disease progression. Virology 1994; 201:285–93.
97. Montefiori DC, Pantaleo G, Fink LM, et al. Neutralizing and infection enhancing antibody responses to human immunodeficiency virus type 1 in long-term nonprogressors. J Infect Dis 1996; 173:60–7.
98. Harper T, Harrer E, Kalams SA, et al. Strong cytotoxic T cell and weak neutralising antibody responses in a subset of persons with stable nonprogressing HIV type 1 infection. AIDS Res Hum Retrovir 1996; 12:585–92.
99. Robinson WE Jr, Montefiori DC, Mitchell WM. Antibody-dependent enhancement of human immunodeficiency virus type I infection. Lancet 1988; i:790–4.
100. Kliks SC, Shioda T, Haigwood NL, Levy JA. V3 variability can influence the ability of an antibody to neutralize or enhance infection by diverse strains of human immunodeficiency virus type 1. Proc Natl Acad Sci USA 1993; 90:11518–22.
101. Klein MR, Van Baalen CA, Holwerda AM, et al. Kinetics of gag-specific cytotoxic T lymphocyte responses during the clinical course of HIV-1 infection: a longitudinal analysis of rapid progressors and long-term asymptomatics. J Exp Med 1995; 181:1365–72.
102. McMichael AJ, Phillips RE. Escape of human immunodeficiency virus from immune control. Annu Rev Immunol 1997; 15:271–96.
103. Harrer T, Harrer E, Kalams SA, et al. Cytotoxic T lymphocytes in asymptomatic long-term nonprogressing HIV-1 infection. Breadth and specificity of the response and relation to in vivo viral quasispecies in a person with prolonged infection and low viral load. J Immunol 1996; 156:2616–23.
104. Bariou C, Genetet N, Ruffault A, Michelet C, Cartier F, Genetet B. Longitudinal study of HIV-specific cytotoxic lymphocytes in HIV type 1-infected patients: relative balance between host immune response and the spread of HIV type 1 infection. AIDS Res Hum Retrovir 1997; 13:1301–12.
105. Pontesilli O, Klein MR, Kerkhof-Garde SR, et al. Longitudinal analysis of human immunodeficiency virus type 1-specific cytotoxic T lymphocyte responses: a predominant gag-specific response is associated with nonprogressive infection. J Infect Dis 1998; 178:1008–18.
106. Pellegrin I, Legrand E, Neau D, et al. Kinetics of appearance of neutralizing antibodies in 12 patients with primary or recent HIV-1 infection and relationship with plasma and cellular viral loads. J AIDS Retrovirol 1997; 11:438–47.
107. Koup RA, Safrit JT, Cao Y, et al. Temporal association of cellular immune response with the initial control of viremia in primary HIV-1 syndrome. J Virol 1994; 68:4650–5.
108. Borrow P, Lewicki H, Wei X, et al. Antiviral pressure exerted by HIV-1-specific cytotoxic T lymphocytes (CTLs) during primary infection demonstrated by rapid selection of CTL escape virus. Nat Med 1997; 3:205–11.

109. Goulder PJR, Phillips RE, Colbert RA, et al. Late escape from an immunodominant cytotoxic T-lymphocyte response associated with progression to AIDS. Nat Med 1997; 3:212–7.
110. Price DA, Goulder PJR, Klenerman P, et al. Positive selection of HIV-1 cytotoxic T-lymphocyte escape variants during primary infection. Proc Natl Acad Sci USA 1997; 94:1890–5.
111. Zhang WH, Hockley DJ, Nermut MV, Jones IM. Functional consequences of mutations in HIV-1 gag p55 selected by CTL pressure. Virology 1994; 203:101–5.
112. Johnson RP, Trocha A, Buchanan TM, Walker BD. Recognition of a highly conserved region of human immunodeficiency virus type 1 gp120 by an HLA-Cw4-restricted cytotoxic T-lymphocyte clone. J Virol 1993; 67:438–45.
113. Nowak MA, May RM, Anderson RM. The evolutionary dynamics of HIV-1 quasispecies and the development of immunodeficiency disease. AIDS 1990; 4:1095–3.
114. Nowak MA, Anderson RM, McLean AR, Wolfs TFW, Goudsmit J, May RM. Antigenic diversity thresholds and the development of AIDS. Science 1991; 254:963–9.
115. McLean AR. The balance of power between HIV and the immune system. Trends Microbiol 1993; 1:9–13.
116. Lukashov VV, Goudsmit J. HIV heterogeneity and disease progression in AIDS: a model of continuous virus adaptation. AIDS 1998; 12:S43–S52.
117. Lukashov VV, Kuiken CL, Goudsmit J. Intrahost human immunodeficiency virus type 1 evolution is related to length of the immunocompetent period. J Virol 1995; 69:6911–6.
118. Wolinsky SM, Korber BTM, Neumann AU, et al. Adaptive evolution of human immunodeficiency virus-type 1 during the natural course of infection. Science 1996; 272:537–42.
119. Shioda T, Oka S, Xin SM, et al. In vivo sequence variability of human immunodeficiency virus type 1 envelope gp120—association of V2 extension with slow disease progression. J Virol 1997; 71:4871–1.
120. Liu SL, Schacker T, Musey L, et al. Divergent patterns of progression to AIDS after infection from the same source—human immunodeficiency virus type 1 evolution and antiviral response. J Virol 1997; 71:4284–95.
121. Salvatori F, Masiero S, Giaquinto C, et al. Evolution of human immunodeficiency virus type 1 in perinatally infected infands with rapid and slow progression to disease. J Virol 1997; 71:4694–706.
122. McDonald RA, Mayers DL, Chung RCY, et al. Evolution of human immunodeficiency virus type 1 env sequence variation in patients with diverse rates of disease progression and T-cell function. J Virol 1997; 71:1871–9.
123. Yamaguchi Y, Gojobori T. Evolutionary mechanisms and population dynamics of the 3rd variable envelope region of HIV within single hosts. Proc Natl Acad Sci USA 1997; 94:1264–9.
124. Zhang LQ, Diaz RS, Ho DD, Mosley JW, Busch MP, Mayer A. Host-specific driving force in human immunodeficiency virus type 1 evolution in vivo. J Virol 1997; 71:2555–61.
125. Ganeshan S, Dickover RE, Korber BTM, Bryson YJ, Wolinsky SM. Human immunodeficiency virus type 1 genetic evolution in children with different rates of development of disease. J Virol 1997; 71:663–77.
126. Delwart EL, Sheppard HW, Walker BD, Goudsmit J, Mullins JI. Human immunodeficiency virus type 1 evolution in vivo tracked by DNA heteroduplex mobility assays. J Virol 1994; 68:6672–83.
127. Halapi E, Leitner T, Jansson M, et al. Correlation between HIV sequence evolution, specific immune response and clinical outcome in vertically infected infants. AIDS 1997; 11:1709–17.
128. Wolinsky SM, Kunstman KJ, Safrit JT, Koup RA, Neumann AU, Korber BTM. HIV-1 evolution and disease progression. Science 1996; 274:1010–11.

13

Polymorphism in HLA and Other Elements of the Class I and II Response Pathways

Richard A. Kaslow and R. Pat Bucy

Vertebrates have evolved a variety of intracellular, cell-surface, and extracellular systems for distinguishing their own biological products from components of unfamiliar intruders such as viruses and other microorganisms. Prominent among the systems for initiating an immune response to these foreign microbes is the machinery of the major histocompatibility complex (MHC), utilized by certain antigen-presenting cells (APCs) including dendritic cells, macrophages, and B cells, to initiate immune surveillance of peptide fragments from both externally introduced and internally derived proteins. The huge array of molecular variants encoded in the MHC, or human leukocyte antigen (HLA) system, mediate events along several major immunologic pathways critical to the control of infection. This chapter summarizes information about HLA and closely related genes, how polymorphisms in these genes influence the course and the control of human immunodeficiency virus type 1 (HIV-1) infection in human populations, and how current knowledge of the major HLA-mediated response mechanisms might inform efforts to reconstitute virus-impaired host immunity.

PATHWAYS OF RESPONSE INVOLVING HLA AND RELATED GENE SYSTEMS—BIOLOGY, ORGANIZATION AND NOMENCLATURE

Genes in the HLA region encode one or both of the two components of the heterodimeric molecules that process, translocate and present to effector cells those peptides continuously being sampled from the synthetic and proteolytic compartments *(1,2)*. These genes making transport proteins for recognition of self and foreign antigen by T cells in the so-called class I and class II pathways are quite distinct from the set of class III genes that encode various mediators of the inflammatory process.

The human class I response pathway (Fig. 1) involves products of a number of MHC loci: the α- and β-chains of HLA-A, -B, and -C; large multicatalytic proteasome (LMP) components responsible for peptide degradation; and transporters associated with antigen processing (TAP). Genes for other essential molecular elements in this pathway (e.g., β_2-microglobulin and chaperone molecules such as calnexin and tapasin) reside outside of the originally defined HLA region or on other chromosomes. Their sequence variations, reflected in slight structural differences, are not as extreme as for the HLA-A, -B, and -C loci; they have not shown enough functional specificity

From: *Retroviral Immunology: Immune Response and Restoration*
Edited by: Giuseppe Pantaleo and Bruce D. Walker © Humana Press Inc., Totowa, NJ

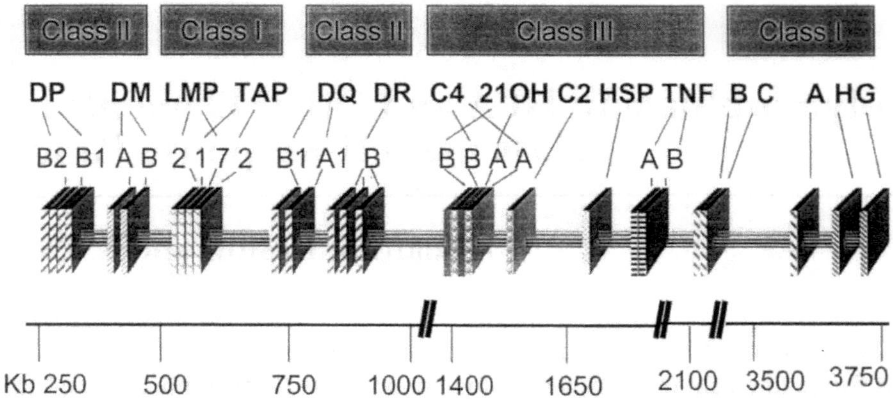

Fig. 1. Schematic diagram of the HLA region showing approximate relative positions of the major class I, II, and III loci.

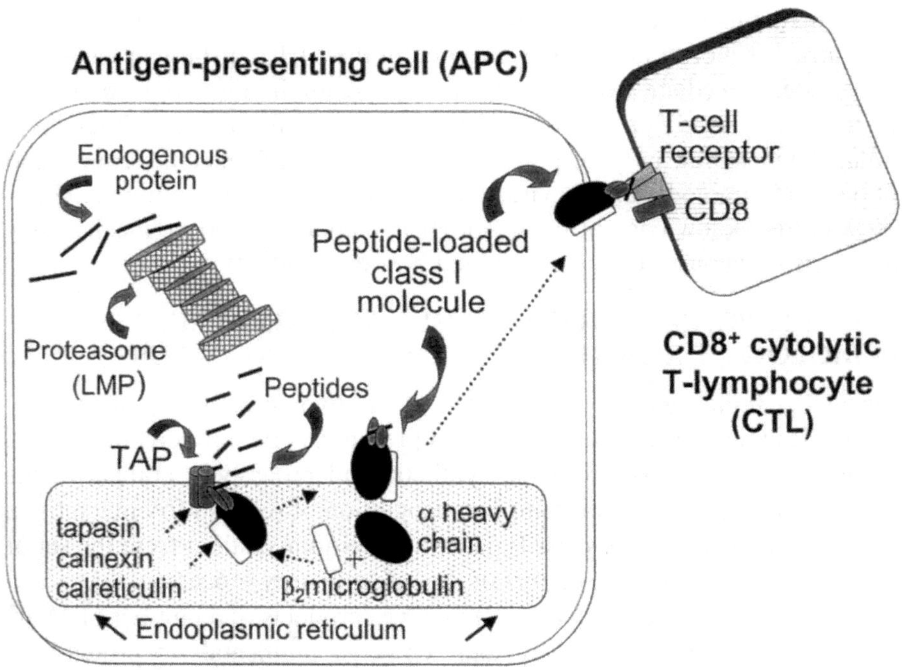

Fig. 2. Schematic view of the antigen presenting cell (APC) and the CTL, the principal molecular components of the class I pathway encoded in the MHC, and the location where the functions take place.

to earn the same intense scrutiny given to the classic HLA genes; and some have been discovered so recently that few data on their variability are available.

In this pathway (Fig. 2) peptides derived from viral or other endogenously produced proteins are catalytically degraded and transported into the endoplasmic reticulum where they are transferred to the binding groove of the HLA heavy chain as it combines with β_2-microglobulin to form a trimolecular (HLA–β_2-microglobulin–peptide) complex. The complex migrates and attaches to the cell membrane, where an encounter with the T-cell receptor (TCR) of a $CD8^+$ cytolytic T lymphocyte (CTL) or interaction with a natural killer (NK) cell triggers a set of defensive biochemical maneuvers for either destroying or sparing the cell that initiated the process.

The class II pathway includes analogous HLA-DR-, DQ-, and DP-locus products, which bind peptides of largely extracellular origin and present them to $CD4^+$ T lymphocytes. Genes in this pathway also encode accessory molecules, such as the invariant chain peptide and its cleavage products that transiently occupy the binding groove in the typical class II HLA heterodimer, and DM, whose atypical class II-like product regulates occupancy of the binding groove by the invariant chain. Interaction of the class II HLA–peptide complex with the $CD4^+$ cell initiates various functions including cytokine regulation of antibody production by B cells and amplification of the CTL response in the class I pathway.

Genes mediating other processes (e.g., tumor necrosis factor [TNF] and heat shock protein [HSP] production as well as certain complement [C2, C4] and enzymatic [21-hydroxylase] functions) are located in the class III HLA region (Fig. 1).

Polymorphism of Genes in the HLA Region

It widely held that throughout vertebrate evolution exposure to infectious agents has driven certain key genes in the HLA system to a degree of variability that is unique. So essential were the functions of products of genes in this region that, as higher species evolved and migrated into more diverse environments, the critical peptide-processing elements of these genes responded to hereditary pressure for survival with exuberant diversification. An exceptionally large number of inherited allelic differences in the codons for amino acids lining the pockets of the HLA peptide binding groove have been produced over millenia by gene duplication, conversion, mutation, and linkage disequilibrium (occurrence of two gene products on the same chromosome more frequently than chance would predict from their individual frequencies). As noted in the preceding, in contrast to HLA, in TAP, LMP, and other genes governing biologic systems of the APC, far less numerous changes are seen.

Through these immunologic pathways humans are well adapted to the phenomenon of continuous encounter with and response to antigens. This process begins early in life as antigenic peptides complexed with HLA molecules literally make topographic impressions on T lymphocytes in the developing thymus via TCRs capable of structural tailoring to fit the composite molecular HLA–peptide facet. The impressions may be stronger or more distinctive or longer lasting (i.e., memorable) for some cells and some peptide motifs than for others. There is also considerable redundancy and overlap throughout the system in binding capability.

Thus, qualitative variability the CTL clonal response to the HLA–peptide complexes among individuals translates into a quantifiable range of response in populations. A single person inherits only a few of the multiple HLA variants, which are capable of binding a moderately broad spectrum of peptides and presenting them to an array of structurally versatile TCRs carrying their own polymorphic domains. Variation between individuals augments the number of potential HLA–peptide–TCR combinations in a given population. Each individual's limited HLA repertoire may withstand different antigenic encounters differently, and some individuals handle a particular encounter better or worse than others.

The enormous diversity of these immune response-"restricting" molecules, compounded across populations, has conferred an evolutionary advantage for survival of past environmental insults. It is now increasingly apparent from the qualitatively and quantitatively preeminent $CD8^+$ CTL response *(3)*, the emerging HIV escape mutants that evade CTL *(4)*, and the $CD4^+$ cell-mediated augmentation of CTL *(5)* that the variability of HLA and TCR molecules represent a crucial evolutionary legacy permitting some parts of some populations now confronting HIV infection to survive its assault.

INFLUENCE OF HLA POLYMORPHISM ON THE RESPONSE TO HIV INFECTION

Epidemiologic Evidence

Early in the epidemic heterogeneity in the clinical course of HIV infection in populations focused attention on the variability in immunity engendered by HLA polymorphism. There were numerous searches for associations of HLA with occurrence of AIDS (reviewed in *6,7*), but often under the erroneous assumption that, as with *Mycobacterium tuberculosis* or hepatitis B virus infection, only a small fraction of HIV-infected individuals would be likely to develop serious immunodeficiency. Comparisons of acquired immune deficiency syndrome (AIDS) cases without regard to the rate at which disease developed could at best suggest HLA relationships with early disease only, and uncertainty about timing often obscured even those relationships. In fact, for HLA associations with disease in general the path to discovery has been tortuous, owing to historically less precise serologic techniques that tended to aggregate different MHC allelic forms into a single assay-dependent "serotype" when, in retrospect, more than one subset of that serotype existed, and the biological phenomenon under study was actually associated with a particular subset. Recent major advances in HLA typing methods (replacement of the microcytotoxicity assay with molecular techniques—oligonucleotide probes, sequence-specific primers, and automated sequencing) have permitted reliable identification of HLA variants, revealing previously inaccessible relationships between HLA alleles and pathogenic processes including HIV-1 infection.

Quests for genetic relationships to disease often focus on family studies because they permit simultaneous formal chromosome-specific (haplotype) analysis of relatively large numbers of known and unknown genes in the vicinity of the indicator marker chosen. Besides revealing a "true" genetic determinant, demonstration of linkage of adjacent genes may be crucial to interpreting apparent genetic relationships to pathophysiologic consequences. The HLA complex is no exception, with both duplicative and distinct but functionally related loci dispersed linearly across a nearly four-megabase landscape. But family studies that permit analysis of haplotype descent in conjunction with a disease state have been especially difficult to conduct in the context of HIV infection because of the natural history of the disease and the sociodemographic features of affected groups. To date there has been only one family study, a sib pair analysis in HIV-infected hemophiliacs, which did demonstrate good concordance between HLA haplotypes and clinical outcome *(8)*.

The difficulty that excessive HLA polymorphism has posed for discovering true relationships without the aid of haplotype-specific data have not always been fully appreciated. Fortunately, the location and variations of major genetic landmarks in the HLA region have been elucidated sufficiently to permit certain strong inferences from popula-

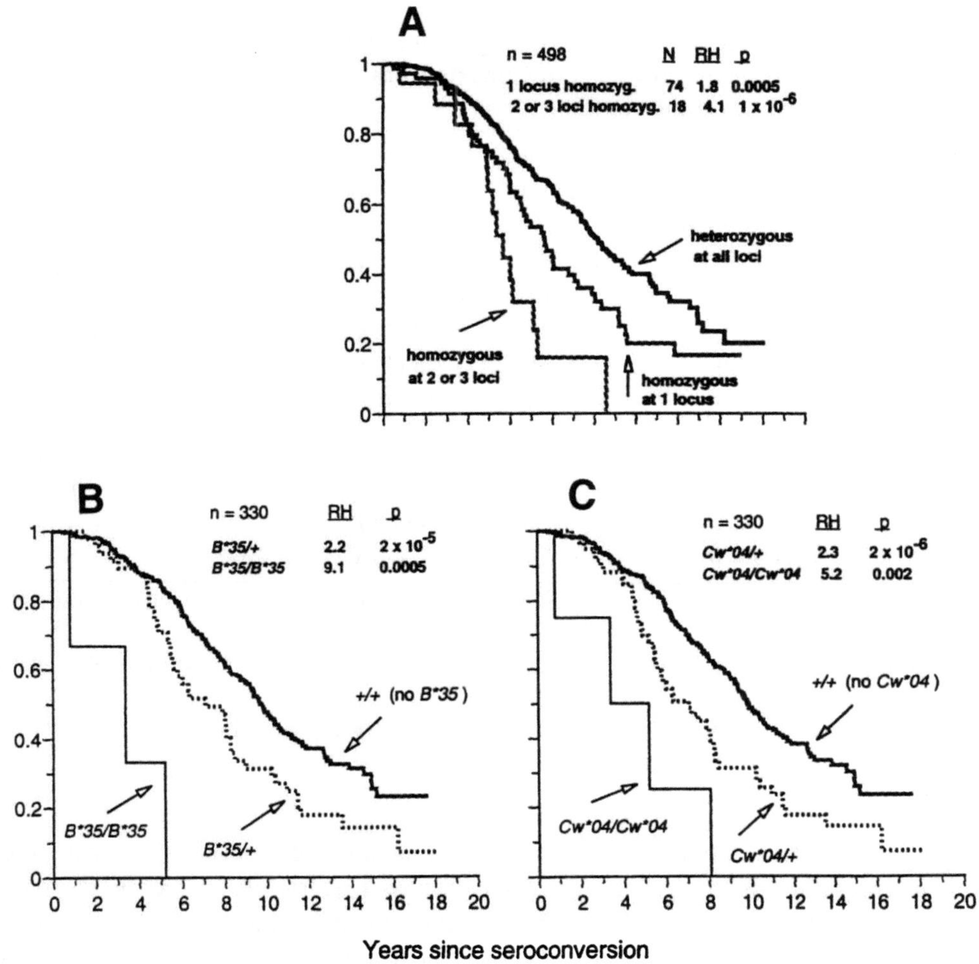

Fig. 3. Kaplan–Meier survival curves of AIDS-free time according to selected characteristics of HLA class I type. Relative hazard (RH) and *p* value were obtained from Cox proportional hazards analysis. **(a)** Comparison of individuals who are homozygous at one or more HLA class I loci (A, B, or C) with those heterozygous at all three loci and **(b)** comparison of individuals heterozygous or homozygous for (1) HLAB*35 and (2) for Cw*04 with those who carry neither. (Adapted with permission from ref. *10,* Carrington et al. Science 1999; 283:1748–52.)

tion studies. The most comprehensive of those studies have been performed principally in assembled cohorts of homosexual men, along with some hemophiliacs and injecting drug users who have also experienced sufficiently long courses of infection under close prospective observation. As other populations with later exposure and initiation of systematic follow-up have matured, they have begun to yield useful comparative information.

The strongest and most consistent differential effect of HLA polymorphism is the advantage conferred by heterozygosity at the class I loci. Three reports covering several separate cohorts with hundreds of subjects uniformly document substantially prolonged median disease progression times or shifts in the distribution of slow and rapid progression according to the degree of homozygosity *(9–11)* (Fig. 3, Table 1). Although whether the risk is equally high for C as for B or A is not yet certain, the

Table 1
Frequencies of HLA-A, -B, -C, and DRB1, DQB1 Homozygosity Among Three Categories of HIV-1-Infected Subjects in Cohorts from Amsterdam, The Netherlands, and Kigali, Rwanda.

Homozygous % (N) HLA loci	Rapid progressors (RPs, *n* = 56)	Intermediate progressors (IPs, *n* = 164)	Slow progressors (SPs, *n* = 122)	RPs vs SPs odds ratio *(p)*	*p* for trend
A	21.4 (12)	23.8 (38)	10.7 (13)	3.2 (0.029)	0.025
B	17.9 (10)	10.4 (17)	9.8 (12)	3.2 (0.018)	0.177
C	12.5 (7)	14.6 (24)	9.0 (11)	1.4 (0.552)	0.331
A only[a]	16.1 (9)	18.9 (31)	9.8 (12)	—	—
B only[a]	8.9 (5)	3.7 (6)	4.9 (6)	—	—
C only[a]	5.4 (3)	6.1 (10)	4.9 (6)	—	—
A or B or both[a]	33.9 (19)	30.5 (50)	19.7 (24)	3.8 (0.003)	0.024
A or B or both[b]	30.4 (17)	26.8 (44)	14.8 (18)	4.0 (0.003)	0.009
DRB1	12.5 (7)	10.4 (17)	13.9 (17)	NS	NS
DQB1	17.9 (10)	17.1 (28)	21.3 (26)	NS	NS

[a] Homozygosity based on intermediate-resolution PCR-SSP that mostly defined specificity at the two-digit level of allele designation.

[b] Homozygosity based on automated sequencing that yielded specificity to the four-digit level of allele designation.

Reproduced with permission from Tang et al. (1999) AIDS Res Hum Retrovir 15:317–24.

effect appears additive (greater for homozygosity at multiple loci). In any case the obvious interpretation is that greater diversity of class I restricting elements affords a broader molecular repertoire for effective binding and presentation of the vast and highly mutable pool of HIV peptides. Zygosity at nearby loci, including DRB1 and DQB1 in one study *(9)*, did not demonstrate the same relationship.

It is equally clear from numerous studies that specificity of class I alleles, in addition to diversity as manifest by heterozygosity, has a profound effect on the response to the virus and the course of infection *(10–15)* (Fig. 3, Table 2). During the early years of the AIDS epidemic, alleles of two common class I haplotypes were consistently although not uniformly associated with a particularly unfavorable course of infection: HLA-B35 with or without Cw4 and B8 with or without its linked A1, Cw7 or DR3 *(12,14,16,17)* (see p. 11, 12). Longer follow-up of larger numbers of infected individuals has subsequently disclosed equally consistent relationships of certain other class I alleles, e.g. B57 *(11,13,15)* and B27 *(11,13,14)*, with favorable outcome. Even more systematic analysis in larger populations *(11,13)*, with adjustment for notorious disequilibrium effects and consideration of interactions, has actually revealed a multiplicity of effects of class I polymorphism fully compatible with the wide spectrum of CTL response generated by those allelic differences. Specific interactions of TAP2 variants with the class I alleles as suggested by earlier analysis *(11,13)* (Table 2) have not been reproduced in subsequent epidemiologic or experimental studies. However, that analysis of interactive effects of multiple class I markers illustrates the importance of a comprehensive analytic approach to the genetics of HIV and other infections.

Table 2
Markers (Class I Alleles, Class I-TAP Combinations, and DRB1-DQB1 Haplotypes) Contributing + or –1 to HLA Profile in Three Cohorts of Caucasian Homosexual HIV-1 Seroconverters

RH[a] ≤ 0.67 $n \geq 15$ = +1				RH[a] ≥ 1.5 $n \geq 15$ = –1			
Marker	n	RH	$p \leq$	Marker	n	RH	$p \leq$
A29-33 (A19) plus TAP2 ala 665[b]	33	0.46	.006	A24	50	1.57	.004
B27	30	0.40	.003	B8 plusTAP2 ile 379	15	1.88	.02
B57	31	0.54	.02	Cw4[c] minus TAP2 ala 665	46	1.79	.001
DRB1*1300-DQB1*0603	45	0.67	.07	DRB1*1200-DQB1*0301	15	1.83	.04
				Homozygosity A or B[d]	68	1.71	.003
RH ≤ 0.55 n = 10–14 = +1				RH ≥ 1.8 n = 10–14 = –1			
Marker	n	RH	$p \leq$	Marker	n	RH	$p \leq$
A25/26 (A10) plus TAP2 ala 665[e]	12	0.31	.02	A23 minus TAP2 ala 665	12	2.04	.02
				A28(68) plus TAP2 ala 665	12	1.88	.08
				B40/60 plus TAP2 ile 379	14	2.24	.005

[a] RH = relative hazard of AIDS-free time in men with and without marker.

[b] Most (A29–32) of the A19 group plus TAP2 ala 665 had similar effects; A33 (A19) (n = 4) did not, but it was included for consistency.

[c] Cw4 is in tight disequilibrium with B35, but neither the single markers nor the combination met criteria; the Cw4-TAP effect shown here appeared stronger than the B35–TAP or the B35–Cw4–TAP effect.

[d] Homozygosity based on molecular typing (n = 64) or serologic identity at A–B–C or B + DRB1–DQB1) (n = 4).

[e] The effect of A25 (A10) plus TAP2 ala 665 explained an ostensible B18 effect, and the closely related A26 (A10) plus TAP2 ala 665 was included because it had a similar effect. [Reproduced with permission from *(11)*.]

The same favorable and unfavorable combinations of primarily class I genetic markers so strongly predictive of time to AIDS in the Multicenter AIDS Cohort Study and other cohorts *(11,13,14)* have also associated with lower and higher plasma viral RNA concentrations during the first 9–15 mo after seroconversion in the multicenter investigation *(18)* (Table 3). More recent analysis of larger numbers of men in that study has reproduced those findings and strengthened the argument that the HLA class I effect operate relatively early in infection, perhaps serving as a principal determinant of the relatively stable level of viral replication achieved by most individuals soon after initiation of infection. If the relationship is further confirmed, the HLA profile may prove

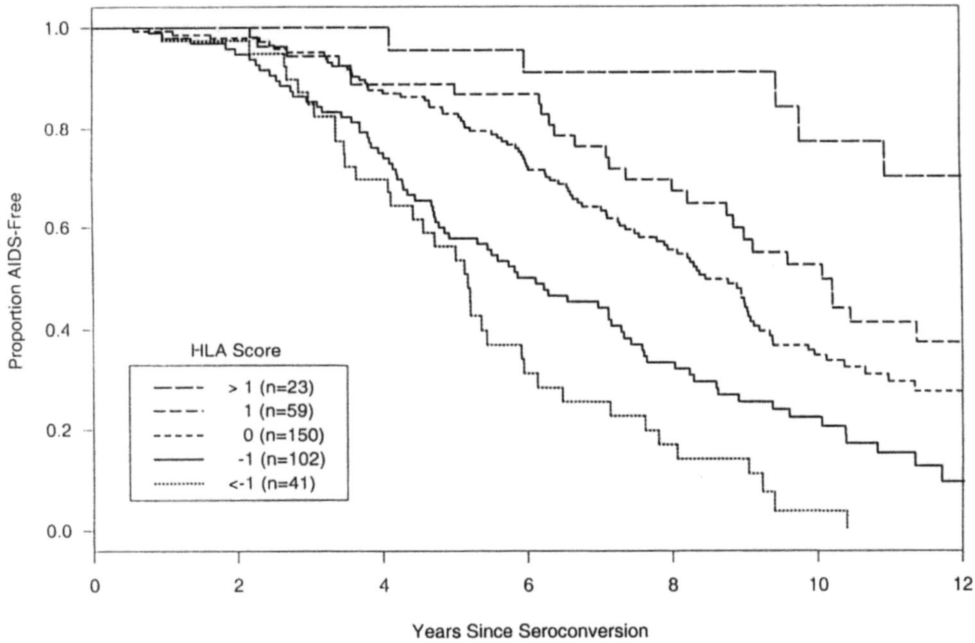

Fig. 4. Kaplan–Meier plots of AIDS-free time in 375 seroconverters aggregated from the Multicenter AIDS Cohort Study, the DC Gay cohort, and the Amsterdam cohort and assigned to 5 categories of HLA profile based on relationships of individual markers in Table 2. Wilcoxon and log rank $p < 10^{-4}$. [Reproduced with permission from *(11)*.]

clinically useful as a prognostic factor in judgments about timing and intensity of intervention and explanations for its failure.

The consequences of diversity and specificity in HLA are profound. The magnitude of the effect of homozygosity at a single locus and the effect of several of the contributing class I markers or combinations are comparable to that seen with any of the chemokine receptor or ligand mutants *(19)*, even without the TAP effect included here (Fig 4), the full HLA profile of individuals probably exerts greater influence *(11)*. Of course, ethnic and other population differences complicate inferences about HLA associations with HIV-1, as with any disease. Early data were drawn preponderantly from Caucasian populations. However, the studies that include subjects of African ethnic origin not only confirm the well known ethnic differences in the frequency distributions of HLA alleles, they also emphasize the unpredictability of their effects on HIV infection. For example, both B35 and Cw4 are common in Caucasians whereas in ethnic Africans the niche B35 occupies is almost completely filled with the nearly identical B53 while Cw4 is at least as common *(10,15)*. In more recent analyses of cohort data, the equally strong association of Cw4 and B35 with rapid progression in Caucasians was not observed in individuals of African origin. Rather, in Caucasians and even more clearly in ethnic Africans, it appeared to be some B35 subtypes more than others and probably B53 that accounted for the associations. Another vain hope for simple explanations of HLA relationships has arisen from a reclassification of class I alleles into a few superfamilies according to binding groove structural relationships *(20,21)*. Although there

Table 3
Associations Between Log_{10} Plasma HIV-1 RNA Viral Load Per Unit Difference in the Predictor Variable

Variable	Univariate (%)	*p*	Multivariate (%)	*p*
Age (per decade)	+12	0.54	+1	0.94
HLA profile (per score unit[a])	–45	0.0001	–39	0.0001
$CD4^+$ cell count (per 100×10^6 cells/L	–17	0.0001	–13	0.002

76.[a] HLA profile based on scoring algorithm from Kaslow et al. Nature M 1996; 2:405–11. Reproduced with permission from Saah et al. AIDS 1998; 12:2107–13.

may be certain pathogenetic relationships to HLA which superfamily clustering may explain more completely, preliminary analysis by superfamily in one large study of HIV-1 infection did not demonstrate any predictive value for the outcomes of interest *(11)*. Despite repeated efforts to distill the effect of polymorphism in the HLA region into a few key relationships, any simple scheme seems unlikely to account fully for the variability in outcome contributed by HLA.

Differential involvement in HIV infection by polymorphic class II gene products has been more difficult to document. Studies in smaller single populations have not been readily reproducible *(8,22)*. The one indication of consistency comes from the reports of protection by certain DRB1*13 suballeles *(11,13,23)*. However, the most promising candidate class II haplotype, DRB1*1301-DQB1*0603, displays linkage disequilibrium with other markers that could explain some if not all of its effect and has not been reported to have distinctive biologic biologic properties that might set it apart from others. The relative paucity of data supporting allele-specific effects of HLA DR or DQ and the inability to detect an advantage of allelic diversity at these loci in attenuating the disease process *(9)* has not been due to technical problems with sequence-specific allele discrimination, which had been solved for DR and DQ well before they had for class I alleles. Nor has effort to identify such relationships been lacking; although technical capability to type at DP has lagged, DR and DQ have been addressed in several cohorts where relationships comparable to those of class I markers were detectable *(9,11)*. These findings could be taken to imply that the control of HIV infection is less dependent on multiplicity of individual class II responses. The biologic plausibility for this distinction between class I and class II effects is discussed later. However, it should be recognized that important population studies have yet to be conducted: typing at additional loci (e.g., DP) and analysis of potential interactions within class II (e.g., with DM); among class I, II, and III markers; and between class II genes within and those outside of the HLA region.

TNF and its promoter genes map to the middle of the HLA region, but polymorphisms in those genes have shown inconsistent relationships to outcome of HIV infection *(24,25)*. Their patterns of disequilibrium linkage to class I and II alleles also make any such relationships contingent on further conjoint analysis of adjacent genes.

Growing epidemiologic evidence for interaction of functionally related HLA gene products and the more recent recognition of involvement of a second polymorphic (chemokine receptor/ligand) gene system advances the paradigm of HIV-1 infection as a pathogenic process under multigenic control. With that paradigm comes the imperative of capturing the multiple genetic contributions to risk in an empirical profile or model—one that will probably require assembly of data from populations larger than most current studies include.

Experimental/Biologic Evidence

Possible Mechanisms of Class I Involvement

Strong empirical association between the highly variable course of HIV-1 infection and the particular inherited profile of HLA gene products is incontrovertible. Its counterpart biologic mechanisms are beginning to be elucidated. The HLA profile represents different combinations of molecules whose polymorphism is precisely defined by amino acids in particular positions of a molecular groove in which antigenic peptide is bound and presented to T lymphocytes. Dominance in this profile by markers in the class I pathway reflects the increasingly apparent critical role of $CD8^+$ T lymphocytes in controlling response to the virus. The most compelling conceptual explanation as well as the preponderance of experimental data support the theory that clones of CTL, driven differentially by HLA-restricted binding of peptide in different individuals, respond to the extraordinarily mutable sequence of HIV quite variably from individual to individual and in the same individual over time. Following is a summary of the experimental findings on the role of HLA in that crucial mechanism as well as others now attracting attention.

CTL Response

Arguments for crucial involvement of HLA class I- restricted CTL response include comparisons of the patterns of mutation in viral genes encoding epitopes preferentially bound by antigen-presenting HLA gene products. Data from a recent cross-sectional study typifies the approach and the thinking *(26)*. A variable number of CTL p17 gag epitopes restricted by specific host HLA type were examined for intra- and interpatient nucleotide variation. The proportion of nonsynonymous greatly outnumbered that of synonymous substitutions in epitopes corresponding to the particular HLA-restricted CTL for each of five patients studied. In the same vein, an elegant study of a macaque sibship experimentally infected with SIVmac 251 produced data remarkably consistent with the epidemiologically-based "profile" concept and with the theory of viral response to differential immune pressure on its HLA allele-specific CTL epitopes *(27)*. Of five animals, two exhibiting poor control of viral replication and rapid clinical deterioration carried the identical two parental class I haplotypes. One slow and one intermediate progressor inherited both of the alternative haplotypes, and the fifth animal carried "reciprocal" haplotypes—one associated with more and the other with less favorable course. Alleles of the most favorable haplotype presented five env and nef epitopes with good CTL recognition. Over time sequenced regions corresponding to those epitopes showed gradual evolution, with highly significant differences in the rate of change between epitope coding compared with adjacent regions. By the late stage of disease the nef sequences recognized by the protective haplotype showed especially high rates of substitution when compared with changes in env sequences. Besides illustrating the phenomenon of cumulative CTL effects depending on combinations of class I alleles, as proposed in human populations *(11,13)*, this successful correlation between indices of variability in both the virus and its nonhuman primate host may presage what will be required in humans to characterize involvement of HLA gene products in host defense.

Human and animal experiments like these form the biologic basis for the belief that certain hypervariable regions defining polymorphic HLA-A, -B, and -C molecules perform the class I processing and presenting functions on HIV peptides more or less effectively than others. However, while numerous laboratories have explored many aspects of class I restricted CTL response in controlling virologic and clinical outcome (i.e. disease intensity and progression), technical difficulties inherent in the available experimental systems have limited investigators' capacity to examine the full spectrum of effects of class I variability. Information has been generated in systems ranging from HLA–peptide elution systems to those using cells and autologous virus of infected individuals who actually displayed extreme (i.e., good or poor) outcomes to those relying on quantification of CTL reaction to a stained HLA molecular carrier (i.e., tetramer) of appropriately bound HIV peptide. Whatever the system, it is usually contrived to measure heavy-chain-binding or CTL-stimulating properties of one or a small number of the many class I alleles complexed with defined peptides.

As new systems have been devised to overcome technical limitations, difficulties imposed by ethnic/geographic diversity and by differences in viral types have also been addressed. Recent experimental as well as epidemiologic studies have begun to replace serologic with sequence-specific allele identification. Molecular typing will accentuate ethnic differences while resolving ambiguities that might have arisen from serologic misidentification. Similarly, although early concentration on clade B virus generated little confidence that results might extend to HIV-1 of other clades and to HIV-2, more recent data from exposed but uninfected Gambian and Kenyan sex workers have been encouraging in that CTLs presumably raised against the local viral type (i.e., HIV-2) or clade (HIV-1 A and D) seem to have provided some cross protection generated by conserved epitopes *(28)*. In analogous work on HIV-1-infected individuals, CTLs stimulated by recombinant vaccinia-expressed clade B gp160 env showed cross-reactivity with gp160 env from clades A and C *(29)*, but the pattern of response appeared to diverge according to HLA B-locus differences.

With regard to HLA allele-specific effects, the most persuasive evidence correlating favorable clinical prognosis with effective specific class I response (broad HIV-1 epitope binding, high proportions of HIV-1 peptide-specific CTLs, or slow evolution of mutant viral quasispecies capable of escape from CTL recognition) have been generated for B27 and for B57. Molecularly subtyped variants of B*27 bind structurally predicted HIV-1 peptide sequences *(30)* and conserved epitopes identified in p24 gag, nef and other proteins well enough to produce strong CTL responses *(31,32)*. B27-induced CTL correlated closely with viral load early in infection *(33)*. Likewise, CTLs from a B57-bearing slow progressor made a strong and broad response to most but not all B57-bound HIV-1 proteins including gag and reverse transcriptase elements, and response to at least one of the same epitopes presented in the context of B58 was similarly strong *(34,35)*. CTLs from B58-positive individuals continued to recognize HIV-1 gag peptide despite extensive amino acid substitution and showed comparable responses to HIV-2 *(36)*.

In contrast to the close correlation between salutary immunologic and clinical effects of B27 and B57-58, no such close immunologic correlation has yet been described for the B8-containing haplotype, noted above as one of the two HLA markers associated with a more aggressive disease course in several epidemiologic studies conducted among Caucasians early in the epidemic. Indeed, the same strong association has not persisted in recent analyses. Precise knowledge of anchor positions and other landmarks within the B8-HIV complex crystal structure has yielded good but not perfect correlation between sequences of predicted binding motifs and those of epitopes actually eluted from B8 molecules. CTL and binding assays for peptides predicted by the structural information have provided more comprehensive picture of the B8 repertoire than eluted peptides alone *(37)*. Moderate effort has been devoted to characterizing distinctive B8 properties, and that allele may not be responsible for the diminution, if any, in CTL response to HIV. It seems increasingly likely that those original associations with unfavorable outcome, in the presence or absence of any specific TAP2 dimorphic variant *(11)*, arose from factors present in B8-posivtive patients independent of peptide binding and presention properties of the B8 allele.

The immunologic basis is no clearer for the occasionally striking, but not especially consistent epidemiologic associations of poor prognosis with B35 and Cw4, or for similar relationships with A24. For B35 there is no indication from studies of CTL response that the allele differs markedly in the number of epitopes bound, in the strength of binding, or in the sensitivity of binding or T-cell recognition to peptide mutations *(38)*. A brief report on a p24 gag epitope presented by Cw*0401, on the other hand, has suggested reduction in efficiency of presentation by cells of one Cw*0401-positive and even absence of that capacity in others *(39)*. The variability from one Cw*0401 cell line to another indicates that suballelic sequence variation or variability in Cw*04-related determinants outside of the hypervariable region may be important. Nor is there any clearer sense from studies of CTLs targeted at numerous and strongly A24-bound gag, pol, nef, or env epitopes why A24-positive individuals should succumb to infection more rapidly *(11,12,40)*, unless specific binding of a nef epitope *(41)* facilitated more efficient class I signal suppression (see p. 14).

Additional data on the role of other allele-specific class I HLA-restricted CTL responses are sparse, but increasing availability and application of allele-specific interferon-γ (IFN-γ)/enzyme-linked immunospot (ELISPOT), tetramer binding and other assays are expected to expand that knowledge rapidly. It will also be important to ascertain whether the substantial prognostic advantage conferred on class I heterozygotes is directly quantifiable in the form of broader or more vigorous CTL responses in those individuals, regardless of the specific alleles they express.

A variety of experimental findings lend credible support to the idea that molecules encoded by class I genes may exert critical control over host–virus interaction by mechanisms other than mediation of CTL response. Because an assay for quantifying CTLs based on the A*0201 tetramer was the first such assay available, studies of peptide binding and presentation dynamics may or may not reflect characteristics peculiar to that allele. For example, highly variable concentrations of the widely used "index" p17 gag peptide SLYNTVATL were needed to stimulate lysis of different target cells in the A*0201 system *(42)*. So highly variable a peptide concentration requirement could reflect a background property of binding to class I alleles in general or further specific genetic heterogeneity present but unrecognized among A*0201^{+} individuals. The implication of the latter would be that apparent "identity" by current molecular HLA typing techniques may not be sufficient to guide allele-specific adjustments in biologics designed to protect via the class I mediated CTL response. Previous indications from SLYNTVATL interaction with A2 that mutant variants of this nonapeptide can antagonize the CTL response *(43)* justifies further caution about extrapolating from experimental results to in vivo events.

The tetramer system is one of several used to study the hypothetical property of immunodominance. In one study, evolution of viral sequences derived from A*0201-positive and -negative individuals actually reflected relatively little immune pressure by different class I alleles against persistence of immunodominant motifs *(42)*. However, again the findings should be interpreted cautiously. Another study of clustering and density of class I peptide motifs across viral protein showed considerable variation from one region to another, with variable regions containing relatively low densities of preferred motifs *(44)*. Dominance may exist, but perhaps only residually in the more fixed domains rather than the variable ones the virus uses to escape effective cytolytic attack. Valid epitopes may be widely dispersed throughout the virus, and their sheer frequency may correlate positively with association of their corresponding class I restriction elements with a favorable response on the clinical/epidemiologic level (i.e., the more frequently the preferred motif occurs in the viral protein sequence, the more protective the allele *(45)*. Thus, intervention in class I dependent immune events may not succeed by merely focusing on the few fixed target motifs that appear dominant and therefore relatively easily attacked.

For other elements dedicated to antigen processing (e.g., TAP and LMP) and for chaperone molecules (e.g. calnexin and tapasin), epidemiologic investigation of polymorphism has not been paralleled by comprehensive laboratory assessment of how the allelic differences contribute to class I regulation of HIV infection. Meager experimental data on differential interaction between allelic forms of TAP and HLA-A, -B, or -C alleles have been generated largely outside of the context of viral infection and may not be generalizable. Dependence of non-HIV peptide loading on tapasin concentration has been reported, with the interesting observation that HLA–B8 exhibits greater dependence than B27, but no information about the existence or impact of allelic variation in tapasin itself is available. Although rats have demonstrated differential transport effects of TAP2 alleles, effects of TAP1 rather than TAP2 polymorphism have been easier to detect in humans *(46)*. In light of the epidemiologic findings, target cells utilizing different combinations of TAP alleles for HIV peptide transport and loading should be used to determine the influence of those differences on surface expression, T-cell receptor engagement and CTL response.

Even less is known about LMP influences on HLA-mediated response to HIV-1, the LMP products encoded in the HLA region, and polymorphism in those genes although there are now indications that proteasomal processing of peptides determines certain features of that response *(47)*. Further exploration of variability in that system may be informative for HIV vaccine development.

CTL-Independent Response

HLA molecules may participate in events other than prototypical binding, translocation, and surface presentation of antigenic peptide, and cognizant CTLs may respond by mechanisms other than target lysis (e.g., interference with early viral protein production, by a B*14 restricted CTL *48*). Whether these other phenomena represent appropriate generic host responses or reflect exploitation by HIV is not always clear, but they could have implications for the evolution and control of HIV infection.

Like other viruses that bud through and coat themselves with host cell membrane, HIV acquires prominent host cell surface features, including both class I and class II HLA molecules *(49)*. Experiments with infected cells lacking HLA on their surface have demonstrated that the virus may be critically dependent on those molecules in order to initiate infection. Complexing of HLA with viral envelope protein at the cell surface has been reported to alter env expression and again may affect cell penetration. However, since the mechanisms of virus-HLA interaction on membranes are obscure *(50)*, it remains to be determined whether polymorphism of HLA heavy chains or other features of the class I peptide binding system differentially regulate cell surface viral functions in any way.

The virus also expropriates the HLA machninery by another potentially critical mechanism. It appears to downregulate surface expression of the HLA molecule by triggering endocytosis of the latter *(51)*. In certain conditions a portion of nef may initiate the process through tyrosine-based sorting of motifs in the cytoplasmic tail of the HLA heavy chain *(52,53)*. Signal by nef is preferentially transmitted to the A- and B- but not the C-locus proteins, a distinction with potentially broad implications if the diminished susceptibility to downregulation of C-locus products is somehow linked to their relatively low degree of polymorphism. Precisely when and under what conditions during viral penetration of the host cell this viral maneuver occurs and how frequent and complete it is will determine whether strategies for circumventing it might assist in recovering class I mediated immunocompetence.

Finally, in addition to the hypervariable regions that form the binding groove of the HLA molecule the nef responsive cytoplasmic tail, other domains in the class I heavy chain mediates activity that may have profound impact on the regulation of HIV infection. These domains can signal immunoglobulin-like proteins belonging to an elaborate molecular system expressed by NK cells to activate or inhibit their killing function *(54)*. Although this system and the cells that operate it are distinct from those involved in classic HLA antigen presentation, the presence of NK receptors on T lymphocytes including CTLs suggests that NK function may be aligned with CTL activity, as does the interruption of HIV-antigen-specific activity in CTLs whose NK receptors are blocked by monoclonal antibody *(55)*. Although the genetics of NK receptor/ligand system is under active investigation, the likelihood is growing that the NK-regulating region of HLA molecules is a further differential determinant of the course of disease and that polymorphism there will deserve attention.

Possible Mechanisms of Class II Involvement

In contrast to the persuasive experimental documentation of the role of HLA class I gene products and their polymorphic variation in host response to HIV infection, far less information is available for products of genes in the class II pathway. An obvious but probably simplistic biological explanation for the failure to observe major differences among class II markers in epidemiologic studies where the class I effects are striking is that the size and shape of the class II binding groove are known to impose less constraint on peptide preference. With relatively little epidemiologic support for

DR or DQ allele-specific differences, and even less for DP, not surprisingly, the meager data that do exist have received relatively little experimental reinforcement. For example, work relating more favorable outcome to one or several DRB1*13 alleles, with or without their haplotypic DQB1 alleles, may have some rationale based on structural features, direct laboratory support is sparse *(23)*. On the other hand, one report of an experimental approach demonstrating concordant binding of multiple gp 120 peptides to both DRB1*0401 and DRB1*1101, two structurally contrasting molecules, strengthens the case for more promiscuous peptide selection *(56)*. Further work on human class II alleles is needed to determine whether more promiscuous binding also implies less restrictive APC–T-helper cell interaction and less prominent influence of polymorphism in those genes.

GENETICALLY REGULATED IMMUNE COMPETENCE IN THE CONTEXT OF HAART

The empirical data implicating polymorphism in class I gene products as major determinants of HIV-1 disease progression are quite convincing. If specific HLA class I alleles influence these late events primarily by generating CTLs that regulate control of viral replication early in HIV infection *(57–61)*, the value of early intervention to restore defective components of immunity may match the urgency for early antiretroviral therapy. During the early acute stage of infection, following introduction of highly aggressive antiretroviral therapy (HAART), antigen-specific CD4 and cytolytic CD8 cell responses can be detected *(5,62–64)*. Those responses and their control of rebound in virus replication and plasma viremia after discontinuation of treatment are different from patient to patient, most likely owing to class I genetic diversity *(63–65)*. Delayed rebound after treatment has even been followed by spontaneous reversal and decline in plasma virus concentration *(63)*, along with measurable increases in effective CTLs, whereas viral variants with mutations that enable escape from CTL lysis *(66–70)* have been found in individuals with progressive disease.

In the natural course of events, because individual effector CTLs controlling viral replication may not survive or act for extended time *(71)*, viral antigen would presumably be continuing to stimulate new $CD8^+$ cells into lytic function required for maintaining steady state viral concentration. How much antigen is needed to stimulate the steady-state lytic response appears to be determined by the cumulative contributions of multiple HLA elements restricting and shaping the CTL repertoire. In the context of effective antiretroviral suppression of virus production, the sequence of events is more obscure. One current view is that once the stimulus is lost, antigen-driven immune clearance may largely subside, permitting resumption of viral replication whenever a small proportion of latently infected cells are incidentally and nonspecifically activated by environmental antigens. With antigenic stimulation rendered insufficient to maintain CTL activity, the capacity of that immune clearance mechanism to eliminate the residual latently infected cell population diminishes. Observed declines in CTL after successful therapeutic viral suppression, coupled with persuasive evidence for the cardinal role of $CD8^+$ effector cells in determining favorable prognosis, provide the rationale for trials of therapeutic immunization with various constructs of HIV antigen. Although the ultimate goal is to develop an agent with universal immunogenicity, it is not yet clear whether the response to agents designed to stimulate class I function will be subject to the same degree of variability conferred by polymorphic class I gene products on the response to natural infection. To the extent that these polymorphisms may predict applicability of immunization strategies, trials of those strategies should concurrently address the role of those potential genetic determinants.

The evidence for antigen-specific response by CD4+ cells, in contrast, emphasizes their augmentation of an effective CD8+ CTL response *(5)* rather than any direct effect on viral replication. Possible reasons for the less allele-specific nature of this class II effect on peptide binding were discussed earlier. However, effects may not be dependent on specific class II binding of HIV-1 antigenic peptide. As with class I gene products, class II (DR) molecules have been found incorporated in the viral membrane, and free virus particles carrying DR1 showed considerably enhanced infectivity *(72)*. The extraordinarily high levels of HIV-1 antigenic protein (i.e., env gene products) during early infection could induce allele-independent tolerance to gp120 *(73)*, impairing CD4+ cell "help" more globally, and thereby mask the more finely tuned CD4 functions sensitive to genetically regulated peptide binding. More speculative is an example of "self" mimicry in which conserved gp120 env sequence closely resembling a motif in the class II DR β-chain actually appeared to be bound and presented in the class I pathway, provoking CTL-mediated damage to DRβ-bearing cells and interrupting class II function *(74)*. Fuller understanding of all of these phenomena should lead to more productive research on immunomodulatory agents.

SUMMARY

Epidemiologic and biologic clues about class I HLA polymorphism-driven differential regulation of both cytolytic and noncytolytic function are sufficient to suggest new and promising approaches to investigation and intervention. By the same token, the difficulty documenting a comparable role for class II polymorphism and the likely interactions among different gene products with complementary function (e.g., class I and class II, class I and TAP) reinforce the impression that resolving these and as yet unrecognized genetic effects and manipulating them in favor of restoration of immunity to HIV will be a formidable task.

REFERENCES

1. Germain R. Antigen processing and presentation. In: Paul WE (ed). Fundamental Immunology, 3rd edit. New York: Raven Press, 1993.
2. Mak T, Simard JJL (eds). Handbook of Immune Response Genes. New York: Plenum, 1998, p. 1–66.
3. Ogg GS, Jin X, Bonhoeffer S, Dunbar PR, Nowak MA, Monard S, et al. Quantitation of HIV-1-specific cytotoxic T lymphocytes and plasma load of viral RNA. Science 1998; 27; 279:2103–6.
4. McMichael AJ, Phillips RE. Escape of human immunodeficiency virus from immune control. Annu Rev Immunol 1997; 15:271–96.
5. Rosenberg ES, Billingsley JM, Caliendo AM, Boswell SL, Sax PE, Kalams SA, Walker BD. Vigorous HIV-1-specific CD4+ T cell responses associated with control of viremia. Science 1997; 278:1447–50.
6. Keet IPM, Klein MR, Just JJ, Kaslow RA. The role of host genetics in the natural history of HIV-1 infection: the needles in the haystack. AIDS 1996; 10:Suppl A, S59–S67.
7. Just JJ. Genetic predisposition to HIV-1 infection and acquired immune deficiency syndrome. A review of the literature examining associations with HLA. Hum Immunol 1995; 44:156–69.

8. Kroner BL, Goedert JJ, Carrington M, Mann DL, Blattner WA. Concordance of haplotype sharing, CD4 decline and AIDS in hemophilic sibling pairs. AIDS 1995; 9:275–80.
9. Tang J, Costello C, Keet IPM, Rivers C, LeBlanc S, Karita E, et al. HLA class I homozygosity accelerates disease progression in human immunodeficiency virus type 1 infection. AIDS Res Hum Retrovir 1999; 15:317–24.
10. Carrington M, Nelson G, Martin MP, Kissner T, Vlahov D, Goedert JJ, et al. HLA and HIV-1: Heterozygote advantage and B*35-Cw*04 disadvantage. Science 1999; 283:1748–52.
11. Keet LPM, Tang J, Klein MR, LeBlanc S, Enger C, Rivers C, et al. Consistent associations of HLA class I, class II and transporter (TAP) gene products with progression of human immunodeficiency virus type 1 infection in homosexual men. J Infect Dis, 1999; 180:299–309.
12. Kaslow RA, Duquesnoy R, VanRaden M, Kingsley L, Marrari M, Su S, et al. Combinations of A1, Cw7, B8, DR3 HLA antigens associated with rapid decline of T-helper lymphocytes in HIV-1-infected homosexual men: a report from the Multicenter AIDS Cohort Study. Lancet 1990; 335:927–30.
13. Kaslow RA, Carrington M, Apple R, Park L, Munoz A, Saah AJ, et al. Influence of combinations of human major histocompatibility complex genes on the course of HIV-1 infection. Nat Med 1996; 2:405–11.
14. McNeil AJ, Yap PL, Gore SM, Brettle RP, McColl M, Wyld R, et al. Association of HLA types A1-B8-DR3 and B27 with rapid and slow progression of HIV disease. Quart J Med 1996; 89:177–85.
15. Costello C, Tang J, Rivers C, Karita E, Meizen-Derr J, Allen S, Kaslow RA. HLA-B*57 Independently associated with slower HIV-1 disease progression in Rwandan women. AIDS 1999; 13:1990–1.
16. Itescu S, Mathur-Wagh U, Skovron ML, Brancato LJ, Marmor M, Zeleniuch-Jacquotte A, Winchester R. HLA-B35 is associated with accelerated progression to AIDS. [Journal Article] AIDS 1992; 5:37–45.
17. Steel CM, Beatson D, Cuthbert RJG, et al. HLA haplotype A1, B8, DR3 as a risk factor for HIV-related disease. Lancet 1988; i:1185–8.
18. Saah AJ, Hoover DR, Weng S, Carrington M, Mellors J, Rinaldo CR Jr, et al. Association of HLA profiles with early plasma viral load, $CD4^+$ cell count and rate of progression to AIDS following acute HIV-1 infection. AIDS 1998; 12:2107–13.
19. Dean M, Carrington M, Winkler C, Huttley G, Smith M, Allikmets R, Goedert J, et al. Genetic restriction of HIV-1 infection and progression to AIDS by a deletion allele of the CKR5 structural gene. Science 1996; 273:1856–62.
20. Sidney J, del Guercio M-F, Southwood S, Engelhard V, Appella E, Rammensee H-G, et al. Several HLA alleles share overlapping peptide specificities. J Immunol 1995; 154:247–59.
21. Threlkeld SC, Wentworth PA, Kalams SA, Wilkes BM, Ruhl DJ, Keogh E, et al. Degenerate and promiscuous recognition by CTL of peptides presented by the MHC class I A3-like superfamily: implications for vaccine development. J Immunol 1997; 159:1648–57.
22. Achord A, Lewis R, Brackin M, Cruse J. HLA-DQB1 markers associated with human immunodeficiency virus type 1 disease progression. Pathobiology 1997; 65:210–5.
23. Itescu S, Rose S, Dwyer E, Winchester R. Certain HLA-DR5 and -DR6 major histocompatibility complex class II alleles are associated with a CD8 lymphocytic host response to human immunodeficiency virus type 1 characterized by low lymphocyte viral strain heterogeneity and slow disease progression. Proc Natl Acad Sci USA 1995; 9:11472–6.
24. Brinkman BMN, Keet IPM, Miedema F, Verweij CL, Klein M. Polymorphisms within the human tumor necrosis factor-promoter region in human immunodeficiency virus type 1-seropositive persons. J Infect Dis 1997; 375:188–90.
25. Khoo SH, Pepper L, Snowden N, Hajeer AH, Vallely P, Wilkins EG, et al. Tumor necrosis factor c2 microsatellite allele is associated with the rate of HIV disease progression. AIDS 1997; 11:423–8.

26. Birk M, Vahlne A, Sonnerborg A, Sallberg M. Nonsynonymous mutations within the human immunodeficiency virus type 1 p17 gene are clustered to sequences binding to the host human leukocyte antigen class I molecules. AIDS Res Hum Retrovir 1998; 14:241–8.
27. Evans D, Jing P, O'connor D, Allen T, Venham J, Rudersdorf R, et al. MHC class I Immunogenetics and CTL escape in a family of MHC-defined macaques infected with SIV. In: 6th Conference on Retroviruses and Opportunistic Infections, Chicago, Jan 31–Feb 4, 1999 (Abstr 255).
28. Rowland-Jones S, Dong T, Krausa P, Sutton J, Newell H, Ariyoshi K, et al. The role of cytotoxic T-cells in HIV infection. Dev Biol Standard 1998; 92:209–14.
29. Wilson S, Pedersen S, Kunich J, Wilkins V, Mann D, Mazzara G, et al. Cross-clade envelope glycoprotein 160-specific $CD8^+$ cytotoxic T lymphocyte responses in early HIV type 1 clade B infection. AIDS Res Hum Retrovir 1998; 14:925–37.
30. De Groot A, George J, Gonzalez M, Jin X, Bond K, Koup R, McNicholl J. Prospective identification of MHC ligands and CTL epitopes from HIV proteins using bioinformatics. In: 6th Conference on Retroviruses and Opportunistic Infections, Chicago, Jan 31–Feb 4, 1999 (Abstr 49).
31. Goulder P, Edwards A, Phillips R, McMichael A. Identification of a novel HLA-B2705-restricted cytotoxic T-lymphocyte epitope within a conserved region of HIV-1 [letter]. AIDS 1997; 11:536–8.
32. Goulder P, Phillips R, Colbert R, McAdam S, Ogg G, Nowak M, et al. Late escape from an immunodominant cytotoxic T-lymphocyte response associated with progression to AIDS. Nat Med 1997; 3:212–7.
33. Wilson JDK, Ogg GS, Kelleher A, Allen RL, Davis C, Shaunak S, et al. A reevaluation of HIV-1 specific CTL precursor frequencies during acute HIV-1 infection. In: 6th Conference on Retroviruses and Opportunistic Infections, Chicago, Jan 31–Feb 4, 1999 (Abstr 25).
34. Goulder P, Bunce M, Krausa P, McIntyre K, Crowley S, Morgan B, et al. Novel, cross-restricted, conserved and immunodominant cytotoxic T lymphocyte epitopes in slow progressors in HIV type 1 infection. AIDS Res Hum Retrovir 1996; 12:1691–8.
35. Klein M, van der Burg S, Hovenkamp E, Holwerda A, Drijfhout J, Melief C, Miedema F. Characterization of HLA-B57-restricted human immunodeficiency virus type 1 Gag- and RT-specific T lymphocyte responses. J Gen Virol 1998; 79:2191–201.
36. Bertoletti A, Cham F, McAdam S, Rostron T, Rowland-Jones S, Sabally S, et al. Cytotoxic T cells from human immunodeficiency virus type-2 infected patients frequently cross-react with different human immunodeficiency virus type 1 clades. J Virol 1998; 72:2439–48.
37. Goulder P, Reid S, Price D, O'Callaghan C, McMichael A, Phillips R, Jones E. Combined structural and immunological refinement of HIV-1 HLA-B8-restricted cytotoxic T lymphocyte epitopes. Eur J Immunol 1997; 27:1515–21.
38. Tomiyama H, Miwa K, Shiga H, Moore Y, Oka S, Iwamoto A, et al. Evidence of presentation of multiple HIV-1 cytotoxic T lymphocyte epitopes by HLA-B*3501 molecules that are associated with the accelerated progression of AIDS. J Immunol 1997; 158:5026–34.
39. Buseyne F, Stevanovic S, Rammensee H, Riviere Y. Characterization of an HIV-1 p24gag epitope recognized by a $CD8^+$ cytotoxic T-cell clone. Immunol Lett 1997; 55:145–9.
40. Ikeda-Moore Y, Tomiyama H, Miwa K, Oka S, Iwamoto A, Kaneko Y, Takiguchi M. Identification and characterization of multiple HLA-A24-restricted HIV-1 CTL epitopes: strong epitopes are derived from V regions of HIV-1. J Immunol 1997; 159:6242–52.
41. Goulder P, Edwards A, Phillips R, McMichael A. Identification of a novel HLA-A24-restricted cytotoxic T-lymphocyte epitope within HIV-1 Nef [letter]. AIDS 1997; 11:1883–4.
42. Brander C, Hartman K, Trocha A, Jones N, Johnson R, Korber B, et al. Lack of strong immune selection pressure by the immunodominant HLA-A*0201-restricted cytotoxic T lymphocyte response in chronic human immunodeficiency virus-1 infection. J Clin Invest 1998; 101:2559–66.
43. Sewell A, Harcourt G, Goulder P, Price D, Phillips R. Antagonism of cytotoxic T lymphocyte-mediated lysis by natural HIV-1 altered peptide ligands requires simultaneous presentation of agonist and antagonist peptides. Eur J Immunol 1997; 27:2323–9.

44. Zhang C, Cornette J, Berzofsky J, DeLisi C. The organization of human leucocyte antigen class I epitopes in HIV genome products: implications for HIV evolution and vaccine design. Vaccine 1997; 15:1291–302.
45. Nelson GW, Goedert JJ, Kaslow RA, Mann DL. Frequency of HLA allele-specific peptide motifs in HIV-1 proteins correlates with the allele's association with relative rates of disease progression after HIV-1 infection. Proc Natl Acad Sci USA 1997; 94:9802–7.
46. Quadri SA, Singal DP. Peptide transport in human lymphoblastoid and tumor cells: effect of transporter associated with antigen presentation (TAP) polymorphism. Immunol Lett 1998; 61:25–31.
47. Goletz TJ, Klimpel KR, Arora N, Leppla SH, Keith JM, Berzofsky JA. Targeting HIV proteins to the major histocompatibility complex class I processing pathway with a novel gp120-anthrax toxin fusion protein. Proc Natl Acad Sci USA 1997; 94:12059–64.
48. Van Baalen C, Schutten M, Huisman R, Boers P, Gruters R, Osterhaus A. Kinetics of antiviral activity by human immunodeficiency virus type 1-specific cytotoxic T lymphocytes (CTL) and rapid selection of CTL escape virus in vitro. J Virol 1998; 72:6851–7.
49. Cantin R, Paquette J-S, Fortin J-F, Tremblay M. The human-derived co-stimulatory molecule CD28 is incorporated into the immunodeficiency virus type 1 envelope and increases its infectivity. In: 6th Conference on Retroviruses and Opportunistic Infections, Chicago, Jan 31–Feb 4, 1999 (Abstr 310).
50. Blanc D, Cosma A, Braun J, Spire B, Klasen S, Pesenti E, et al. HIV Infectivity Depends upon Virion-Associated HLA-Class I Heavy Chains. In: 6th Conference on Retroviruses and Opportunistic Infections, Chicago, Jan 31–Feb 4, 1999 (Abstr 31).
51. Collins KL, Chen BK, Kalams SA, Walker BD, Baltimore D. HIV-1 Nef protein protects infected primary cells against killing by cytotoxic T lymphocytes. Nature 1998; 391:397–401.
52. Le Gall S, Erdtmann L, Benichou S, Berlioz-Torrent C, Liu L, Benarous R, et al. Nef interacts with the mu subunit of clathrin adaptor complexes and reveals a cryptic sorting signal in MHC I molecules. Immunity 1998; 8:483–95.
53. Le Gall S, Erdtmann L, Benichou S, Berlioz-Torrent C, Liu L, Benarous R, et al. Analysis of Nef-induced MHC-I modulation. In: 6th Conference on Retroviruses and Opportunistic Infections, Chicago, Jan 31–Feb 4, 1999 (Abstr S22).
54. Colonna M. Specificity and function of immunoglobulin superfamily NK cell inhibitory and stimulatory receptors. Immunol Rev 1997; 155:127–33.
55. DeMaria A, Ferraris A, Guastella M, Pilia S, Cantoni C, Polero L, et al. Expression of HLA class I-specific inhibitory natural killer cell receptors in HIV-specific cytolytic T lymphocytes: impairment of specific cytolytic functions. Proc Natl Acad Sci USA 1997; 94:10285–8.
56. Gaudebout P, Zeliszewski D, Golvano J, Pignal C, Le Gac S, Borras-Cuesta F, Sterkers G. Binding analysis of 95 HIV gp 120 peptides to HLA-DR1101 and -DR0401 evidenced many HLA-class II binding regions on gp120 and suggested several promiscuous regions. J AIDS Hum Retrovir 1997; 14:91–101.
57. Saah AJ, Hoover DR, Weng S, Carrington M, Mellors J, Rinaldo CR Jr, et al. Association of HLA profiles with early plasma viral load, $CD4^+$ cell count and rate of progression to AIDS following acute HIV-1 infection. Multicenter AIDS Cohort Study. AIDS 1998; 12:2107–13.
58. Borrow P, Lewicki H, Hahn BH, Shaw GM, Oldstone MB. Virus-specific CD8+ cytotoxic T-lymphocyte activity associated with control of viremia in primary human immunodeficiency virus type 1 infection. J Virol 1994; 68:6103–10.
59. Koup RA, Safrit JT, Cao Y, Andrews CA, McLeod G, Borkowsky W, et al. Temporal association of cellular immune responses with the initial control of viremia in primary human immunodeficiency virus type 1 syndrome. J Virol 1994; 68:4650–5.
60. Musey L, Hughes J, Schacker T, Shea T, Corey L, McElrath MJ. Cytotoxic-T-cell responses, viral load, and disease progression in early human immundeficiency virus 1 infection. N Engl J Med 1997; 337:1267–74.

61. Pantaleo G, Demarest JF, Schacker T, Vaccarezza M, Cohen OJ, Daucher M, et al. The qualitative nature of the primary immune response to HIV infection is a prognosticator of disease progression independent of the initial level of plasma viremia. Proc Natl Acad Sci USA 1997; 94:254–8.
62. Dalod M, Harzic M, Pellegrin I, Dumon B, Hoen B, Sereni D, et al. Evolution of cytotoxic T lymphocyte responses to human immunodeficiency virus type 1 in patients with symptomatic primary infection receiving antiretroviral triple therapy. J Infect Dis 1998; 178:61–9.
63. Ortiz GM, Jin X, Demoite MA, Donahoe S, Kuebler PJ, Bonhoeffer S, et al. Containment of breakthrough HIV plasma viremia in the absence of antiretorviral drug therapy is associated with a borad and vigorous HIV specific cytotoxic T lymphocyte (CTL) response. In: 6th Conference on Retroviruses and Opportunistic Infections, Chicago, Jan 31–Feb 4, 1999 (Abstr 256).
64. Lisziewicz J, Rosenberg ES, Lieberman J, Jessen H, Lopalco L, Siliciano R, et al. Immune control of HIV after suspension of therapy. In: 6th Conference on Retroviruses and Opportunistic Infections, Chicago, Jan 31–Feb 4, 1999 (Abstr 351).
65. Lori F, Zinn D, Varga G, Maserati R, Seminari E, Timpone J, et al. Intermittent drug therapy increases the time to HIV rebound in humans and induces the control of SIV after treatment interruption in monkeys. In: 6th Conference on Retroviruses and Opportunistic Infections, Chicago, Jan 31–Feb 4, 1999 (Abstr LB5).
66. Rosenberg ES. Preserving HIV-1 specific T-cell help: Will it prevent progression? In: 6th Conference on Retroviruses and Opportunistic Infections, Chicago, Jan 31–Feb 4, 1999 (Abstr S41).
67. Haas G, Plikat U, Debre P, Lucchiari M, Katlama C, Dudoit Y, et al. Dynamics of viral variants in HIV-1 Nef and specific cytotoxic T lymphocytes in vivo. J Immunol 1996; 157:4212–21.
68. Klenerman P, Phillips RE, Rinaldo CR, Wahl LM, Ogg GS, May RM, et al. Cytotoxic T lymphocytes and viral turnover in HIV type 1 infection. Proc Natl Acad Sci USA 1996; 93:15323–8.
69. Borrow P, Lewicki H, Wei X, Horwitz MS, Peffer N, Meyers H, et al. Antiviral pressure exerted by HIV-1-specific cytotoxic T lymphocytes (CTLs) during primary infection demonstrated by rapid selection of CTL escape virus. Nat Med 1997; 3:205–11.
70. Haas G, Hosmalin A, Hadida F, Duntze J, Debre P, Autran B. Dynamics of HIV variants and specific cytotoxic T-cell recognition in nonprogressors and progressors. Immunol Lett 1997; 57:63–8.
71. McMichael A. T cell responses and viral escape. Cell 1998; 93:673–6.
72. Bucy RP. Immune clearance of HIV-1 replication active cells: a model of two patterns of steady state HIV infection. AIDS Res Hum Retrovir 1999; 15:223–7.
73. Cantin R, Fortin J, Lamontagne G, Tremblay M. The presence of host-derived HLA-DR1 on human immunodeficiency virus type 1 increases viral infectivity. J Virol 1997; 71:1922–30.
74. Wilson S, Habeshaw J, Addawe M, Hounsell E, Oxford J. HIV type 1 envelope glycoprotein 120 carboxy-terminal peptide-induced human T cell lines selectively suppress heterogeneous proliferative T cell responses to soluble antigens. AIDS Res Hum Retrovir 1997; 13:1313–24.

14
Immunologic Approaches to the Therapy of Patients with HIV Infection

H. Clifford Lane and Scott Seeley

INTRODUCTION

The primary modality of therapy for patients with human immunodeficiency virus (HIV) infection is the use of combination antiretroviral chemotherapy to suppress HIV replication. As has been clearly established by a number of studies, effective suppression of HIV replication leads to an immediate improvement in immune function as evidenced by a marked decrease in opportunistic infections and increases in the naïve and memory CD4 T cell pools *(1–4)*. Unfortunately, it has also been clearly established that as a single approach, antiretroviral therapy only suppresses but does not eradicate HIV infection and thus life-long therapy is likely to be required in many patients *(5)*. Given the concerns about long-term toxicities and the development of resistance there remains an interest in looking at alternatives to antiretroviral therapy alone. Immunologic approaches to therapy involve interventions that directly modulate the immune system.

Immune-based therapies can take the form of strategies designed to sustain or modify the overall CD4 T cell pool or strategies geared toward decreasing the level of HIV replication. Among the strategies that are aimed at sustaining or modifying the CD4 T cell pool are the use of cytokines with T-cell growth factor activity and the adoptive transfer of lymphocytes. Inhibition of HIV replication has been attempted through strategies designed to enhance HIV-specific immunity or suppress the activity of proinflammatory cytokines such as tumor necrosis factor-α (TNF-α).

Compared to the efforts that have been expended in the development of antiretroviral therapies, relatively little has been done in the area of immune-based therapies. This is beginning to change as the limitations of antiretroviral therapy become better appreciated and as new immunologic strategies emerge. Greater commitment on the part of the pharmaceutical industry is also apparent as phase III trials of active immunotherapy with HIV immunogens have recently been completed and phase III trials of interleukin-2 (IL-2) have been initiated.

NONSPECIFIC EXPANSION OF THE CD4 POOL

The hallmark of HIV infection is a progressive decline in the number of CD4 T lymphocytes. This decline is seen in both "naïve" and "memory" phenotypes. Once the

From: *Retroviral Immunology: Immune Response and Restoration*
Edited by: Giuseppe Pantaleo and Bruce D. Walker © Humana Press Inc., Totowa, NJ

number of antigen-specific CD4 T cells for a given opportunistic pathogen declines below a critical threshold the patient becomes at increased risk for disease with that agent. T-cell growth factors such as IL-2 and the adoptive transfer of lymphocytes have been studied as ways to directly maintain the size of the T-cell pool in the face of the destructive forces of HIV infection.

Cytokine-Based Therapies

IL-2 is a 15-KDa protein that is produced by T lymphocytes. It has a variety of effects on the immune system including induction of CD4 and CD8 T cell proliferation, induction of natural killer (NK) and B-cell proliferation, enhancement of cytolytic activity, and induction of immunoglobulin and cytokine secretion. Among the cytokines produced in response to IL-2 alone are granulocyte-macrophage colony stimulating factor (GM-CSF), TNF-α, IL-6, IL-7 and IL-10. IL-2 has been studied as a potential therapy for patients with HIV infection since 1983. It is licensed in the United States for treatment of metastatic renal cell cancer and malignant melanoma.

A main activity of IL-2 is to promote T-cell growth as indicated by its original name, T-cell growth factor. In patients with untreated HIV infection, the rate of CD4 T cell destruction exceeds the rate of CD4 T-cell production. The net result is the progressive development of immunodeficiency. When given as a 5-d intermittent administration approx every 8 wk, IL-2 is able to intermittently increase the production of CD4 T lymphocytes by approximately sixfold. Over the course of 1 yr of intermittent therapy one may see up to a doubling of the CD4 T cell count *(6)*. These increases can be seen, regardless of the plasma level of HIV-1, although lower levels of virus seem to be associated with better responses (particularly in patients with CD4 counts <200 cells/μL).

The expansion of T cells induced by intermittent IL-2 is selective for the CD4 T-cell pool. It is an expansion of both naïve and memory phenotype cells with a preferential expansion of the naïve pool *(4)*. IL-2 is capable of binding to the low-affinity IL-2 receptor complex (β/γ chains) on the surface of the cell. This binding leads to expression of the α-chain of the IL-2 receptor, thus creating a high-affinity heterotrimer on the surface of the cell *(4a)*.

A series of phase II studies carried out over the past 8 yr have clearly delineated that intermittent administration of IL-2 (5 d every 8 wk) consistent leads to substantial increases in CD4 T cells in the majority of patients with HIV infection and CD4 counts >200 *(7–10)*. With the use of protease-inhibitor containing antiretroviral regimens similar results have been seen in patients with more advanced disease, albeit in a lower percentage of patients *(11)*. IL-2 is most effective in expanding CD4 T cells when it is given for 5 d (as opposed to 3 or 4) every 8 wk. While the initial studies were done with continuous intravenous administration of drug at doses ranging from 6 to 18 minimum inhibitory units (MIU)/24 h, the majority of the current trials utilize subcutaneous administration at doses ranging from 1.5 to 7.5 MIU bid *(12)*.

In addition to causing expansion of CD4 T cells, intermittent IL-2 administration may also lead to transient increases in plasma levels of HIV-1 RNA *(6)*. These increases typically represent a sixfold increase above baseline, are seen in approx 50% of patients on dual nucleoside therapy and under 25% of patients on nuclease and protease inhibitor therapy. They do not appear to be associated with long-term increases in viral burden. These transient increases typical last for 3–7 d and are rarely seen in the setting of potent antiretroviral therapy. It has been suggested that these bursts of virus may represent expression of virus from latent reservoirs and that IL-2 may serve to purge HIV from these reservoirs *(13)*. Studies exploring this strategy as a means of decreasing the pool of infected cells have thus far been disappointing *(13a)*.

A meta-analysis of the first three randomized, controlled trials of intermittant IL-2 has demonstrated that patients randomized to IL-2 had lower levels of virus, higher CD4 T cell counts, and a trend toward fewer acquired immune deficiency syndrome (AIDS)-defining illnesses *(13b)*. Two Phase III trials are currently underway to determine the magnitude of the clinical benefit associated with IL-2. One study (Subcutaneous IL-2 in combination with highly active antiretrovival therapy in patients with low CD4 T-cell counts [SILCAA]) is enrolling patients with CD4 T-cell counts under 300. The other (Evaluation of subcutaneous Proleukin® in a randomized international trial [ESPRIT]) is enrolling patients with CD4 T-cell counts over 300. Such trials are of considerable importance, especially when one considers that IL-2 administration is associated with a series of significant side effects. Among these are severe flulike symptoms, diarrhea, nausea, and elevations in serum bilirubin. Hypothyroidism occurs in approx 10% of patients treated with IL-2.

A variety of other cytokines also possess some degree of T-cell growth factor activity. Among those that have been in clinical trials in patients with HIV infection are granulocyte-colony stimulating factor (G-CSF) and IL-4.

GM-CSF is an 18-kDa glycoprotein naturally produced by monocytes, fibroblasts, and endothelial cells. Its primary activity is to regulate the production and function of neutrophils. A nonglycosylated recombinant form, filgrastim, containing an amino (N)-terminal methionine is licensed in the United States for treatment of patients with chemotherapy or bone marrow transplantation associated neutropenia, for increased mobilization of hematopoietic progenitor cells for collection by leukapheresis, and for treatment of patients with severe chronic neutropenia. In addition, it is licensed in Australia, Canada, and Japan for the treatment and prevention of HIV-associated neutropenia. The majority of studies of G-CSF in patients with HIV infection have been in patients with advanced disease and have been focused on having an impact on the incidence of secondary infections and survival *(14,15)*. In clinical trials in patients with HIV infection, treatment with G-CSF has been associated with transient increases in numbers of peripheral blood $CD4^+$ T lymphocytes bearing surface characteristics of "memory" T cells *(16)*. Although the mechanisms involved remain unclear it is interesting to note that, in vitro, G-CSF can lead to increases in IL-2 production.

IL-4, originally named B-cell growth factor, is a 129-amino-acid glycoprotein with a molecular mass of 15–19,000 daltons. It is primarily produced by activated T cells and, in addition to facilitating B-cell growth and differentiation, is capable of inducing T-cell proliferation. It is a prototypic T helper-2 (Th2) type cytokine and is a potent inducer of immunoglobulin E (IgE) synthesis. Due to its antagonist effects on IL-6–induced growth of Kaposi's sarcoma cells it has been studied in patients with Kaposi's sarcoma and HIV infection. The majority of clinical experience with IL-4 in HIV infection has been in patients with advanced disease. In these studies, IL-4 when given for periods of time up to 6 mo, was found to cause a transient elevation in CD4 T cell counts that was not sustained beyond 2 wk. This may indicate the development of a tachyphylaxis to the T-cell growth factor effects of IL-4 in the setting of chronic administration. It is possible that greater effects on T-cell growth might be seen with intermittent administration in patients with earlier stages of disease. In contrast to in vitro studies that indicated IL-4 increased HIV replication, if anything there was a decrease in plasma levels of HIV RNA in the clinical trials. Only minimal antitumor effects were seen and little work is currently ongoing with this agent *(17)*.

Adoptive Transfer of Lymphocytes

The infusion of lymphocytes has been studied as a potential form of therapy for patients with HIV infection since the beginning of the epidemic. These approaches have involved the passive transfer of lymphocytes from healthy individuals to their HIV-infected syngenic twins *(18)* and the ex vivo expansion and subsequent reinfusion of autologous cells *(19,20)*. These studies have clearly demonstrated that it is possible to adoptively transfer specific immunity to a neoantigen such as keyhole limpet hemocyanin. However, aside from yielding transient increases in CD4 T-cell counts that appear to be proportional to the baseline counts of the recipient there is little evidence of substantial alteration in the course of HIV disease as a result of these interventions. The use of CD3/CD28 has allowed for approximately a 40-fold ex vivo expansion of purified CD4 T cells. Of interest is the fact that cells activated and expanded in this manner appear less susceptible to HIV infection due to downregulation of coreceptors for HIV. The long-term impact of infusions of cells expanded in this fashion is under investigation.

Additional work in the area of lymphocyte therapy involves the transfer of lymphocytes genetically engineered to be resistant to HIV infection, selected to have specificity toward HIV antigens, or transduced with a second T-cell receptor to confer specificity to HIV antigens. Among the strategies that have been employed for genetically protecting cells against HIV infection have been the introduction of transdominant *rev* mutants and/or *tar* decoys. Preliminary data suggest that such modifications may provide a survival advantage over cells modified with control vectors *(21,22)*. As in the case of the adoptive transfer of CD3/CD28-stimulated cells, the potential role of this form of intervention remains a topic of active investigation. Studies of lymphocytes with specificity for HIV-1 are discussed in the following section.

STRATEGIES DIRECTED TOWARD DECREASING THE LEVEL OF HIV REPLICATION

A variety of immune based therapeutic strategies have been utilized in an attempt to decrease the levels of HIV replication. These include manipulation of the proinflammatory cytokine network, active immunotherapy through immunization with recombinant HIV proteins or inactivated viral particles and passive immunotherapy through the adoptive transfer of HIV-specific T cells.

Inhibition of Pro-inflammatory Cytokines

The pro-inflammatory cytokines GM-CSF, TNF-α and IL-6 are well described inducers of HIV replication in a variety of tissue culture systems *(23)*. The bursts of HIV replication seen in the setting of IL-2 therapy are associated with increases in the levels of these cytokines as well. A great deal of effort has been directed at trying to ascertain the potential benefit of inhibiting these agents in patients with HIV infection.

Among the agents that have been studied are corticosteroids, thalidomide, humanized anti-TNF antibodies, soluble TNF receptor, and IL-10.

Corticosteroids have potent antiinflammatory and immunosuppressive properties. As such, they can be viewed as a double-edged sword in the setting of HIV infection. While clearly shown to confer a survival benefit to patients with severe cases of Pneumocystis carinii pneumonia, chronic use of corticosteroids in HIV infected patients has also been associated with an increased incidence of oropharyngeal candidiasis, cytomegalovirus diseases, and Kaposi's sarcoma. When given to patients with HIV infection and CD4 counts in the 200–799 cells/μL range, oral prednisolone (0.5 mg/kg for 6 mo followed by 0.3 mg/kg) was found to increase the peripheral blood CD4 count by 119 cells/μL (median) *(24)*. The mechanism was postulated to be via decreasing activation-induced apoptosis. In a separate study, four patients with advanced HIV disease were treated with corticosteroids for wasting syndrome and found to have a mean weight gain of 3.5 kg and a transient 0.5 log decrease in levels of HIV RNA *(25)*. Taken together these data suggest that in certain cases brief courses of corticosteroids may be of benefit. Randomized, controlled trials will be needed to better assess the overall risks and benefits of this approach as a primary intervention.

Given that TNF-α has been shown to be a potent inducer of HIV replication in vitro several studies have attempted to evaluate the impact of TNF blockade on plasma HIV RNA levels. Studies of anti-TNF antibody and soluble TNF receptor have been conducted *(26)*. At the doses studied, these agents were unable to significantly impact either serum TNF-α levels or plasma levels of HIV-1 RNA. The best studied agent in this area is thalidomide; an immunomodulatory agent licensed in the United States for treatment of erythema nodosum leprosum. It is felt to work via inhibition of TNF-α synthesis and has been shown to inhibit HIV replication in peripheral blood mononuclear cells, but not in the ACH-2 T-cell line *(27)*. In a placebo controlled 4-wk trial of 200 mg once daily, healing of aphthous ulcers was noted in 16/29 patients in the thalidomide group compared to 2/28 patients in the placebo group ($p < 0.001$). In contrast to what was expected, thalidomide therapy was also associated with increases in TNF-α levels and increases in HIV RNA levels *(28)*. In a separate study evaluating the effects of thalidomide in the setting of wasting associated with coinfection with HIV and tuberculosis, patients treated with thalidomide were found to have decreases in levels of TNF-α, decreases in plasma HIV-1 RNA levels, and an average weight gain of 6.5% compared to patients receiving a placebo. A marked correlation was noted between HIV RNA levels and plasma levels of TNF-α *(29)*. Given the significant side effects of drowsiness, hypersensitivity reactions, and teratogenicity associated with thalidomide one should be judicious in its use *(30)*.

IL-10 is a 16-kDa, potent antiinflammatory cytokine produced by monocytes, $CD4^+$ lymphocytes, $CD8^+$ lymphocytes, B lymphocytes, and keratinocytes. The antiinflammatory properties of IL-10 include the inhibition of IL-1, IL-2, IL-5, IL-6, IL-12, GM-CSF, G-CSF, and TNF-α, the downregulation of surface expression of MHC-II and co-stimulatory molecules, and the inhibition of proinflammatory chemoattractants including MIP-1α and IL-8 *(31,32)*. IL-10 is expressed late (6–8 h) following endotoxin administration and is thought to be important in modulating the deleterious effects of prolonged systemic inflammation. The effects of IL-10 on HIV replication are variable and likely depend to a great extent on the presence or absence of other cytokines, especially T-cell growth and activation factors, and upon the pretreatment activation state of the cell. Its greatest anti-HIV effects have been demonstrated in systems employing the acute infection of monocyte derived macrophages *(33)*. IL-10 has been studied in a phase I clinical trial in patients with HIV infection. Following a bolus infusion of IL-10, no significant decreases in plasma HIV RNA levels were observed (D. Weissman and A. S. Fauci, *personal communication*). Data demonstrating that IL-10 levels are elevated in patients with HIV infection and potentially responsible for the polyclonal hypergammaglobulinemia in these patients suggest that the therapeutic utility of this cytokine, despite its antiinflammatory properties, may be limited *(34)*.

Enhancement of HIV-Specific Immunity

In addition to cytokine-based strategies, efforts have been made to decrease levels of HIV-1 through enhancement of the adaptive immune response to HIV-1. These studies include trials of active immunotherapy with HIV-1 antigens as well as the passive transfer of lymphocytes with specificity for HIV-1 antigens. Although these studies have provided interesting insights as to some of the pathophysiologic mechanisms involved in HIV infection, they have yet to demonstrate any impact on clinical disease.

The development of anti-HIV specific immune-based therapies has been hampered, as have efforts in the development of an HIV vaccine, by a lack of precise understanding of the nature of the protective immune response to HIV infection. As in the case of HIV vaccine development, an empiric approach has been taken with the development of strategies that enhance a variety of T-cell responses to a variety of HIV antigens. These have included immunization with recombinant envelope proteins, envelope-depleted, inactivated virions, DNA encoding HIV proteins, and/or recombinant pox viruses containing HIV genes; the adoptive transfer of HIV-specific T-cell lines or clones; and the adoptive transfer of syngeneic T cells transduced with retroviral vectors to express a second receptor with specificity for HIV gp120.

Active Immunotherapy

In 1986, it was suggested by Jonas Salk and others that it might be possible to prevent the reactivation of latent HIV by boosting the immune response to HIV with HIV antigens during the latent phase of the disease. Based on this hypothesis, two major efforts were launched. One was directed toward testing the effect of immunization with recombinant HIV envelope antigens (VaxSyn®). The other examined the role of inactivated virions (Remune®). Of note was the fact that in the process of viral purification of this latter product envelope proteins were lost from the viral particle. This resulted in a product (Remune®) that was enriched for structural proteins. As a consequence, studies involving VaxSyn tended to evaluate the role of envelope-specific responses while studies involving Remune tended to evaluate the role of gag-specific responses.

A series of randomized, placebo controlled trials of gp160 were carried out in the United States *(35)*, in Canada *(36)*, and in Scandinavia *(37)*. In all, a total of 1721 patients were enrolled in these trials and patients were followed for anywhere from 3 to 5 yr. Each of these studies enrolled patients with relatively early HIV infection (CD4 T cell counts >400, >500, and >200 respectively for the three studies). In each trial there was clear evidence that immunization with the recombinant envelope protein led to substantial increases in lymphocyte blast transformation responses to gp160. Despite this there was no evidence of a significant impact on viral load or disease progression.

Although these studies did not identify a new therapy for patients with early HIV disease, they did clearly demonstrate that the induction of CD4 T-cell responses to the HIV envelope alone was not adequate to have an impact on the host's ability to contain viral replication.

Among the criticisms that have been directed toward the aforementioned studies are that they did not deal with the correct antigen and that the ability of the immune system to make a better immune response may require the type of virologic control possible only since the utilization of combination antiretroviral therapy including protease inhibitors or non-nucleoside reverse transcriptase inhibitors. The demonstration that patients treated early in the course of their HIV infection as well as long-term nonprogressors with low levels of plasma HIV RNA have in vitro lymphocyte blast transformation responses to the p24 antigen of HIV has made this an attractive candidate for immunotherapy studies *(38)*. This response has been seen following immunization with Remune® in a series of well-designed studies *(39)*. As in the case of gp160, however, clinical efficacy could not be demonstrated in the setting of a large phase III trial involving Remune® *(39a)*. In this later study, many of the patients were on potent combination regimens. It has been suggested that the inability to see a difference between placebo and control patients in this trial may have been the result of too few endpoints as a result of the widespread use of highly active antiretroviral therapy. Whatever the ultimate mechanisms underlying this observation are determined to be, the fact remains that active immunotherapy has been able to induce CD4 T-cell responses to either gp160 or p24 without demonstrating a significant impact on disease progression.

A variety of additional attempts at active immunotherapy are currently underway including the use of DNA-based vaccines and recombinant canarypox vaccines. The hope is that these approaches, in contrast to the approaches outlined above, may lead to the generation of cytotoxic T-cell responses that may be more effective than the cytotoxic T-cell responses generated in the course of natural infection. Several studies have evaluated the immunogenicity and safety of DNA vaccines encoding either envelope *(40,41)* or regulatory protein genes *(42)*. Studies of the envelope-containing construct have demonstrated increases in anti-gp 120 antibody levels and some increases in cytotoxic T cell activity. Administration of nef, rev or tat containing constructs led to newly measurable HIV-specific cytotoxicity in eight of nine patients. At present, it is not known whether or not any of these immunologic responses to the DNA immunizations will translate to improved immunity to HIV-1. A randomized controlled trial comparing immunization with a recombinant canarypox virus encoding HIV-1 gp160 (ALVAC-HIV) to immunization with a recombinant canarypox encoding for rabies antigen (ALVAC-RG) in a cohort of 20 patients with HIV infection and CD4 T cell counts >500 cells/μL has been conducted *(43)*. In this study no differences were seen between the groups with respect to either proliferative or T-cell responses to HIV antigens or levels of HIV virus or provirus. Given the fact that HIV infection is characterized by ongoing viral replication and thus continued exposure of the immune system to at least some HIV antigen it remains a considerable challenge to develop a form of active immunotherapy that will improve the host immune response to the virus.

Passive Immunotherapy

While active immunotherapy refers to strategies in which the immune system is stimulated to make an immune response, passive immunotherapy describes those approaches in which elements of HIV-specific immunity are directly administered to the infected patient. This may take the form of hyperimmune immunoglobulin or HIV-specific T cells. As with the efforts in active immunotherapy, studies of passive immunotherapy have provided some interesting insights as to the workings of the immune system: however, have had little impact on viral replication.

The antibody response to HIV infection is directed towards multiple antigens of the virus. While a variety of assays have been developed that are capable of measuring different qualitative aspects of the antibody response, it has been difficult to use either quantitative or qualitative measures of the antibody response as prognostic markers. A series of studies have evaluated the potential role of HIV-specific antibodies in the treatment of patients with HIV infection. These studies have involved hyperimmune plasma as well as humanized monoclonal antibodies. Prior to the development of highly active antiretroviral therapy regimens, several randomized controlled trials of hyperimmune plasma were carried out in patients with HIV infection. In one of these trials, patients with AIDS randomized to receive hyperimmune plasma were noted to have higher CD4 T cell counts than patients randomized to infusions of albumin *(44)*. In another study there were fewer deaths or AIDS defining events in the hyperimmune plasma treated patients compared to controls receiving HIV-seronegative plasma (18 vs 29 events). Patients received their assigned treatment every 14 d for 1 yr. Of note was the fact that this difference was only seen at the 1-yr evaluation despite continued infusions of 300 mL of plasma every 4 wk after the first year *(45)*. In an effort to improve upon the activity of polyclonal antibodies, monoclonal antibodies have been developed with high titer neutralizing activity against a variety of HIV isolates. While these antibodies have proven to be quite potent in preventing primary HIV infection in animal models *(46)* they have not been shown to have substantial activity in the setting of established infection in either animal models or patients with HIV infection *(47–49)*.

Given that T-cell immunity is an important component of host defense against viral infections and the fact that T-cell immunity is compromised by HIV infection, a considerable effort has been directed toward the passive transfer of T cells with specificity for HIV antigens. These trials have employed lymphocytes from HIV uninfected syngeneic twin donors immunized with HIV antigens, autologous cytotoxic T-cell clones and lines and genetically engineered CD4 and CD8 T cells.

In syngeneic twin studies, lymphocytes from healthy twins immunized with recombinant vaccinia virus expressing HIV gp160 protein and/or recombinant gp160 protein *(50)* have been transferred to HIV-infected recipients. The results from these studies were similar to what had been seen following the transfer of nonprimed lymphocytes, namely transient increases in both CD4 T cells and plasma levels of HIV. More recent work has examined the effects of the adoptive transfer of syngeneic or autologous CD8 and/or CD4 T lymphocytes transduced with a retroviral vector to express a second T cell receptor capable of binding HIV-1 gp120 *(51a)*. Of note thus far from these studies has been the observation that the survival of the genetically engineered CD8 T cells is greatly enhanced by the coadministration of CD4 T cells transduced with the same T cell receptor. Such data demonstrate the possible requirement for antigen-specific CD4 T cell help in maintaining an antigen-specific CD8 T-cell response.

In addition to the transfer of syngeneic T cells, autologous T-cell lines and clones have been generated from the peripheral blood T cells of patients with HIV infection, expanded to large numbers and infused back into the donors. In one study, infusion of large numbers of a nef-specific T-cell clone was unexpectedly associated with a decline in the CD4 T cell count and an increase in plasma levels of HIV-1 *(52)*. Analysis of HIV quasispecies in this patient suggested that the infusion of the cytotoxic T cells led to selection of viral variants lacking the nef-epitope of the clone. In another series of studies, $CD8^+$ HIV-specific cytotoxic T cells were generated from six patients with HIV infection and transduced with a gene to permit positive and negative selection. Following receipt of these cells, five of the six donors developed cytotoxic T cells directed toward the foreign gene product that led to rapid elimination of the infused cells *(53)*. In a more recent study, HIV-1 gag-specific $CD8^+$ cytotoxic T-cell clones were adoptively transferred to HIV-infected individuals. Studies of lymphoid tissues in these recipients indicated that these cytotoxic T cells retained their lytic function in vivo and migrated to sites of HIV infection *(54)*. While none of these studies have demonstrated a major sustained effect on levels of plasma virus or reservoirs of HIV-1 this area remains one of the more promising areas of immune based therapy research.

SUMMARY

Combination antiretroviral therapy has changed the outlook for patients with HIV disease. Despite these advances HIV infection remains a chronic illness that provides an ongoing challenge to identify better therapeutic strategies. Studies of immune-based therapies have helped to further our understanding of the pathogenesis of HIV infection, however, have not yet led to improved treatments. It is hoped that as our knowledge of the pathogenesis of HIV infection expands so will our ability to discover and develop novel approaches to treatment that will complement the successes of antiretrovirals alone.

REFERENCES

1. Mocroft A, Vella S, Benfield T, et al. Changing patterns of mortality across Europe in patients in fected with HIV-1. EuroSIDA Study Group. Lancet 1998; 352:1725–30.
2. Palella FJ Jr, Delaney KM, Moorman AC, et al. Declining morbidity and mortality among patients with advanced human immunodeficiency virus infection. HIV Outpatient Study Investigators. New Engl J Med 1998; 338:853–60.
3. Kelleher AD, Carr A, Zaunders J, Cooper DA. Alterations in the immune response of human immunodeficiency virus (HIV)-infected subjects treated with an HIV-specific protease inhibitor, ritonavir. J Infect Dis 1996; 173:321–9.
4. Connors M, Kovacs JA, Krevat S, Gea-Banacloche JC, Sneller MC, Flanigan M, et al. HIV infection induces changes in $CD4^+$ T-cell phenotype and depletions within the $CD4^+$ T-cell repertoire that are not immediately restored by antiviral or immune-based therapies. Nat Med 1997; 3:533–40.

4a. Sereti I, Gea-Banacloche JC, Kan M-Y, Hallahan CW, and Lane HC. Interleukin-2 leads to dose dependent expression of the alpha chain of the IL-2 receptor on CD25 negative T lymphocytes in the absence of antigenic stimulation. Clin Immunol 2000; 97:266–76.

5. Harrigan PR, Whaley M, Montaner JS. Rate of HIV-1 RNA rebound upon stopping antiretroviral therapy. AIDS 1999; 13:F59–62.
6. Kovacs JA, Baseler M, Dewar RJ, Vogel S, Davey RT Jr, Falloon J, et al. Increases in CD4 T lymphocytes with intermittent courses of interleukin-2 in patients with human immunodeficiency virus infection. A preliminary study. N Engl J Med 1995; 332:567–75.

7. Kovacs JA, Vogel S, Albert JM, Falloon J, Davey RT Jr, Walker RE, et al. Controlled trial of interleukin-2 infusions in patients infected with the human immunodeficiency virus. N Engl J Med 1996; 335:1350–6.
8. Carr A, Emery S, Lloyd A, Hoy J, Garsia R, French M, et al. Outpatient continuous intravenous interleukin-2 or subcutaneous, polyethyleneglycol-modified interleukin-2 in human immunodeficiency virus-infected patients: arandomized, controlled, multicenter study. Australian IL-2 Study Group. J Infect Dis 1998; 178:992–9.
9. Levy Y, Capitant C, Houhou S, Carriere I, Viard JP, Goujard C, et al. Comparison of subcutaneous and intravenous interleukin-2 in asymptomatic HIV-1 infection: a randomised controlled trial. ANRS 048 study group. Lancet 1999; 353:1923–9.
10a. Levy Y, Capitant C, Houhou S, Carriere I, Viard JP, Goujard C, Gastaut JA, Oksenhendler E, Boumsell L, Gomard E, Rabian C, Weiss L, Guillet JG, Delfraissy JF, Aboulker JP, Seligmann M. Comparison of subcutaneous and intravenous interleukin-2 in asymptomatic HIV-1 infection: a randomized controlled, trial. ANRS 048 study group. Lancet. 1999 Jun 5; 353(9168):1923–9.
10b. Losso MH, Belloso, WH, Emery S, Benetucci JA, Cahn PE, Lasala MC, Lopardo G, Salomon H, et al. A randomized, controlled, phase II trial comparing escalating doses of subcutaneous Interleukin-2 plus antiretrovirals versus antiretrovirals alone in human immunodeficiency virus infected patients with $CD4^+$ cell counts ≥ 350/mm^3. J Inf Dis 2000; 181:1614–21.
10c. Ruxrungtham K, Suwanagool S, Tavel JA, Chuenyam M, Kroon E, Ubolyam S, Buranapraditkun S, Techasathit W, Li Y, Emery S, Davey DR, Fosdick L, Kunanusont C, Lane HC, Phanuphak P, and the Vanguard Study Group. A randomized, controlled 24 week study of intermittent subcutaneous interleukin-2 (scIL-2) in HIV-1 infected patients in Thailand. AIDS 14:2509–13.
10. Hengge UR, Goos M, Esser S, Exner V, Dotterer H, Wiehler H, et al. Randomized, controlled phase II trial of subcutaneous interleukin-2 in combination with highly active antiretroviral therapy (HAART) in HIV patients. AIDS 1998; 12:F225–34.
11. Arn A, Ruiz L, Juan M, Jou A, Balagu M, Zayat MK, et al. Efficacy of low-dose subcutaneous interleukin-2 to treat advanced human immunodeficiency virus type 1 in persons with ≤/=250/µL CD4 T cells and undetectable plasma virus load. J Infect Dis 1999; 180:56–60.
12. Davey RT Jr, Chaitt DG, Albert JM, Piscitelli SC, Kovacs JA, Walker RE, et al. A randomized trial of high- versus low-dose subcutaneous interleukin-2 outpatient therapy for early human immunodeficiency virus type 1 infection. J Infect Dis 1999; 179:849–58.
13. Chun TW, Engel D, Mizell SB, Hallahan CW, Fischette M, Park S, et al. Effect of interleukin-2 on the pool of latently infected, resting $CD4^+$ T cells in HIV-1-infected patients receiving highly active anti-retroviral therapy. Nat Med 1999; 5:651–5.
13a. Davey RT, Bhat N, Yoder C, Chun TW, Metcalf JA, Dewar R, et al. HIV-1 and T cell dynamics after interruption of highly active antiretroviral therapy (HAART) in patients with a history of sustained viral suppression. Proc Natl Acad Sci USA 1999 Dec 21; 96(26):15109–14.
13b. Emery S, Capra WB, Cooper DA, Mitsuyasu RT, Kovacs JA, Vig P, Smolskis M, Saravolatz LD, Lane HC, Fyfe GA, and Curtin PT for the International IL-2 Study Group. Pooled-analysis of three, randomised, controlled trials of interleukin-2 therapy in adult HIV disease. J Inf Dis 2000; 182:428–34.
14. Keiser P, Rademacher S, Smith JW, Skiest D, Vadde V. Granulocyte colony stimulating factor use is associated with decreased bacteremia and increased survival in neutropenic HIV-infected patients. Am J Med 1998; 104:48–55.
15. Kuritzkes DR, Parenti D, Ward Dj, et al. Filgrastim prevents severe neutropenia and reduces infective morbidity in patients with advanced HIV infection: results of a randomized, multicenter, controlled trial. AIDS 1998; 12:65–78.
16. Nielsen SD, Afzelius P, Dam-Larsen S, et al. Effect of G-CSF in HIV-infected patients: increase in numbers of naïve CD4+ cells and CD34+ cells. AIDS 1998; 12:Suppl 4, S64.

17. Tulpule A, Joshi B, DeGuzman N, Espina BM, Mocharnuk R, Prakash O, et al. Interleukin-4 in the treatment of AIDS-related Kaposi's sarcoma. Ann Oncol 1997; 8:79–83.
18. Lane HC, Masur H, Long DL, Klein HG, Rook AH, Quinnan GV, et al. Partial immune reconstruction in a patient with the acquired immunodeficiency syndrome. N Engl J Med 1984; 311:1099–103.
19. Levine BL, Cotte J, Small CC, Carroll RG, Riley JL, Bernstein WB, et al. Large-scale production of $CD4^+$ T cells from HIV-1 infected donors aftner CD3/CD28 costimulation. J Hematother 1998; 7:437–48.
20. Trickett AE, Kelly M, Cameron BA, Lloyd A, French RA, Dwyer JM. A preliminary study to determine the effect of an infusion of cryopreserved autologous lymphocytes on immunocompetence and viral load in HIV-infected patients. J Acquir Immune Defic Hum Retrovirol 1998; 17:129–36.
21. Woffendin C, Ranga U, Yang Z, Xu L, Nabel GJ. Expression of a protective gene-prolongs survival of T cells in human immunodeficiency virus-infected patients. Proc Natl Acad Sci USA 1996; 93:2889–94.
22. Morgan RA, Walker R. Gene therapy for AIDS using retroviral mediated gene transfer to deliver HIV-1 antisense TAR and transdominant Rev protein genes to syngeneic lymphocytes in HIV-1 infected identical twins. Hum Gene 1996; 7:1281–306.
23. Poli G, Kinter AL, Vicenzi E, Fauci AS. Cytokine regulation of acute and chronic HIV infection in vitro: from cell lines to primary mononuclear cells. Res Immunol 1994; 145:578–82.
24. Andrieu JM, Lu W, Levy R. Sustained increases in CD4 cell counts in asymptomatic human immuodeficiency virus type 1-seropositive patients treated with prednisolone for 1 year. J Infect Dis 1995; 171:523–30.
25. Kilby JM, Tabereaux PB, Mulanovich V, Shaw GM, Bucy RP, Saag MS. Effects of tapering doses of oral prednisone on viral load among HIV-infected patients with unexplained weight loss. AIDS Res Hum Retrovir 1997; 13:1533–7.
26. Walker RE, Spooner KM, Kelley G, McCloskey RV, Woody JN, Falloon J, et al. Inhibition of immunoreactive tumor necrosis factor-alpha by a chimeric antibody in patients infected with human immunodeficiency virus type 1. J Infect Dis 1996; 174:63–8.
27. Makonkawkeyoon S, Limson-Pobre RN, Moreira AL, Schaur V, Kaplan G. Thalidomide inhibits the replication of human immunodeficiency virus type 1. Proc Natl Acad Sci USA 1993; 90:5974–8.
28. Jacobson JM, Greenspan JS, Spritzler J, Ketter N, Fahey JL, Jackson JB, et al. Thalidomide for the treatment of oral aphthous ulcers in patients with human immunodeficiency virus infection. N Eng J Med 1997; 336:1487–93.
29. Klausner JD, Makonkawkeyoon S, Akarasewi P, Nakata K, Kasinrerk W, Corral L, et al. The effect of thalidomide on the pathogenesis of human immunodeficiency virus type I and M. tuberculosis infection. J AIDS Hum Retrovirol 1996; 11:247–57.
30. Haslett P, Tramontana J, Burroughs M, Hempstead M, Kaplan G. Adverse reactions to thalidomide in patients infected with human immunodeficiency virus. Clin Infect Dis 1997; 24:1223–7.
31. deWaal-Malefyt R, Abrams J, Bennett B, Fidgor C, deVries J. IL-10 inhibits cytokine synthesis by human monocytes: an autoregulatory role of IL-10 produced by monocytes. J Exp Med 1991; 174:1209–20.
32. Chen WF, Zlotnik A. IL-10: a novel cytotoxic T cell differentiation factor. J Immunol 1991; 147:528–34.
33. Weissman D, Poli G, Fauci AS. Interleukin-10 blocks HIV replication in macrophages by inhibiting the autocrine loop of TNF-α and IL-6 induction of virus. AIDS Res Hum Retrovir 1994; 10:1199–206.
34. Muller F, Aukrust P, Nordoy I, Froland SS. Possible role of interleukin-10 and CD40 ligand expression in the pathogenesis of hypergammaglobulinemia in human immunodeficiency virus infection: modulation of IL-10 and Ig production after intravenous Ig infusion. Blood 1998; 92:3721–29.

35. Birx DL, Davis C, Ruiz N, et al. Results of phase II double-blinded, multicenter, placebo controlled HIV therapeutic vaccine trial. In: XI International Conference on AIDS, Vancouver, July, 1996 (Abstr TuA275).
36. Tsoukas CM, Raboud J, Bernard NF, Montaner JS, Gill MJ, Rachlis A, et al. Active immunization of patients with HIV infection: a study of the effect of VaxSyn, a recombinant HIV envelope subunit vaccine, on progression of immunodeficiency. AIDS Res Hum Retrovir 1998; 14:483–90.
37. Sandstrom E, Wahren B, the Nordic VAC-04 Study Group. Therapeutic immunisation with recombinant gp160 in HIV-1 infection: a randomised double-blind placebo-controlled trial. Lancet 1999; 353:1735–42.
38. Rosenberg ES, Billingsley JM, Caliendo AM, Boswell SL, Sax PE, Kalams SA, Walker BD. Vigorous HIV-1-specific $CD4^+$ T cell responses associated with control of viremia. Science 1997; 278:1447–50.
39. Kahn JO, Cherng DW, Mayer K, Murray H, Lagakos S. Evaluation of HIV-1 immunogen, an immunologic modiffier, administered to patients infected with HIV having 300 to 549 x 10(6)/L CD4 cell counts: A randomized controlled trial. JAMA 2000; 284(17):2193–202.
40. Ugen KE, Nyland SB, Boyer JD, Vidal C, Lera L, Rasheid S, et al. DNA vaccination with HIV-1 expressing constructs elicits immune responses in humans. Vaccine 1998; 16:1818–21.
41. MacGregor RR, Boyer JD, Ugen KE, Lacy KE, Gluckman SJ, Bagarazzi ML, et al. First human trial of a DNA-based vaccine for treatment of human immunodeficiency virus type 1 infection: safety and host response. J Infect Dis 1998; 178:92–100. Lancet 1998; May 2;351:1320–5.
42. Calarota S, Bratt G, Nordlund S, Hinkula J, Leandersson AC, Sandstrom E, Wahren B. Cellular cytotoxic response induced by DNA vaccination in HIV-1-infected patients. Lancet 1998; 351:1320–5.
43. Tubiana R, Gomard E, Fleury H, Gougeon ML, Mouthon B, Picolet H, Katlama C. Vaccine therapy in early HIV-1 infection using a recombinant canarypox virus expressing gp160MN (ALVAC-HIV): a double-blind controlled randomized study of safety and immunogenicity. AIDS 1997; 11:819–20.
44. Levy J, Youvan T, Lee ML. Passive hyperimmune plasma therapy in the treatment of acquired immunodeficiency syndrome: results of a 12-month multicenter double-blind controlled trial. The Passive Hyperimmune Therapy Study Group. Blood 1994; 84:2130–5.
45. Vittecoq D, Chevret S, Morand-Joubert L, Heshmati F, Audat F, Bary M, et al. Passive immunotherapy in AIDS: a double-blind randomized study based on transfusions of plasma rich in anti-human immunodeficiency virus 1 antibodies vs.transfusions of seronegative plasma. Proc Natl Acad Sci USA 1995; 92:1195–9.
46. Gauduin MC, Parren PWHI, Weir R, Barbas CF, Burton DR, Koup RA. Passive immunization with a human monoclonal antibody protects hu-PBL-SCID mice against challenge by primary isolates of HIV-1. Nat Med 1997; 3:1389–93.
47. Poignard P, Sabbe R, Picchio GR, Wang M, Gulizia RJ, Katinger H, et al. Neutralizing antibodies have limited effects on the control of established HIV-1 infection in vivo. Immunity 1999; 10:431–8.
48. Cavacini LA, Samore MH, Gambertoglio J, Jackson B, Duval M, Wisnewski A, et al. Phase I study of a human monoclonal antibody directed against the CD4-binding site of HIV type 1 glycoprotein 120. AIDS Res Hum Retrovir 1998; 14:545–50.
49. Gunthard HF, Gowland PL, Schupbach J, Fung MS, Boni J, Liou RS, et al. A phase I/IIA clinical study with a chimeric mouse-human monoclonal antibody to the V3 loop of human immunodeficiency virus type 1 gp120. J Infect Dis 1994; 170:1384–93.
50. Bex F, Hermans P, Sprecher S, Achour A, Badjou R, Desgranges C, et al. Syngeneic adoptive transfer of anti-human immunodeficiency virus (HIV-1)-primedlymphocytes from a vaccinated HIV-seronegative individual to his HIV-1-infected identical twin. Blood 1994; 84:3317–26.

51. Walker RE, Bechtel CM, Natarajan V, Baseler M, Hege KM, Metcalf JA, Stevens R, Hazen A, Blaese RM, Chen CC, Leitman SF, Palensky J, Wittes J, Davey RT, Falloon J, Polis MA, Kovacs JA, Broad DF, Levine BL, Roberts MR, Masur H, Lane HC. Long-term in vivo survival of receptor-modified syngeneic T cells in patients with human immunodeficiency virus infection. Blood 200 Jul 15; 96(2):467–74.

51a. Mitsuyasu RT, Anton PA, Deeks SG, Scadden DT, Connick E, Downs MT, Bakker A, Roberts MR, June CH, Jalali S, Lin AA, Pennathur-Das R, Hege KM. Prolonged survival and tissue trafficking following adoptive transfer of CD4zeta gene-modified autologous CD4(+) and CD8(+) T cells in human immunodeficiency virus-infected subjects. Blood 2000 Aug 1; 96(3):785–93.

52. Koenig S, Conley AJ, Brewah YA, Jones GM, Leath S, Boots LJ, et al. Transfer of HIV-1-specific cytotoxic T lymphocytes to an AIDS patient leads to selection for mutant HIV variants and subsequent disease progression. Nat Med 1995; 1:330–6.

53. Riddell SR, Elliott M, Lewinsohn DA, Gilbert MJ, Wilson L, Manley SA, et al. T-cell mediated rejection of gene-modified HIV-specific cytotoxic T lymphocytes in HIV-infected patients. Nat Med 1996; 2:216–23.

54. Brodie SJ, Lewinsohn DA, Patterson BK, Jiyamapa D, Krieger J, Corey L, et al. In vivo migration and function of transferred HIV-1-specific cytotoxic T cells. Nat Med 1999; 5:34–41.

Index

D

E

F

MIX
Papier aus verantwortungsvollen Quellen
Paper from responsible sources
FSC® C105338

If you have any concerns about our products,
you can contact us on
ProductSafety@springernature.com

In case Publisher is established outside the EU,
the EU authorized representative is:
Springer Nature Customer Service Center GmbH
Europaplatz 3, 69115 Heidelberg, Germany

Printed by Libri Plureos GmbH
in Hamburg, Germany